Pancreatic Cancer: An Issue of the Oncology Clinics

Pancreatic Cancer: An Issue of the Oncology Clinics

Edited by Malcolm Stark

hayle
medical

New York

Hayle Medical,
750 Third Avenue, 9th Floor,
New York, NY 10017, USA

Visit us on the World Wide Web at:
www.haylemedical.com

ISBN: 978-1-63241-688-9

Cataloging-in-Publication Data

    Pancreatic cancer : an issue of the oncology clinics / edited by Malcolm Stark.
       p. cm.
    Includes bibliographical references and index.
    ISBN 978-1-63241-688-9
    1. Pancreas--Cancer. 2. Pancreas--Cancer--Treatment. 3. Oncology.
    I. Stark, Malcolm.
RC280.P25 P36 2019
616.994 37--dc23

Table of Contents

Preface

The main aim of this book is to educate learners and enhance their research focus by presenting diverse topics covering this vast field. This is an advanced book which compiles significant studies by distinguished experts in the area of analysis. This book addresses successive solutions to the challenges arising in the area of application, along with it; the book provides scope for future developments.

The condition that arises when cells in the pancreas begin to multiply uncontrollably and form a mass is called pancreatic cancer. Such cancerous cells can start to invade other parts of the body with time. There are different kinds of pancreatic cancer, principal among which are adenocarcinomas and non-adenocarcinomas. Pancreatic adenocarcinoma is not easily diagnosed in the early stages, as symptoms do not appear. Unexplained weight loss, nausea, tiredness and vomiting characterize the disease. More than 50% of all pancreatic adenocarcinomas occur in people over the age of 70. The risk factors associated with pancreatic cancer are smoking, obesity, diabetes mellitus and certain dietary and genetic factors. This book explores all the important aspects of pancreatic cancer in the present day scenario. It provides significant information of this type of cancer to help develop a good understanding of the challenges of this condition. It will help the readers in keeping pace with the rapid changes in this field.

It was a great honour to edit this book, though there were challenges, as it involved a lot of communication and networking between me and the editorial team. However, the end result was this all-inclusive book covering diverse themes in the field.

Finally, it is important to acknowledge the efforts of the contributors for their excellent chapters, through which a wide variety of issues have been addressed. I would also like to thank my colleagues for their valuable feedback during the making of this book.

Editor

FRAX597, a PAK1 inhibitor, synergistically reduces pancreatic cancer growth when combined with gemcitabine

Dannel Yeo[1], Hong He[1], Oneel Patel[1], Andrew M. Lowy[2], Graham S. Baldwin[1] and Mehrdad Nikfarjam[1*]

Abstract

Background: Pancreatic ductal adenocarcinoma remains one of the most lethal of all solid tumours. Treatment options are limited and gemcitabine-based chemotherapy remains the standard of care. Although growing evidence shows that p21-activated kinase 1 (PAK1) plays a crucial role in pancreatic cancer, its role has not been fully elucidated. This study aimed to characterise the expression and functional relevance of PAK1 in pancreatic cancer.

Methods: PAK1 expression was measured in pancreatic cancer specimens by immunohistochemistry and in pancreatic cancer cell lines by western blotting. The effect of inhibition of PAK1 by either shRNA knock-down (KD), or by a selective inhibitor, FRAX597, alone or in combination with gemcitabine, on cell proliferation and migration/invasion was measured by thymidine uptake and Boyden chamber assays, respectively. The effect on tumour growth and survival was assessed in orthotopic murine models.

Results: PAK1 was expressed in all human pancreatic cancer samples tested, an7d was upregulated in all pancreatic cancer cell lines tested. PAK1 KD inhibited pancreatic cancer cell growth and survival, and increased sensitivity to gemcitabine treatment. AKT activity and HIF1α expression were also inhibited. FRAX597 inhibited pancreatic cancer cell proliferation, survival, and migration/invasion. When combined with gemcitabine, FRAX597 synergistically inhibited pancreatic cancer proliferation in vitro and inhibited tumour growth in vivo.

Conclusions: These results implicate PAK1 as a regulator of pancreatic cancer cell growth and survival. Combination of a PAK1 inhibitor such as FRAX597 with cytotoxic chemotherapy deserves further study as a novel therapeutic approach to pancreatic cancer treatment.

Keywords: Pancreatic adenocarcinoma, PAK1, Gemcitabine, Proliferation, Orthotopic murine model

Background

Pancreatic ductal adenocarcinoma remains one of the most lethal of all solid tumours. It is the fourth leading cause of cancer-related mortality in Australia and the United States and is expected to become the second leading cause of cancer-related deaths by 2030, based on current management with no significant treatment improvements [1]. The 5-year survival rate is less than 5 % and has not improved over the past few decades [2]. Although combinational chemotherapies exist such as

FOLFIRINOX and gemcitabine with nab-paclitaxel, as a single agent, gemcitabine remains the standard of care for the treatment of pancreatic cancer in most countries [3]. Gemcitabine targets rapidly replicating cells by inhibiting DNA synthesis, but intrinsic and acquired chemoresistance is common. The limited treatment regimens and predicted increase in cancer-related mortality highlight the urgent need for the development of effective therapies based on our understanding of the molecular mechanisms involved in pancreatic cancer.

The most frequent and earliest mutation in pancreatic cancer is the Kras mutation, present in over 95 % of pancreatic cancer patients [4]. This mutation results in a constitutively active p21 protein, Ras, which can activate

* Correspondence: mehrdad.nikfarjam@gmail.com
[1]Department of Surgery, Austin Health, University of Melbourne, Heidelberg, VIC, Australia
Full list of author information is available at the end of the article

a number of signalling pathways, including other p21 proteins such as Cdc42 and Rac, through direct and indirect mechanisms [5]. These p21 proteins can then activate the p21-activated kinases (PAKs). Although there is evidence for the activation of PAKs by Kras-driven pathways, other non-Kras-driven pathways or indirect Kras mechanisms may also activate PAKs.

PAKs are a family of non-receptor serine/threonine kinases, which mediate many effector functions from cell cycle and DNA transcription to cell adhesion and motility [6]. There are six isoforms of PAKs, divided into two groups: Group 1 contains PAK1, 2 and 3, and Group 2 contains PAK4, 5 and 6. Of the six isoforms, PAK1 is the best documented and has been found to be up-regulated in a number of cancers [7], including pancreatic cancer [8]. PAK1 is also up-regulated in pancreatic cancer cell lines when expression of MUC13, a transmembrane mucin, is increased [9]. We have previously found that a non-selective PAK inhibitor, glaucarubinone, reduced pancreatic cancer growth, and that treatment in combination with gemcitabine resulted in synergistic inhibition [10]. The role of PAK1 in pancreatic cancer and its therapeutic potential have not been fully elucidated.

FRAX597 is a small-molecule pyridopyrimidinone that targets group 1 PAKs through binding to the ATP-binding site [11]. Although it has been found to preferentially target group 1 PAKs, FRAX597 also inhibits other kinases such as RET, YES1, TEK, and CSF1R [12]. Of the group 1 PAKs, FRAX597 selectively inhibits PAK1 with a kinase IC_{50} of 8 nM, compared to 13 nM and 19 nM with PAK2 and PAK3, respectively. No inhibition of the group 2 PAKs was observed [11]. FRAX597 inhibits proliferation in neurofibromatosis type 2 (NF2)-associated schwannomas [12], but has not been tested previously in pancreatic cancer. This study aimed to elucidate the role of PAK1 in pancreatic cancer, by examining the effects of reduction of PAK1 expression by shRNA knock-down, or PAK1 activity with the selective inhibitor FRAX597, on the growth and migration/invasion of pancreatic cancer cell lines in vitro, and in orthotopic murine models in vivo, alone and in combination with gemcitabine.

Methods

Cells and reagents

The human PANC-1, MiaPaCa-2 and BxPC-3 pancreatic cancer cell lines (American Type Culture Collection, Manassas, VA) and the murine Pan02 (Division of Cancer Treatment and Diagnosis Tumor Repository, NCI, Frederick, MD), and LM-P (obtained from Andrew Lowy (Moores Cancer Center, University of California, San Diego, CA) [13]) pancreatic cancer cell lines were cultured in Dulbecco's Modified Eagle's Medium (DMEM) supplemented with 10 % FBS (fetal bovine

serum: Hyclone Laboratories Inc., Scoresby, Australia). Normal immortalised human pancreatic duct epithelial (HPDE) cells (obtained from M.S Tsao (Ontario Cancer Institute, Ontario, Canada)) were cultured in Keratinocyte serum-free medium supplemented with bovine pituitary extract (BPE) and epidermal growth factor (EGF). All cells were cultured in a 37 °C incubator with 5 % CO_2. Cells were tested regularly for mycoplasma contamination and were not passaged more than 30 times or for more than 6 months after resuscitation.

FRAX597 was purchased from SYNthesis (Parkville, Australia) and gemcitabine was purchased from Sigma-Aldrich (Castle Hill, Australia).

Immunohistochemistry (IHC) on human pancreatic cancer samples

Human tissue collection was approved by the Austin Health Human Research Ethics Committee (H2013/04953) and informed consent was obtained from all participants. Samples of 10 human pancreatic cancers and adjacent normal pancreas were collected from patients undergoing pancreatic cancer resection at Austin Health, and confirmed to have pancreatic ductal adenocarcinoma by two independent pathologists. For PAK1 IHC, sample sections were incubated with 3 % hydrogen peroxide in methanol for 10 min at room temperature to quench endogenous peroxidase activity. Antigens were retrieved by incubation in 10 mM citrate buffer and blocked in 5 % horse serum. Sections were incubated with antibody against PAK1 (Santa Cruz Biotechnology, Dallas, TX) or IgG. Sections were visualised using an ENvision Plus polymer-based detection kit (Dako, Botany, Australia). The slides were then counter-stained and images were taken with a NIKON Coolscope (Coherent Scientific, Hilton, Australia).

shRNA transfection

To obtain PAK1 knock-down (KD) clones, PANC-1 and MiaPaCa-2 cells were transfected with SureSilencing shRNA plasmids for human PAK1 (SABioscience, Doncaster, Australia), or with a scrambled sequence as a negative control (NC), using Lipofectamine2000 (Invitrogen, Mulgrave, Australia), according to the manufacturer's instructions. Stable clones were selected with geneticin (G418; 1 mg/ml). PAK1 protein expression was detected by western blot.

Western blot

Proteins in cell lysates were detected with antibodies against phospho-PAK1 (Santa Cruz Biotechnology), PAK1, phospho-AKT, AKT, HIF1α (BD Biosciences, North Ryde, Australia), and GAPDH. Antibodies were from Cell Signalling Technology (Arundel, Australia), unless otherwise stated. Bound antibodies were visualised using ECL reagents (GE Healthcare, Amersham, UK), and the density of each band was analysed using Multigauge computer software (Berthold, Bundoora, Australia). HIF1α expression was determined in cells cultured under normoxia or hypoxia (1 % O_2).

Cell proliferation, cell survival and combination index

Cell proliferation and survival was measured using ^{3}H-thymidine incorporation and withdrawal assays, respectively, as previously described [14]. Growth curves were fitted based on a log-scale using MATLAB (MathWorks, Natick, MA) and differences in proliferation were evaluated by comparison of growth rates (expressed as %/h). Assessment of proliferation with FRAX597 and the combination of FRAX597 with gemcitabine was measured as previously described [10]. For assessment of cell survival with FRAX597, cells were seeded with increasing concentrations of FRAX597 for 24 h without serum.

The combined effects of FRAX597 and gemcitabine were evaluated using the Chou-Talalay method [15] as previously described [10]. The CalcuSyn program (Biosoft, Cambridge, UK) was used to calculate the combination index (CI) for each drug affected fraction (Fa). The CI value is interpreted as: <1, synergistic; =1, additive; >1, antagonistic.

Cell migration/invasion

Cell migration/invasion was measured using the Transwell Boyden chamber assay as previously described [14]. Cells were seeded into the upper chambers of the inserts (ThinCert™, 8 µm pore size; Greiner Bio-One, Frickenhausen, Germany) with increasing concentrations of FRAX597. After 24 h, membranes were fixed and stained with Quick-Dip (Fronine, Riverstone, Australia) and 24 fields were counted at 40 times magnification using a NIKON Coolscope.

Murine orthotopic pancreatic cancer model

All mice experiments were approved by the Austin Health Animal Research Ethics Committee (A2013/04898). Pan02 cells were implanted orthotopically in the pancreatic head or tail as previously described [16]. For assessment of tumour growth, 28 mice were implanted with cells in the pancreatic tail and monitored for 30 days. 7 mice per treatment group were randomly allocated to the four treatment groups: control, intraperitoneal (i.p.) injection of saline every other day; FRAX597 alone, FRAX597 (3 mg/kg) i.p. every other day; gemcitabine alone, gemcitabine (40 mg/kg) i.p. twice weekly; and combination of FRAX597 and gemcitabine, following the individual treatments as described above. A single investigator measured the dimensions of all tumours, at the endpoint, using micro-calipers, in a double-blinded manner. Tumour volume was calculated using

the formula for ellipsoid tumours: $V = L \times W \times H \times (\pi/6)$ where L was the longest distance from right to left; W, the largest dorsal/ventral diameter; and H, the largest rostral/caudal diameter. For assessment of survival, 54 mice were implanted with cells in the head of the pancreas. Mice were monitored based on health score for up to 45 days and euthanased when a poor health score was reached. Mice were treated with either control, gemcitabine alone, or combination of FRAX597 and gemcitabine, as described above. An initial study was undertaken with 24 mice, with 12 mice per group for control or gemcitabine treatment alone. A second study was undertaken with 30 mice, with 13 mice per group for gemcitabine alone or combination treatment, and the remaining 4 mice allocated to the control group. A collated Kaplan-Meier survival curve was plotted, and the two studies were analysed together using stratified Cox regression analysis (SPSS; IBM, New York, NY).

Statistical analysis

All values are expressed as means ± standard error. Experiments were done in duplicate and data collated from three independent experiments. Results were analysed using student's t-test or one-way ANOVA (SPSS). Differences between two means with $p < 0.05$ were considered significant.

Results

PAK1 is expressed in human pancreatic cancer and upregulated in pancreatic cancer cell lines

PAK1 staining of pancreatic ductal adenocarcinoma cells was observed in all 10 human pancreatic cancer samples tested (Fig. 1a). In corresponding normal pancreas samples, islet cells stained for PAK1, however, staining was absent in acinar and ductal epithelial cells. Expression of PAK1, and of the phosphorylated, active form of PAK1, was detected in low levels in the normal HPDE cell line and was significantly lower when compared to all the pancreatic cancer cell lines. All human and murine pancreatic cancer cell lines tested expressed phosphorylated and total PAK1 (Fig. 1b).

Inhibition of PAK1 by shRNA knock-down decreases proliferation and survival of pancreatic cancer cells

The PAK1 protein concentrations in two PANC-1 PAK1 KD clones (2.05 and 2.10) were decreased to 22 % and 24 %, respectively, of the PAK1 protein concentrations of the corresponding NC cells, which had been transfected with scrambled sequences (Fig. 2a). Similarly, the PAK1 protein concentrations in two MiaPaCa-2 PAK1 KD clones (3.09 and 3.12) were decreased to 11 % and 9 %, respectively, of the PAK1 protein expression of the corresponding NC cells (Fig. 2b). The proliferation rate

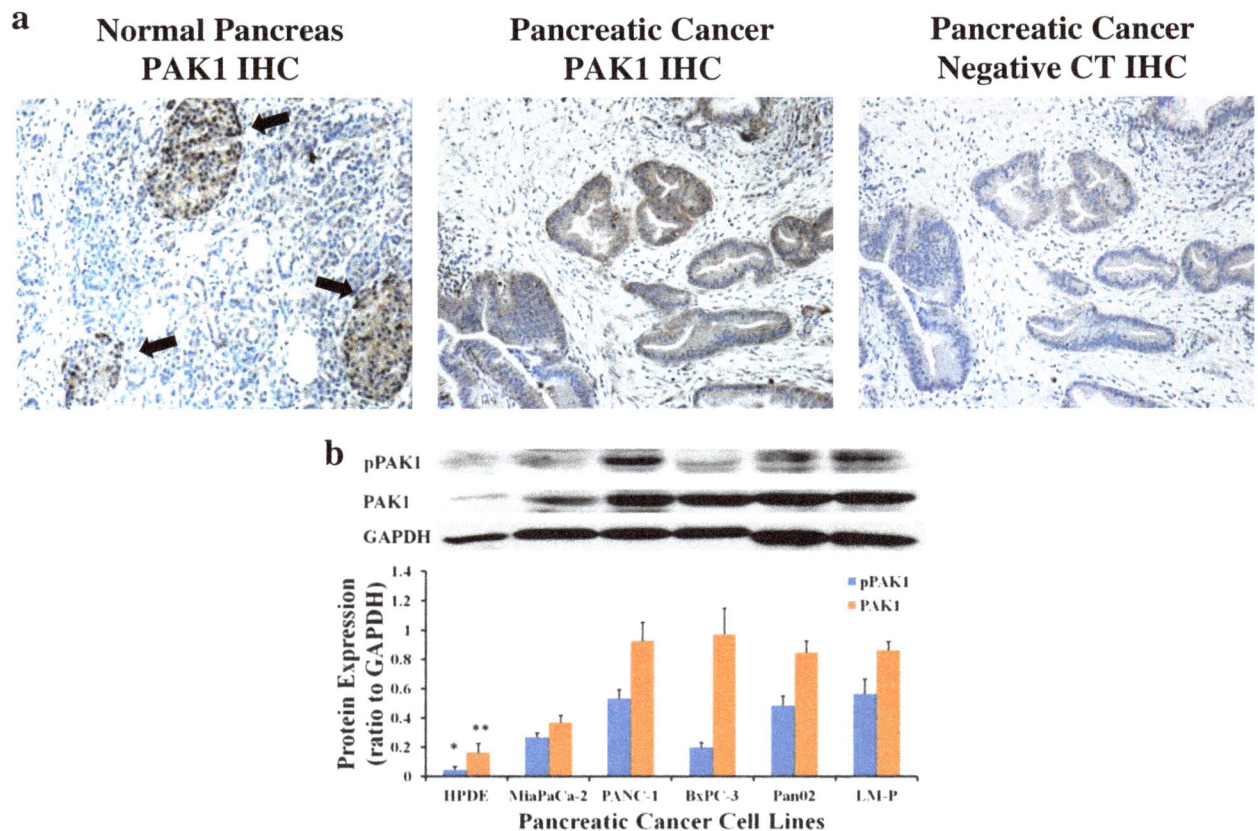

Fig. 1 PAK1 is up-regulated in pancreatic cancer specimens and pancreatic cancer cell lines. (**a**) Acinar and ductal cells in normal pancreas are not stained for PAK1 by immunohistochemistry (IHC), but islet cells (arrow) are positive. Magnification: x200. Pancreatic ductal adenocarcinomas stain more strongly for PAK1 than the negative control (CT). Magnification: x100. (**b**) The normal pancreas cell line, HPDE, expressed low levels of phospho-PAK1 (active form) and PAK1 as detected by western blotting. All pancreatic cancer cell lines, MiaPaCa-2, PANC-1, BxPC-3, Pan02 and LM-P expressed phospho-PAK1 and PAK1. The data represent mean ± SEM, summarised from three independent experiments. * $p < 0.05$; ** $p < 0.01$, compared to all other pancreatic cancer cell lines

was significantly reduced in both PANC-1 (Fig. 2c) and MiaPaCa-2 (Fig. 2d) PAK1 KD cells compared to the corresponding NC cells. The growth rate of two clones of PANC-1 PAK1 KD cells (1.9 %/h and 2.1 %/h) was significantly less than two clones of NC cells (2.4 %/h and 2.6 %/h) (Table 1). A similar difference was observed in the MiaPaCa-2 PAK1 KD cells.

Inhibition of PAK1 by shRNA knock-down sensitises pancreatic cancer cells to gemcitabine

Proliferation of PANC-1 (Fig. 2e) and MiaPaCa-2 (Fig. 2f) PAK1 KD cells in the presence of gemcitabine at concentrations of 20 nM and 50 nM was inhibited to a greater extent than the corresponding NC cells. The IC_{50} values of two clones of PANC-1 PAK1 KD cells (20 nM and 21 nM) (Table 1), were significantly less than the values for NC cells (26 nM and 39 nM). Similarly, the IC_{50} values of two clones of MiaPaCa-2 PAK1 KD cells (26 nM and 25 nM) (Table 1) were

significantly less than the values for NC cells (29 nM and 28 nM).

Inhibition of PAK1 by shRNA knock-down reduces AKT activity and HIF-1α expression

AKT activity was significantly reduced in two clones of PANC-1 PAK1 KD cells, by 22 % and 31 % (Fig. 3a), and in two clones of MiaPaCa-2 PAK1 KD cells by 24 % and 33 % (Fig. 3b). HIF1α expression was significantly reduced in two clones of both PANC-1 (Fig. 3c) and MiaPaCa-2 (Fig. 3d) PAK1 KD cells compared to the NC cells under either normoxia or hypoxia.

FRAX597 decreases proliferation and migration/invasion in pancreatic cancer cell lines

FRAX597 inhibited proliferation in all pancreatic cancer cell lines in a dose-dependent manner (Fig. 4a), with IC_{50} values between 650 nM for BxPC-3 cells and 2.0 μM for PANC-1 cells (Table 2). Similarly, FRAX597

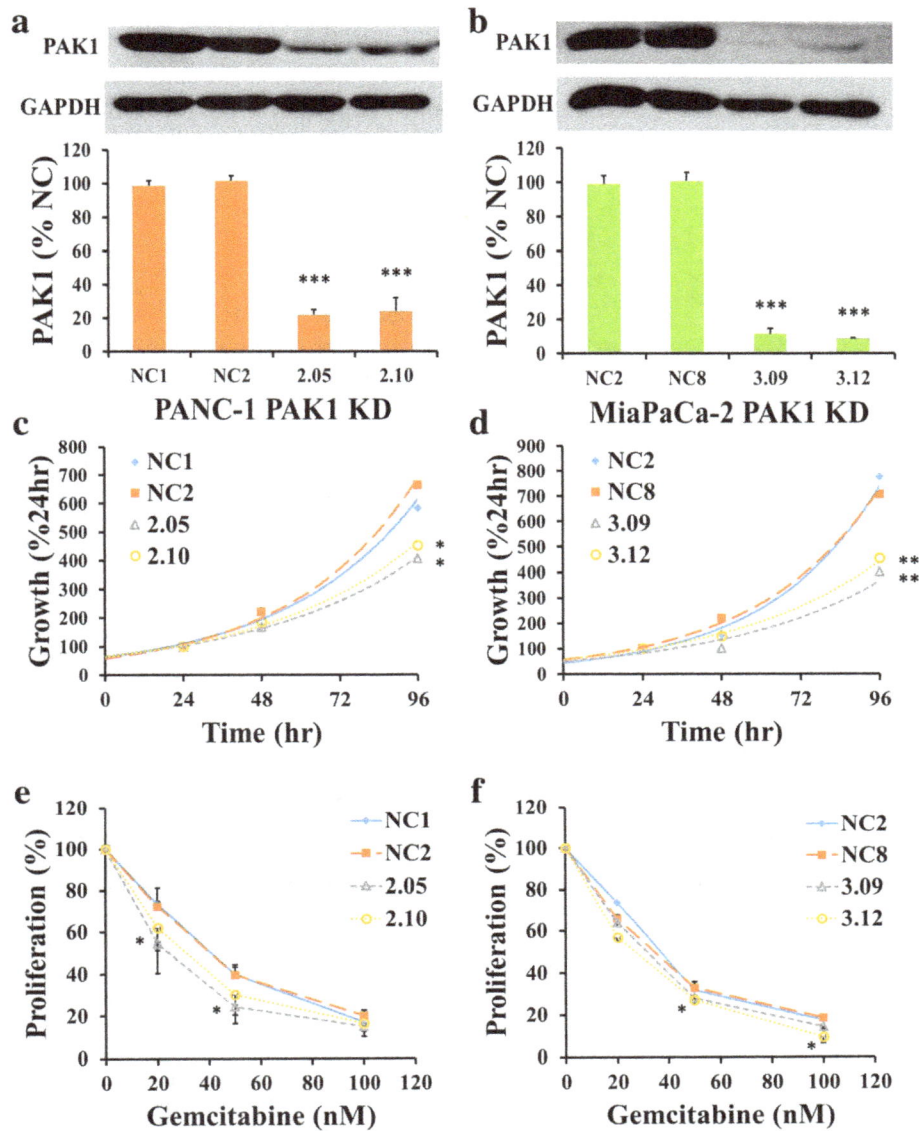

Fig. 2 PAK1 knock-down (KD) inhibits proliferation and increases gemcitabine sensitivity. PANC-1 (**a**) and MiaPaCa-2 (**b**) PAK1 KD cells were generated using shRNA transfection. As detected by western blot, clones 2.05 and 2.10; and clones 3.09 and 3.12 for PANC-1 and MiaPaCa-2, respectively, expressed significantly less PAK1 than negative control (NC) clones, which had been transfected with a scrambled shRNA. The proliferation rate of the KD clones for both PANC-1 (**c**) and MiaPaCa-2 (**d**), measured by thymidine incorporation, was significantly lower after 96 h. Sensitivity of the KD clones to gemcitabine (20 nM and 50 nM for PANC-1 (**e**), and 50nM and 100nM for MiaPaCa-2 (**f**)) was significantly increased. The data represent mean ± SEM, summarised from three independent experiments. * $p < 0.05$; ** $p < 0.01$, *** $p < 0.001$, compared to either NC clone (only the higher p value of the two is presented)

inhibited migration and invasion in all pancreatic cancer cell lines in a dose-dependent manner (Fig. 4b), with IC_{50} values between 105 nM for MiaPaCa-2 cells and 605 nM for Pan02 cells (Table 2). FRAX597 inhibited survival of LM-P cells in the absence of FBS in a dose-dependent manner with an IC_{50} value of 1.10 μM (Fig. 4c). Significant inhibition of survival of PANC-1, MiaPaCa-2, BxPC-3, and Pan02 cells was only observed at concentrations greater than 1 μM.

FRAX597 synergises with gemcitabine in inhibiting pancreatic cancer cell growth

Gemcitabine alone inhibited proliferation in all pancreatic cancer cell lines (Fig. 5a-e) in a dose-dependent manner, with IC_{50} values between 5 nM for BxPC-3 cells and 80 nM for Pan02 cells (Table 2). A further reduction in proliferation was observed in all pancreatic cancer cell lines (Fig. 5a-e) when FRAX597 was combined with gemcitabine, compared to gemcitabine alone. The

Table 1 PAK1 knock-down (KD) inhibits proliferation and increases gemcitabine sensitivity

	Growth rate (%/h)		Gemcitabine IC$_{50}$ (nM)	
	PANC-1	MiaPaCa-2	PANC-1	MiaPaCa-2
NC1	2.4	2.9	26 ± 2	29 ± 1
NC2	2.6	2.7	39 ± 1	28 ± 1
KD1	1.9 *	2.0 **	20 ± 2 **	26 ± 1 *
KD2	2.1 *	2.1 **	21 ± 2 *	25 ± 2 *

NC1 and NC2 indicate PANC-1 NC clones NC1 and NC2; and MiaPaCa-2 NC clones NC2 and NC8 respectively. KD1 and KD2 indicate PANC-1 KD clones 2.05 and 2.10; and MiaPaCa-2 KD clones 3.09 and 3.12 respectively. * $p < 0.05$; ** $p < 0.01$, compared to either NC clone (only the higher p value of the two is presented)

combination index, calculated for all pancreatic cancer cell lines (Fig. 5f), was less than 1, indicating that the effect was synergistic.

Inhibition of pancreatic cancer cell growth by FRAX597 and gemcitabine is associated with reduced amounts of active PAK1

The total amount of PAK1 and the amount of active phospho-PAK1 were measured using western blot after treatment with FRAX597 or gemcitabine, or the combination of FRAX597 and gemcitabine. The amount of active PAK1 was significantly reduced when treated with FRAX597 alone compared to control in all pancreatic cancer cell lines without affecting the amount of total PAK1 (Fig. 6a-e). No effect on PAK1 expression was observed after treatment with gemcitabine alone. For MiaPaCa-2 cells (Fig. 6b) and BxPC-3 cells (Fig. 6c), combined treatment with FRAX597 and gemcitabine resulted in significant further reduction of active PAK1 compared to the FRAX597 treatment alone. In contrast, in the other cell lines PANC-1 (Fig. 6a), Pan02 (Fig. 6d) and LM-P (Fig. 6e), no further reduction in active PAK1 expression was observed following the combination treatment.

FRAX597 and gemcitabine inhibit pancreatic tumour growth in an orthotopic murine model

The tumour take rate was 100 % for both pancreatic head and pancreatic tail models. The survival rate following surgery was 100 % for the pancreatic tail model and over 95 % for the pancreatic head model. No difference in tumour volume was observed for mice treated

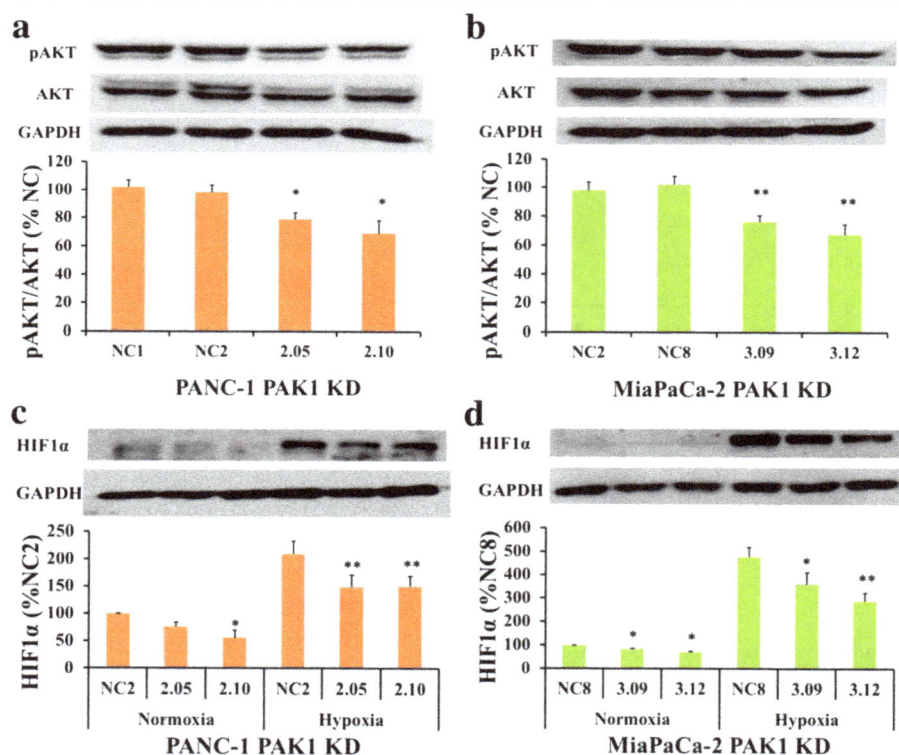

Fig. 3 PAK1 knock-down (KD) inhibits expression of AKT and HIF1α. Expression of phospho-AKT (pAKT) was significantly reduced in the PAK1 KD clones: 2.05 and 2.10 (PANC-1 (**a**)); and 3.09 and 3.12 (MiaPaCa-2 (**b**)), compared to the negative controls (NC), as assessed by western blot. HIF1α expression was reduced in PANC-1 (**c**) and MiaPaCa-2 (**d**) PAK1 KD clones under normoxia and hypoxia (1 % O$_2$) conditions. The data represent mean ± SEM, summarised from three independent experiments. * $p < 0.05$; ** $p < 0.01$, *** $p < 0.001$, compared to either NC clone (only the higher p value of the two is presented)

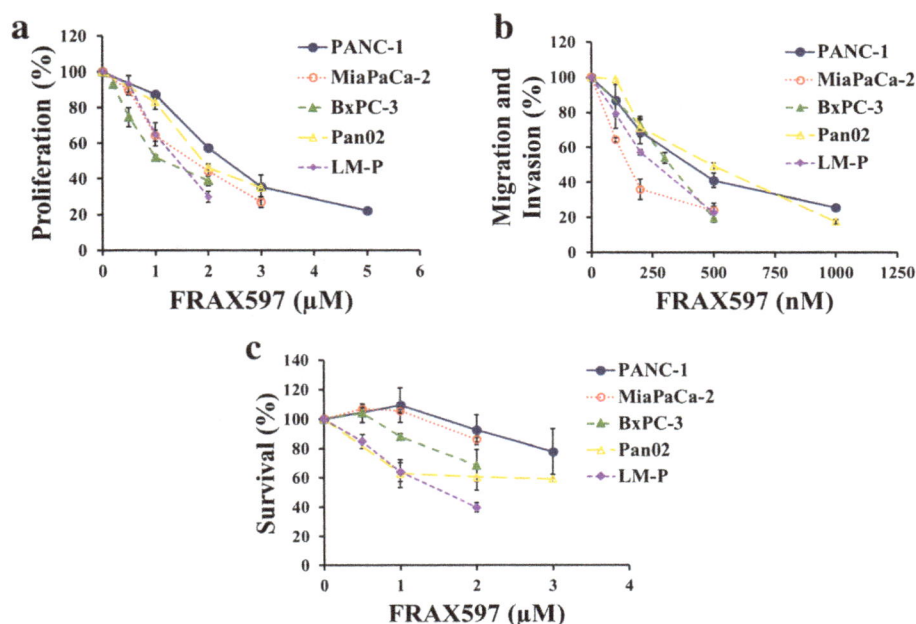

Fig. 4 FRAX597 inhibits proliferation, migration/invasion, and survival. The effect of the selective group 1-PAK inhibitor FRAX597 on cell proliferation (**a**), cell migration/invasion (**b**) and cell survival (**c**) of the indicated human pancreatic cancer cell lines was measured using the thymidine-incorporation method, the Transwell Boyden chamber assay, and the thymidine-withdrawal method, respectively. The values for the untreated cells were taken as 100 %. The data represent mean ± SEM, summarised from three independent experiments. Significance is not shown for clarity

with control or FRAX597 alone. Mice treated with gemcitabine alone had significantly reduced tumour volume when compared to control or FRAX597 alone, and a further significant reduction in tumour volume was observed for the mice treated with the combination of FRAX597 and gemcitabine (Fig. 7a). A similar trend was found when mice were evaluated for the presence of peritoneal carcinomatosis. 43 % of mice in the combined treatment group had peritoneal carcinomatosis compared to 71 % of mice in the gemcitabine treatment group, and 100 % of mice in the control and FRAX597 treatment groups (Fig. 7b).

Survival of mice in the combination treatment group was significant increased compared to the control group,

as assessed by a stratified Cox regression analysis (Fig. 7c). A rates ratio of 7 was calculated, indicating that mice in the control group had a mortality rate 7 times greater than mice in the combination treatment group (Table 3). The rates ratio of 2.7 for mice in the gemcitabine alone group, compared to mice in the combination treatment group, was not statistically significant ($p = 0.09$).

Discussion

Our finding that PAK1 is expressed in pancreatic cancer is in agreement with previous studies [8, 17]. We confirmed that PAK1 was not expressed in normal pancreatic acinar or ductal cells, which are the likely progenitors of pancreatic cancer [18]. In contrast, PAK1 was expressed in the tumour tissue, in which the pancreatic ductal adenocarcinomas cells stained positive (Fig. 1a). All pancreatic cancer cell lines showed upregulation of PAK1 compared to the normal pancreas cell line, HPDE, regardless of Kras mutational status. The observation from BxPC-3 and Pan02, that are Kras wildtype cell lines, indicates that non-Kras mechanisms may result in the activation of PAK1. Further investigation will be required to elucidate those mechanisms [19, 20]. The emergence of PAK1 expression implies that PAK1 is involved in pancreatic carcinogenesis, however, its role and therapeutic potential have not been fully elucidated.

Table 2 IC$_{50}$ values for inhibition of proliferation and migration/invasion by FRAX597, and of proliferation by gemcitabine

	FRAX IC$_{50}$ proliferation (µM)	FRAX IC$_{50}$ migration/invasion (nM)	Gemcitabine IC$_{50}$ proliferation (nM)
PANC-1	2.0 ± 0.2	290 ± 70	33 ± 3
MiaPaCa-2	1.4 ± 0.4	105 ± 10	30 ± 3
BxPC-3	0.65 ± 0.1	330 ± 45	5 ± 1
Pan02	1.4 ± 0.1	605 ± 80	80 ± 10
LM-P	1.1 ± 0.2	150 ± 25	16 ± 2

IC$_{50}$ values were obtained by fitting the data in Fig. 3 and Additional file 2: Figure S2 using Sigmaplot

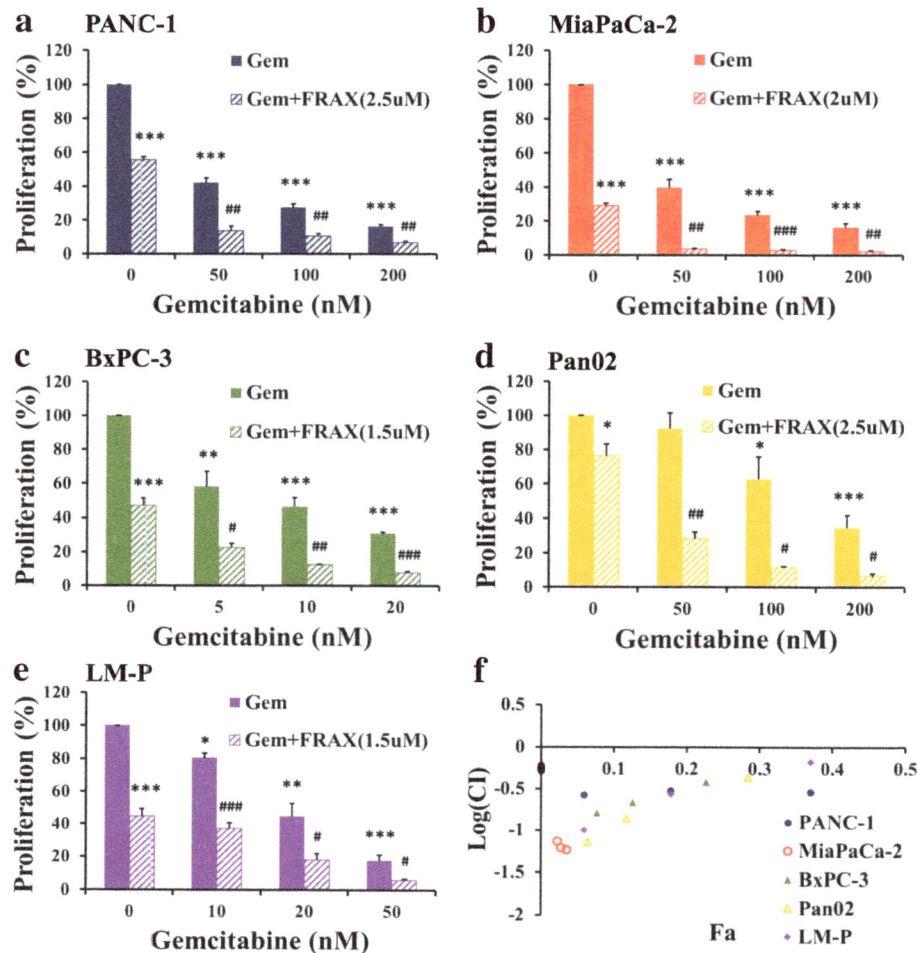

Fig. 5 FRAX597 synergises with gemcitabine to inhibit proliferation. The effects of gemcitabine alone (Gem, solid bars), and gemcitabine after 20 h pre-treatment with FRAX597 (Gem + FRAX, striped bars), on proliferation of PANC-1 (**a**), MiaPaCa-2 (**b**), BxPC-3 (**c**), Pan02 (**d**), and LM-P (**e**) cells were assessed by thymidine incorporation. The concentration of FRAX597 used was based on the IC_{50} value determined in Fig. 4a. The combination index (CI), calculated by the Chou-Ta alay method, was used to determine the mechanism of action of FRAX597 and gemcitabine (**f**). A value < 1 indicates synergistic inhibition. The data represent mean ± SEM, summarised from three independent experiments. * $p < 0.05$, ** $p < 0.01$, *** $p < 0.001$, compared to control or untreated cells. # $p < 0.05$, ## $p < 0.01$, ### $p < 0.001$ compared to the corresponding gemcitabine treatment

Reduction of PAK1 expression by shRNA knock-down (Fig. 2a-b) inhibited proliferation of the PANC-1 and MiaPaCa-2 pancreatic cancer cell lines (Fig. 2c-d), likely through modulation of the AKT pathway. These two human cell lines were chosen based on the PAK1 activity where PANC-1 is considered 'high' activity whilst MiaPaCa-2 is considered 'low' activity (Fig. 1b). This difference may contribute to the contrasting results in cell survival where a reduction was observed in PANC-1 PAK1 KD cells (Additional file 1: Figure S1A) but not in MiaPaCa-2 PAK1 KD cells (Additional file 1: Figure S1B). The suggestion that 'high' PAK1 expressing cells may be driving cell survival whereas 'low' PAK1 expressing cells may rely on other mechanisms to drive cell survival requires further investigation. The reduction in cell growth

in PAK1 KD cells was associated with a decrease in AKT activity (Fig. 3a-b), but not in ERK activity (Additional file 1: Figure S1C-D). Our group has previously found that PAK1 mediated growth of colorectal cancer cell lines by both ERK and AKT pathways [14], while another group has found that PAK1 signalled preferentially through the ERK pathway to control skin cancer growth [11]. Thus, PAK1 signalling through AKT and ERK pathways is dependent on the cancer type, and our study suggests that PAK1 mediates pancreatic cancer cell growth through the AKT pathway rather than the ERK pathway.

PAK1 may play a role in the resistance of pancreatic cancer to hypoxia through regulation of HIF1α. The transcription factor HIF1α regulates oxygen delivery and

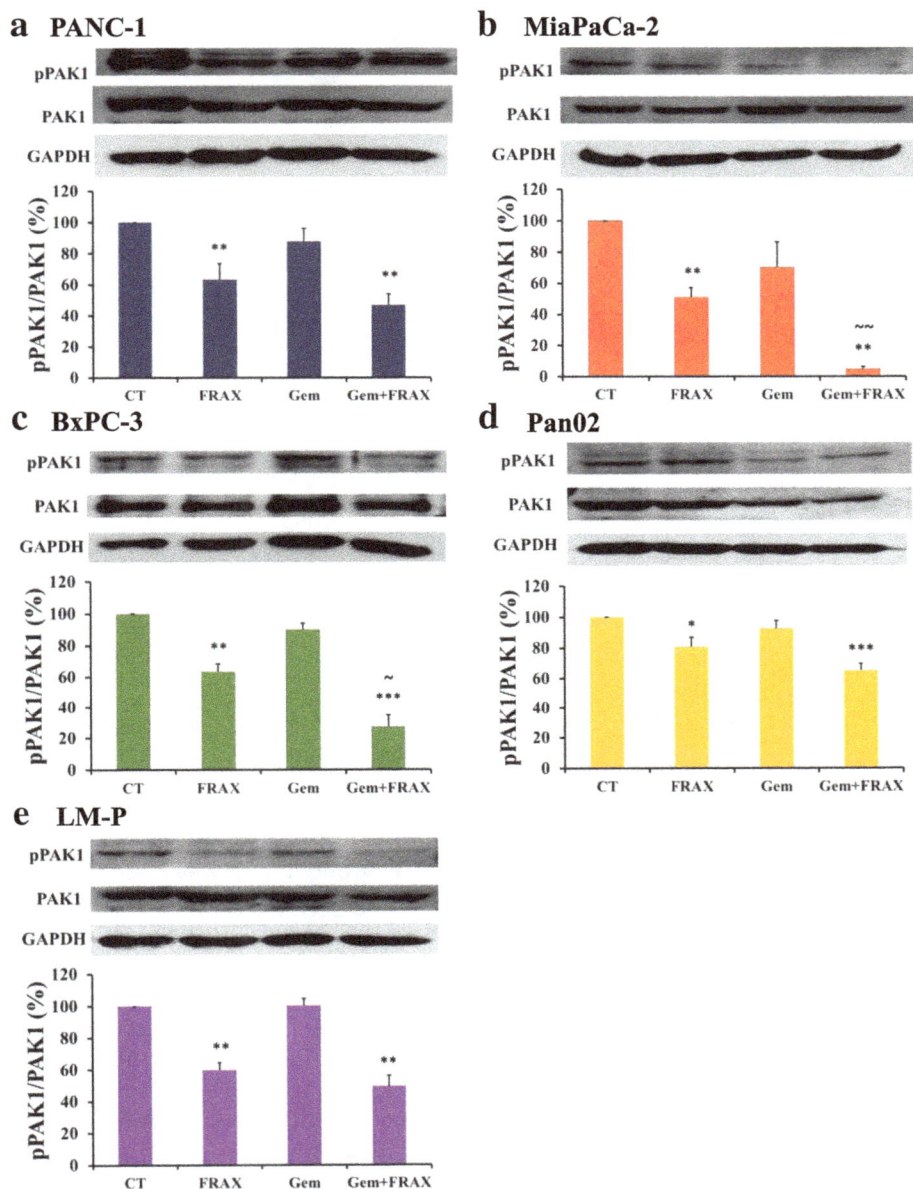

Fig. 6 FRAX597 and gemcitabine reduce PAK1 activity. Expression of phospho-PAK1 (pPAK1) and PAK1 was measured in PANC-1 (**a**), MiaPaCa-2 (**b**), BxPC-3 (**c**), Pan02 (**d**), and LM-P (**e**) cells in the presence of FRAX597 (FRAX), gemcitabine (Gem), or the combination of FRAX597 and gemcitabine (Gem + FRAX) using western blot. Variations in protein loading were corrected by GAPDH expression, and the values for untreated control cells were taken as 100 %. The data represent mean ± SEM, summarised from three independent experiments. ** $p < 0.01$, *** $p < 0.001$, compared to control or untreated cells. ~ $p < 0.05$, ~ ~ $p < 0.01$ compared to FRAX597 treatment

metabolic adaptation to hypoxia and has been found to be a prognostic marker for pancreatic cancer [21]. Pancreatic tumours are known to be highly hypoxic, as they feature a dense desmoplastic reaction (stroma), which may contribute to pancreatic cancer invasion, metastasis, and resistance to therapy [22]. Thus, mediators of survival in response to a hypoxic challenge are attractive therapeutic targets for pancreatic cancer. Although, as far as we are aware, this is the first study to examine

HIF1α as a downstream effector of PAK1 in pancreatic cancer, PAK1 has previously been linked to HIF1α in colorectal cancer [23]. The ability of PAK1 to contribute to pancreatic carcinogenesis via multiple signalling pathways enhances its potential as a therapeutic target.

PAK1 knock-down also enhanced the sensitivity of PANC-1 and MiaPaCa-2 cells to gemcitabine (Fig. 2e-f), as revealed by comparison of the IC$_{50}$ values for inhibition of proliferation between control and knock-down

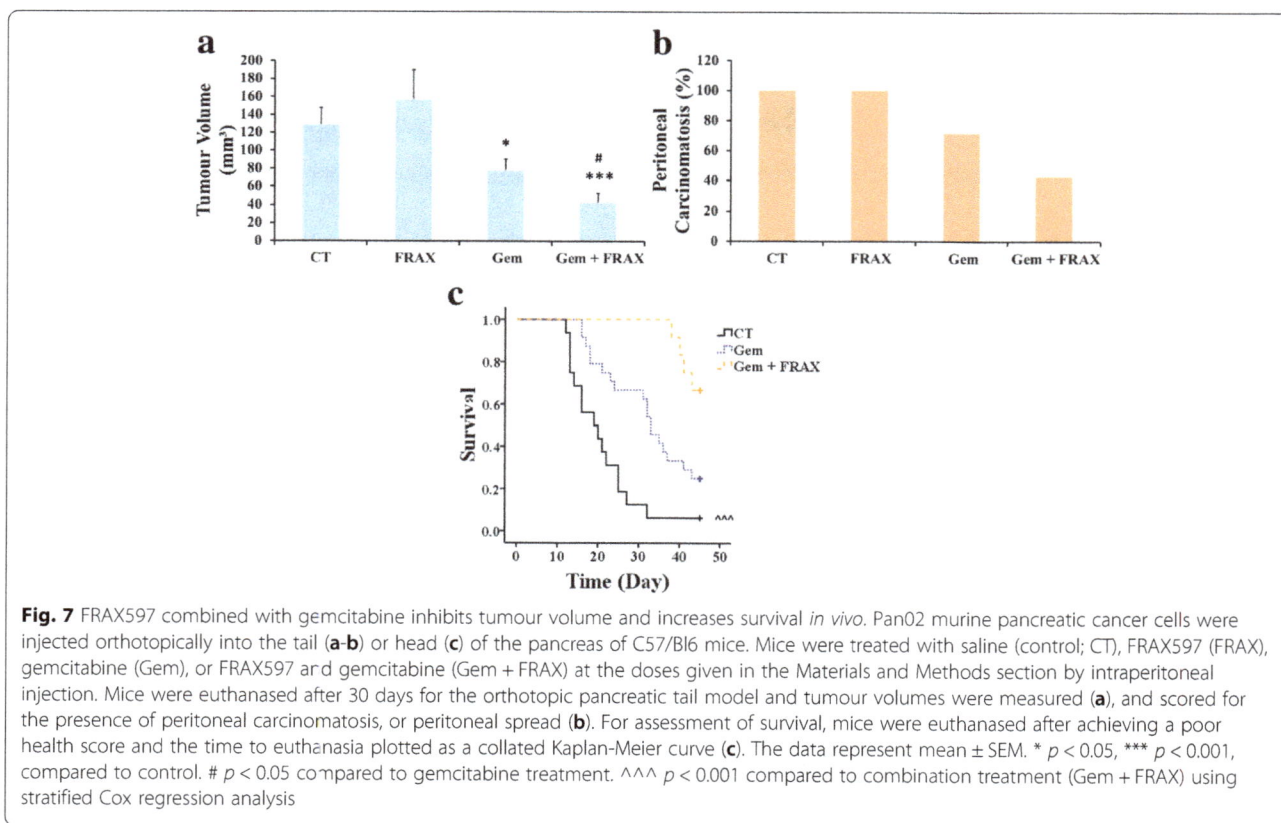

Fig. 7 FRAX597 combined with gemcitabine inhibits tumour volume and increases survival *in vivo*. Pan02 murine pancreatic cancer cells were injected orthotopically into the tail (**a-b**) or head (**c**) of the pancreas of C57/Bl6 mice. Mice were treated with saline (control; CT), FRAX597 (FRAX), gemcitabine (Gem), or FRAX597 and gemcitabine (Gem + FRAX) at the doses given in the Materials and Methods section by intraperitoneal injection. Mice were euthanased after 30 days for the orthotopic pancreatic tail model and tumour volumes were measured (**a**), and scored for the presence of peritoneal carcinomatosis, or peritoneal spread (**b**). For assessment of survival, mice were euthanased after achieving a poor health score and the time to euthanasia plotted as a collated Kaplan-Meier curve (**c**). The data represent mean ± SEM. * $p < 0.05$, *** $p < 0.001$, compared to control. # $p < 0.05$ compared to gemcitabine treatment. ^^^ $p < 0.001$ compared to combination treatment (Gem + FRAX) using stratified Cox regression analysis

clones (Table 1). Although gemcitabine remains a standard monotherapy treatment for pancreatic cancer patients, combining treatments with gemcitabine with the goal of decreasing chemotherapy-associated cytotoxicity and chemo-resistance and increasing survival has had varied results [3]. Previous studies have found that the PAK1 downstream effectors AKT and HIF1α could play a role in gemcitabine resistance through NFκB which limits gemcitabine uptake by decreasing nucleoside transporters such as hENT and hCNT [3]. Furthermore, PAK1 has been shown to regulate NFκB transcription upstream of fibronectin regulation in pancreatic cancer [8]. Although further investigation is required, the data presented herein supports the use of a PAK1 inhibitor combined with gemcitabine to limit gemcitabine cytotoxicity and chemo-resistance.

Table 3 FRAX597 combined with gemcitabine increases survival in a mouse orthotopic pancreatic cancer model

Treatment	Rates ratio	95 % CI	P value
Control	7.0	1.8 ± 27.0	0.005
Gemcitabine	2.7	1.0 ± 8.7	0.09
Gemcitabine + FRAX	1.0 (ref)		

The overall statistics for the stratified Cox regression analysis were: χ^2 (2) = 9.9, $p = 0.007$

The group 1 PAK-selective inhibitor FRAX597 inhibited proliferation, migration/invasion, and survival of all pancreatic cancer cell lines tested (Fig. 4a-c). Although FRAX597 also inhibits other kinases such as RET, YES1, TEK, and CSF1R [12], the similar results obtained in the PAK1 knock-down experiments suggest that in this case PAK1 is indeed the relevant target. Furthermore, the IC_{50} values for proliferation are similar to the value observed in NF2-null Schwann cells [12]. However, the IC_{50} values for either proliferation or migration/invasion did not significantly correlate with the amount of active PAK1 in the pancreatic cancer cells (data not shown). This observation suggests that there may be a barrier (e.g. uptake at the cell membrane) that prevents realisation of the full potential for inhibition in intact cells. The presence of such a barrier could have contributed to the failure to detect any difference in tumour volume between the FRAX597-treated mice and the control mice in our *in vivo* study. Furthermore, the dense desmoplastic reaction may have also prevented the drug's uptake by the tumour. These observations illustrate the importance of the microenvironment in assessment of a drug's efficacy, as the *in vitro* cell culture conditions may not fully mimic the clinical setting.

Combination of the PAK1 inhibitor, FRAX597, with gemcitabine resulted in increased inhibition of PAK1 activity in some, but not all, of the pancreatic cancer cell lines tested (Fig. 6a-e). In all the pancreatic cancer cell lines tested, PAK1 activity was significantly decreased after treatment with FRAX597 alone, but no change in activity was observed after treatment with gemcitabine alone. Thus, combined treatment with FRAX597 and gemcitabine might be expected to inhibit PAK1 to the same extent as FRAX597 treatment alone, as was observed for PANC-1, Pan02 and LM-P cells. The significantly greater inhibition observed in MiaPaCa-2 and BxPC-3 cells after combination treatment provided clear evidence for synergy, although the mechanism for this is unclear. Interestingly, these two pancreatic cancer cell lines had the lowest phospho-PAK1 expression of all the pancreatic cancer cell lines tested. This observation suggests that phospho-PAK1 may be a predictive marker for gemcitabine response, as has recently been shown for PAK4 in pancreatic cancer [24].

Treatment with FRAX597 combined with gemcitabine significantly decreased tumour volume *in vivo* (Fig. 7a) and revealed a promising trend towards decreasing metastasis (Fig. 7b) and increasing survival (Fig. 7c). Furthermore, Ki67 staining of the tumours indicated that the difference in tumour volume was due to inhibition of proliferation (Additional file 2: Figure S2). Although liver metastasis is often observed in the orthotopic pancreatic tail murine model, a total of only three mice, from control and FRAX treatment groups, had liver metastases at sacrifice, so no comparison could be undertaken [16]. However, peritoneal carcinomatosis, or peritoneal spread, was present and was compared. As a difference in tumour volume was observed between animals treated with gemcitabine alone or with the combination of FRAX597 and gemcitabine, a decrease in peritoneal carcinomatosis and an increase in survival was expected, but significance was not reached. This may be due to the fact that the study was stopped early, before all mice were euthanised because of tumour-related illness. Although the potential clinical value of FRAX597 and the likely therapeutic benefit of targeting PAK1 are clearly established by the data in Fig. 4, longer studies are needed for a complete picture of the possible survival benefits of combination treatment.

Conclusion

PAK1 is upregulated in human pancreatic cancer. Knock-down experiments indicated that PAK1 is required for proliferation and survival of human pancreatic cancer cell lines through AKT- and/or HIF1α-dependent pathway(s). Furthermore, PAK1 knock-down sensitised pancreatic cancer cells to gemcitabine. A group 1 PAK-specific inhibitor, FRAX597, inhibited proliferation, migration/invasion, and survival of human pancreatic cancer cell lines. When combined with gemcitabine, FRAX597 synergistically inhibited pancreatic cancer growth *in vitro* and *in vivo*. This study suggests the promise of inhibiting PAK1 function and defines areas for further investigation to clarify its potential value as a target for pancreatic cancer therapy.

Ethics approval and consent to participate and publication

Human ethics approval was obtained from the Austin Health Human Research Ethics Committee (H2013/04953) and all participants gave consent to participate and for publication. All mice experiments were approved by the Austin Health Animal Research Ethics Committee (A2013/04898).

Additional files

Additional file 1: Figure S1. PAK1 Knock-down (KD) effects on survival and ERK expression. PAK1 KD cells were measured in the presence (darker bars) and absence (lighter bars) of FBS to measure survival, using thymidine-withdrawal. Survival in PANC-1 PAK1 KD clones (A) was significantly lower but no difference was observed in MiaPaCa-2 PAK1 KD clones (B). No reduction in the expression of either phospho-ERK (pERK1/2) or total ERK (ERK1/2) was detected in either PANC-1 (C) or MiaPaCa-2 (D) PAK1 KD cells, as assessed by western blot. The data represent mean ± SEM, summarised from three independent experiments. *** $p < 0.001$, compared to the corresponding clone with FBS.

Additional file 2: Figure S2. FRAX597 and gemcitabine decreased Ki67 staining on orthotopic pancreatic tail tumours. Pan02 murine pancreatic tumours from the orthotopic pancreatic tail tumour model treated with saline (control; CT), FRAX597 (FRAX), gemcitabine (Gem), or FRAX597 and gemcitabine (Gem + FRAX) at the doses given in the Materials and Methods section, were fixed and stained for the proliferative marker, Ki67. Three representative images were taken from each treatment group.

Abbreviations
BPE: bovine pituitary extract; CI: combination index; EGF: epidermal growth factor; Fa: affected fraction; HPDE: human pancreatic duct epithelial cells; IHC: immunohistochemistry; i.p.: intraperitoneal; KD: knock-down; NC: negative control; NF2: neurofibromatosis type 2; PAK1: p21-activated kinase 1; shRNA: short hairpin RNA.

Competing interests
The authors declare that they have no competing interests.

Authors' contributions
DY, HH, GSB, and MN designed the experimental settings. DY carried out all the *in vitro* experimental studies and drafted the manuscript. HH, OP, AML and MN carried out the animal studies. HH, GSB, and MN helped to draft the manuscript. All authors read and approved the final manuscript.

Acknowledgements
We thank Prof. Ian Gordon, Statistical Consulting Centre, The University of Melbourne, Parkville, Australia for his assistance with statistical analysis, and Chelsea Dumesny, Nhi Huynh, and Marie Laval for skilled assistance with the animal experiments. D.Y. is supported by Australian Rotary Health (The Ian Loxton Pancreatic Cancer Research PhD Scholarship).
This work was supported by National Health and Medical Research Council of Australia Grants [508908 to H.H] and [1020983 to G.S.B]; National Institutes of Health [CA155620-01 to A.M.L]; Austin Hospital Medical Research Foundation (M.N); and Sir Edward Dunlop Foundation Grant (M.N).

Author details

[1]Department of Surgery, Austin Health, University of Melbourne, Heidelberg, VIC, Australia. [2]Department of Surgery, Division of Surgical Oncology, University of California at San Diego, Moores Cancer, La Jolla, CA, USA.

References

1. Rahib L, Smith BD, Aizenberg R, Rosenzweig AB, Fleshman JM, Matrisian LM. Projecting cancer incidence and deaths to 2030: the unexpected burden of thyroid, liver, and pancreas cancers in the United States. Cancer Res. 2014;74(11):2913–21.

2. Bosetti C, Bertuccio P, Negri E, La Vecchia C, Zeegers MP, Boffetta P. Pancreatic cancer: overview of descriptive epidemiology. Mol Carcinog. 2012;51(1):3–13.

3. de Sousa CL, Monteiro G. Gemcitabine: metabolism and molecular mechanisms of action, sensitivity and chemoresistance in pancreatic cancer. Eur J Pharmacol. 2014;741:8–16.

4. Zavoral M, Minarikova P, Zavada F, Salek C, Minarik M. Molecular biology of pancreatic cancer. World J Gastroenterol. 2011;17(24):2897–908.

5. Yeo D, He H, Baldwin G, Nikfarjam M. The role of p21-activated kinases in pancreatic cancer. Pancreas. 2015;44(3):363–9.

6. Rane CK, Minden A. P21 activated kinases: structure, regulation, and functions. Small GTPases. 2014; doi:10.4161/sgtp.28003

7. Ye DZ, Field J. PAK signaling in cancer. Cell Logist. 2012;2(2):105–16.

8. Jagadeeshan S, Krishnamoorthy YR, Singhal M, Subramanian A, Mavuluri J, Lakshmi A, et al. Transcriptional regulation of fibronectin by p21-activated kinase-1 modulates pancreatic tumorigenesis. Oncogene. 2014;34(4):455–64.

9. Chauhan SC, Ebeling MC, Maher DM, Koch MD, Watanabe A, Aburatani H, et al. MUC13 mucin augments pancreatic tumorigenesis. Mol Cancer Ther. 2012; 11(1):24–33.

10. Yeo D, Huynh N, Beutler JA, Christophi C, Shulkes A, Baldwin GS, et al. Glaucarubinone and gemcitabine synergistically reduce pancreatic cancer growth via down-regulation of p21-activated kinases. Cancer Lett. 2014;346(2):264–72.

11. Chow HY, Jubb AM, Koch JN, Jaffer ZM, Stepanova D, Campbell DA, et al. p21-Activated kinase 1 is required for efficient tumor formation and progression in a Ras-mediated skin cancer model. Cancer Res. 2012;72(22):5966–75.

12. Licciulli S, Maksimoska J, Zhou C, Troutman S, Kota S, Liu Q, et al. FRAX597, a Small Molecule inhibitor of the p21-activated kinases, inhibits tumorigenesis of Neurofibromatosis Type 2 (NF2)-associated Schwannomas. J Biol Chem. 2013;288(40):29105–14.

13. Tseng WW, Winer D, Kenkel JA, Choi O, Shain AH, Pollack JR, et al. Development of an orthotopic model of invasive pancreatic cancer in an immunocompetent murine host. Clin Cancer Res. 2010;16(14):3684–95.

14. Huynh N, Liu KH, Baldwin GS, He H. P21-activated kinase 1 stimulates colon cancer cell growth and migration/invasion via ERK- and AKT-dependent pathways. Biochim Biophys Acta. 2010;1803(9):1106–13.

15. Chou TC, Talalay P. Quantitative analysis of dose-effect relationships: the combined effects of multiple drugs or enzyme inhibitors. Adv Enzyme Regul. 1984;22:27–55.

16. Nikfarjam M, Yeo D, He H, Baldwin G Fifis T, Costa P, et al. Comparison of two syngeneic orthotopic murine models of pancreatic adenocarcinoma. J Invest Surg. 2013;26(6):352–9.

17. Han J, Wang F, Yuan SQ, Guo Y, Zeng ZL, Li LR, et al. Reduced expression of p21-activated protein kinase 1 correlates with poor histological differentiation in pancreatic cancer. BMC Cancer. 2014;14:650.

18. Zhu L, Shi G, Schmidt CM, Hruban RH, Konieczny SF. Acinar cells contribute to the molecular heterogeneity of pancreatic intraepithelial neoplasia. Am J Pathol. 2007;171(1):263–73.

19. Deer EL, Gonzalez-Hernandez J, Coursen JD, Shea JE, Ngatia J, Scaife CL, et al. Phenotype and genotype of pancreatic cancer cell lines. Pancreas. 2010;39(4):425–35.

20. Wang Y, Zhang Y, Yang J, Ni X, Liu S, Li Z, et al. Genomic sequencing of key genes in mouse pancreatic cancer cells. Curr Mol Med. 2012;12(3):331–41.

21. Hoffmann AC, Mori R, Vallbohmer D, Brabender J, Klein E, Drebber U, et al. High expression of HIF1a is a predictor of clinical outcome in patients with pancreatic ductal adenocarcinomas and correlated to PDGFA, VEGF, and bFGF. Neoplasia. 2008;10(7):674–9.

22. Yuen A, Diaz B. The impact of hypoxia in pancreatic cancer invasion and metastasis. Hypoxia. 2014; doi: 10.2147/HP.S52636

23. Liu KH, Huynh N, Patel O, Shulkes A, Baldwin G, He H. P21-activated kinase 1 promotes colorectal cancer survival by up-regulation of hypoxia-inducible factor-1alpha. Cancer Lett. 2013;340(1):22–9.

24. Moon SU, Kim JW, Sung JH, Kang MH, Kim SH, Chang H et al. P21-activated kinase 4 (PAK4) as a predictive marker of gemcitabine sensitivity in pancreatic cancer cell lines. Cancer Res Treat. 2014; doi:10.4143/crt.2014.054

2

Regulation of pancreatic stellate cell activation by Notch3

Haiyan Song and Yuxiang Zhang[*] (iD)

Abstract

Background: Activated pancreatic stellate cells (PaSCs) are the key cellular source of cancer-associated fibroblasts in the pancreatic stroma of patients with pancreatic ductal adenocarcinoma (PDAC), however, the activation mechanism of PaSCs is not yet known. The Notch signaling pathway, components of which are expressed in stromal cells, is involved in the fibrosis of several organs, including the lung and liver. In the current study, we investigated whether Notch signal transduction is involved in PaSC activation in PDAC.

Methods: The expression of Notch signaling pathway components in human PDAC was examined via immunohistochemical staining and assessed in mouse PaSCs using RT-qPCR and western blotting. Notch3 expression in both PDAC stromal cells and activated mouse PaSCs was evaluated using immunofluorescence, RT-qPCR and western blotting. The impact of siRNA-mediated Notch3 knockdown on PaSC activation was detected with RT-qPCR and western blotting, and the impact on PaSC proliferation and migration was detected using CCK-8 assays and scratch experiments. The effect of conditioned medium from PaSCs activated with Notch3 siRNA on pancreatic cancer (LTPA) cells was also detected with CCK-8 assays and scratch experiments. The data were analyzed for statistical significance using Student's t-test.

Results: Notch3 was overexpressed in both human PDAC stromal cells and activated mouse PaSCs, and Notch3 knockdown with Notch3 siRNA decreased the proliferation and migration of mouse PaSCs. The levels of markers related to PaSC activation, such as α-smooth muscle actin (α-SMA), collagen I and fibronectin, decreased in response to Notch3 knockdown, indicating that Notch3 plays an important role in PaSC activation. Furthermore, we confirmed that inhibition of PaSC activation via Notch3 siRNA reduced the proliferation and migration of PaSC-induced mouse pancreatic cancer (LTPA) cells.

Conclusions: Notch3 inhibition in PaSCs can inhibit the activation, proliferation and migration of PaSCs and reduce the PaSC-induced pro-tumorigenic effect. Therefore, Notch3 silencing in PaSCs is a potential novel therapeutic option for patients with PDAC.

Keywords: Pancreatic ductal adenocarcinoma, Pancreatic stellate cells, Notch3, Activation

Background

Pancreatic stellate cells (PaSCs) are myofibroblast-like cells found in exocrine areas of the pancreas, and they play an important role in the pathogenesis of pancreatitis and pancreatic cancer [1–3]. Fibrosis is a major feature of chronic pancreatitis and desmoplasia, a stromal reaction characteristic of pancreatic ductal carcinoma cancer (PDAC) [4]. In a normal pancreas, PaSCs constitute 4–7% of all pancreatic cells and are quiescent [5–7], however, PaSCs can switch between quiescent and activated phenotypes. In their quiescent state they have abundant vitamin-A-containing lipid droplets in their cytoplasm and express specific markers, such as desmin and glial fibrillary acidic protein (GFAP) [6]. When the pancreatic cells are injured, PaSCs transform into their active state, which is characterized by loss of the cytoplasmic vitamin-A-containing lipid droplets and upregulated expression of the cytoskeletal protein α-smooth muscle actin (α-SMA) [6, 7]. Activated PaSCs subsequently synthesize excessive extracellular matrix

* Correspondence: yxzhang@ccmu.edu.cn
Department of Biochemistry and Molecular Biology, Cancer Institute, Beijing Key Laboratory for Cancer Invasion and Metastasis Research, Capital Medical University, No. 10 Xitoutiao, You An Men, Fengtai District, Beijing 100069, People's Republic of China

(ECM) proteins, such as collagen, fibronectin and laminin, and the proliferation and migration of PaSCs increases [8].

Recently, attention has been focused on the desmoplastic reaction in pancreatic cancer, specifically how it regulates cancer progression. This desmoplastic reaction occurs because activated PaSCs secrete large quantities of ECM proteins, including collagen types I, III, and IV, into the tumor microenvironment [7, 8]. There is strong evidence of a correlation between activated PaSCs and PDAC [9–11]. Thus, elucidation of the mechanism underlying PaSC transformation from a quiescent to an activated phenotype has many important implications.

Several signaling pathways and molecules that mediate PaSC activation have been identified, including Sonic hedgehog [12, 13], mitogen-activated protein kinases [14], peroxisome proliferator activated receptor γ [15, 16], the Janus kinase/signal transducer and activator of transcription pathway, and the transcription factor nuclear factor-kappa B [17–20].

However, more research is required to understand the details of PaSC activation. The Notch signaling family is an evolutionarily highly conserved signaling pathway. Notch activation plays critical roles in embryonic development, cell differentiation, cell proliferation and apoptosis [21, 22]. The canonical Notch signaling pathway is known as the CSL-dependent pathway. Notch receptor proteins can be activated by interacting with a family of ligands on adjacent cells. Upon activation, the Notch receptor is cleaved, and the intracellular domain of the Notch receptor (NICD) is released from the membrane into the cytoplasm and translocates into the nucleus. NICD in the nucleus binds with CSL (CBF1/Su(H)/LAG-1, also known as RBP-Jκ) and forms a transcriptional activation complex that acts as a potent transcriptional activator of CSL target genes, such as Hes1, and thus promotes downstream gene expression [23]. Notch signaling pathway components are highly expressed in PDAC [24–26], and inhibition of the Notch signaling pathway inhibits PDAC progression [27, 28]. These results indicate that the Notch signaling pathway plays an important role in PDAC occurrence and progression. In addition, the Notch pathway is involved in stromal cell activation during lung and hepatic fibrosis [29–32], however, the role of the Notch pathway in PaSC activation remains undefined. We hypothesized that components of the Notch pathway are present in PaSCs and that Notch signaling regulates the activation of these cells. To date, four Notch receptors have been identified in mammals, and the presence of multiple Notch receptors and ligands suggests that different receptors play different roles in PaSC activation. In the present study, we investigate the role of Notch signaling in PaSC activation.

Methods

Pancreatic tissues and animals

Human pancreatic cancer tissue microarrays were purchased from Xi'an Alena Biotechnology Co., Ltd. of China. For this study, male C57BL/6 J wild-type mice (6 weeks old, weight range 20–25 g) were supplied by the Laboratory Animal Services Center of Capital Medical University. Mouse LTPA cells (ATCC Number: CRL-2389™) were obtained from American Type Culture Collection (ATCC).

Cell isolation and culture conditions

We isolated normal mouse PaSCs from the pancreas using the outgrowth method described by Apte and Bachem [5, 6]. PaSCs were cultured in DMEM/F12 (Gibco, New York, USA) containing 20% fetal bovine serum (FBS) (Gibco, New York, USA) and antibiotics (1% penicillin and streptomycin) (Beyotime, Haimen, China). PaSCs were confirmed by their fibroblast-like morphology and immunocytochemical positivity for PaSC markers such as α-SMA, collagen I and fibronectin.

Immunohistochemical staining

Xylene and a graded alcohol series (ZSGB-BIO, Beijing, China) were used for dewaxing and rehydration. Subsequently, sections were treated with citrate salt buffer (pH 6.0) in the microwave for 15 min for antigen retrieval, followed by 3% hydrogen peroxide (ZSGB-BIO, Beijing, China) for 15 min to block endogenous peroxidase activity. Then, the samples were blocked with 5% donkey blood serum (Jackson, West Grove, USA) in phosphate-buffered saline (PBS) for 1 h at room temperature. The primary antibodies used in our experiments are listed in Table 1. The samples were then incubated with primary antibodies (against Notch1, Notch2, Notch3, Notch4, Jagged1, Jagged2, Delta1, Delta3 and Delta4) at 4 °C overnight, followed by incubation with secondary horseradish peroxidase (HRP)-conjugated antibodies (ZSGB-BIO, Beijing, China) for 1 h at room temperature. Next, diaminobenzidine (DAB) and hematoxylin (ZSGB-BIO, Beijing, China) were applied for staining and counterstaining. After dehydration with a graded alcohol series and xylene, the samples were sealed with coverslips and neutral gum.

Immunofluorescence

Following dewaxing, rehydration and antigen retrieval, the samples were immunostained with mouse monoclonal anti-α-SMA (1:100) and rabbit polyclonal anti-Notch3 (1:50) antibodies at 4 °C overnight. The sections were then incubated with Alexa Fluor 594-conjugated donkey anti-rabbit IgG (Invitrogen, Chicago, USA) (1:1000) and Alexa Fluor 488-conjugated anti-mouse IgG (Invitrogen, Chicago, USA) (1:1000) for 1 h at room

Table 1 List of antibodies

	Host species	Dilution		Source/catalog no.
		IHC	WB	
Notch1	Rabbit	1:50	1:500	Santa Cruz/ sc-6014R
Notch2	Rabbit	1:500	1:2000	Lifespan/ LS-B399
Notch3	Rabbit	1:50	1:500	Santa Cruz/sc-5593
Notch4	Rabbit	1:50	1:500	Santa Cruz/sc-5594
HES1	Rabbit		1:200	Santa Cruz/ sc-25392
Jagged1	Rabbit	1:50		Santa Cruz/ sc-8303
Jagged2	Rabbit	1:50		Santa Cruz/ sc-5604
DLL1	Rabbit	1:50		Santa Cruz/ sc-9102
DLL3	goat	1:50		Santa Cruz/ sc-66513
DLL4	goat	1:50		Santa Cruz/ sc-18640
α-SMA	Mouse	1:100		Dako/M0851
α-SMA	Rabbit	1:100	1:1000	Abcam/ab5694
Fibronectin	Rabbit	1:50	1:1000	Proteintech/15613–1-AP
Collagen I	Rabbit	1:50	1:1000	Proteintech/14695–1-AP
CSL	Rabbit		1:1000	Cell Signaling/5313
GAPDH	Rabbit		1:10000	Sigma/G9545

temperature. Nuclei were counterstained with 4′, 6-diamidino-2-phenylindole (DAPI; Sigma-Aldrich, Munich, Germany) for 5 min. The stained tissues were visualized using a laser scanning confocal microscope (Olympus, Postfach, Hamburg, Germany).

Immunocytochemical staining

Mouse PaSCs from adherent cultures were digested with 0.25% trypsin/EDTA and centrifuged at 800 rpm for 3 min. The cell pellets were resuspended in complete medium. After preparing 6-well plates with coverslips, cell suspension was added into each well. The cells were cultured at 37 °C in 5% CO_2 for 48 h, washed with PBS and fixed with 4% paraformaldehyde (PFA) (ZSGB-BIO, Beijing, China) for 15 min. Then, cells were treated with 10% donkey serum at room temperature for 1 h and incubated with the following primary antibodies: mouse monoclonal anti-α-SMA (1:100), rabbit polyclonal anti-fibronectin (1:50), and rabbit polyclonal anti-collagen I (1:50) at 4 °C overnight. The cells were then incubated with Alexa 594-conjugated anti-rabbit IgG (Invitrogen, Chicago, USA) (1:1000) or Alexa 488-conjugated anti-mouse IgG (Invitrogen, Chicago, USA) (1:1000) for 1 h at room temperature. Nuclear staining was performed with 4′,6-diamidino-2-phenylindole (DAPI; Sigma-Aldrich Munich, Germany) for 5 min. The stained coverslips were visualized using a Nikon 80i fluorescence microscope.

siRNA-mediated Notch3 knockdown in PaSCs

One Notch3 siRNA (sc-37,136) was purchased from Santa Cruz and another was synthesized by Shanghai

Genepharma Co. Ltd. (Shanghai, China). The Notch3 siRNA sequence was (5′-3′)GCCAGAACUGUGAAGU-CAATT, and the control siRNA sequence was (5′-3′) UUCUCCGAACGUGUCACGUTT. PaSCs transfection was performed using the following steps. PaSCs were seeded into 6-well plates and transfected with Notch3 siRNA (50 nM) or negative siRNA using Lipofectamine 2000. After 48 h of transfection, mRNA and protein were extracted from the cells. Quantitative real-time reverse transcription polymerase chain reaction (RT-qPCR) and western blotting were used to confirm the Notch3 knockdown efficiency.

Cell proliferation

Cells (2×10^5) were seeded in a 24-well plate in 800 µl of DMEM/F12 containing 20% FBS and incubated at 37 °C in 5% CO_2 for 24 h. Mouse PaSCs in serum-free medium were transfected with Notch3 siRNA using Lipofectamine 2000 transfection reagent (Invitrogen, Chicago, USA) in accordance with the manufacturer's instructions. Five h after transfection, serum-free medium was replaced with complete medium. At 24, 48 and 72 h after transfection, cell growth was measured using a CCK-8 cell viability assay (AAT Bioquest, USA) according to the manufacturer's instructions.

To study the effect of PaSCs on mouse pancreatic cancer cells (LTPA cells), conditioned medium from mouse PaSCs was collected. Mouse PaSCs were seeded into a 6-well plate in complete medium for 24 h and then transfected with Notch3 siRNA. Forty-eight hours after transfection, the medium conditioned by PaSCs was collected. LTPA cells were incubated in the PaSC-conditioned medium for 24, 48 and 72 h, and their growth was measured using the CCK-8 cell viability assay (AAT Bioquest, USA) according to the manufacturer's instructions.

Cell migration assay

Mouse PaSCs were seeded in a 6-well plate $(2 \times 10^5$ cells) and incubated for 24 h. A scratch was made using a 1 ml pipette tip before the cells were transfected with Notch3 siRNA. Images were captured at 0, 24 and 48 h after transfection under an inverted microscope. ImageJ software was used to calculate the area of the scratch. Then, the percentage of wound closure was calculated and compared with that of the negative control.

To study the effect of PaSCs on mouse LTPA tumor cell migration, conditioned medium from mouse PaSCs was collected as described above. Mouse LTPA cells were seeded into the top of transwell chambers at 3×10^5 cells/ml. The bottom of the transwell chambers contained 600 µl of PaSC-conditioned medium. After 24 h, LTPA cells in the top chambers were swabbed away with a Q-tip. The membranes were washed three times with

PBS and then fixed with 4% PFA for 20 min and with 0.1% crystal violet (Sigma-Aldrich, Munich, Germany) for 15 min. LTPA cells were counted in at least in five random fields and photographed via microscopy (×200).

RT-qPCR

Total RNA was isolated from non-activated and activated mouse PaSCs 48 h after transfection with either Notch3 siRNA or control siRNA using TRIzol reagent (Invitrogen, Chicago, USA). The RNA concentration was measured using a NanoDrop® ND-1000 Spectrophotometer (Wilmington, DE). cDNA was synthesized with a RevertAid first strand cDNA synthesis kit (k1622, Thermo Scientific, Waltham, USA). RT-qPCR primers were synthesized by Sangong Biotech (Shanghai) and are listed in Table 2. RT-qPCR was conducted using a Mx3000p RT-PCR detection system and TransStart Top Green qPCR SuperMix (AQ131–02, Transgen Biotech, Beijing, China). The relative gene expression levels were normalized to glyceraldehyde 3-phosphate dehydrogenase (GAPDH) levels.

Western blotting

Proteins were isolated from non-activated and activated mouse PaSCs 48 h after transfection with either Notch3 siRNA or control siRNA using radioimmunoprecipitation assay buffer (Beyotime Bio, Haimen, China) containing a protease inhibitor cocktail and PMSF. Cells were centrifuged at 12,000 g for 30 min, and supernatant fractions were collected. Protein was measured with a Pierce™ BCA protein assay kit according to the manufacturer's instructions (Prod #23225, Thermo Scientific, Waltham, USA). Equal amounts of protein were loaded and separated on 8% or 10% PAGE gels and transferred onto nitrocellulose filter membranes (Millipore, Darmstadt, Germany). The membranes were incubated with 5% milk for 1 h at room temperature and then probed with primary antibodies overnight at 4 °C. The primary antibodies are shown in Table 1. Subsequently, the membranes were incubated with peroxidase-conjugated AffiniPure goat anti-rabbit

IgG (H + L) (ZB-2301, ZSGB-Bio) for 1 h at room temperature. The proteins were detected with enhanced chemiluminescence (Millipore, Darmstadt, Germany) using an LAS3000 System (Fujifilm, Japan). Protein levels were normalized to GAPDH levels and quantified using ImageJ software (NIH).

Statistical analysis

The data are presented as the mean ± SD. Comparisons between two groups were analyzed with a two-sided Student's t-test using SPSS16.0 software. $P < 0.05$ was considered statistically significant. All experiments were repeated three to six times.

Results
Expression of notch receptors and ligands in human PDAC stroma

To investigate the expression of Notch signaling components in human PDAC, we performed an immunohistochemistry (IHC) analysis. We found that both Notch receptors and ligands were expressed in PDAC tumor cells, but the degree of expression varied. Notch1 and Notch3 and the Notch ligands DLL1, DLL3 and DLL4 were highly expressed, and Notch2 and Notch4 and the Notch ligands Jagged1 and Jagged2 were slightly expressed (Fig. 1a). We also identified Notch3 and Notch1 expression in PDAC stroma (Fig. 1b). The results of immunofluorescence co-localization demonstrated that Notch3 was expressed in α-SMA-positive activated PaSCs (Fig. 1c).

Primary culture and identification of non-activated and activated mouse PaSCs

According to the literature, PaSCs in the normal pancreas have similar function compared to PaSCs in PDAC, such as promoting tumor cell growth and metastasis [33, 34]. We used primary normal mouse PaSCs as a model to study the possible activation mechanism of PaSC, and we used oil red O staining [33] to identify non-activated and activated PaSCs. We identified numerous lipid droplets in early-passage primary cells, indicating that these cells were non-activated PaSCs (Fig. 2a). After growth on a plastic surface for 5 days, the lipid droplets in these primary cells disappeared, and the morphology of the cells changed, the cells became flattened and developed long cytoplasmic extensions, which are characteristics of activated PaSCs (Fig. 2a). The transition of quiescent PaSCs to an activated myofibroblastic phenotype was accompanied by changes in the cytoskeleton.

The activated PaSCs were positive for α-SMA, collagen I and fibronectin (Fig. 2b). Quantitative reverse transcription polymerase chain reaction (RT-qPCR) and sodium dodecyl sulfate polyacrylamide gel electrophoresis

Table 2 Primers used for RT-qPCR

Primer	Forward sequence 5'-3'	Reverse sequence 5'-3'
Notch1	TCGTGCTCCTGTTCTTTGTG	CTCTCCGCTTCTTCTTGCTG
Notch2	GCAGGAGCAGGAGGTGATAG	ATGAGAAGCCAGGAGAGCAG
Notch3	TGGCTATGCTGGTGACAGTT	AGGGGGACAGGAACAGAGAT
Notch4	AATGCCAAGGTCAGGAACAC	AGCCCTCATCACACACACAC
α-SMA	AATGGCTCTGGGCTCTGTAA	CTCTTGCTCTGGGCTTCATC
Fibronectin	GAAGTCGCAAGGAAACAAGC	GTAGGTGAACGGGAGGACAC
CollagenI	TGACTGGAAGAGCGGAGAGT	GACGGCTGAGTAGGGAACAC
HES1	GGCGAAGGGCAAGAATAAAT	TGCTTCACAGTCATTTCCAGA
GAPDH	GGTTGTCTCCTGCGACTTCA	TGGTCCAGGGTTTCTTACTCC

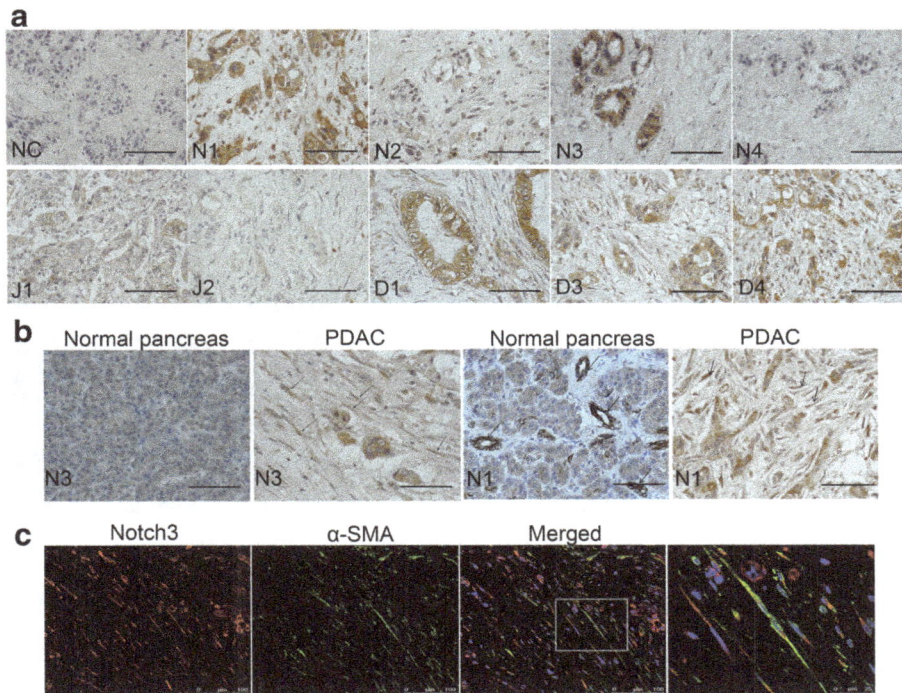

Fig. 1 Expression of Notch1-Notch4 and the Notch ligands Jagged1, Jagged2, DLL1, DLL3, and DLL4 in PDAC. **a** Representative immunohistochemistry images of Notch1-Notch4 receptors (N1,N2,N3,N4) and Jagged1 (J1), Jagged2 (J2), DLL1 (D1), DLL3 (D3), and DLL4 (D4) ligands in PDAC. NC: negative control. **b** Representative immunohistochemistry images of Notch1 and Notch3 protein expression in PDAC and in normal pancreas. **c** Representative double immunofluorescence staining of α-SMA (green) and Notch3 (red) in PDAC stroma. High magnification image is shown on the right. Scale bars: 50 μm in (**a**) and (**b**)

(SDS-PAGE) followed by western blotting were used to detect α-SMA, collagen I and fibronectin mRNA and protein, respectively. Densitometry analyses revealed that compared to non-activated PaSCs activated PaSCs had higher mRNA and protein levels of α-SMA (1.000 ± 0 vs 8.854 ± 5.485 and 0.6738 ± 0.0668 vs 1.604 ± 0.1725, respectively), collagen I (1.000 ± 0 vs 3.803 ± 2.154 and 0.4138 ± 0.09837 vs 0.7192 ± 0.1449, respectively) and fibronectin (1.000 ± 0 vs 11.20 ± 5.890 and 0.08677 ± 0.00979 vs 0.4358 ± 0.0366, respectively) ($n = 4$, $P < 0.001$; Fig. 2c-d). Taken together, these results indicate that we cultivated PaSCs.

The expression of notch signaling pathway components in non-activated and activated PaSCs

Western blotting and RT-qPCR were used to detect changes in the expression of Notch family proteins induced by PaSCs activation. Levels of Notch1 (0.7169 ± 0.03594 vs 0.2761 ± 0.008455, $P < 0.001$), Notch2 (0.2378 ± 0.05646 vs 0, $P < 0.01$), Notch3 (1.061 ± 0.01039 vs 0.1033 ± 0.03333, $P < 0.001$), the transcription factor CSL (0.6074 ± 0.07683 vs 0.2139 ± 0.01509, $P < 0.01$) and the Notch target gene HES1 (0.4100 ± 0.02194 vs 0.2035 ± 0.004786, $P < 0.001$) were upregulated in activated PaSCs compared to non-activated PaSCs ($n = 4$; Fig. 3a).

Notch4 was not detectable (Fig. 3a). The mRNA levels of Notch1 (1.587 ± 0.5973 vs 1.000 ± 0, $P < 0.01$), Notch2 (2.858 ± 1.352 vs 1.000 ± 0, $P < 0.001$), Notch3 (2.291 ± 0.4797 vs 1.000 ± 0, $P < 0.001$) and HES1 (1.992 ± 0.9125 vs 1.000 ± 0, $P < 0.001$) were upregulated in activated PaSCs compared to non-activated PaSCs, respectively ($n = 4$; Fig. 3b), which is consistent with the trend in protein levels. In addition, Notch4 mRNA was downregulated (0.7216 ± 0.2144 vs 1.000 ± 0, $P < 0.001$) ($n = 4$). Using immunofluorescence double-staining, we demonstrated that the Notch3 protein was highly expressed in α-SMA-positive but not α-SMA-negative PaSCs (Fig. 3c). Taken together, these results demonstrate Notch3 expression in activated PaSCs.

Effect of Notch3 inhibition on PaSC activation

To investigate whether Notch3 downregulation inhibits mouse PaSC activation, Notch3 siRNA (50 nM) was used to knock down Notch3 expression. Cytoplasmic lipid droplets reappeared in activated PaSCs 48 h after transfection with Notch3 siRNA (Fig. 4a). We observed a significant downregulation of Notch3 protein in cells transfected with Notch3 siRNA but not in those transfected with control siRNA (0.1117 ± 0.1368 vs 0.9938 ± 0.6741; $P < 0.01$; $n = 4$) (Fig. 4b). α-SMA, collagen I and

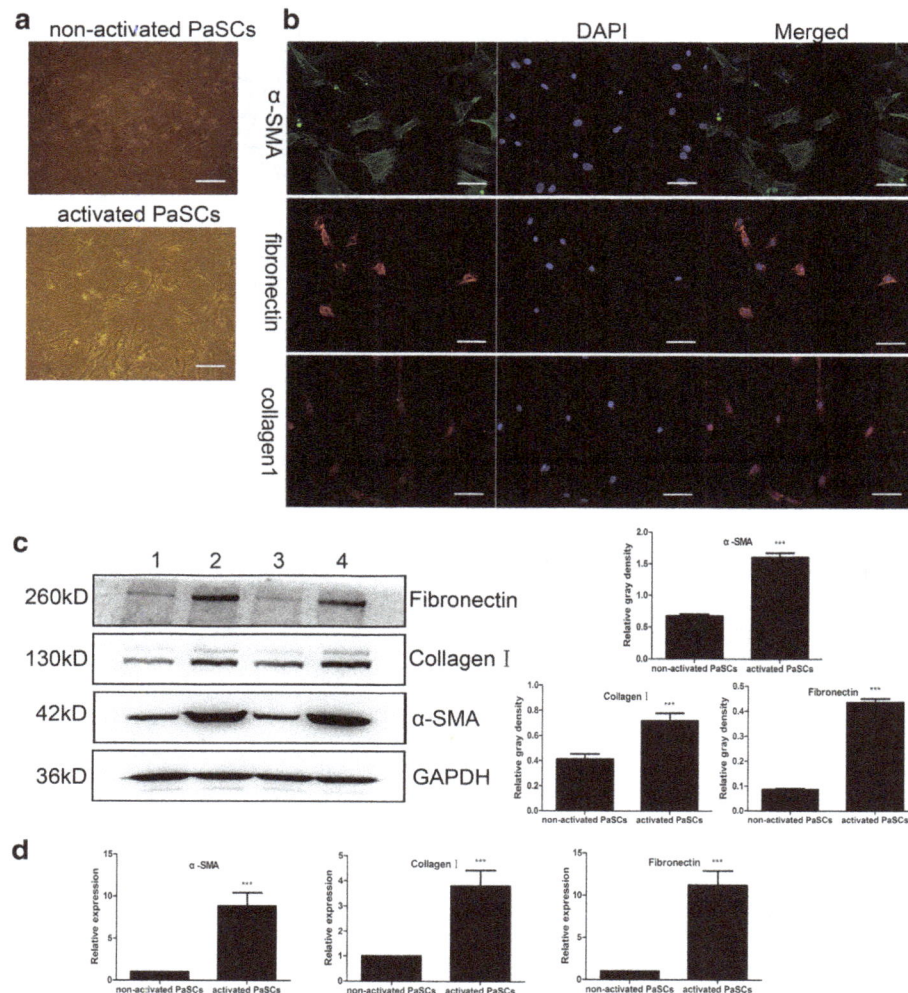

Fig. 2 Culture and identification of primary mouse PaSCs. **a** Representative oil red O staining in mouse non-activated and activated PaSCs. **b** Immunofluorescence staining of α-SMA, collagen I and fibronectin in mouse PaSCs. Nuclei were counterstained with DAPI. **c** Representative western blotting images showing the α-SMA, collagen I and fibronectin expression in non-activated and activated PaSCs; densitometry analyses of the blots are also shown (groups 1 and 3 represent non-activated PaSCs; groups 2 and 4 represent activated PaSCs). **d** Representative RT-qPCR results showing the α-SMA, collagen I and fibronectin mRNA expression in non-activated and activated PaSCs. Scale bars: 50 μm in (**a**) and (**b**). The data are presented as the mean ± SD. ***$P < 0.001$; $n = 4$; (t-test); Student's t-test

fibronectin are markers of activated PaSCs, and α-SMA, collagen I and fibronectin were all significantly lower in PaSCs treated with Notch3-specific siRNA. In control-siRNA-treated cells, α-SMA, collagen I and fibronectin levels were 1.028 ± 0.01647, 0.8719 ± 0.007824 and 1.032 ± 0.02623, respectively, and in Notch-3-siRNA-treated cells, these levels were reduced to 0.8252 ± 0.01324 ($P < 0.001$), 0.0000 ($P < 0.001$) and 0.6397 ± 0.03654 ($P < 0.01$), respectively (Fig. 4b). The protein expression level of the Notch target gene HES1 was also downregulated by Notch3 siRNA (0.9155 ± 0.03396 vs 0.6038 ± 0.01053, $P < 0.01$; Fig. 4b).

We also confirmed downregulation of α-SMA, collagen I and fibronectin mRNA in PaSCs treated with Notch3-specific siRNA. The mRNA levels of α-SMA, collagen I

and fibronectin fell from 0.7513 ± 0.1846, 0.9198 ± 0.3538, and 1.145 ± 0.7626 in cells treated with control siRNA to 0.3620 ± 0.09951 ($P < 0.001$), 0.3762 ± 0.1392 ($P < 0.001$), and 0.4260 ± 0.2995 ($P < 0.01$), respectively, in cells treated with Notch3 siRNA (Fig. 4c). The mRNA of the Notch target gene HES1 was significantly downregulated in PaSCs transfected with Notch3 siRNA compared to PaSCs transfected with control siRNA (0.2637 ± 0.1776 vs 0.7092 ± 0.1991, $P < 0.05$, $n = 4$; Fig. 4c).

PaSCs are activated by culture in conditioned medium from PDAC cells

The activation of PaSCs by treatment with mouse PDAC tumor cell (LTPA cell)-conditioned medium (2 ml) was

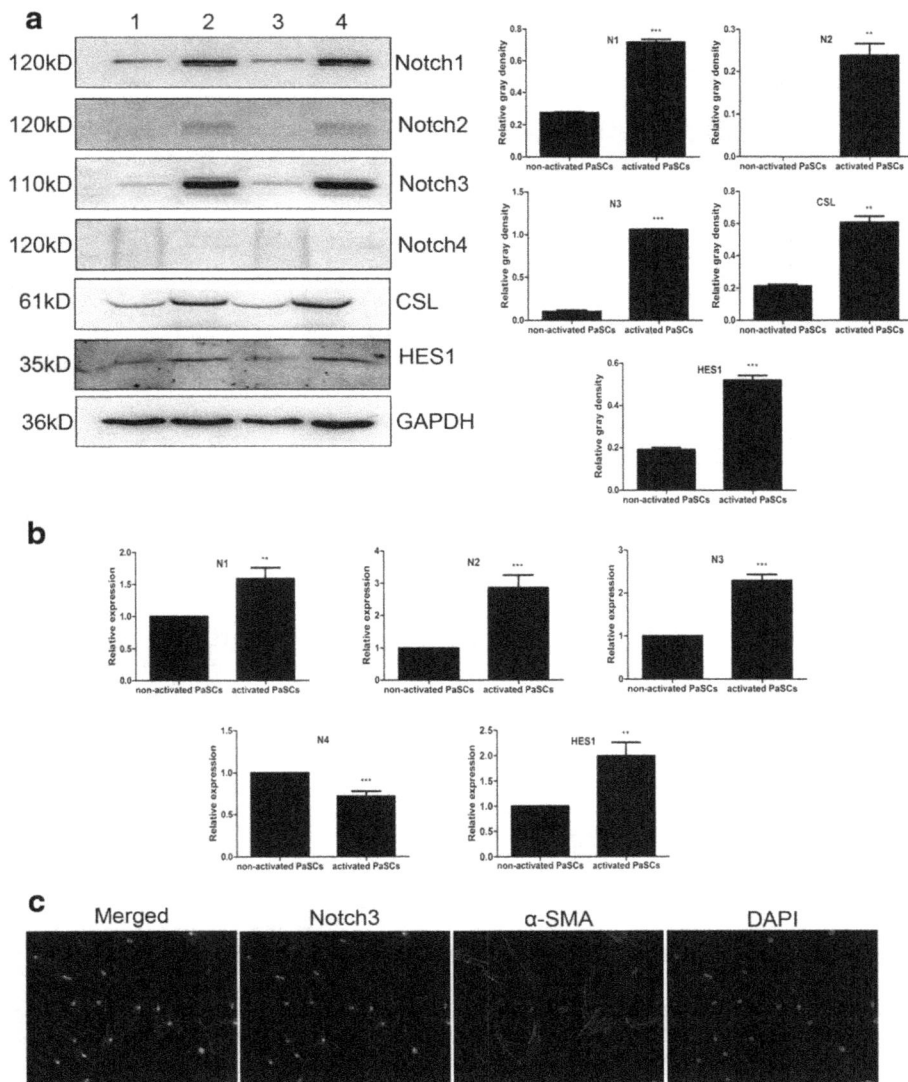

Fig. 3 Notch receptor expression in primary mouse PaSCs. **a** Representative western blotting images showing the Notch1–4, CSL and HES1 protein expression in non-activated and activated PaSCs; densitometry analyses of the blots are also shown (groups 1 and 3 represent non-activated PaSCs; groups 2 and 4 represent activated PaSCs). **b** RT-qPCR results showing the Notch1–4 and HES1 mRNA expression in non-activated and activated PaSCs. **c** Representative double immunofluorescence staining of α-SMA (red) and Notch3 (green) in primary mouse PaSCs. Scale bars: 50 μm in (**c**). The data are presented as the mean ± SD, **$P < 0.01$ and ***$P < 0.001$; $n = 4$; Student's t-test

assessed by analyzing the expression of markers of activated PaSCs. After 3 days of standard culture, PaSCs were further cultured with LTPA-conditioned medium for 24 h and then transfected with either Notch3 siRNA or control siRNA for 48 h to determine if Notch3 siRNA suppressed the PaSC activation induced by LTPA-conditioned medium. We found that Notch3-specific siRNA downregulated the expression of PaSC activation markers (Additional file 1: Figure S1). These results collectively demonstrate that Notch3 plays an important role in the transition of PaSCs from a quiescent to an activated state.

Effect of Notch3 siRNA on migration and proliferation of PaSCs

We examined whether Notch3 plays a role in the migration and proliferation of PaSCs. We used a scratch assay (wound healing assay) and a cholecystokinin-8 (CCK-8) assay to measure the effect of Notch3 siRNA on migration and proliferation, respectively, of mouse PaSCs (see Methods). The scratch assay showed that Notch3 siRNA (50 nM) inhibited wound closure (scratch gap), and therefore migration of PaSCs, compared to control siRNA. As shown in Fig. 5a, mock-control PaSCs (non-transfected) and control-siRNA-treated PaSCs migrated

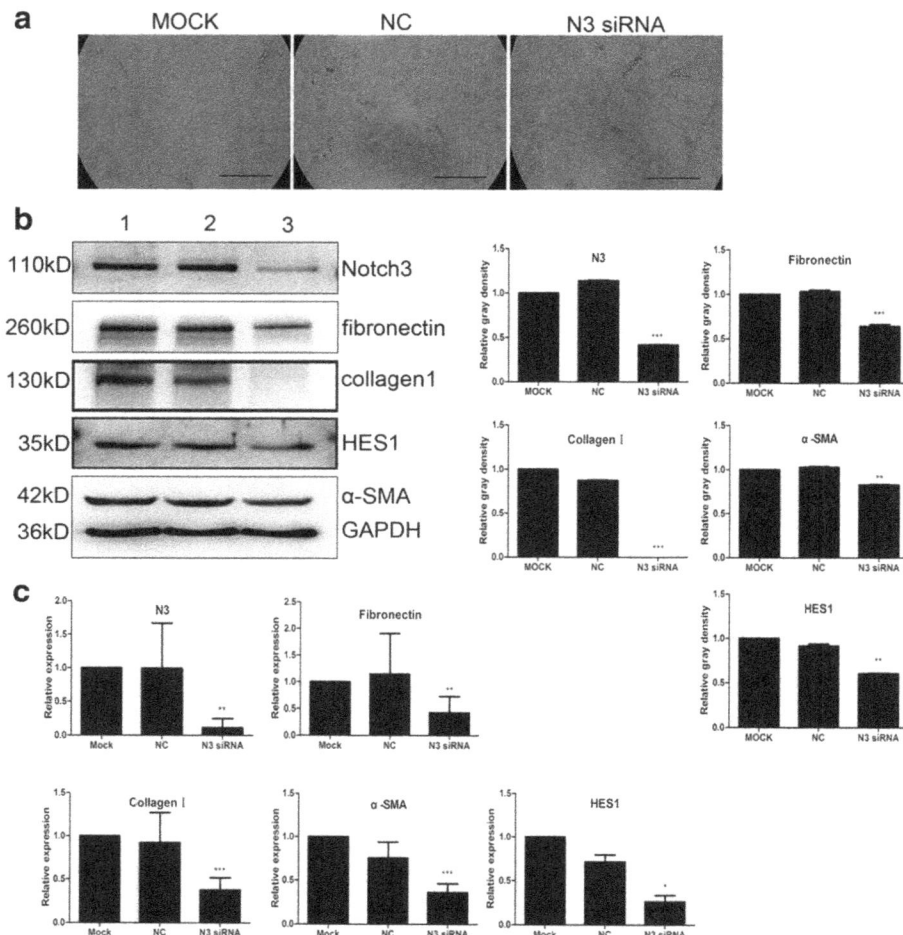

Fig. 4 Effect of siRNA-mediated Notch3 inhibition on mouse PaSC activation. **a** Transfection of Notch 3 siRNA in mouse PaSCs activation after 48 h, the morphological changes in PaSCs. **b** Representative western blotting images showing the effect of siRNA-mediated Notch3 inhibition on PaSC activation markers, such as α-SMA, fibronectin and collagen I, and on the Notch target gene HES1; densitometry analyses of the blots are also shown. **c** RT-qPCR results showing the effect of siRNA-mediated Notch3 inhibition on PaSC activation markers, such as α-SMA, fibronectin and collagen I, and on the Notch target gene HES1 at the transcriptional level. Scale bars: 100 μm in (**a**). The data are presented as the mean ± SD, *$P < 0.05$, **$P < 0.01$, and ***$P < 0.001$; $n = 4$; Student's t-test

into the gap formed by the scratch made in the cell monolayer and covered 40.25% and 36.44% of the gap surface area 24 h after transfection and 58% and 55.07% 48 h after transfection, respectively. In contrast, PaSCs transfected with Notch3 siRNA migrated much more slowly than both mock-control-treated and siRNA-control-treated PaSCs, filling only 15.48% and 18.02% of the gap at 24 h and 48 h, respectively (Notch3 siRNA-treated PaSCs vs control-siRNA-treated PaSCs at 24 h: 15.48 ± 0.9891 vs 36.44 ± 0.7617, $P < 0.001$; and at 48 h: 18.02 ± 1.340 vs 55.07 ± 1.441, $P < 0.001$; $n = 4$).

These results indicate that Notch3 knockdown severely inhibits the migratory activity of PaSCs.

We further investigated whether downregulation of Notch3 by siRNA inhibited PaSC proliferation and found that Notch3 knockdown significantly inhibited

PaSC proliferation (Fig. 5b) (24 h: 0.2440 ± 0.02298 vs 0.3022 ± 0.02005, $P < 0.01$; 48 h: 0.3838 ± 0.03224 vs 0.4732 ± 0.03949, $P < 0.01$; 72 h: 0.4692 ± 0.01975 vs 0.5704 ± 0.01991, $P < 0.001$; $n = 6$). These data suggest that Notch3 regulates PaSC migration and proliferation.

Effect of PaSC-conditioned medium on migration and proliferation of tumor cells

Control-siRNA-treated and Notch3-siRNA-treated PaSCs were cultured for 48 h, and then, the culture medium was collected and used to culture LTPA (mouse PDAC) cells. The migration and proliferation of LTPA cells were then examined. Transwell experiment results showed that the migration of LTPA cells cultured in the conditioned medium from Notch3 siRNA-treated PaSCs was significantly reduced compared with that of LTPA

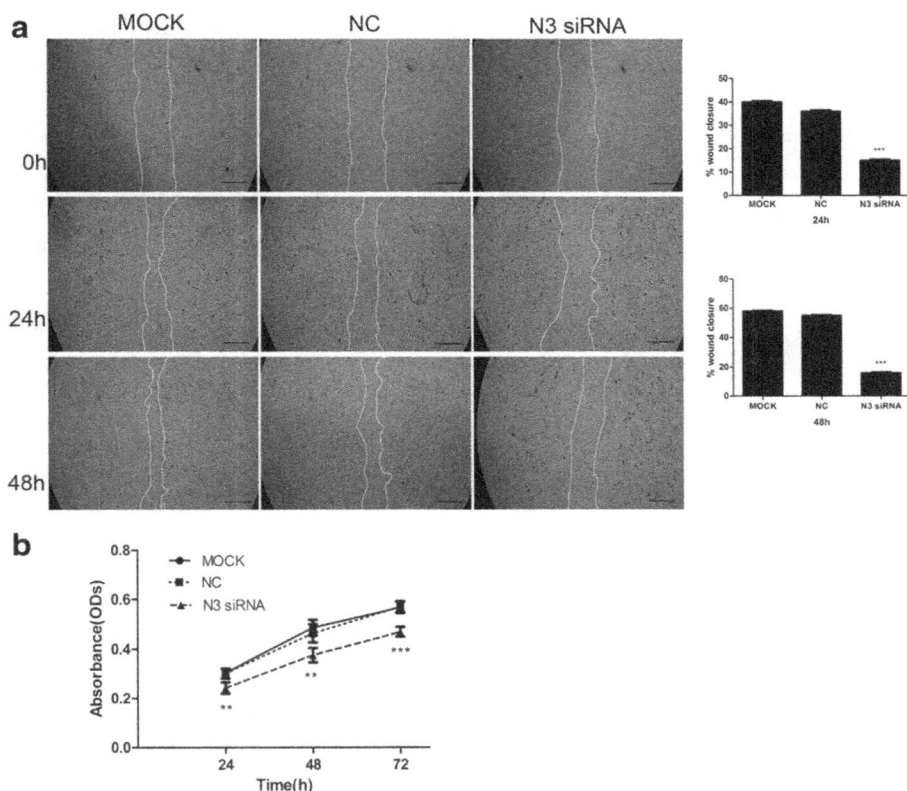

Fig. 5 Effect of Notch3 siRNA on migration and proliferation of mouse PaSCs. **a** Representative microscopic images showing the effect of Notch3 siRNA on the migration of mouse PaSCs; the semi-quantitative image analysis is also presented ($n = 4$). **b** Cell growth curve showing that transfection of mouse PaSCs with Notch3 siRNA significantly reduced PaSC proliferation compared to negative control siRNA. Scale bars: 100 μm in (**a**). The data are presented as the mean ± SD, $**P < 0.01$ and $***P < 0.001$; $n = 6$; Student's t-test

cells cultured in conditioned medium from the control-siRNA-transfected PaSCs (Fig. 6a; 199.3 ± 14.05 vs 654.7 ± 49.14, $P < 0.01$; $n = 4$). We also used CCK-8 assays to determine the effect of PaSC-conditioned medium on LTPA cell proliferation. We observed that the proliferation of LTPA cells cultured with conditioned medium from Notch3-siRNA-transfected PaSCs was decreased compared with that of the LTPA cells cultured with conditioned medium from control-siRNA-transfected PaSCs (Fig. 6b; 48 h: 1.234 ± 0.03753 vs 1.422 ± 0.08884, $P < 0.01$; 72 h: 1.359 ± 0.03249 vs 1.577 ± 0.07606, $P < 0.01$; $n = 6$). These data indicate that inhibition of PaSC activation by Notch3 siRNA reduces tumor cell migration and proliferation, presumably by releasing currently unidentified factors into the medium.

Discussion

One of the features of PDAC is the presence of extensive desmoplasia. The desmoplastic stroma consists of ECM and stromal cells [35]. PaSCs are the most numerous stromal cells and are responsible for ECM production. Thus, they play an important role in regulating the PDAC tumor microenvironment [2, 36, 37]. In a healthy

pancreas, PaSCs remain in a quiescent state, exhibit abundant lipid droplets rich in vitamin A in their cytoplasm [1], and express desmin and glial fibrillary acidic protein (GFAP) [6]. However, when the pancreas is injured by either inflammation or tumor growth, the PaSCs are activated by growth factors, cytokines or oxidative stress [38]. Activated PaSCs transdifferentiate into myofibroblast-like cells, express the fibroblast activation marker α-SMA, acquire proliferative capacity, and increase the synthesis of collagen and fibronectin [7]. Although a number of studies have shown that growth factors (such as platelet-derived growth factor (PDGF) and transforming growth factor (TGF-β1), cytokines (such as interleukin-6, interleukin-8 and tumor necrosis factor (TNF-α) and oxidative stress products activate PaSCs [39–43], the activation mechanism is not yet fully understood.

Recently, Notch1 has been shown to be involved in myofibroblast activation and to regulate α-SMA expression in lung fibrosis [32]. In addition, the Notch3 receptor plays a critical role in the transition of quiescent hepatic stellate cells (HSCs) into myofibroblastic HSCs in hepatic fibrosis [29–31]. In the present study, we

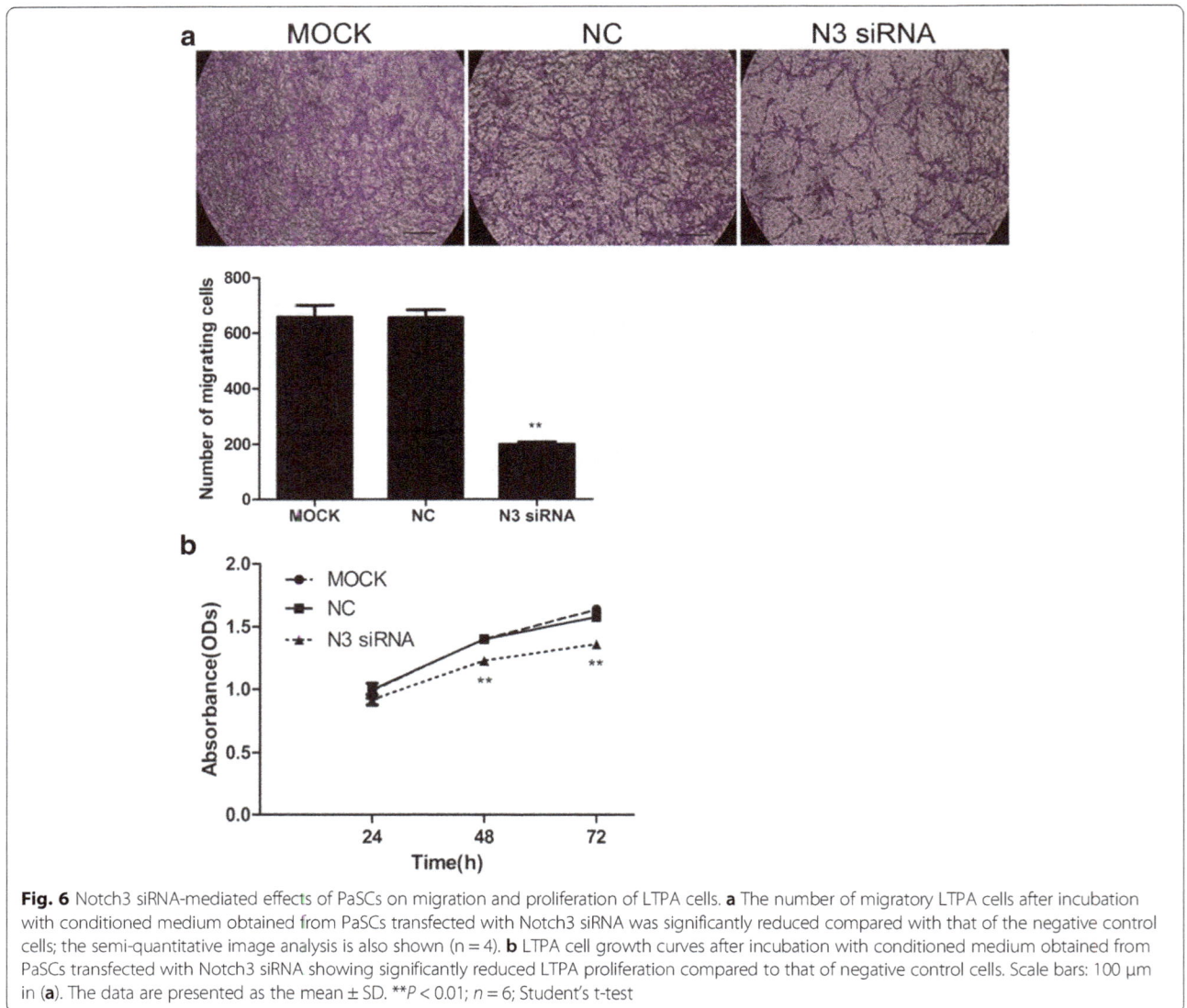

Fig. 6 Notch3 siRNA-mediated effects of PaSCs on migration and proliferation of LTPA cells. **a** The number of migratory LTPA cells after incubation with conditioned medium obtained from PaSCs transfected with Notch3 siRNA was significantly reduced compared with that of the negative control cells; the semi-quantitative image analysis is also shown (n = 4). **b** LTPA cell growth curves after incubation with conditioned medium obtained from PaSCs transfected with Notch3 siRNA showing significantly reduced LTPA proliferation compared to that of negative control cells. Scale bars: 100 μm in (**a**). The data are presented as the mean ± SD. **$P < 0.01$; $n = 6$; Student's t-test

found that Notch3 was highly expressed in α-SMA-positive cells in human pancreatic tumor tissue but not in normal pancreatic cells, suggesting that Notch3 participates in PaSC activation.

Quiescent PaSCs can be activated when PaSCs in normal pancreatic tissue are cultured in vitro. Although gene microarray analysis has shown gene expression differences between cultured cancer-associated PaSCs and normal PaSCs, the cells exert the same effects on pancreatic cancer cells [34]. Primary PaSCs isolated from normal pancreatic specimens are qualitatively indistinguishable from pancreatitis- and pancreatic cancer-derived PaSCs [33]. Furthermore, immortalized PaSCs have the same response to TGF-β1 and PDGF as their cultured primary cell counterparts [44, 45]. In the present study, we investigated the role of Notch signaling in PaSC activation using primary cultured PaSCs from normal mouse pancreas.

We observed that Notch3 is highly expressed in activated PaSCs, but not in non-activated PaSCs. Moreover, the levels of PaSC markers, such as α-SMA, collagen I and fibronectin were reduced by knocking down Notch3 expression in PaSCs. This suggests that Notch3 plays a crucial role in PaSC activation. In addition, we showed that Notch3 knockdown reduced migration and proliferation of PaSCs, which are required for the formation of desmoplasia [46]. We also found that conditioned medium from cultures of activated PaSCs enhanced the proliferation of LTPA PDAC cells. Thus, Notch3 is a potential target for inhibition of PaSC activation and thus desmoplasia.

Conclusions

In summary, we have demonstrated for the first time that Notch3 plays an important role in PaSC activation, migration and proliferation, and thus, the canonical Notch signaling pathway is involved in desmoplastic stroma formation in PDAC.

Abbreviations
CP: Chronic pancreatitis; DAB: Diaminobenzidine; ECM: Extracellular matrix; GFAP: Glial fibrillary acidic protein; MAPK: Mitogen-activated protein kinase; PaSCs: Pancreatic stellate cells.; PBS: Phosphate-buffered saline.; PDAC: Pancreatic ductal adenocarcinoma.; α-SMA: α-smooth muscle actin.

Acknowledgments
The authors would like to thank the financial support from the National Natural Science Foundation of China. The authors also thank Hong Lan for technical assistance.

Funding
The research was supported by the National Natural Science Foundation of China, grant number 81372156 (Yu-xiang Zhang). The funding agency only financially supported this study and did not participate in either the design of the study, collection, analysis and interpretation of data or in writing the manuscript.

Authors' contributions
YXZ and HYS conceived and designed the experiments. HYS conducted the experiments. YXZ and HYS wrote and revised the manuscript. Both authors have read and approved the final version of this manuscript.

Authors' information
HYS is a PhD student at Capital Medical University (shy80825@163.com). YXZ is a full professor at Capital Medical University (yxzhang@ccmu.edu.cn).

Competing interests
The authors declare that they have no competing interests.

References
1. Apte MV, Pirola RC, Wilson JS. Pancreatic stellate cells: a starring role in normal and diseased pancreas. Front Physiol. 2012;3:344.
2. Omary MB, Lugea A, Lowe AW, Pandol SJ. The pancreatic stellate cell: a star on the rise in pancreatic diseases. J Clin Invest. 2007;117(1):50–9.
3. Masamune A, Watanabe T, Kikuta K, Shimosegawa T. Roles of pancreatic stellate cells in pancreatic inflammation and fibrosis. Clin Gastroenterol Hepatol. 2009;7(11 Suppl):S48–54.
4. Longnecker DS. Pathology and pathogenesis of diseases of the pancreas. Am J Pathol. 1982;107(1):99–121.
5. Apte MV, Haber PS, Applegate TL, et al. Periacinar stellate shaped cells in rat pancreas: identification, isolation, and culture. Gut. 1998;43(1):128–33.
6. Bachem MG, Schneider E, Gross H, et al. Identification, culture, and characterization of pancreatic stellate cells in rats and humans. Gastroenterology. 1998;115(2):421–32.
7. Wehr AY, Furth EE, Sangar V, Blair IA, Yu KH. Analysis of the human pancreatic stellate cell secreted proteome. Pancreas. 2011;40(4):557–66.
8. Bachem MG, Zhou S, Buck K, Schneiderhan W, Siech M. Pancreatic stellate cells–role in pancreas cancer. Langenbeck's Arch Surg. 2008;393(6):891–900.
9. Apte MV, Wilson JS. Dangerous liaisons: pancreatic stellate cells and pancreatic cancer cells. J Gastroenterol Hepatol. 2012;2(27 Suppl):69–74.
10. Kikuta K, Masamune A, Watanabe T, Ariga H, Itoh H, Hamada S, Satoh K, Egawa S, Unno M, Shimosegawa T. Pancreatic stellate cells promote epithelial-mesenchymal transition in pancreatic cancer cells. Biochem Biophys Res Commun. 2010;403:380–4.
11. Hamada S, Masamune A, Yoshida N, Takikawa T, Shimosegawa T. IL-6/STAT3 plays a regulatory role in the interaction between pancreatic Stellate cells and cancer cells. Dig Dis Sci. 2016;61:1561–71.
12. Li X, Wang Z, Ma Q, et al. Sonic hedgehog paracrine signaling activates stromal cells to promote perineural invasion in pancreatic cancer. Clin Cancer Res. 2014;20(16):4326–38.
13. Rhim AD, Oberstein PE, Thomas DH, et al. Stromal elements act to restrain, rather than support, pancreatic ductal adenocarcinoma. Cancer Cell. 2014; 25(6):735–47.
14. McCarroll JA, Phillips PA, Santucci N, Pirola RC, Wilson JS, Apte MV. Vitamin a inhibits pancreatic stellate cell activation: implications for treatment of pancreatic fibrosis. Gut. 2006;55(1):79–89.
15. Masamune A, Kikuta K, Satoh M, Sakai Y, Satoh A, Shimosegawa T. Ligands of peroxisome proliferator-activated receptor-gamma block activation of pancreatic stellate cells. J Biol Chem. 2002;277(1):141–7.
16. Jaster R, Lichte P, Fitzner B, et al. Peroxisome proliferator-activated receptor gamma overexpression inhibits pro-fibrogenic activities of immortalised rat pancreatic stellate cells. J Cell Mol Med. 2005;9(3):670–82.
17. Shimada M, Andoh A, Hata K, et al. IL-6 secretion by human pancreatic periacinar myofibroblasts in response to inflammatory mediators. J Immunol. 2002;168(2):861–8.
18. Andoh A, Takaya H, Saotome T, et al. Cytokine regulation of chemokine (IL-8, MCP-1, and RANTES) gene expression in human pancreatic periacinar myofibroblasts. Gastroenterology. 2000;119(1):211–9.
19. Masamune A, Sakai Y, Kikuta K, Satoh M, Satoh A, Shimosegawa T. Activated rat pancreatic stellate cells express intercellular adhesion molecule-1 (ICAM-1) in vitro. Pancreas. 2002;25(1):78–85.
20. Masamune A, Kikuta K, Watanabe T, Satoh K, Satoh A, Shimosegawa T. Pancreatic stellate cells express toll-like receptors. J Gastroenterol. 2008; 43(5):352–62.
21. Artavanis-Tsakonas S, Rand MD, Lake RJ. Notch signaling: cell fate control and signal integration in development. Science. 1999;284(5415):770–6.
22. Gazave E, Lapébie P, Richards GS, et al. Origin and evolution of the notch signalling pathway: an overview from eukaryotic genomes. BMC Evol Biol. 2009;9:249.
23. Ranganathan P, Weaver KL, Capobianco AJ. Notch signalling in solid tumours: a little bit of everything but not all the time. Nat Rev Cancer. 2011; 11:338–51.
24. Mann CD, Bastianpillai C, Neal CP, et al. Notch3 and HEY-1 as prognostic biomarkers in pancreatic adenocarcinoma. PLoS One. 2012;7(12):e51119.
25. Mullendore ME, Koorstra JB, Li YM, et al. Ligand-dependent notch signaling is involved in tumor initiation and tumor maintenance in pancreatic cancer. Clin Cancer Res. 2009;15(7):2291–301.

26. Doucas H, Mann CD, Sutton CD, et al. Expression of nuclear Notch3 in pancreatic adenocarcinomas is associated with adverse clinical features, and correlates with the expression of STAT3 and phosphorylated Akt. J Surg Oncol. 2008;97(1):63–8.

27. Yao J, Qian C. Inhibition of Notch3 enhances sensitivity to gemcitabine in pancreatic cancer through an inactivation of PI3K/Akt-dependent pathway. Med Oncol. 2010;27(3):1017–22.

28. Palagani V, Bozko P, El KM, et al. Combined inhibition of notch and JAK/STAT is superior to monotherapies and impairs pancreatic cancer progression. Carcinogenesis. 2014;35(4):859–66.

29. Zhang QD, Xu MY, Cai XB, Qu Y, Li ZH, Lu LG. Myofibroblastic transformation of rat hepatic stellate cells: the role of notch signaling and epithelial-mesenchymal transition regulation. Eur Rev Med Pharmacol Sci. 2015;19(21):4130–8.

30. Zheng SP, Chen YX, Guo JL, et al. Recombinant adeno-associated virus-mediated transfer of shRNA against Notch3 ameliorates hepatic fibrosis in rats. Exp Biol Med (Maywood). 2013;238(6):600–9.

31. Chen Y, Zheng S, Qi D, et al. Inhibition of notch signaling by a γ-secretase inhibitor attenuates hepatic fibrosis in rats. PLoS One. 2012;7(10):e46512.

32. Liu T, Hu B, Choi YY, et al. Notch1 signaling in FIZZ1 induction of myofibroblast differentiation. Am J Pathol. 2009;174(5):1745–55.

33. Han S, Delitto D, Zhang D, et al. Primary outgrowth cultures are a reliable source of human pancreatic stellate cells. Lab Investig. 2015;95(11):1331–40.

34. Xu Z, Vonlaufen A, Phillips PA, et al. Role of pancreatic stellate cells in pancreatic cancer metastasis. Am J Pathol. 2010;177(5):2585–96.

35. Neesse A, Algül H, Tuveson DA, Gress TM. Stromal biology and therapy in pancreatic cancer: a changing paradigm. Gut. 2015;64(9):1476–84.

36. Feig C, Gopinathan A, Neesse A, Chan DS, Cook N, Tuveson DA. The pancreas cancer microenvironment. Clin Cancer Res. 2012;18(16):4266–76.

37. Neesse A, Michl P, Frese KK, et al. Stromal biology and therapy in pancreatic cancer. Gut. 2011;60(6):861–8.

38. Masamune A, Shimosegawa T. Signal transduction in pancreatic stellate cells. J Gastroenterol. 2009;44(4):249–60.

39. Apte MV, Haber PS, Darby SJ, et al. Pancreatic stellate cells are activated by proinflammatory cytokines: implications for pancreatic fibrogenesis. Gut. 1999;44(4):534–41.

40. Luttenberger T, Schmid-Kotsas A, Menke A, et al. Platelet-derived growth factors stimulate proliferation and extracellular matrix synthesis of pancreatic stellate cells: implications in pathogenesis of pancreas fibrosis. Lab Investig. 2000;80(1):47–55.

41. Schneider E, Schmid-Kotsas A, Zhao J, et al. Identification of mediators stimulating proliferation and matrix synthesis of rat pancreatic stellate cells. Am J Physiol Cell Physiol. 2001;281(2):C532–43.

42. Shek FW, Benyon RC, Walker FM, et al. Expression of transforming growth factor-beta 1 by pancreatic stellate cells and its implications for matrix secretion and turnover in chronic pancreatitis. Am J Pathol. 2002;160(5):1787–98.

43. Mews P, Phillips P, Fahmy R, et al. Pancreatic stellate cells respond to inflammatory cytokines: potential role in chronic pancreatitis. Gut. 2002; 50(4):535–41.

44. Sparmann G, Hohenadl C, Tornøe J, et al. Generation and characterization of immortalized rat pancreatic stellate cells. Am J Physiol Gastrointest Liver Physiol. 2004;287(1):G211–9.

45. Jesnowski R, Fürst D, Ringel J, et al. Immortalization of pancreatic stellate cells as an in vitro model of pancreatic fibrosis: deactivation is induced by matrigel and N-acetylcysteine. Lab Investig. 2005;85(10):1276–91.

46. Yang C, Zeisberg M, Mosterman B, et al. Liver fibrosis: insights into migration of hepatic stellate cells in response to extracellular matrix and growth factors. Gastroenterology. 2003;124(1):147–59.

3

Innovative substance 2250 as a highly promising anti-neoplastic agent in malignant pancreatic carcinoma - in vitro and in vivo

M. Buchholz[1*], B. Majchrzak-Stiller[1], S. Hahn[2], D. Vangala[2,4], R. W. Pfirrmann[3], W. Uhl[1], C. Braumann[1] and A. M. Chromik[1]

Abstract

Background: Former studies already revealed the anti-neoplastic properties of the anti-infective agent Taurolidine (TRD) against many tumor species in vitro and in vivo. Its anti-proliferative and cell death inducing capacity is largely due to its main derivative Taurultam (TRLT). In this study it could be demonstrated, that substance 2250 - a newly defined innovative structural analogue of TRLT - exhibits an anti-neoplastic effect on malignant pancreatic carcinoma in vitro and in vivo.

Methods: The anti-neoplastic potential of substance 2250 as well as its mode of action was demonstrated in extensive in vitro analysis, followed by successful and effective in vivo testings, using xenograft models derived from established pancreatic cancer cell lines as well as patient derived tissue.

Results: Our functional analysis regarding the role of oxidative stress (ROS) and caspase activated apoptosis showed, that ROS driven programmed cell death (PCD) is the major mechanisms induced by substance 2250 in pancreatic carcinoma. What is strongly relevant towards clinical practice is especially the observed inhibition of patient derived pancreatic cancer tumor growth in mice treated with this new substance in combination with its sharply higher metabolic stability.

Conclusion: These encouraging results provide new therapeutical opportunities in pancreatic cancer treatment and build the basis for further functional analysis as well as first clinical studies for this promising agent.

Keywords: Taurolidine, Apoptosis, Chemotherapy, Cancer, Substance 2250

Background

Pancreatic ductal adenocarcinoma (PDAC) is the most lethal common cancer, usually diagnosed at an advanced stage when curative therapy is almost impossible [1]. It is the fourth most common cause of cancer-related death in Europe [2] and in the US [3]. The pancreatic adenocarcinoma typically has a poor prognosis with a five year relative survival rate of 4–5% [4]. In fact, incidence and mortality of PDAC are almost equal. Surgical resection is the only potentially curative therapy for pancreatic cancer. Because of the poor outcome associated with surgery only, the role of adjuvant therapies has been extensively evaluated. A series of studies revealed, that chemotherapy with gemcitabine or fluorouracil improves the overall survival of patients with pancreatic adenocarcinoma [5–8]. In the majority of cases a complete resection of the tumor is impossible. Therefore a palliative chemotherapy may be conducted to prolong survival and improve the quality of life. In these cases new combination therapies like FOLFIRINOX are investigated in clinical trials or are in use [7, 8] However, current chemotherapeutic agents are still disappointing due to their poor response

* Correspondence: marie.buchholz-a7y@rub.de
[1]Division of Molecular and Clinical Research, St. Josef-Hospital, Ruhr-University Bochum, Bochum, Germany
Full list of author information is available at the end of the article

and high toxicity. New and innovative agents have to be found to expand the therapeutic opportunities.

Taurolidine (TRD) is a substance derived from the aminosulfonacid taurine. Owing to its anti-inflammatory and its anti-microbial qualities, it has been clinically used primarily in peritonitis and catheter related blood stream infections [9]. 1997 Jacobi et al. could show for the first time, that TRD also applied an anti-proliferative and anti-neoplastic activity in vitro and in vivo [10]. This anti-neoplastic and apoptosis inducing effect could also be verified by other research groups [11] in a variety of cell lines derived from malignant tumors e.g. glioblastoma [12], melanoma [13], mesothelioma [14] and colon carcinoma [15]. Furthermore, latest reports about the systemic application of TRD in patients with gastric carcinoma and glioblastoma revealed promising results with almost absence of toxicity [16, 17].

The favorable safety profile of TRD renders this compound to a promising novel agent for the oncological care. However, the metabolic stability of TRD is limited due to its short half-life [18].

This study was designed to analyze a novel compound related to Taurultam (TRLT), the main derivative of TRD. Substance 2250 is a structural analogue of TRLT and is an oxathiazine derivative (Fig. 1). The respective Sulfonamides are promising substances due to their antibacterial and anti-neoplastic activity. The 1.4.5-Oxathiazin derivatives, like the new substance 2250, are almost unexplored whereas 1.2.3-Oxathiazin derivatives are already identified, mainly as artificial sweeteners [19]. However, no representative studies are published analyzing the anti-neoplastic effects of the substance 2250 so far. The aim of this study was to investigate the anti-neoplastic activity on malignant pancreatic cancer in vitro and in vivo.

Methods
Cell lines and culture conditions
Six different human pancreatic cancer cell lines were used for our experiments: AsPC-1 (CLS Cell Lines Service,

Eppenheim, Germany), BxPC-3 (ATCC – LGC Standards GmbH, Wesel, Germany), MiaPaca-2 (ATCC – LGC Standards GmbH, Wesel, Germany), Panc-1 (CLS Cell Lines Service, Eppenheim, Germany) and Panc-TuI (ATCC – LGC Standards GmbH, Wesel, Germany). Cells were passaged fewer than 6 months after receiving from the mentioned cell banks. Authentication was analyzed by STR analysis. MiaPaca-2, Panc-1 and Panc-TuI cells were cultured in Dulbecco's Modified Eagle Medium (DMEM). The remaining cell lines (AsPC-1, BxPC-3) were maintained in RPMI 1640. All cultures were supplemented with the antibiotics penicillin (100 U/ml), streptomycin (100 U/ml) and 2 mM L-Glutamine. AsPC-1 cells were further supplemented with 1 mM Sodium Pyruvate. Cells were grown as monolayer and cultured in $25cm^2$ flasks at 37 °C and 5% CO_2 in humidified atmosphere.

Tissue
Different human pancreatic cancer tissues were used for the in vivo experiments:

Bo70, adenocarcinoma, UICC IIb.

Bo 80, adenocarcinoma, UICC IIb.

Reagents
The 2250 and TRLT ultrapure powder (kindly provided by Geistlich Pharma AG, Wohlhusen, Switzerland) was dissolved in double distilled Water (ddH$_2$O), sterile filtered, set to a physiological pH and freshly prepared once per week.

MTT cytotoxicity assay
Cells were seeded to a density of 3.5×10^4 cells/well in 96-well plates and incubated for 24 h to obtain a sub confluent monolayer. To examine the dose-response of 2250 and TRLT regarding its anti-neoplastic activity, cells were incubated with increasing concentrations (100, 200, 500, 1000, 1500, 2000 µmol/l) and ddH$_2$O as control for 6, 12, 24 and 48 h. 4 h before the measurement 10 µl yellow MTT (3-(4,5-Dimethylthiazol-2-yl)-2,5-diphenyltetrazoliumbromid) reagent (5 mg/ml) was added to the test media. Yellow MTT is converted by viable cells into violet Formazan crystals. The test media was discarded and 50 µl DMSO (Dimethylsulfoxide) was applied. After an incubation time of 5–10 min the viability of cells could be analyzed by using a microplate absorbance reader by measuring the OD (optical density) (Tecan trading AG, Switzerland). The amount of violet Formazan is directly proportional to the amount of viable cells. The assay was performed in 4–6 independent experiments with consecutive passages.

BrdU proliferation assay
Cells were seeded to a density of 4×10^4 cells/well in 96-well plates and incubated for 24 h to obtain a sub

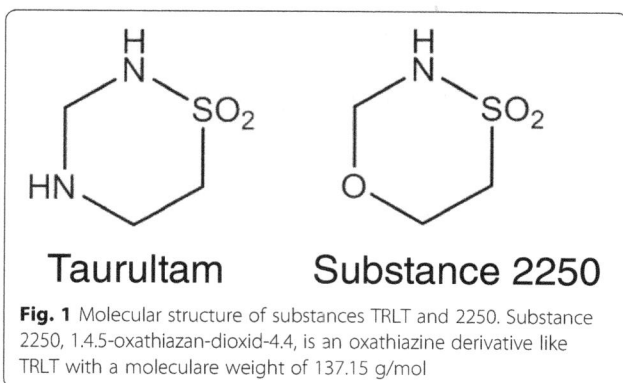

Fig. 1 Molecular structure of substances TRLT and 2250. Substance 2250, 1.4.5-oxathiazan-dioxid-4.4, is an oxathiazine derivative like TRLT with a moleculare weight of 137.15 g/mol

confluent monolayer. To examine the dose-response of 2250 and TRLT regarding its anti-proliferative activity, cells were incubated with increasing concentrations of 2250 (100, 200, 500, 1000, 1500, 2000 µmol/l) and ddH$_2$O as control for 6 h and submitted to BrdU proliferation assay (5-bromo-2-deoxyuridine)-ELISA (Roche Applied Science, Mannheim, Germany) according to the manufacturer's instructions. Based on the incorporation of the thymidine analogue BrdU during DNA synthesis, the amount of synthesized DNA is detected using a microplate absorbance reader (Tecan trading AG, Switzerland). BrdU assays were performed with 8 replicates of three independent experiments with consecutive passages. The incubation time of 6 h has been shown to be appropriate for the BrdU proliferation assay in previous experiments.

Flow Cytometry analysis

Cells were seeded to a density of 2×10^5 cells/well in 6-well plates and incubated for 24 h to obtain a subconfluent monolayer. Different concentrations of 2250 (200, 500, 1000, 1500, 2000 µmol/l) and ddH$_2$O as control were used for 24 h and 48 h before analyzed by FACS analysis. FACS analysis was performed in 4–6 independent experiments with 2–4 consecutive passages. Cells were fixed in 200 µl binding buffer (Bender MedSystems, Vienna, Austria). Subsequently, 5–10 µl Annexin V-FITC (BD Biosciences, Heidelberg, Germany) was added to the cell suspension and incubated for 15 min at room temperature in the dark. Thereafter, 10 µl Propidiumiodide (PI) (Bender MedSystems, Vienna, Austria) was added. Cells were analyzed immediately using a flow cytometer (FACS Calibur BD Biosciences, Heidelberg, Germany) for Annexin V-FITC (apoptotic) and PI (necrotic) binding. Dot plots and histograms were analyzed by CellQuest Pro software (BD Biosciences, Heidelberg, Germany).

Functional mechanisms

To get insights into functional mechanisms of drug effects cells were additionally treated with the radical scavenger N-acetylcysteine NAC (5 mmol/l) (Sigma Aldrich, Munich, Germany) or the pan caspase inhibitor-zVad (2 µmol/l) (Enzo Life Sciences, Lörrach, Germany) before analysis by FACS or MTT standard procedure as already described. Concentrations of 500 and 1000 µmol/l 2250 with an incubation time of 24 h were used for co-incubation assays in all cell lines.

The direct impact of 2250 on the cellular level of reactive oxygen species (ROS) was analyzed using the Cellular ROS/Superoxide Detection Assay KIT (Abcam, Cambridge, UK) following the manufactures instructions.

Analysis of the maximal tolerable dose
Acute toxicity

For determining the acute toxicity of substance 2250 in nude mice, mice (each group $n = 8–10$) were treated intraperitoneal (ip) with different concentrations (500, 1000, 1500, 2000 mg/kg*BW) once, followed by control of body weight and general vital function. A loss of 20% of body weight over 48 h was classified as toxic.

Chronic toxicity

To assess the chronic toxicity mice were treated with different concentrations of substance 2250 (500, 1000, 1500 mg/kg*BW) on alternating days for 3 weeks. Control of body weight and general vital function were measured as well. A loss of 20% of body weight over 48 h was classified as toxic.

Analysis of metabolic half-life in blood

For determining the metabolic half-life of the new substance 2250 in the blood of nude mice, a colorimetric assay using NASH-Reagent and protein free serum was used. The serum level was analyzed 1 h and 25 h after treatment with the substance 2250 (500 mg/kg*BW).

Animal studies

Five-week-old female NMRI Foxn1nu/Foxn1nu mice (Janvier, France) were acclimated into a 12-h light cycle-controlled environment 1 week before initiation of the study. The animals were allowed standard laboratory food and water ad libitum. Mice were anesthetized by inhalation of Isofluran. 5×10^6 cells of different pancreatic adenocarcinoma cell lines (MiaPaca-2 and PancTU-I) or tumor tissue fragments were administered subcutaneously in the flank region. After implantation, the recipient mice were monitored for general health status and the presence of subcutaneous tumors. Tumor volume was determined by measuring tumor diameters (measurement of 2 perpendicular axes of tumor) using a caliper and calculated as.

$$V = \frac{1}{2}\left(ab^2\right),$$

(a = larger axe, b = smaller axe).

Following randomization (two groups, $n = 10$) the systemic influence of 2250 on tumor growth after intraperitoneal (ip) application were investigated. As the metabolic half-life of 2250 in nude mice was found to be 13.8 h, a dosing schedule of every second day was chosen for the in vivo experiments. Group1: substance 2250 500 mg/kg*BW on alternating days, group 2: control group Ringer's solution 300 µl was applied ip on alternating days. The treatment was initiated when the tumor volume reached

200 mm^3 and the tumor volume was measured every second day for 2–3 weeks. The experiment was terminated either after an application period of 3 weeks or when the tumor reached a volume of 1000 mm^3.

Statistics and calculations

Results of FACS-analysis (percentage of viable, apoptotic and necrotic cells) as well as results of MTT and BrdU assay (percentage of living/proliferating cells) are expressed as means ± SEM. Comparison between experimental groups with normal distribution was performed using one-way ANOVA followed by Tukey's post-hoc test. For categorical data Fisher's exact test used if appropriate. P-values ≤0.05 were considered as statistically significant

and indicated in the figures as follows: *** $p \leq 0.001$, ** $p \leq 0.01$, * $p \leq 0.05$.

For the calculation of metabolic half-life the following formula was used: $G(x) = Go \times \left(\frac{1}{2}\right)^{\frac{x}{t}}$

(G(x) = serum concentration (24 h), G_0 = serum concentration (0 h), x = 24 h, t = metabolic half-time)

Results

2250 has a cytotoxic effect on all cell lines in a dose dependent manner

To determine the effect of substance 2250 on the cell viability the OD (optical density), MTT tests were conducted. As indicated in Fig. 2, incubation with 2250 in increasing concentrations (100, 200, 500, 1000, 1500, 2000 μmol/l)

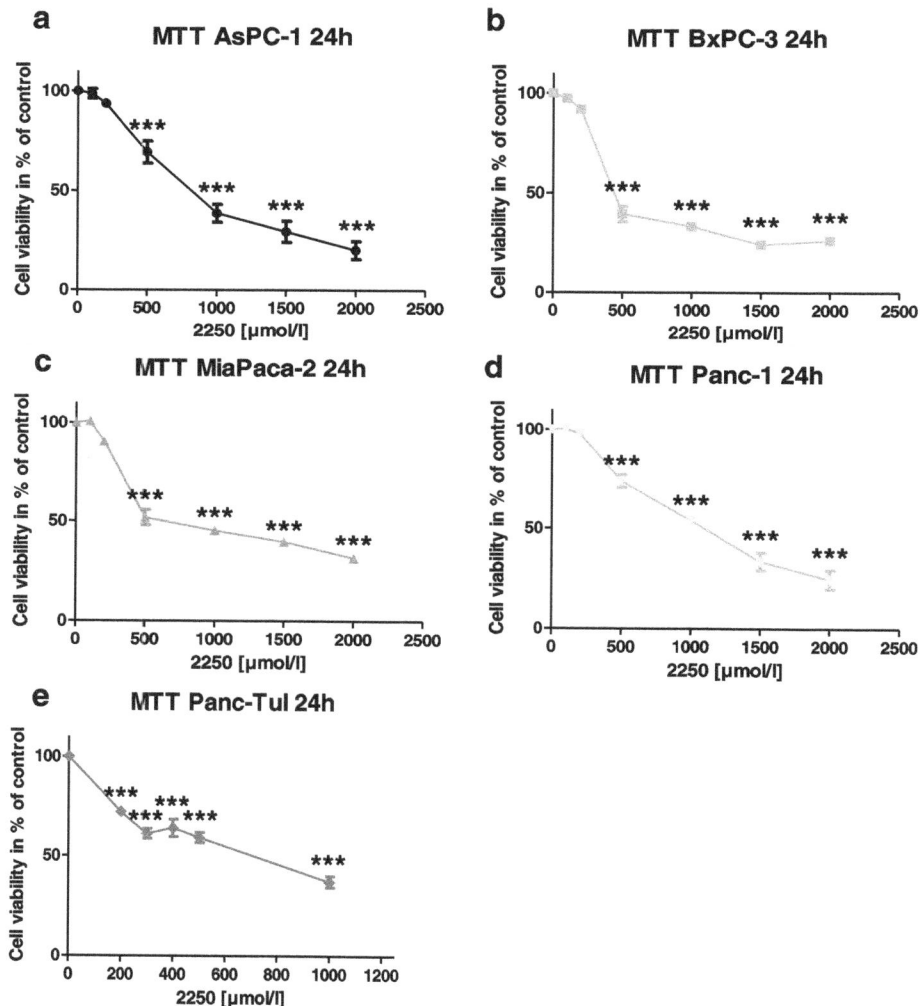

Fig. 2 Effects of 2250 in different malignant cell lines measured by MTT-assay. AsPC-1 (**a**), BxPC-3 (**b**), MiaPaca-2 (**c**), Panc-1 (**d**) and Panc Tul cells (**e**) were incubated with 2250 (100, 200, 500, 1000, 1500, 2000 μmol/l) and ddH$_2$O (control) for 24 h and submitted to a MTT-assay. Values are means ± SEM of 6 replicates of three independent experiments with consecutive passages. Asterisk symbols indicate differences between control, which was adjusted to 100% and 2250 treatment. *** $p \leq 0.001$, ** $p \leq 0.01$, * $p \leq 0.05$, n.s. $p > 0.05$ (one-way ANOVA followed by Tukey's post-hoc test)

for 24 h resulted in a dose dependent reduction of living cells - as measured by MTT assay. The substance 2250 in the cell line Panc-TuI was only analyzed up to a concentration of 1000 µmol/l, because this cell line was used additionally for in vivo treatment. The concentrations used in vitro were the important ones for in vivo treatment.

In all cell lines, even the lowest concentration of 500 µmol/l led to a significant reduction of cell viability ranging between 39.4% (± 3.8%) (BxPC-3) and 73.8% (± 3.3%) (Panc-1) which was significantly lower compared to untreated controls (100%) with ddH$_2$O (Fig. 2). However, at the following concentration of 1000 µmol/l 2250, the monitored reduction of cell viability was more than 50% in four out of five cell lines. This pronounced reduction, mediated by 2250 in a concentration

of 1000 µmol/l resulted in values of living cells between 33.3% (± 1.2%) for BxPC-3 and 59.1% (± 2.6%) for PancTuI (Fig. 2b, e). The maximum dose of 2000 µmol/l led to an intense cytotoxic effect in all cell lines. As a result, in three cell lines a proportional doses-effect curve and in BxPC-3 as well as in MiaPaca2 a sigmoid character was observed (Fig. 2). The effective doses (ED) 50 were varying between the different cell lines from 221 µmol/l (BxPC-3) to 1100 µmol/l (Panc-1) within an incubation time of 24 h.

2250 inhibits proliferation of all cell lines in a dose dependent manner

To examine the effect of substance 2250 on cell proliferation in a culture model, BrdU assays were conducted. As indicated in Fig. 3, incubation with substance 2250 in

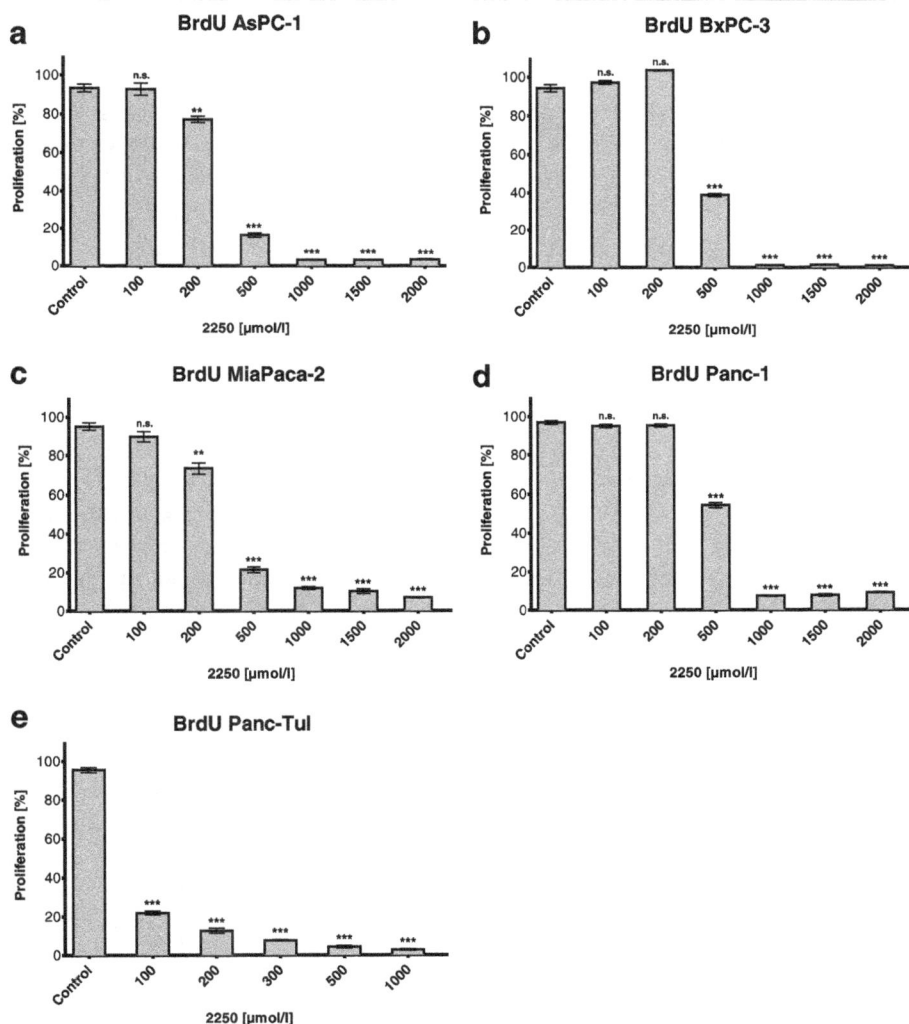

Fig. 3 Effects of Taurolidine (TRD) on cell proliferation in different malignant cell lines measured by BrdU-assay. AsPC-1 (**a**), BxPC-3 (**b**), MiaPaca-2 (**c**), Panc-1 (**d**) and Panc TuI cells (**e**) were incubated with 2250 (100, 200, 500, 1000, 1500, 2000 µmol/l) and ddH$_2$O (control) for 6 h and submitted to a BrdU-assay. Values are means ± SEM of 8 replicates of three independent experiments with consecutive passages. Asterisk symbols on columns indicate differences between control, which was adjusted to 100% and 2250 treatment. *** $p \leq 0.001$, ** $p \leq 0.01$, * $p \leq 0.05$, n.s. $p > 0.05$ (one-way ANOVA followed by Tukey's post-hoc test)

increasing concentrations (100, 200, 500, 1000, 1500, 2000 µmol/l) for 6 h resulted in a dose dependent reduction of proliferating cells. In three cell lines, even a concentration of 200 µmol/l 2250 was capable of inhibiting proliferation leading to values of proliferating cells ranging between 12.7% (± 1.3%) (Panc-TuI) and 77.2% (± 1.6%) (AsPC-1) which was significantly lower compared to untreated controls (100%) with ddH$_2$O (Fig. 3). The concentration of 500 µmol/l 2250 significantly inhibited proliferation in all analyzed cell lines. This inhibition resulted in amounts of proliferating cells between 4.3% (± 0.6%) for Panc-TuI and 54.3% (± 1.2) for Panc-1 (Fig. 3 d, e). The maximum dose of 2000 µmol/l implicated an extended inhibition of proliferation in all cell lines, so the dose response for cell proliferation could be characterized as proportional in all five pancreatic cancer cell lines (Fig. 3).

Table 1 shows the relative amounts of cell viability and cell proliferation of three different cell lines upon treatment with substances TRLT and 2250 (2000 µmol/l each). In all analyzed cell lines substance 2250 shows a substantial higher impact on cell viability as well as on cell proliferation. In AsPC-1 and Panc-1 substance 2250 is even twice as effective as TRLT.

2250 induces apoptotic cell death in all cell lines

Additional FACS analysis revealed the impact of substance 2250 on apoptotic-, as well as on necrotic cell death. As summarized in Fig. 4, incubation of three cell lines for 24 h with substance 2250 with a concentration of 1000 µmol/l and 1500 µmol/l resulted in a significant reduction of viable cells compared to control treatment with ddH$_2$O as evaluated by FACS analysis with Annexin V-FITC and PI. The significant reduction of cell viability by 1000 µmol/l 2250 was paralleled by a significant increase of apoptotic cells in all cell lines (Fig. 4). Cell viability following incubation with 1000 µmol/l was varying between 41.1% (±0.7%) for BxPC-3 and 59.0% (±1.9%) for AsPC-1 cells. The strong impact on cell viability was paralleled by a significant apoptotic effect in all cell lines ranging between 14.2% (± 1.5%) apoptotic cells for AsPC-1 and 35.0% (± 2.01%) for Panc-TuI. The contribution of necrosis to the loss of cell viability was smaller. However, a significant increase in necrotic cells between 16.4% (± 2.5%) for Panc-TuI and 28.9% (± 1.0%) for BxPC-3 was observed (Fig. 4).

The following incubation with 1500 µmol/l of 2250 showed a pronounced and significant reduction in cell viability between 28.5% (± 1.5%) for Panc-TuI and 7.6% (± 0.8%) for BxPC-3 cells. This reduction in cell viability was also paralleled by a significant increase of apoptotic cells – but only in two of three cell lines (AsPc-1, Panc-TuI). In BxPc-3 no significant apoptotic alteration was detected. However, BxPc-3 cells responded towards 1500 µmol/l with a strong necrotic effect 80.6% (± 1.1%) which was highest observed among all cell lines and concentrations (Fig. 4).

The radical scavenger N-acetylcysteine (NAC) and pancaspase inhibitor z-VAD show divergent effects on 2250 induced cell death

To evaluate the contribution of Caspase or reactive oxygen species mediated cell death to the observed effects of substance 2250 co-incubation experiments with substance 2250 and NAC or z-VAD were performed.

In AsPc-1 and Panc-1 cells, co-incubation of 2250 with NAC for 24 h led to a complete protection towards 2250 induced cell death. NAC entirely abrogated the 2250 induced reduction of viable cells leading to cell viability, equal to untreated controls (Fig. 5a, d). In BxPC-3, MiaPaca-2 and Panc-TuI, the co-incubation of 2250 with NAC was characterized by a strong protection of cell viability. However, there was no complete protection in the amount of viable cells compared to untreated controls. The effect could only be characterized as a partial protection (Fig. 5b, c, e).

Further data of FACS analysis of AsPC-1 co-incubated with 2250 and NAC for 24 h shown in Fig. 5 confirmed previous results. In contrast to the MTT assay, the FACS analysis shows this effect on the different cell populations more in detail. The co-incubation was characterized by a completely protection against the 2250 induced reduction of viable cells leading to a significant increase of viable cells (Fig. 6a). No differences from untreated controls were detected. Together with a small but significant reduction of apoptotic cells under treatment with a concentration of 500 µmol/l 2250, a complete reduction of necrotic cells could be achieved under treatment with 1000 µmol/l 2250 (Fig. 6b, c). Furthermore the cellular level of ROS is significantly increased in cells treated with substance 2250. Fig. 5f provides an exemplary presentation of tested cell lines. This effect can be reversed by additional treatment with NAC.

Table 1 Results of MTT and BrdU assay of substance 2250 compared with TRLT in three different cell lines

	AsPC-1		BxPC-3		Panc-1	
	TRLT	2250	TRLT	2250	TRLT	2250
MTT assay cell viability (%)	48.78 ± 2.8	21.00 ± 3.8	36.01 ± 7.3	26.24 ± 0.3	65.24 ± 1.5	24.4 ± 4.6
BrdU Assay cell proliferation (%)	8.5 ± 0.9	3.34 ± 0.2	6.66 ± 0.7	1.0 ± 0.2	16.32 ± 1.2	9.14 ± 0.3

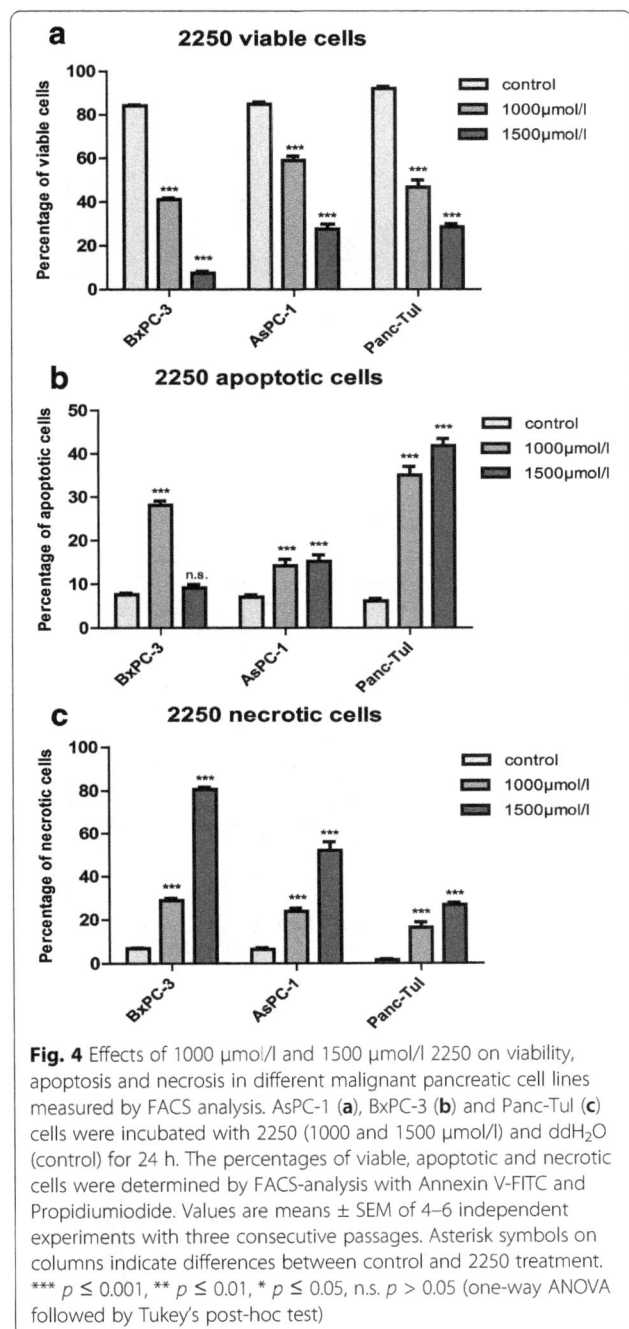

Fig. 4 Effects of 1000 µmol/l and 1500 µmol/l 2250 on viability, apoptosis and necrosis in different malignant pancreatic cell lines measured by FACS analysis. AsPC-1 (**a**), BxPC-3 (**b**) and Panc-TuI (**c**) cells were incubated with 2250 (1000 and 1500 µmol/l) and ddH$_2$O (control) for 24 h. The percentages of viable, apoptotic and necrotic cells were determined by FACS-analysis with Annexin V-FITC and Propidiumiodide. Values are means ± SEM of 4–6 independent experiments with three consecutive passages. Asterisk symbols on columns indicate differences between control and 2250 treatment. *** $p \leq 0.001$, ** $p \leq 0.01$, * $p \leq 0.05$, n.s. $p > 0.05$ (one-way ANOVA followed by Tukey's post-hoc test)

All pancreatic cancer cell lines which were analyzed did not show any detectable effect on cell viability after z-VAD co-incubation (data not shown).

Detection of the maximal tolerable dose of substance 2250

By analyzing the acute toxicity, the highest concentration of 2000 mg/kg*BW was toxic in nude mice. The body weight was reduced about 1 g in 48 h and the mouse died 5 days after treatment. For the other concentrations no changes in body weight and vital function could be observed.

Determining the chronic toxicity it could be observed that concentrations higher than 1000 mg/kg*BW are toxic in nude mice. While treatment with 500 mg/kg*BW no changes in body weight and vital function could be monitored.

Analysis of metabolic half-life in blood

For determining the metabolic half-life of the new substance 2250 in blood of nude mice a colorimetric assay using NASH reagent was used. The alignment of the measured values of substance 2250 in mice serum after 1 h and 25 h with the calibration curve yielded a metabolic half-life of 13.8 h (Fig. 7, Table 2).

2250 induces reduction of subcutaneous tumor growth in vivo

Finally, to elucidate the effect of substance 2250 in vivo, we tested the impact of the treatment of xenografts derived from cancer cell lines and patient tissue in different tumor mouse models.

As indicated in Fig. 8, the intraperitoneal (ip) application of 2250 (500 mg/kg*BW) reduced the subcutaneous tumor growth in vivo in tumors induced by established pancreatic cancer cell lines (MiaPaca-2, Panc-TuI) as well as in xenograft models from patient tissue. The ip application of 2250 led to a significant reduction of 57% of relative tumor volume in comparison to the control group after an application period of 3 weeks in tumors caused by the established cell line MiaPaca-2 (Fig. 8a). In a second tumor model evoked by the established cell line Panc-TuI (Fig. 8b) almost the same inhibition of tumor growth was observed by ip application of 2250 (500 mg/kg*BW). A significant reduction of 49.7% of relative tumor growth was detected after an application period of 2 weeks. The tumor volume endpoint of 1000 mm^3 was reached after this treatment period and the experiment was terminated. The subcutaneous tumor, derived from patient tissue (Bo 70) was analyzed in a separate tumor model in which a significant reduction of tumor growth of 36.8% under the treatment with substance 2250 could be observed (Fig. 8c). In a second patient derived xenograft (Bo 80) almost the same inhibition of approximately 30% could be detected (Fig. 8d).

Discussion

The anti-neoplastic effects of the recently developed, novel substance 2250 have not been published yet. During development of the compound, a cytotoxicity test was performed in the glioma cell line LN 229 which indicated a promising anti-neoplastic capacity of the substance 2250 (EC 50 = 55 µg/ml after 24 h) [unpublished data], similar in potency to TRD. The anti-neoplastic activity of the parent compound TRD

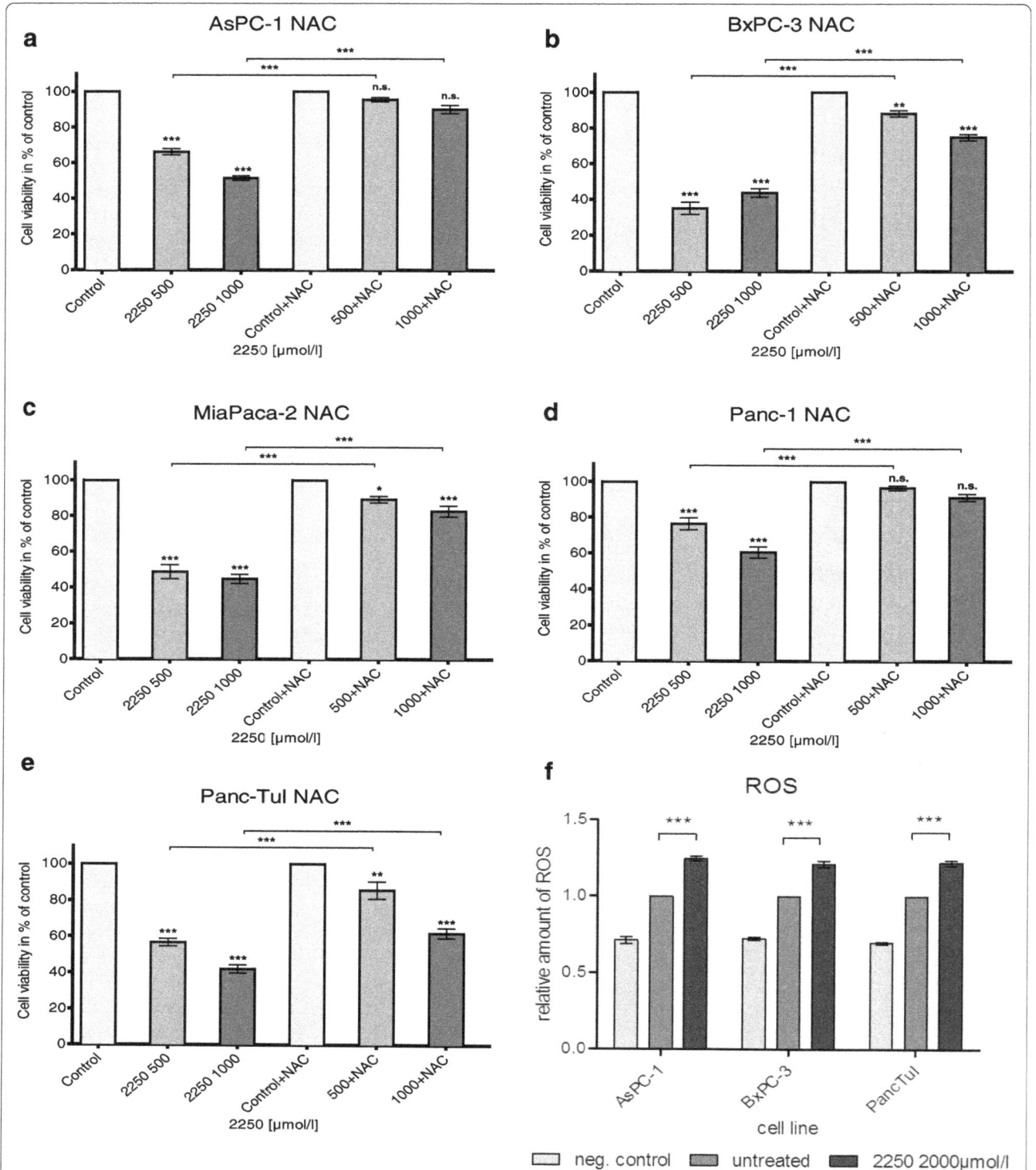

Fig. 5 Effects of NAC on 2250 induced cell death in different malignant cell lines measured by MTT (**a-e**); impact of 2250 on the cellular level of ROS (f). AsPC-1 (**a**), BxPC-3 (**b**), MiaPaca-2 (**c**), Panc-1 (**d**) and Panc Tul (**e**) cells were incubated with either 2250 (500, 1000 µmol/l), NAC (5 mmol/l) or the combination of both agents (2250 500, 1000 µmol/l + NAC 5 mmol/l) and ddH$_2$O as control for 24 h and submitted to a MTT-assay. The level of ROS was analyzed in untreated compared to 2250 treated cells, additional NAC treatment served as a neg. Control (**f**). Values are means ± SEM of 6 replicates of three independent experiments with consecutive passages. Asterisk symbols indicate differences between control, which was adjusted to 100% and 2250 treatment. *** $p \leq 0.001$, ** $p \leq 0.01$, * $p \leq 0.05$, (one-way ANOVA followed by Tukey's post-hoc test)

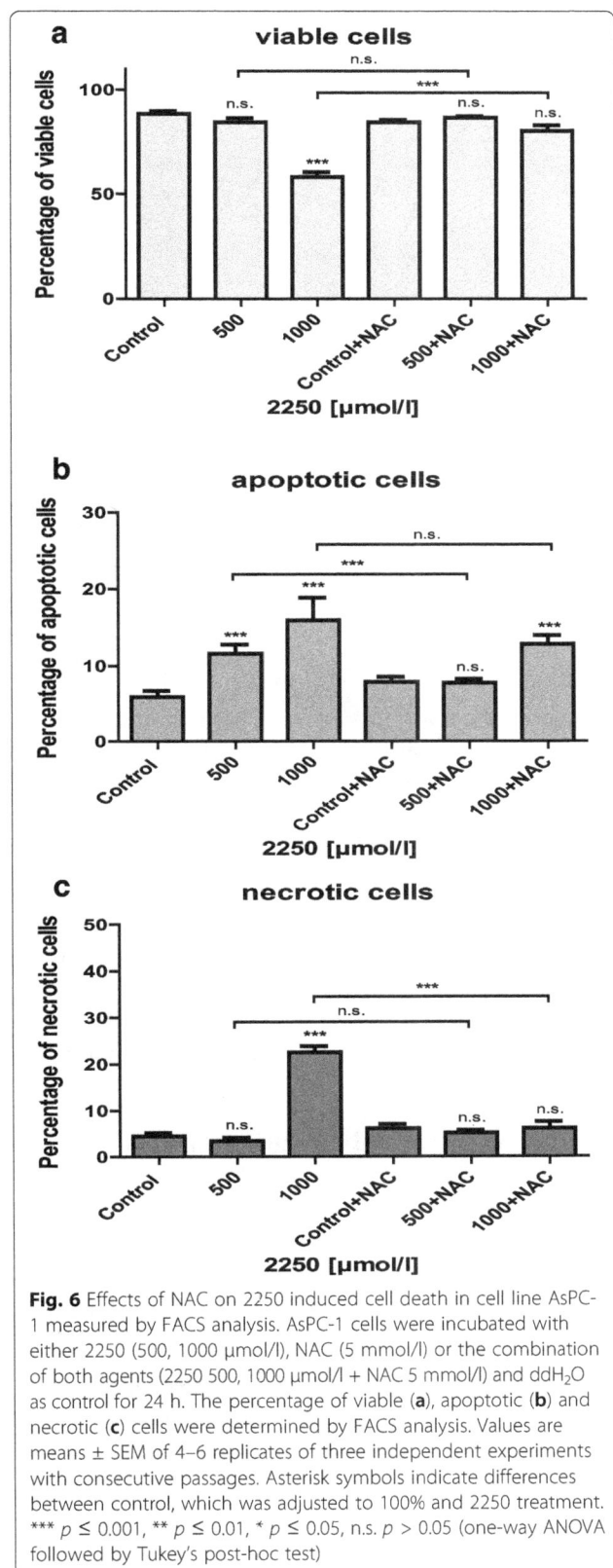

Fig. 6 Effects of NAC on 2250 induced cell death in cell line AsPC-1 measured by FACS analysis. AsPC-1 cells were incubated with either 2250 (500, 1000 µmol/l), NAC (5 mmol/l) or the combination of both agents (2250 500, 1000 µmol/l + NAC 5 mmol/l) and ddH$_2$O as control for 24 h. The percentage of viable (**a**), apoptotic (**b**) and necrotic (**c**) cells were determined by FACS analysis. Values are means ± SEM of 4–6 replicates of three independent experiments with consecutive passages. Asterisk symbols indicate differences between control, which was adjusted to 100% and 2250 treatment. *** $p \leq 0.001$, ** $p \leq 0.01$, * $p \leq 0.05$, n.s. $p > 0.05$ (one-way ANOVA followed by Tukey's post-hoc test)

has been demonstrated in many studies on different cancer entities in vitro as well as in vivo [18, 20, 21]. Even pilot clinical studies confirmed previous results [16, 18, 22]. Therefore, the aim of this study was to analyze anti-neoplastic effects of substance 2250 in comparison to its structural analogue TRLT, the main derivative of its effective parent compound TRD.

In the first part of this study we determined dose-response characteristics and analyzed the relative contribution of apoptosis and necrosis during substance 2250 induced cell death. In all five different malignant pancreatic cancer cell lines the dose response effects of substance 2250 were nearly homogenous. We found a pattern which is characterized by a *proportional or sigmoidal dose effect* where increasing concentrations of substance 2250 led to an increase of cell death after 24 and 48 h. This pattern could be observed for the cytotoxicity of the substance via MTT assay, as well as for the anti-proliferative effect by BrdU analysis. This *proportional dose effect* pattern, observed during this study, is analog to those described in several previous studies for the treatment with TRD [23–26].

Three pancreatic cancer cell lines (AsPC-1, BxPC-3 and PancTuI) also displayed a dose-response relationship concerning the relative distribution of viable, apoptotic and necrotic cells determined by FACS analysis, where the amount of viable cells decreased with increasing concentration of substance 2250. The incubation with 1000 µmol/l of substance 2250 was characterized by apoptotic as well as necrotic cell death whereby the apoptotic effect was the predominant characteristic. In contrast, the incubation with 1500 µmol/l of substance 2250 was characterized by a pronounced necrotic effect in BxPC-3. This effect became more obvious in AsPC-1. Opposite to this, in PancTuI cells treated with 1500 µmol/l the amount of apoptotic cells prevailed. This dose depending ratio of viable, apoptotic and necrotic cells is according to previous studies with TRD in our group [15] and by others [13, 26]. Regarding the pronounced necrotic effect of rising concentrations of substance 2250, only speculations are possible. Whereby, cell culture models could reveal a potential explanation. Generally, apoptosis is due to caspase-dependent or independent cell destruction and to phagocytosis of the apoptotic cells. In a cell culture setting, which lacks phagocytosis a secondary necrosis follows, which is characterized by the same appearance of primary necrosis [27].

In our in vitro studies there is no possibility of phagocytosis by inflammatory cells, because they are not present in our cell culture model. The marker, used for necrosis (PI) could ultimately not differentiate between a substance-induced primary necrosis and a secondary necrosis - due to the lack of phagocytosis. Another possible explanation

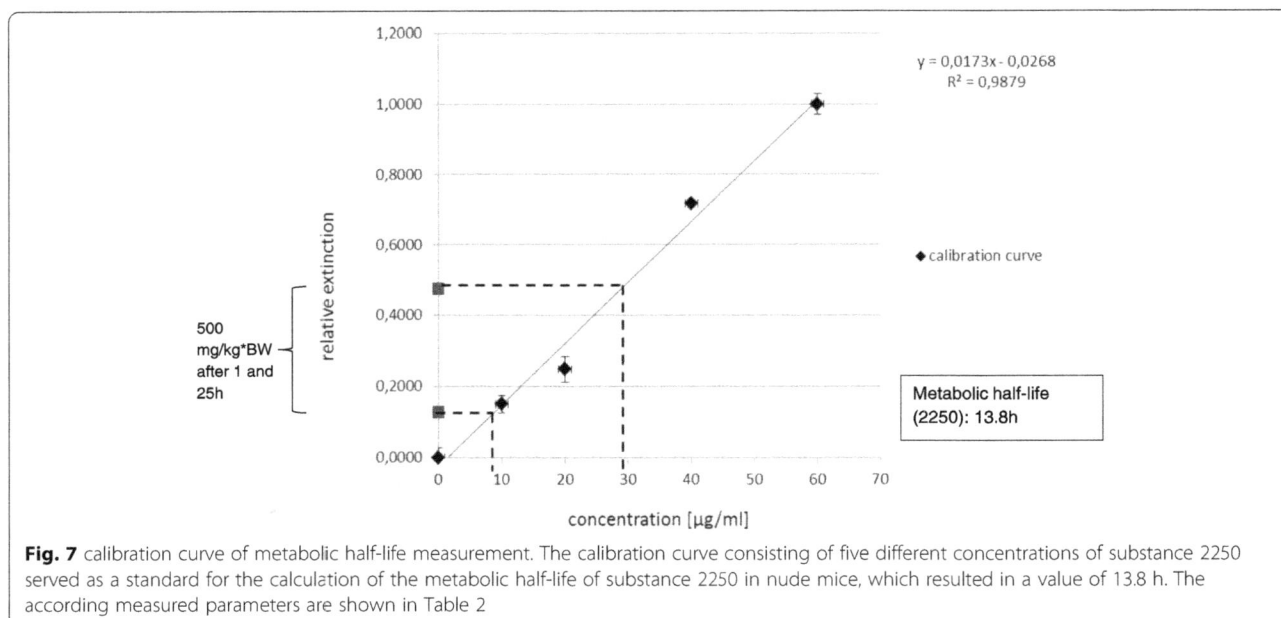

Fig. 7 calibration curve of metabolic half-life measurement. The calibration curve consisting of five different concentrations of substance 2250 served as a standard for the calculation of the metabolic half-life of substance 2250 in nude mice, which resulted in a value of 13.8 h. The according measured parameters are shown in Table 2

might be the induction of a programmed necrosis by substance 2250 itself, as shown previously for Taurolidine [26]. Programmed necrosis is, besides apoptosis and autophagy, the third type of programmed cell death, which involves cell swelling, organelle dysfunction and cell lysis. Programmed necrosis can be induced by different signaling pathways a. o. via activation of death receptors or cell stress can induce activation of receptor- interacting-protein kinases RIP1 and RIP3, which influence mitochondria to induce ROS increase [27, 28]. Further work is required to clarify whether substance 2250 lead to the induction of programmed necrosis on such a high level, at least in BxPC-3 and AsPC-1 at high concentrations.

The second part of this study deals with the contribution of reactive oxygen species (ROS) to substance 2250 induced cell death and the analysis of another major cell death associated pathway, the caspase pathway. Previous studies with TRD revealed an involvement of ROS 12, 40 [29], triggering apoptosis via caspase-independent pathways [12, 20], caspase-dependent pathways 40 [15, 20, 25] as well as necroptosis and autophagy [26]. Furthermore, cell death, induced by ROS, has been shown to be prevented by applying the radical scavenger N-acetycysteine (NAC) [12, 25, 29]. Hence,

in this study both the cellular ROS induction upon treatment and co-incubation experiments with either the radical scavenger NAC for inhibition of oxidative stress or the pan caspase inhibitor z-VAD for involvement of the caspase pathway were performed. Substance 2250 clearly induced ROS production in all tested cell lines. This effect could be completely canceled by the radical scavenger NAC. In line with this result, all analyzed pancreatic cancer cell lines responded to NAC co-incubation with an attenuated cell death, induced by substance 2250. Nevertheless, the extent of protection from cell death was divergent between the analyzed cell lines, ranging from partial protection (BxPC-3, MiaPaca-2, PancTuI) to complete protection (AsPC-1, Panc-1). In general, ROS is regarded as being an ambiguous compound in terms of antineoplastic activity [30]. On the one hand, it is able to support tumor cell proliferation and survival [14, 30]. On the other hand, excessive ROS generation in tumor cells can induce cell death. This therapeutic effect is used by many chemotherapeutics as platinum, arsenic, ascorbate or piperlongumine [13, 30–32]. In conclusion, the generation of ROS and the consequent activation of following pathways is an obvious explanation of the induction of cell death by substance 2250 in pancreatic cancer cell lines. Thus, ROS induced cell death may not be the universal mechanism of substance 2250, but our experiments highlight its central role in programmed cell death (PCD).

We also analyzed another major cell death associated pathway mentioned in the literature referring TRD induced cell death - the caspase pathway [20, 25, 33]. Among the literature, the activation of the caspase

Table 2 Measured parameters of metabolic half-life calculation

Time of blood sampling	Relative extinction	Concentration in serum [µg/ml]
1 h	0.475	29.044
25 h	0.128	8.954

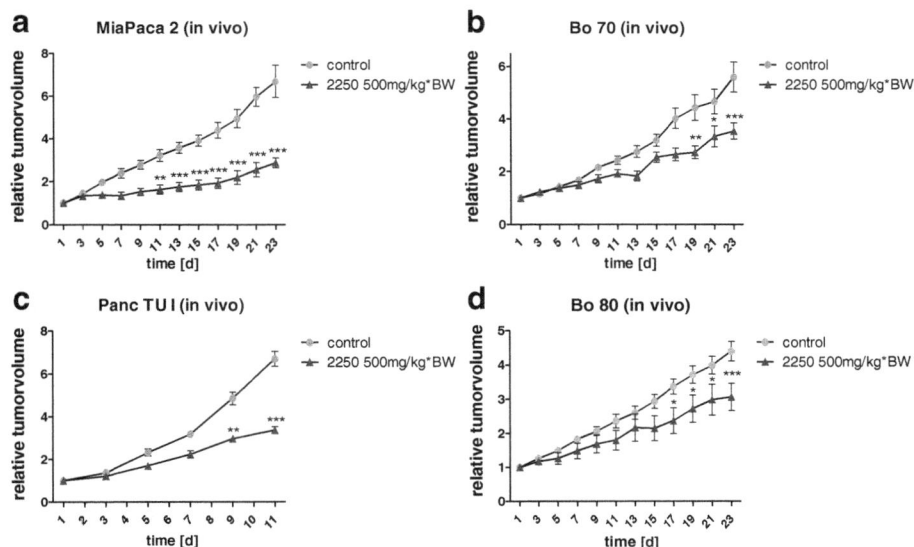

Fig. 8 Effects of 500 mg/kg*BW 2250 on the subcutaneous tumor growth in nude mice in vivo. Nude mice with tumors of MiaPaca-2 (**a**), Panc-TuI (**c**) or patient tissue (**b**, **d**) were incubated with 2250 (500 mg/kg*BW) and ddH$_2$O (control) for up to 3 weeks. The tumor volume was measured on alternating days for up to 3 weeks. Asterisk symbols indicate differences between control and 2250 treatment. *** $p \leq 0.001$, ** $p \leq 0.01$, * $p \leq 0.05$, n.s. $p > 0.05$ (one-way ANOVA followed by Tukey's post-hoc test)

pathway by TRD has been mentioned for several cell lines, but the findings were divergent between different tumor entities. Furthermore, caspase independent PCD induced by TRD was reported in the literature as well [12, 20]. The analyzed pancreatic cancer cell lines (AsPC-1, BxPC-3) were not protected via inhibition of pan-caspases from PCD induced by substance 2250 in our experiments. Previous studies of our group determined that pancreatic cancer cell lines were not protected from PCD caused by TRD, via inhibition of pan caspases, either [15]. The response observed in pancreatic cancer cell lines regarding the inhibition of 2250 induced cell death, via the pan-caspase inhibitor zVAD, leads to the assumption, that especially for pancreatic cancer cell lines the caspase dependent PCD plays only a minor role. Therefore, other pathways like necroptosis or caspase independent programmed cell death may play a more considerable role. These pathways are well discussed in the latest literature related to cancer therapies [34–37]. Further studies in this field are necessary to clarify the involvement of caspase independent types of programmed cell death following the treatment with the substance 2250.

On the basis of this foregone promising in vitro results, we analyzed the anti-neoplastic effects of substance 2250 in vivo. Prior to the in vivo studies the metabolic half-life of the new substance 2250 was determined, due to the fact that Taurolidine shows a very short metabolic half-life of only 1–2 h in healthy human volunteers [22]. Our analysis yielded a metabolic half-life of substance 2250 of 13.8 h in nude mice, displaying a

much higher metabolic stability compared to TRD. Based on the fact that mice have a higher metabolism than humans, it can be assumed, that the metabolic half-life of substance 2250 in humans is even higher. TRD was previously found to suppress tumor growth of different tumor entities in rodents [10, 11, 20, 21, 38–45]. The ip application of TRD inhibits the ip tumor growth of colonic carcinoma [42], mesothelioma [31], malignant melanoma [13, 45] and pancreatic carcinoma [43, 44]. It could also be shown that the intravenous (iv) application of TRD decreases the ip tumor growth as well [38, 40, 41, 46]. Existing studies also have experiences with the effect of TRD application on subcutaneous tumor growth. In colon carcinoma the subcutaneous tumor growth was not influenced by TRD application [38, 40], whereas the subcutaneous tumor growth in malignant melanoma [13, 47] and prostate carcinoma [48] was inhibited by TRD instillation ip and iv.

Therefore our experimental in vivo study was based on the hypothesis that substance 2250 could also inhibit the growth of pancreatic cancer after ip administration in an established cell line model and a xenograft model with patient tissue in nude mice. We observed a significant reduction of subcutaneous tumor growth in tumors induced by established pancreatic cancer cell lines (MiaPaca 2, PancTuI) as well as in xenograft models from patient tissue (Bo70, Bo80). In tumors caused by established pancreatic cell lines, the ip application led to a significant reduction by approximately 50% of relative tumor volume in comparison to the controls. These results were confirmed by the xenograft models derived from patient tissue, where a reduction of relative subcutaneous tumor volume by 30–40% was observed after treatment with substance 2250.

Conclusion

In conclusion, this is the first study providing an evaluation of substance 2250 induced cell death among several pancreatic cancer cell lines in vitro and inhibition of pancreatic tumor growth in vivo. Substance 2250 is characterized by a clear dose response relationship due to the fact that all analyzed cells lines were susceptible to substance 2250 induced cell death. Functional analysis of the involvement of ROS driven and caspase activated PCD showed, that ROS plays a fundamental role inducing cell death in pancreatic carcinoma. In contrast, PCD by caspase activation was less important. Furthermore substance 2250 seems to effectively inhibit pancreatic cancer tumor growth in mice, simultaneously displaying a higher metabolic stability, which will be a strong benefit towards clinical practice. These encouraging results are the basis for further functional analysis and initial clinical studies for this promising agent. It remains to be seen whether 2250, in analogy to TRD, also exerts anti-inflammatory activity by reducing pro-inflammatory cytokines.

Abbreviations

Annexin V-FITC: Annexin V-Fluorescein; BrdU: 5-bromo-2-deoxyuridine; DMEM: Dulbecco's modified eagle medium; DMSO: Dimethylsulfoxide; ELISA: Enzyme Linked Immunosorbent Assay; FACS: Fluoreszcence-activated cell scanning; Ip: Intraperitoneal; NAC: N-acetylcysteine; OD: Optical density; PCD: Programmed cell death; PDAC: Pancreatic ductal adenocarcinoma; PI: Propidiumiodide; ROS: Reactive oxygen species; RPMI 1640: Roswell park memorial institute medium 1640; TRD: Taurolidine; TRLT: Taurultam; UICC: Union international contre le cancer; z-VAD: carbobenzoxy-valyl-alanyl-aspartyl-[O- methyl]- fluoromethylketone

Acknowledgements
The substance 2250 was granted by Geistlich, a company in Wolhusen, Switzerland.

Funding
Our working group has not received any financial support. This study was only financially supported by University Research funding.

Authors' contributions
MB made substantial contributions to conception and design, acquisition of data as well as analysis and interpretation of data. AC made substantial contributions to conception and design. SH and DV guided the in vivo experiments. RP synthesized the analyzed agent. BMS, CB and WU revised the manuscript. All authors have read and approved the manuscript and take public responsibility for it.

Competing interests
Dr. Pfirrmann had indeed a scientific advising function at Geistlich Pharma AG, and was not participating on any profits of this firm. However, he left the firm and is no longer part of Geistlich Pharma. Therefore, no conflict of interest was disclosed.

Author details
[1]Division of Molecular and Clinical Research, St. Josef-Hospital, Ruhr-University Bochum, Bochum, Germany. [2]Department of Molecular Gastrointestinal Oncology, Ruhr-University Bochum, Bochum, Germany. [3]Geistlich Pharma AG, Wolhusen, Switzerland. [4]Department of Internal Medicine, Knappschaftskrankenhaus, Ruhr-University Bochum, Bochum, Germany.

References

1. Ryan DP, Hong TS, Bardeesy N. Pancreatic Adenocarcinoma. N Engl J Med. 2014;371:1039–49.
2. Malvezzi M, Bertuccio P, Levi F, La Vecchia C, Negri E. European cancer mortality predictions for the year 2013. Ann Oncol. 2013;24:792–800.
3. Cancer Facts and Figures | American Cancer Society. 2015. http://old.cancer.org/acs/groups/content/@editorial/documents/document/acspc-044552.pdf.
4. Stewart BW, Wild CP. World Cancer Report. 2014. ISBN: 978-92-832-0443-5.
5. Burris HA, Moore MJ, Andersen J, Green MR, Rothenberg ML, Modiano MR, et al. Improvements in survival and clinical benefit with gemcitabine as first-line therapy for patients with advanced pancreas cancer: a randomized trial. J Clin Oncol. 1997;15:2403–13.
6. Ueno H, Ioka T, Ikeda M, Ohkawa S, Yanagimoto H, Boku N, et al. Randomized phase III study of gemcitabine plus S-1, S-1 alone, or gemcitabine alone in patients with locally advanced and metastatic pancreatic cancer in Japan and Taiwan: GEST study. J Clin Oncol. 2013;31:1640–8.
7. Conroy T, Desseigne F, Ychou M, Bouché O, Guimbaud R, Bécouarn Y, et al. FOLFIRINOX versus gemcitabine for metastatic pancreatic cancer. N Engl J Med. 2011;364:1817–25.
8. Von Hoff DD, Ervin T, Arena FP, Chiorean EG, Infante J, Moore M, et al. Increased survival in pancreatic cancer with nab-paclitaxel plus gemcitabine. N Engl J Med. 2013;369:1691–703.
9. Jurewitsch B, Lee T, Park J, Jeejeebhoy K. Taurolidine 2% as an antimicrobial lock solution for prevention of recurrent catheter-related bloodstream infections. JPEN J Parenter Enteral Nutr. 1998;22:242–4.
10. Jacobi CA, Ordemann J, Böhm B, Zieren HU, Sabat R, Müller JM. Inhibition of peritoneal tumor cell growth and implantation in laparoscopic surgery in a rat model. Am J Surg. 1997;174:359–63.
11. McCourt M, Wang JH, Sookhai S, Redmond HP. Taurolidine inhibits tumor cell growth in vitro and in vivo. Ann Surg Oncol. 2000;7:685–91.
12. Rodak R, Kubota H, Ishihara H, Eugster H-P, Könü D, Möhler H, et al. Induction of reactive oxygen intermediates-dependent programmed cell death in human malignant ex vivo glioma cells and inhibition of the vascular endothelial growth factor production by taurolidine. J Neurosurg. 2005;102:1055–68.
13. Sun BS, Wang JH, Liu LL, Gong SL, Redmond HP. Taurolidine induces apoptosis of murine melanoma cells in vitro and in vivo by modulation of the Bcl-2 family proteins. J Surg Oncol. 2007;96:241–8.
14. Aceto N, Bertino P, Barbone D, Tassi G, Manzo L, Porta C, et al. Taurolidine and oxidative stress: a rationale for local treatment of mesothelioma. Eur Respir J. 2009;34:1399–407.
15. Chromik AM, Daigeler A, Bulut D, Flier A, May C, Harati K, et al. Comparative analysis of cell death induction by Taurolidine in different malignant human cancer cell lines. J Exp Clin Cancer Res. 2010;29:21.
16. Stendel R, Picht T, Schilling A, Heidenreich J, Loddenkemper C, Jänisch W, et al. Treatment of glioblastoma with intravenous taurolidine. First clinical experience. Anticancer Res. 2004;24:1143–7.
17. Braumann C, Gutt CN, Scheele J, Menenakos C, Willems W, Mueller JM, et al. Taurolidine reduces the tumor stimulating cytokine interleukin-1beta in patients with resectable gastrointestinal cancer: a multicentre prospective randomized trial. World J Surg Oncol. 2009;7:32.
18. Gong L, Greenberg HE, Perhach JL, Waldman SA, Kraft WK. The pharmacokinetics of taurolidine metabolites in healthy volunteers. J Clin Pharmacol. 2007;47:697–703.
19. Clauss K, Lück E, von Rymon Lipinski GW. Acetosulfam, a new sweetener. 1. Synthesis and properties (author's transl). Zeitschrift für Leb und -forsch. 1976;162:37–40.
20. Jacobi CA, Sabat R, Ordemann J, Wenger F, Volk HD, Müller JM. Peritoneal instillation of taurolidine and heparin for preventing intraperitoneal tumor growth and trocar metastases in laparoscopic operations in the rat model. Langenbecks Arch für Chir. 1997;382:S31–6.
21. Jacobi CA, Peter FJ, Wenger FA, Ordemann J, Müller JM. New therapeutic strategies to avoid intra- and extraperitoneal metastases during laparoscopy: results of a tumor model in the rat. Dig Surg. 1999;16:393–9.

22. Stendel R, Scheurer L, Schlatterer K, Stalder U, Pfirrmann RW, Fiss I, et al. Pharmacokinetics of taurolidine following repeated intravenous infusions measured by HPLC-ESI-MS/MS of the derivatives taurultame and taurinamide in glioblastoma patients. Clin Pharmacokinet. 2007;46:513–24.

23. Gorman SP, McCafferty DF, Woolfson AD, Jones DS. Reduced adherence of micro-organisms to human mucosal epithelial cells following treatment with Taurolin, a novel antimicrobial agent. J Appl Bacteriol. 1987;62:315–20.

24. Bedrosian I, Sofia RD, Wolff SM, Dinarello CA. Taurolidine, an analogue of the amino acid taurine, suppresses interleukin 1 and tumor necrosis factor synthesis in human peripheral blood mononuclear cells. Cytokine. 1991;3:568–75.

25. Leithäuser ML, Rob PM, Sack K. Pentoxifylline, cyclosporine a and taurolidine inhibit endotoxin-stimulated tumor necrosis factor-alpha production in rat mesangial cell cultures. Exp Nephrol. 1997;5:100–4.

26. Stendel R, Biefer HRC, Dékány GM, Kubota H, Münz C, Wang S, et al. The antibacterial substance taurolidine exhibits anti-neoplastic action based on a mixed type of programmed cell death. Autophagy. 2009;5:194–210.

27. Vanden Berghe T, Vanlangenakker N, Parthoens E, Deckers W, Devos M, Festjens N, et al. Necroptosis, necrosis and secondary necrosis converge on similar cellular disintegration features. Cell Death Differ. 2010;17:922–30.

28. Ouyang L, Shi Z, Zhao S, Wang F-T, Zhou T-T, Liu B, et al. Programmed cell death pathways in cancer: a review of apoptosis, autophagy and programmed necrosis. Cell Prolif. 2012;45:487–98.

29. Stendel R, Scheurer L, Stoltenburg-Didinger G, Brock M, Möhler H. Enhancement of Fas-ligand-mediated programmed cell death by taurolidine. Anticancer Res. 2003;23:2309–14.

30. Shrayer DP, Lukoff H, King T, Calabresi P. The effect of Taurolidine on adherent and floating subpopulations of melanoma cells. Anti-Cancer Drugs. 2003;14:295–303.

31. Nici L, Monfils B, Calabresi P. The effects of taurolidine, a novel antineoplastic agent, on human malignant mesothelioma. Clin Cancer Res. 2004;10:7655–61.

32. Möhler H, Pfirrmann RW, Frei K. Redox-directed cancer therapeutics: Taurolidine and Piperlongumine as broadly effective antineoplastic agents. Int J Oncol. 2014;45:1329–36.

33. Opitz I, Sigrist B, Hillinger S, Lardinois D, Stahel R, Weder W, et al. Taurolidine and povidone-iocine induce different types of cell death in malignant pleural mesothelioma. Lung Cancer. 2007;56:327–36.

34. Tait SWG, Ichim G, Green DR. Die another way–non-apoptotic mechanisms of cell death. J Cell Sci. 2014;127:2135–44.

35. Kroemer G, Martin SJ. Caspase-independent cell death. Nat Med. 2005;11:725–30.

36. Kim E-A, Jang J-H, Lee Y-H, Sung E-G, Song I-H, Kim J-Y, et al. Dioscin induces caspase-independent apoptosis through activation of apoptosis-inducing factor in breast cancer cells. Apoptosis. 2014;19:1165–75.

37. Leon LJ, Pasupuleti N, Gorin F, Carraway KL. A cell-permeant amiloride derivative induces caspase-independent. AIF-mediated programmed necrotic death of breast cancer cells PLoS One. 2013;8:e63038.

38. Braumann C, Ordemann J, Kilian M, Wenger FA, Jacobi CA. Local and systemic chemotherapy with taurolidine and taurolidine/heparin in colon cancer-bearing rats undergoing laparotomy. Clin. Exp. Metastasis. 2003;20:387–94.

39. Opitz I, van der Veen HC, Braumann C, Ablassmaier B, Führer K, Jacobi CA. The influence of adhesion prophylactic substances and taurolidine/heparin

40. Bobrich E, Braumann C, Opitz I, Menenakos C, Kristiansen G, Jacobi CA. Influence of intraperitoneal application of taurolidine/heparin on expression of adhesion molecules and colon cancer in rats undergoing laparoscopy. J Surg Res. 2007;137:75–82.

41. Braumann C, Stuhldreier B, Bobrich E, Menenakos C, Rogalla S, Jacobi CA. High doses of taurolidine inhibit advanced intraperitoneal tumor growth in rats. J Surg Res. 2005;129:129–35.

42. Nestler G, Schulz HU, Schubert D, Krüger S, Lippert H, Pross M. Impact of taurolidine on the growth of CC531 coloncarcinoma cells in vitro and in a laparoscopic animal model in rats. Surg Endosc. 2005;19:280–4.

43. Raue W, Kilian M, Braumann C, Atanassow V, Makareinis A, Caldenas S, et al. Multimodal approach for treatment of peritoneal surface malignancies in a tumour-bearing rat model. Int J Color Dis. 2010;25:245–50.

44. Kilian M, Mautsch I, Braumann C, Schimke I, Guski H, Jacobi CA, et al. Effects of taurolidine and octreotide on tumor growth and lipid peroxidation after staging-laparoscopy in ductal pancreatic cancer. Prostaglandins Leukot Essent Fatty Acids. 2003;69:261–7.

45. Braumann C, Jacobi CA, Rogalla S, Menenakos C, Fuehrer K, Trefzer U, et al. The tumor suppressive reagent taurolidine inhibits growth of malignant melanoma–a mouse model. J Surg Res. 2007;143:372–8.

46. Braumann C, Ordemann J, Wildbrett P, Jacobi CA. Influence of intraperitoneal and systemic application of taurolidine and taurolidine/heparin during laparoscopy on intraperitoneal and subcutaneous tumour growth in rats. Clin Exp Metastasis. 2000;18:547–52.

47. Da Costa ML, Redmond HP, Bouchier-Hayes DJ. Taurolidine improves survival by abrogating the accelerated development and proliferation of solid tumors and development of organ metastases from circulating tumor cells released following surgery. J Surg Res. 2001;101:111–9.

48. Darnowski JW, Goulette FA, Cousens LP, Chatterjee D, Calabresi P. Mechanistic and antineoplastic evaluation of taurolidine in the DU145 model of human prostate cancer. Cancer Chemother Pharmacol. 2004;54:249–58.

on local recurrence and intraperitoneal tumor growth after laparoscopic-assisted bowel resection of colon carcinoma in a rat model. Surg Endosc. 2003;17:1098–104.

4

^{18}F- FDG PET/CT helps differentiate autoimmune pancreatitis from pancreatic cancer

Jian Zhang[1,2†], Guorong Jia[2†], Changjing Zuo[2†], Ningyang Jia[3] and Hui Wang[1*]

Abstract

Background: ^{18}F-FDG PET/CT could satisfactorily show pancreatic and extra-pancreatic lesions in AIP, which can be mistaken for pancreatic cancer (PC). This study aimed to identify ^{18}F-FDG PET/CT findings that might differentiate AIP from PC.

Methods: FDG-PET/CT findings of 26 AIP and 40 PC patients were reviewed. Pancreatic and extra-pancreatic lesions related findings, including maximum standardized uptake values (SUVmax) and patterns of FDG uptake, were identified and compared.

Results: All 26 patients with AIP had increased pancreatic FDG uptake. Focal abnormal pancreatic FDG activities were found in 38/40 (95.00%) PC patients, while longitudinal were found in 18/26 (69.23%) AIP patients. SUVmax was significantly different between AIP and PC, both in early and delayed PET/CT scans ($p < 0.05$). AUCs were 0.700 (early SUVmax), 0.687 (delayed SUVmax), 0.683 (early lesions/liver SUVmax), and 0.715 (delayed lesion/liver SUVmax). Bile duct related abnormalities were found in 12/26 (46.15%) AIP and 10/40 (25.00%) PC patients, respectively. Incidentally, salivary and prostate gland SUVmax in AIP patients were higher compared with those of PC patients ($p < 0.05$). In males,an inverted "V" shaped high FDG uptake in the prostate was more frequent in AIP than PC patients (56.00%, 14/25 vs. 5.71%, 2/35). Increased FDG activity in extra-pancreatic bile duct was present in 4/26 of AIP patients, while was observed in none of the PC patients. Only in AIP patients, both diffuse pancreatic FDG accumulation and increased inverted "V" shaped FDG uptake in the prostate could be found simultaneously.

Conclusions: ^{18}F-FDG PET/CT findings might help differentiate AIP from PC.

Keywords: Autoimmune pancreatitis, Pancreatic cancer, Positron-emission tomography

Background

Autoimmune pancreatitis (AIP) is a chronic pancreatitis characterized by pancreatic enlargement, irregular pancreatic duct stenosis, and increased serum IgG4 levels, mediated by autoimmune mechanisms [1]. Although AIP responds well to steroid therapy, it has no characteristic clinical manifestation(s) and may easily be misdiagnosed as pancreatic cancer (PC) or cholangiocarcinoma, with patients having to undergo unnecessary surgeries and sustaining hardship and high expenses [2, 3]. About 2.2% of lesions resected with suspected pancreatic carcinoma

are histologically proven AIP [4]. Vice versa, 95.7% (22/23) of AIP patients are misdiagnosed with pancreatic cancer or bile duct cancer [5], with up to 91.3% (21/23) operated. FDG PET/CT imaging, with high sensitivity, can show characteristic glucose metabolism that reflects the inflammatory activity of pancreatic lesions [6]. It has been reported that FDG PET/CT could satisfactorily show pancreatic and extra-pancreatic lesions in AIP patients, providing more specific information for diagnosis and facilitating the understanding of AIP's pathological features [7–11]. Besides, in previous studies [12, 13], we found that more than half of AIP patients show inverted "V" shaped high FDG uptake in the prostate. Further research is needed to determine whether the metabolic characteristics of the

---
* Correspondence: wanghui@xinhuamed.com.cn
†Equal contributors
[1]Department of Nuclear Medicine, Xinhua Hospital Affiliated to Shanghai Jiaotong University School of Medicine, Shanghai 200092, China
Full list of author information is available at the end of the article

pancreas and extra-pancreatic organs could be used for the differential diagnosis of AIP and PC.

Methods

Patient population

In this retrospective study, the patients in our study were selected from the population who were suspected of having pancreatic mass and underwent FDG PET/CT. Consecutive patients diagnosed with AIP from August 2010 to March 2014 at Changhai hospital were analyzed. The PC group comprised randomly selected age and sex matched patients to match the AIP group.

Inclusion criteria were: (1) confirmed diagnosis of AIP based on the 14th International Association of Pancreatology diagnostic criteria (which include 5 aspects, namely pancreatic and main pancreatic duct images, serology, EPLs, histology, and hormone therapeutic reaction) and ^{18}F-FDG PET/CT imaging results before treatment for AIP; (2) confirmed diagnosis of pancreatic cancer based on histological findings or liquid based cytology.

Exclusion criteria were: (1) invasive examinations such as aspiration biopsy, ERCP, and stent placement before the PET/CT examination; (2) treatment for inflammation or cancer.

Of the 36 enrolled AIP patients, 10 were excluded (5, 2, and 3 had a history of acute pancreatitis within prior 6 months, incomplete PET/CT, and a recent history of ERCP and/or biliary stent placement, respectively). Median age of the 26 AIP patients included was 60 years, ranging from 40 to 83 years; there was one female. Meanwhile, a total of 40 patients with pancreatic cancer (35 men and 5 women, aged 34-82 years, median age of 60 years) were enrolled. The study was approved by the ethics committee of Chnaghai hospital.

Each of the 66 patients (26 AIP and 40 PC) underwent a whole body PET/CT. Meanwhile, 22/26 AIP patients and 36/40 PC patients had additional delayed PET-CT scans of the abdomen at 120 min after tracer injection.

PET/CT scan

The Siemens Biograph64 PET/CT (52 LSO crystal and 64-slice spiral CT) was used for the PET/CT. ^{18}F-FDG (radiochemical purity >95%) was provided by Shanghai Atomic Sinovac Pharmaceutical Co., Ltd. Subjects were instructed to fast for more than 6 h, and 3.70-5.55 MBq/kg of ^{18}F-FDG was intravenously injected when blood glucose (BG) < 11.1 mmol/L. Then, after resting in the waiting room for 60 min, a body topogram scan was performed using an electric current of 35 mA at a voltage of 120 kV, a scan time of 10.5-15.6 s and a scan thickness of 0.6 mm. Then, whole-body CT scans were performed using an electric current of 170 mA at a voltage of 120 kV, with a scan time of 18.67-21.93 s and scan thickness of 3 mm. Then, whole-body PET scans were performed covering 5-6 bed positions, with an acquisition time of 2.0-2.5 min per bed position. The 3D scanning of the head was performed additionally. Delayed PET scans of the pancreas were carried out with 1-2 bed positions,120 min after injection with ^{18}F-FDG, using the same parameters described above. Images were reconstructed by the post-processing workstation TureD System, including the direction of cross-sectional, coronal, and sagittal tomographic images and three-dimensional projection images.

Image analysis

^{18}F-FDG PET/CT images were interpreted by two experienced nuclear medicine physicians blinded to clinical and histopathological data. Images were evaluated by visual, subjective and semi-quantitative (SUVmax) methods. Any disagreement was resolved by discussions. Mean values from both physicians were considered as final results. The mean retention index (RI) was calculated as RI = ([PET$_{120min}$ SUVmax] – [PET$_{60min}$ SUVmax] ÷ PET$_{60min}$ SUVmax ×100%.

The SUVmax values of lesions of the pancreas, hilar lymph nodes, peri-pancreatic lymph nodes, liver, salivary gland, and prostate were measured. SUVmax ratio of prostate to liver background ratio (PBR) was calculated. Pancreatic lesions were grouped into three categories: a) diffuse, b) focal, and c) multifocal. The multifocal type was defined as more than 1 foci of non-continuous pancreatic lesions were present. The presence or absence of each of the following parameters was determined as "yes" (present) or "no" (absent) by the reviewers: (1) increased FDG activity in the pancreatic lesion; (2) dilated main pancreatic duct; (3) biliary duct abnormalities, including increased FDG activity in the extra-pancreatic bile duct and gallbladder, dilation and wall thickening of intra and extra-hepatic bile ducts; (4) abnormal mediastinal, pulmonary hilar, peri-pancreatic or retroperitoneal lymph nodes; (5) retroperitoneal fibrosis; (6) inverted "V" shaped high FDG uptake in the prostate.

Statistical analysis

Statistical analyses were performed with SPSS version 17.0. Measurement data with normal distribution were shown as $\bar{x} \pm$ SD, and compared by independent samples t-test. Data with abnormal distribution were presented in median and interquartile range (IQR), and compared by rank-sum test. Using statistically significant data of the above parameters, ROC curves were generated and areas under the curves (AUCs) were calculated. Cut-off values were determined by the Youden index. The corresponding sensitivity, specificity, and positive predictive value were calculated. Differences in SUVmax between PET$_{60min}$ and PET$_{120min}$ scans were analyzed by t-test, and the corresponding SUVmax retention index calculated. Differences in detection rates between the two groups were determined using chi-squared analysis or Fisher's exact test.

Results

The 26 AIP patients included 25 men and 1 woman with a median age of 60.0 ± 10.7; two patients were diagnosed based on IgG4-positive plasma cells found by submandibular lymph node and pancreatic biopsies, respectively. In 17 patients, endoscopic ultrasonography assisted fine-needle aspiration revealed no malignant cells. Meanwhile, 22 patients had abnormally elevated serum IgG4 levels. All 26 patients had clinical follow-up with imaging studies at least 6 months.

The forty pancreatic cancer patients included 35 men and 5 women with a median age of 60.7 ± 10.6; final diagnosis was confirmed by surgical pathology ($n = 23$) and endoscopic ultrasonography assisted fine-needle aspiration (FNA) and/or laparoscopy ($n = 17$). In PC group, diameter of the tumour was 30.9 ± 12.2 mm, and 57.5% (23/40) located in the pancreatic head, 22.5% (9/40) located in the pancreatic body, 10% (4/40) located in the pancreatic tail, 10% (4/40) located in the junction of pancreatic body and tail; 20% (8/40) was classified as Stage T1, 10% (4/40) was classified as Stage T2, 30% (12/40) was classified as Stage T3, 40% (4/40) was classified as Stage T4; 50% (20/40) was classified as Stage N0, 50% (20/40) was classified as Stage N1; 72.5% (29/40) was classified as Stage M0, 27.5% (11/40) was classified as Stage M1.

Clinical characteristics of AIP and PC groups were shown in Table 1. There was no statistical difference between the two groups, except for CA19-9 and ALP.

Findings of whole body ^{18}F-FDG PET/CT studies
Pancreatic lesions (Tables 2, 3 and 4)
All patients had increased FDG activity of pancreatic lesions on early PET/CT scan ($\mathrm{PET}_{60\mathrm{min}}$). Eighteen patients with a diffuse pattern of increased pancreatic FDG uptake, six patients with a focal FDG uptake lesion and two patients with multifocal pattern were observed in 26 AIP patients. Average SUVmax was 5.24 ± 1.81.

In the PC group ($n = 40$), the patterns of increased FDG metabolic activity included: focal ($n = 38$), diffuse ($n = 1$), multifocal ($n = 1$) types, with an average SUVmax of 7.30 ± 3.21. FDG activity of the lesions in PC patients was higher than that of the AIP group, with a statistically significant difference ($t = -3.32$, $P < 0.05$).

Twenty-two patients with AIP and 36 patients with PC had delayed PET/CT scans ($\mathrm{PET}_{120\mathrm{min}}$), with a statistically significant difference ($t = -2.967$, $P < 0.05$) between average SUVmax between the two groups.

We also compared liver SUVmax and the ratio of pancreatic lesion SUVmax to liver SUVmax between the two groups in both early and delayed scans. The results showed that SUVmax of pancreatic lesion and above

Table 1 Clinical characteristics of patients with autoimmune pancreatitis and pancreatic cancer

	AIP group $n = 26$	PC group $n = 40$	P value
Women / men	1/25	5/35	NS
Age (years)	60.03 ± 10.72	60.73 ± 10. 60	NS
Fasting blood sugar (mmol/L)	5.90 ± 1.40	6.10 ± 1.47	NS
CRP (mg/L)	5.66(3.32, 8.69)	11.15 ± 7.44	NS
White blood cells (×10⁹/L)	6.15 ± 1.37	5.65 ± 2.12	NS
BUN (mmol/L)	5.24 ± 2.51	5.26 ± 1.80	NS
Creatinine (μmol/L)	70.00(57.25, 79.25)	72.87 ± 16.01	NS
Total bilirubin (μmol/L)	11.60(7.00, 23.90)	14.10(10.60, 21.60)	NS
ALP (U/L)	214.95 ± 164.52	84.00(61.00, 118.00)	P < 0.05
Amylase (U/L)	130.63 ± 157.74	49.00(39.75, 135.00)	NS
CA19-9 (U/ml)	18.30(7.72, 71.63)	406.81 ± 352.09	P < 0.05
Serum total protein(g/L)	62.88 ± 19.99	68.69 ± 5.72	NS
Serum albumin(g/L)	33.59 ± 6.63	39.54 ± 3.87	P < 0.05
Serum globulin(g/L)	33.41 ± 8.97	29.15 ± 4.08	NS
Albumin/Globulin	1.05 ± 0.28	1.38 ± 0.20	P < 0.05
ALT(U/L)	80.71 ± 104.02	23.00(14.00,39.00)	NS
AST(U/L)	62.23 ± 60.98	23.00(19.00,27.00)	P < 0.05

CRP C-reactive protein, *BUN* blood urea nitrogen, *ALP* alkaline phosphatase, *ALT* Alanine aminotransferase, *AST* Aspartate aminotransferase

Table 2 Comparison of quantitative metabolic parameters between the AIP and PC groups

Groups	AIP group	PC group	P value
Early SUVmax of pancreatic lesions	5.24 ± 1.81	7.30 ± 3.21	0.001*
Early SUVmax of Liver	2.84 ± 0.50	2.90 ± 0.40	0.64
Pancreas lesion/liver in early scan	1.91 ± 0.83	2.57 ± 1.17	0.015*
Delayed SUVmax of pancreatic lesions	6.54 ± 2.41	9.15 ± 4.89	0.004*
Delayed SUVmax of Liver	2.73 ± 0.52	2.61 ± 0.53	0.407
Pancreas lesion/liver in delayed scan	2.48 ± 1.10	3.48 ± 1.49	0.005*
RI of Pancreas lesion	21.32 ± 13.11	21.23 ± 24.94	0.986
RI of liver	−1.81 ± 6.46	−6.71(−9.90,-1.18)	0.047*
SUVmax of salivary gland	2.36(1.95,3.41)	2.02 ± 0.76	0.003*
Mediastinal/hilar lymph node	3.52(2.46,4.67)	2.77(2.48,3.99)	0.198
Peri-pancreatic lymph node	2.03 ± 1.23	2.28(1.31,3.78)	0.27
SUVmax of prostate	3.11 ± 1.27	2.11 ± 0.44	0.01*
Prostater/liver	1.10 ± 0.45	0.73 ± 0.15	0.001*

*$P < 0.05$

Table 3 Performance of multiple metabolic parameters in differential diagnosis of AIP and PC

Diagnostic parameters	AUC	Cutoff value	Sensitivity	Specificity	Accuracy
Early SUVmax of pancreatic lesions	0.700	5.94	70.0%	76.9%	72.7%
Pancreas lesion/liver in early scan	0.683	2.16	70.0%	73.1%	71.2%
Delayed SUVmax of pancreatic lesions	0.687	8.13	63.9%	86.4%	72.4%
Pancreas lesion/liver in delayed scan	0.715	3.14	69.4%	90.9%	77.6%
SUVmax of salivary gland	0.716	1.92	84.6%	57.5%	68.2%
SUVmax of prostate	0.776	2.94	56.0%	97.1%	80.0%
RI of liver	0.657	−5.87%	72.7%	58.3%	63.8%
Prostater/liver	0.729	1.02	56.0%	97.1%	80.0%

SUVmax ratio were statistically different. However, SUVmax of the liver were not significantly different between AIP and PC patients (Table 1).

ROC curves showed that the AUC of the ratio of pancreatic lesion SUVmax to liver SUVmax in delayed scan was the largest (0.715) to diagnose PC.

AIP patients' pancreatic lesion SUVmax RI was 21.32 ± 13.11%, while 21.23 ± 24.94% was obtained for PC patients. Liver SUVmax RI values were −1.81 ± 6.46 and −6.71% (−9.90, −1.18%) in AIP and PC patients, respectively. There was statistically significant difference between the two groups in the RI values of the liver (Mann-Whitney U test, $P < 0.05$), but not of pancreatic lesions ($P > 0.05$) (Table 1).

Pancreatic duct dilatation was observed in only 6 of 26 (23.1%) AIP patients, and in 22 of the 40 (55.0%) patients with PC. Fisher's exact test confirmed the statistically significant difference between the two groups ($P < 0.05$).

Table 4 Common PET-CT findings in patients with autoimmune pancreatitis and pancreatic cancer

PET/CT findings	AIP group	PC group	P value
Dilated pancreatic duct	6/26	22/40	$P < 0.05$
Changes of biliary system	12/26	10/40	$P < 0.05$
High uptake of extra-pancreatic bile duct	4/26	0/40	$P < 0.05$
Mediastinal & hilar lymph node	17/26	20/40	NS
Peri-pancreatic and peritoneal lymph node	20/26	31/40	NS
Inverted "V" shape high prostate FDG uptake	14/25	2/35	$P < 0.001$
Retroperitoneal fibrosis	2	0	NS

Extra-pancreatic lesions (EPLs) on PET/CT
Morphological and metabolic features of EPLs (Table 3)

Fisher's exact test showed statistical differences in the positive rates of high FDG uptake of extra-pancreatic bile duct ($P < 0.05$) and inverted "V" shaped high FDG uptake in the prostate ($P < 0.001$); however, there was no statistically significant difference in the positive rate of retroperitoneal fibrosis, FDG uptake of mediastinal and hilar lymph node, or peri-pancreatic peritoneum lymph nodes. Increased FDG activity of the extra pancreatic portion of the bile duct was only observed in the AIP group (4/26 of patients), but not in PC patients (0/40); with pancreatic lesions showing diffuse FDG accumulation, inverted "V" shaped high FDG uptake in the prostate was observed in 11 of the 20 patients with AIP, while none of the 2 patients with PC showed this feature (Figs. 1, 2 and 3).

Quantitative analysis of PET/CT in extra-pancreatic lesions (Tables 1, 2)
Salivary glands

Median SUVmax of salivary glands in AIP patients was 2.36 (range: 1.95- 3.41), and was 2.02 ± 0.76 in PC patients, indicating a statistically significant difference between the two groups ($P < 0.05$). The AUC of the SUVmax of salivary glands in diagnosing AIP was 0.716; with a cut-off value of 1.92, sensitivity and specificity were 84.6 and 57.5%, respectively.

Lymph nodes

Median SUVmax of mediastinal and hilar lymph nodes in AIP patients was 3.52 (range: 2.46-4.67) and was 2.77 (range: 2.48-3.99) in PC patients. No significant difference between the two groups was found (Mann-Whitney U test; $P > 0.05$). No significant difference in the average SUVmax of peri-pancreatic and retroperitoneum lymph nodes was observed between the two groups (2.28 (1.31-3.78) for patients with PC, 2.03 ± 1.23 for patients with AIP, $P > 0.05$).

Prostate

Mean SUVmax of the prostate was higher in the AIP group (3.11 ± 1.27) than that in the PC group (2.11 ± 0.44, $P < 0.05$). The AUC of prostate SUVmax in diagnosing AIP was 0.776; with a cut-off value of 2.94; sensitivity, specificity, and accuracy value were 56.0, 97.1, and 97.1%, respectively.

The ratios of prostate SUVmax to liver SUVmax (prostate/liver) were also evaluated. Compared with the PC group (0.73 ± 0.15), AIP patients showed significantly higher values (1.10 ± 0.45; $t = -4.584$, $P < 0.05$). AUC of this ratio in diagnosing AIP was 0.729; with a cut-off value of 1.02, sensitivity, specificity, and accuracy value were 56.0, 97.1, and 97.1%, respectively.

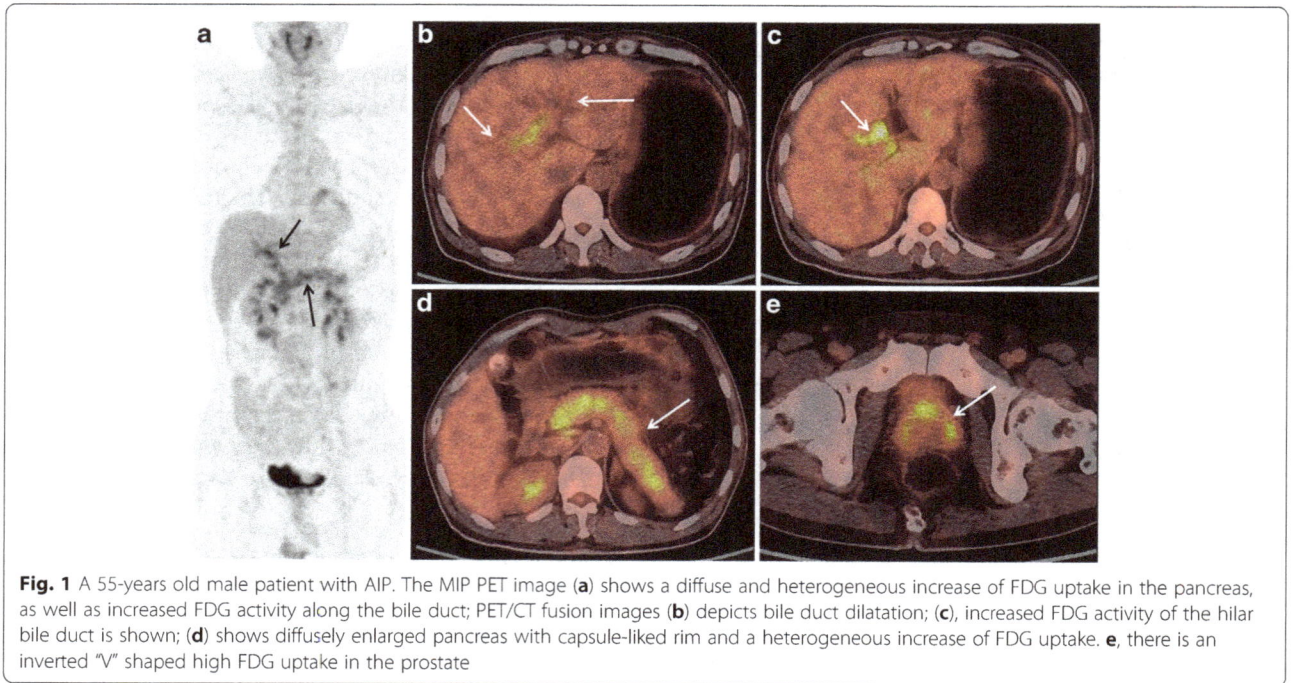

Fig. 1 A 55-years old male patient with AIP. The MIP PET image (**a**) shows a diffuse and heterogeneous increase of FDG uptake in the pancreas, as well as increased FDG activity along the bile duct; PET/CT fusion images (**b**) depicts bile duct dilatation; (**c**), increased FDG activity of the hilar bile duct is shown; (**d**) shows diffusely enlarged pancreas with capsule-liked rim and a heterogeneous increase of FDG uptake. **e**, there is an inverted "V" shaped high FDG uptake in the prostate

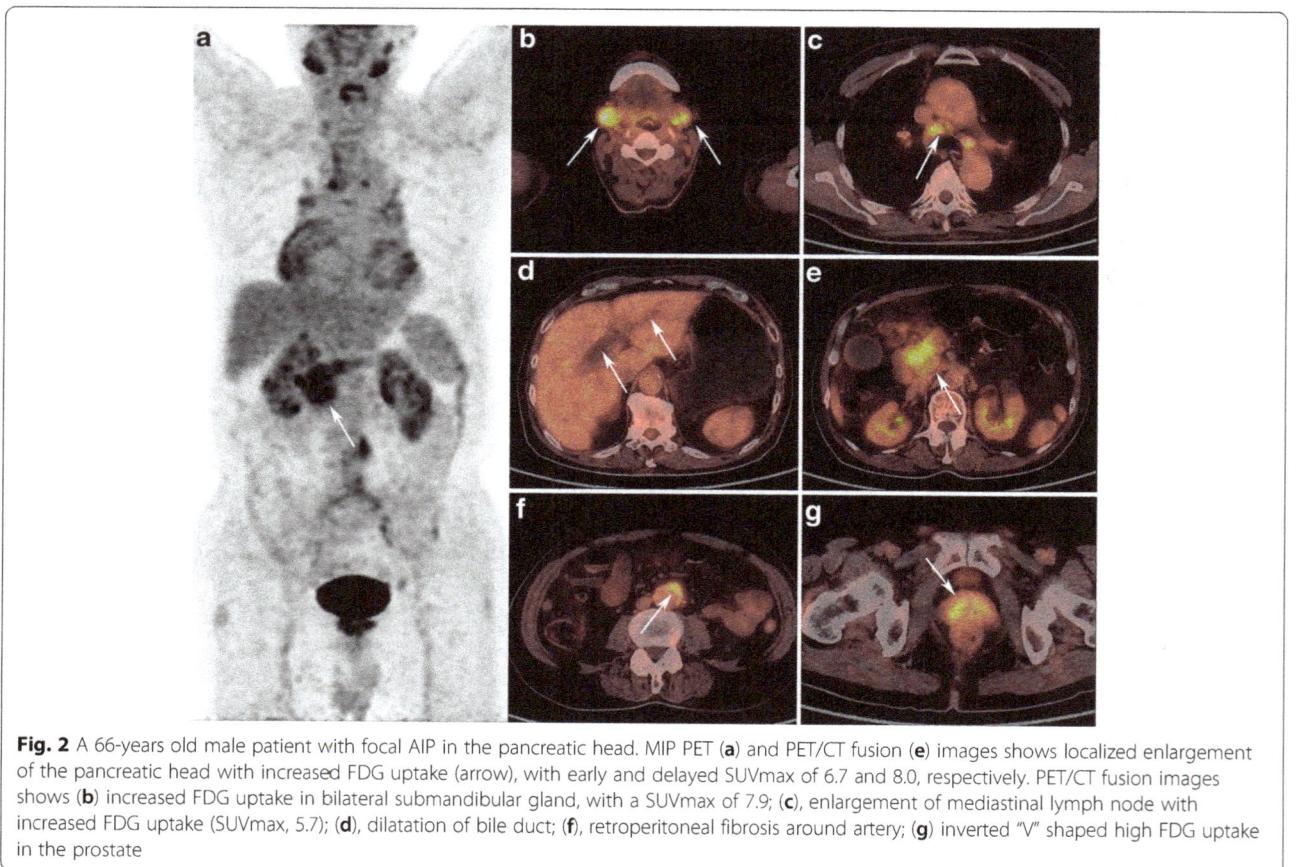

Fig. 2 A 66-years old male patient with focal AIP in the pancreatic head. MIP PET (**a**) and PET/CT fusion (**e**) images shows localized enlargement of the pancreatic head with increased FDG uptake (arrow), with early and delayed SUVmax of 6.7 and 8.0, respectively. PET/CT fusion images shows (**b**) increased FDG uptake in bilateral submandibular gland, with a SUVmax of 7.9; (**c**), enlargement of mediastinal lymph node with increased FDG uptake (SUVmax, 5.7); (**d**), dilatation of bile duct; (**f**), retroperitoneal fibrosis around artery; (**g**) inverted "V" shaped high FDG uptake in the prostate

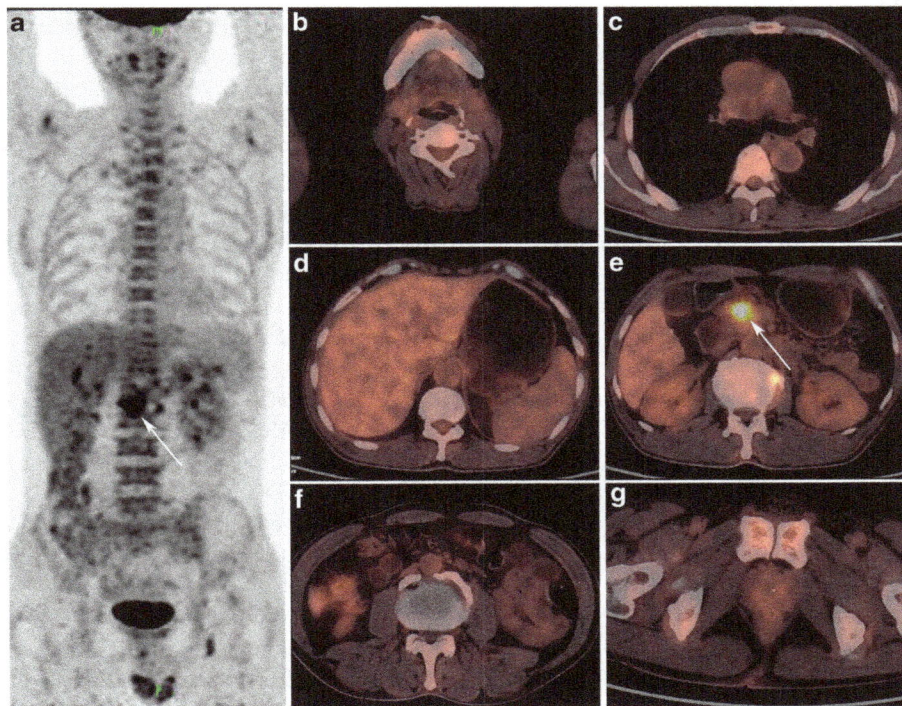

Fig. 3 A 59-years old male patient with pancreatic cancer. MIP PET (**a**) and PET/CT fusion (**e**) images show a mass in the pancreatic head with increased FDG uptake (arrow), with early and delayed SUVmax of 9.3 and 10.8, respectively. Compared with AIP patients in Fig. 2, no increased FDG uptake foci in the salivary gland **b**), mediastinal lymph nodes (**c**), retroperitoneal space (**f**), and prostate (**g**) are observed, as well as no bile duct expansion (**d**)

Discussion

Autoimmune pancreatitis (AIP) is a specific type of chronic pancreatitis, including two subtypes, which might be identified using tissue pathology, clinical features and/or diagnostic criteria [14–16]. Type-I AIP is more prevalent in elderly Asian males and characterized by lymphoplasmacytic sclerosing pancreatitis, which commonly involves other organs as well.

In the early years, due to the lack of awareness of AIP, it was often misdiagnosed as PC. In a study of 37 AIP patients utilizing conventional imaging modalities, six patients were misdiagnosed as PC and two cases as cholangiocarcinoma [17]. Another study found that 9 of 17 AIP cases were misdiagnosed as pancreatic cancer, and they proposed a few reasons: demographics, clinical manifestations, serology and bile duct stenosis [18]. With the wide application and development in recent years, contrast-enhanced CT and MR have played an important role in the differential diagnosis of AIP and PC. Some manifestation, such as "sausage-like" pancreatic enlargement, capsule-like rim, segmental stricture of pancreatic duct, and delayed enhancement were known as the characteristics of AIP. In this study, we found some parameters and imaging characteristics of FDG PET/CT could help to differentially diagnose AIP from PC.

It is well documented that increased FDG accumulation might be used as a marker of inflammatory lesions [19–21]. Thus, FDG PET/CT might play a critical role in revealing pancreatic and extra-pancreatic lesions in patients with AIP. Ozaki et al., [9] showed that high FDG activity was observed in all AIP patients, while only 73.1% PC patients had increased FDG activity in lesions.

A focal, nodular pattern of increased FDG activity was significantly more frequent in patients with pancreatic cancer, whereas an longitudinal abnormal pancreatic FDG activities was more suggestive of AIP [8, 9]. In this study a longitudinal pattern of increased FDG accumulation along the pancreas was found in 69.2% of AIP patients, and only in 2.5% of PC cases. On the other hand, a focal nodular pattern of increased FDG activity was found in 23.1 and 95% patients with AIP and PC, respectively.

Previous studies suggested that FDG SUV of a lesion was usually greater than 4.0 in patients with PC, 3.0 - 4.0 in chronic pancreatitis patients and below 3 in healthy volunteers [22]. Although AIP is a subtype of chronic pancreatitis, Ozaki et al. [9] found no significant difference in SUV of lesions between patients with AIP and PC, either on early or delayed phase images; similar SUVmax ratio between early and delayed phases were also found. Lee et al. [8] compared the frequency of increased

FDG uptake of pancreatic lesions in patients with AIP and PC, and overall frequency showed no significant differences as well. Our study, including age and sex matched AIP ($n = 26$) and PC ($n = 40$) patients, suggested that both SUVmax and the SUVmax ratio of pancreas to liver in the early and delayed phases were significantly different. On early PET/CT scans with a cut-off value of SUVmax of 5.94, diagnostic sensitivity and specificity were 70.0 and 76.9%, respectively, for PC diagnosis. The larger sample size of AIP in the present study might be the reason for disagreement with prior reports. In addition, the following reasons could be considered as well. (1) Technical differences between previously used PET scanners and modern PET-CT scanners, which could account for discrepant SUV values. (2) In the current study, FDG SUV were compared in age and sex matched two groups, unlike previous studies [8, 9]. (3) In the current study, the AIP patient population comprised consecutive patients, which was not the case in Lee et al. [8]. (4) The number of pancreatic cancer patients in Lee's [8] study was distinctly larger than that of AIP patients, which might have impaired the power of statistical tests. (5) Invasive diagnostic procedures were performed prior to PET/CT scan in some cases, which might have influenced FDG metabolism and the SUV value. In the current study such factors were well controlled and eliminated. However, the diagnostic sensitivity of SUV in the PC group was lower (70.0%) in the current study. We tentatively put forward that diversity of PC metabolism results in varied SUV values in a large range. For example, FDG uptake may increase slightly in some small, low-malignant or mucinous pancreatic cancer cases. Furthermore, a quite remarkable metabolism was detected in some patients with AIP, with the highest SUVmax of 11.8, leading to false positivity and decreased specificity.

Patients with AIP may have autoimmune inflammation involving the liver and biliary tract [23, 24]; inflammation induces abnormal hepatobiliary function and decreases the liver clearance of FDG. Our results revealed that FDG retention index values of the AIP and PC groups were 1.8 and 6.7%, respectively, suggesting that liver clearance of FDG activity is slower in the AIP group than in PC patients. Thus, the AIP SUVmax ratio of lesion to liver was lower compared with that of the PC group in the delayed phase.

When pancreatic cancer invades the bile duct, the main manifestation is direct compression of the bile duct, stenosis, or even an obstruction. In pancreatic cancer, the bile duct can also be compressed by a metastatic lymph node. In AIP patients, the inflammatory swelling of the pancreatic head could also cause narrowing and occlusion of the distal common bile duct, eventually

leading to secondary expansion/dilatation of the upstream bile duct. In the current study, 46.2% patients in the AIP group showed biliary duct changes, which was only present in 25.0% of PC patients. The higher positive rate for the AIP group is possibly related to frequent involvement of the pancreatic head (88.5 AIP vs 52.5% PC). Besides concomitant bile duct inflammation might result in higher proportion of biliary system change in AIP patients. Moreover, this study revealed that FDG accumulation in the extra pancreatic portion of the bile duct was only observed in AIP patients.

A number of studies have shown that AIP also involves salivary glands, and is characterized by increased FDG hyper metabolism on PET/CT. Ozaki's comparative study [9] found that 13.3% (2/15) of AIP patients have FDG accumulation in the salivary gland, with the PC group showing no increased FDG accumulation in the salivary gland. Lee et al. [8] showed that 35.3% (6/17) of AIP patients have high FDG accumulation in the salivary gland, with statistically significant difference between the two groups. In this study, considering physiological FDG uptake of normal salivary gland, we measured the SUVmax of the salivary gland, and found higher values in the AIP group compared with PC patients (2.36 vs 2.02, $P < 0.05$). At a threshold value for salivary gland's FDG SUVmax of greater than 1.92, diagnostic sensitivity was 84.6% in the AIP group, for a specificity of 57.5%. These results suggested the involvement of the salivary gland in patients with AIP.

Our previous studies demonstrated that over half of AIP male patients show inverted "V" shaped high FDG uptake in the region of the prostate gland [12, 13]. This characteristic may be related to inflammatory infiltration of the prostatic transitional and central zones, which shaped like a inverted "V". However, whether this characteristic can be used to differentiate AIP from PC remains unclear. This study found that the positive rate of inverted "V" shaped high FDG uptake was significantly different in AIP and PC patients (56.0 vs 2.9%). This result provided more evidence that inverted "V" shaped high FDG uptake in the prostate can contribute to AIP diagnosis. The previous reports [9, 23] of complicated prostatitis of AIP patients, but the frequency is low. Reasons may include: (1) due to normal prostate also can uptake FDG physiologically, previous reports defined prostatic involvement usually based on FDG metabolism increased significantly in prostate, and symptoms associated with prostatitis. While in our research, it is based on whether there is inverted "V" shaped high FDG accumulation, which might with slightly increased FDG metabolism, most of these patients had not symptoms associated with prostatitis. Two PC patients were detected with inverted "V" shaped high FDG uptake. Given their advanced ages, we speculated that these patients may have autoimmune prostatitis [25]. However, only in

AIP patients, both diffuse pancreatic FDG accumulation and increased inverted "V" shaped FDG uptake in the prostate could be found simultaneously. We also found that prostate SUVmax in the AIP group was higher than in PC patients; with a cut-off value of 2.94, a specificity of 97.1% was obtained. Although previous studies [8, 9] suggested that retroperitoneal fibrosis is commonly observed in AIP patients, the current study population had a very limited number of such cases, namely 2 patients.

In contrast to prior reports [8, 9], no significant differences in SUVmax and the frequency of increased FDG uptake of mediastinal and hilar lymph nodes were found between the two groups. A possible reason is that patients with pancreas cancer sometimes suffer from mediastinal and hilar lymph node metastasis; besides, elder patients could show non-tumorous FDG accumulation in mediastinal and hilar lymph nodes [26]. This study found no statistically significant difference in SUVmax and number of para-pancreatic lymph nodes. A possible reason is that metastatic lymph nodes in pancreatic cancer might have small volume and low FDG uptake; another explanation is that AIP patients could have peri-pancreatic lymph node involvement.

Conclusions

Diffuse uptake of FDG in the pancreas might be used to differentiate AIP from PC. Furthermore, some parameters including the ratio of pancreatic lesion/liver SUV, the SUV of salivary glands, the SUV of prostate might help to differentiate, and some morphological and metabolic features of EPLs including inverted "V" shaped high FDG uptake in the prostate and increased FDG activity in extra-pancreatic bile duct have high specificity for diagnosing AIP. FDG PET/CT could provide various findings as supplements to CECT and MR, which might improve the diagnostic accuracy.

Abbreviations
AIP: Autoimmune pancreatitis; AUCs: Areas under the curves; EPLs: Extra-pancreatic lesions; FNA: Fine-needle aspiration; IQR: Interquartile range; PBR: prostate-to-background ratio; PC: Pancreatic cancer; RI: Retention index; SUVmax: Maximum standardized uptake values

Acknowledgements
The authors are grateful to Pro. Cahid Civelek of NIH Clinical Center helped polish the manuscript.

Funding
This study was supported by Shanghai Science and Technology Committee (grant number 10410708800); National Natural Science Foundation of China (grant number 81170435, 81471714).

Authors' contributions
JZ, GRJ and CJZ contributed equally to this work; JZ and GRJ collected and analyzed the data, and drafted the manuscript; CJZ and JZ designed and supervised the study; HW provided analytical oversight and revised the manuscript for important intellectual content; NYJ, GRJ offered technical or material support. All authors read and approved the final manuscript.

Competing interests
The authors declare that they have no competing interests.

Author details
[1]Department of Nuclear Medicine, Xinhua Hospital Affiliated to Shanghai Jiaotong University School of Medicine, Shanghai 200092, China. [2]Department of Nuclear Medicine, Changhai Hospital, Second Military Medical University, Shanghai 200433, China. [3]Department of Radiology, Eastern Hepatobiliary Surgery Hospital, Second Military Medical University, Shanghai 200433, China.

References
1. Finkelberg DL, Sahani D, Deshpande V, Brugge WR. Autoimmune pancreatitis. N Engl J Med. 2006;355:2670–6.
2. Nakazawa T, Ohara H, Sano H, Ando T, Imai H, Takada H, et al. Difficulty in diagnosing autoimmune pancreatitis by imaging findings. Gastrointest Endosc. 2007;65:99–108.
3. Kamisawa T, Egawa N, Nakajima H, Tsuruta K, Okamoto A, Kamata N. Clinical difficulties in the differentiation of autoimmune pancreatitis and pancreatic carcinoma. Am J Gastroenterol. 2003;98:2694–9.
4. Hardacre JM, Iacobuzio-Donahue CA, Sohn TA, Abraham SC, Yeo CJ, Lillemoe KD, et al. Results of pancreaticoduodenectomy for lymphoplasmacytic sclerosing pancreatitis. Ann Surg. 2003;237:853–8. discussion 8-9
5. Wu LL, Li W. An analysis of clinical characteristics of autoimmune pancreatitis. Zhonghua Nei Ke Za Zhi. 2010;49:943–6.
6. Dong A, Dong H, Zhang L, Zuo C. Hypermetabolic lesions of the pancreas on FDG PET/CT. Clin Nucl Med. 2013;38:e354–66.
7. Shigekawa M, Yamao K, Sawaki A, Hara K, Takagi T, Bhatia V, et al. Is (18)F-fluorodeoxyglucose positron emission tomography meaningful for estimating the efficacy of corticosteroid therapy in patients with autoimmune pancreatitis? J Hepatobiliary Pancreat Sci. 2010;17:269–74.
8. Lee TY, Kim MH, Park DH, Seo DW, Lee SK, Kim JS, et al. Utility of 18F-FDG PET/CT for differentiation of autoimmune pancreatitis with atypical pancreatic imaging findings from pancreatic cancer. AJR Am J Roentgenol. 2009;193:343–8.
9. Ozaki Y, Oguchi K, Hamano H, Arakura N, Muraki T, Kiyosawa K, et al. Differentiation of autoimmune pancreatitis from suspected pancreatic cancer by fluorine-18 fluorodeoxyglucose positron emission tomography. J Gastroenterol. 2008;43:144–51.
10. Nakajo M, Jinnouchi S, Fukukura Y, Tanabe H, Tateno R, Nakajo M. The efficacy of whole-body FDG-PET or PET/CT for autoimmune pancreatitis and associated extrapancreatic autoimmune lesions. Eur J Nucl Med Mol Imaging. 2007;34:2088–95.
11. Sato M, Okumura T, Shioyama Y, Imura J. Extrapancreatic F-18 FDG accumulation in autoimmune pancreatitis. Ann Nucl Med. 2008;22:215–9.
12. Jian Z. Imaging characteristics of autoimmune pancreatitis: F-18-FDG PET/CT versus Contrast Enhanced CT. J Nucl Med. 2015;56
13. Zhang J, Shao C, Wang J, Cheng C, Zuo C, Sun G, et al. Autoimmune pancreatitis: whole-body 18F-FDG PET/CT findings. Abdom Imaging. 2013; 38:543–9.
14. Zhang L, Chari S, Smyrk TC, Deshpande V, Kloppel G, Kojima M, et al. Autoimmune pancreatitis (AIP) type 1 and type 2: an international consensus study on histopathologic diagnostic criteria. Pancreas. 2011;40:1172–9.
15. Shimosegawa T, Chari ST, Frulloni L, Kamisawa T, Kawa S, Mino-Kenudson M, et al. International consensus diagnostic criteria for autoimmune pancreatitis: guidelines of the International Association of Pancreatology. Pancreas. 2011;40:352–8.
16. Lee LK, Sahani DV. Autoimmune pancreatitis in the context of IgG4-related disease: review of imaging findings. World J Gastroenterol. 2014;20:15177–89.
17. Kamisawa T, Okamoto A. Autoimmune pancreatitis: proposal of IgG4-related sclerosing disease. J Gastroenterol. 2006;41:613–25.
18. Sugumar A, Chari S. Autoimmune pancreatitis: an update. Expert Rev Gastroenterol Hepatol. 2009;3:197–204.

19. Sperti C, Pasquali C, Decet G, Chierichetti F, Liessi G, Pedrazzoli S. F-18-fluorodeoxyglucose positron emission tomography in differentiating malignant from benign pancreatic cysts: a prospective study. J Gastrointest Surg. 2005;9:22–8. discussion 8-9

20. Shreve PD. Focal fluorine-18 fluorodeoxyglucose accumulation in inflammatory pancreatic disease. Eur J Nucl Med. 1998;25:259–64.

21. Balink H, Tan SS, Veeger NJ, Holleman F, van Eck-Smit BL, Bennink RJ, et al. (1)(8)F-FDG PET/CT in inflammation of unknown origin: a cost-effectiveness pilot-study. Eur J Nucl Med Mol Imaging. 2015;42:1408–13.

22. Imdahl A, Nitzsche E, Krautmann F, Hogerle S, Boos S, Einert A, et al. Evaluation of positron emission tomography with 2-[18F]fluoro-2-deoxy-D-glucose for the differentiation of chronic pancreatitis and pancreatic cancer. Br J Surg. 1999;86:194–9.

23. Nakatani K, Nakamoto Y, Togashi K. Utility of FDG PET/CT in IgG4-related systemic disease. Clin Radiol. 2012;67:297–305.

24. Horiuchi A, Kawa S, Hamano H, Hayama M, Ota H, Kiyosawa K. ERCP features in 27 patients with autoimmune pancreatitis. Gastrointest Endosc. 2002;55:494–9.

25. Murphy SF, Schaeffer AJ, Thumbikat P. Immune mediators of chronic pelvic pain syndrome. Nat Rev Urol. 2014;11:259–69.

26. Jian Z. Comparsion of Positron Emission Tomography/Computed Tomography and Contrast-Enhanced Computed Tomography in Lung Cancer Lymph Node Staging. J Nucl Med. 2015;56:1385.

5

Histone profiling reveals the H1.3 histone variant as a prognostic biomarker for pancreatic ductal adenocarcinoma

Monika Bauden[1†], Theresa Kristl[2†], Agata Sasor[3], Bodil Andersson[1], György Marko-Varga[2], Roland Andersson[1] and Daniel Ansari[1*] ⓘD

Abstract

Background: Epigenetic alterations have been recognized as important contributors to the pathogenesis of PDAC. However, the role of histone variants in pancreatic tumor progression is still not completely understood. The aim of this study was to explore the expression and prognostic significance of histone protein variants in PDAC patients.

Methods: Liquid chromatography-tandem mass spectrometry (LC-MS/MS) was employed for qualitative analysis of histone variants and histone related post-translational modifications (PTMs) in PDAC and normal pancreatic tissues. Survival analysis was conducted using the Kaplan-Meier method and Cox proportional hazards regression.

Results: Histone variant H1.3 was found to be differentially expressed ($p = 0.005$) and was selected as a PDAC specific histone variant candidate. The prognostic role of H1.3 was evaluated in an external cohort of patients with resected PDAC using immunohistochemistry. Intratumor expression of H1.3 was found to be an important risk factor for overall survival in PDAC, with an adjusted HR value of 2.6 (95% CI 1.1–6.1), $p = 0.029$.

Conclusion: We suggest that the intratumor histone H1.3 expression as reported herein, may serve as a new epigenetic biomarker for PDAC.

Keywords: Biomarkers, Epigenetics, Histone variants, H1.3, LC-MS/MS, Immunohistochemistry, Pancreatic Ductal Adenocarcinoma

Background

Pancreatic ductal adenocarcinoma (PDAC) is the most frequent histologic subtype of pancreatic cancer and accounts for one of the most aggressive malignancies. With an extremely low five-year survival rate, PDAC represents the fourth leading cause of cancer-related deaths in the United States and Europe [1, 2]. At the time of diagnosis, most patients have developed a locally advanced or metastatic disease, which limits the possibilities for therapeutic intervention and contributes to the poor prognosis [3, 4]. Detailed understanding of the biology behind pancreatic cancer is crucial for the improvement of clinical outcome as well as for the

discovery of new biomarkers for early diagnosis, prognosis, and therapeutic targeting.

It is now apparent that, besides the extensive genetic alterations, an aberrant epigenetic regulation, including modifications of the chromatin structure, also significantly contributes to the pathogenesis of PDAC [5–7]. Chromatin depositions of histone variants have been implicated in the establishment and maintenance of the epigenetic states. Variants of histone proteins are further involved in fundamental cellular processes, such as regulation of transcriptional activity or DNA repair, hence considered as contributors to tumor progression [8, 9].

Histone proteins constitute nucleosomes, which are the basic structural and functional components of the chromatin. The nucleosomes consist of superhelical DNA wrapped around a histone octamer composed of two copies of each histone protein H2A, H2B, H3 and

---

* Correspondence: daniel.ansari@med.lu.se
†Equal contributors
[1]Department of Surgery, Clinical Sciences Lund, Lund University, Skåne University Hospital, SE-221 85 Lund, Sweden
Full list of author information is available at the end of the article

H4. The higher order chromatin stabilization is facilitated by the linker histone H1 variants [10].

Histone proteins are usually divided into conventional, canonical histones that function mainly in the packaging of the newly replicated DNA and histone variants that replace the canonical histones when nucleosomes are disrupted, at any phase of the cell cycle. Histone isoforms within each histone family are distinguished from each other by a specific primary amino acid sequence, differing often with only a few amino acids. The incorporation of diverse histone variants can influence the functional properties of the nucleosome and thus affect the chromatin conformation and the accessibility of the genome. The nucleosomal assembly of histone variants, together with histone related post-translational modifications, is essential for the transition between active and silent chromatin states and thus plays a significant role in the epigenetic regulation of gene transcription [11–13]. Alteration of epigenetic processes involved in chromatin dynamics may ultimately promote cancer development and tumor progression [14, 15]. The availability of biobank materials and advanced proteomic analysis tools makes it possible to investigate the changes in chromatin-related epigenetics, including histone variants coinciding with the malignant transformation [16, 17]. The profile of histone variants, as the regulators of chromatin, should therefore be explored in order to provide further insights regarding PDAC pathobiology and guide new approaches for disease management to ameliorate the poor prognosis of PDAC.

Here, we report the profile of histone protein variants in PDAC tissue in relation to normal pancreas, assessed by high-resolution nano-liquid chromatography-tandem mass spectrometry (LC-MS/MS). The intratumor distribution of the PDAC specific histone variant candidate was verified by immunohistochemistry (IHC). The prognostic value of H1.3 expression in PDAC was explored using survival analysis.

Methods
Materials
Unless stated otherwise, the following chemicals and solvents were purchased from Sigma-Aldrich St. Louis, MO, USA; Tris-HCl, guanidine-HCl, ammonium bicarbonate (AMBIC), dithiothreitol (DTT), iodoacetamide (IAA), formic acid (FA), acetonitrile (ACN), sodium chloride (NaCl), sodium citrate, Tween 20, Triton X-100 and bovine serum albumin (BSA). Xylene, Pertex and hematoxylin were obtained from Histolab Products AB, Gothenburg, Sweden and ethanol (EtOH) from Solveco, Rosenberg, Sweden. Protein determination assay, peptide determination kit and Pierce LC-MS grade water was obtained from Thermo Scientific, Rockford, IL, USA. Milli-Q water was produced using an in-house installed purification system Q-POD Millipore (EMD Millipore,

Billerica, MA, USA). Thermo-Fisher Scientific, Bremen, Germany was the supplier of analytical instruments used in this study, including EASY-nLC™ 1000 nanoflow liquid chromatography system and Q Exactive™ Plus Hybrid Quadrupole-Orbitrap™ mass spectrometer equipped with a Thermo Scientific™ EASY-Spray™ source. The table centrifuge 5415R, speed vacuum concentrator plus, and thermomixer Comfort were provided by Eppendorf AG, Hamburg, Germany.

Analysis of the histone profile in PDAC using LC-MS/MS
Tissue acquisition
Fresh frozen PDAC tissue ($n = 10$) used for LC-MS/MS analysis was acquired from patients undergoing pancreaticoduodenectomy between July 2013 and April 2015 at the department of Surgery, Skåne University Hospital in Lund, Sweden. PDAC specimens were selected retrospectively from a local biobank, using information recorded in the hospital patient registry to obtain a study population as homogeneous as possible. The inclusion criteria were based on following parameters: histopathological diagnosis of low to moderately differentiated PDAC with a primary tumor located in the pancreatic head, stage T3 N1 (AJCC, 7th edition), no diabetes mellitus and no neoadjuvant therapy undertaken. The accepted co-morbidity was limited to cardiovascular associated disease, kidney stone and age-related conditions as e.g. benign prostate hyperplasia.

Fresh frozen pancreatic head biopsies ($n = 10$) were obtained from organ donors and acquired through the Lund University Diabetes Center (LUDC), a part of the national consortium Excellence of Diabetes Research in Sweden (EXODIAB) and co-analyzed as comparative healthy control.

Tissue processing
Respective fresh frozen specimens were separately pulverized in liquid N_2 using dry ice chilled mortar and pestle and homogenized in extraction buffer (500 mM Tris-Cl, [pH 8] and 6 M guanidine-HCl in 50 mM AMBIC), supplemented with protease and phosphatase inhibitor. The crude homogenates were then subjected to four thaws and freeze cycles, followed by ultrasonic bath treatment for 20 min on ice and a short centrifugation to remove debris. The soluble proteins in the supernatant were reduced with 15 mM DTT for 60 min at 60 °C, alkylated for 30 min at room temperature (RT) using 50 mM IAA and precipitated overnight with ice cold absolute ethanol, with the ratio of one part sample and nine parts 99.5% EtOH. The precipitated proteins were dissolved in 50 mM AMBIC and quantified using the BCA assay. To increase the sequence coverage and the probability to identify the highly divergent subtypes among the conserved histone families, 130 μg of the precipitated protein fraction from respective tissue sample digested overnight at 37 °C using either

Mass Spec Grade Trypsin/Lys-C Mix or Sequencing grade Glu-C (both from Promega, Madison, WI, USA), at a final protein enzyme ratio of 1:100. The next day, the digests were evaporated using a SpeedVac and dissolved in 50 µl mobile phase A (0.1% FA). The peptides were quantified using the Pierce quantitative colorimetric peptide assay. For a possible normalization and control of the chromatographic performance, the Thermo Scientific Pierce Peptide Retention Time Calibration Mixture consisting of 15 peptides was added to each sample.

LC-MS/MS analysis

The LC-MS/MS analysis was performed using high-performance liquid chromatography (HPLC) system, EASY-nLC™ 1000, connected to Q Exactive quadrupole Orbitrap mass spectrometer with a nanospray ion source.

Each sample, containing 1.00 µg of the Trypsin or Glu-C digested peptides in mobile phase A and 25 fmol of the retention time kit was injected at a flow rate of 300 nl/min and separated with a 132 min gradient of 5–22% ACN in 0.1% FA, followed by a 18 min gradient of 22–38% ACN in 0.1% FA. For the separation, a two-column setup was used, including the EASY-Spray analytical column (25 cm × 75 µm ID, particle size 2 µm, pore size 100 Å, PepMap C18) and the Acclaim pre-column (2 cm × 75 µm ID, particle size 3 µm, pore size 100 Å, PepMap C18). Each sample was measured in duplicate in a random order. The raw files obtained from the four measurements (Trypsin and Glu-C, replicate 1 and 2) of each sample were combined and evaluated using Proteome Discoverer targeting high confident peptides only.

The Q Exactive Plus system was operated in the positive data-dependent acquisition (DDA) mode to automatically switch between the full scan MS and MS/MS acquisition. For the peptide identification, full MS survey scan was performed in the Orbitrap detector. Fifteen data-dependent higher energy collision dissociation MS/MS scans were performed on the most intense precursors. The MS1 survey scans of the eluting peptides were executed with a resolution of 70,000, recording a window between m/z 400.0 and 1600.0. The automatic gain control (AGC) target was set to 1×10^6 with an injecting time of 100 ms. The normalized collision energy (NCE) was set at 27.0% for all scans. The resolution of the data dependent MS2 scans was fixed at 17500 and the values for the AGC target and inject time were 5×10^5 and 80 ms, respectively.

Identification of histone proteins and histone related post-translational modifications

The acquired MS/MS raw data files obtained from the combined randomized measurements were processed with Proteome Discoverer software, Version1.4 (Thermo Fisher), to identify the histone proteins including information regarding a number of unique peptides, sequence coverages and modifications.

The selection of spectra was based on the following settings: min precursor mass 350 Da; max precursor mass 5000 Da; s/n threshold 1.5. Parameters for Sequest HT searches were as follows: precursor mass tolerance 10 ppm; fragment mass tolerance 0.02 Da; depending on the sample type, trypsin or Glu-C was used as enzyme; 1 missed cleavage site; UniProt human database; dynamic modifications: acetyl (+42.011 Da; K), methyl (+14.016 Da; K, R), dimethyl (+28.031 Da; K, R), trimethyl (+42.047 Da; K, R), glygly (+114.043 Da; K) and oxidation (+15.995 Da; M, P) fixed modification: carbamidomethyl (+57.021 Da; C). The percolator was used for the processing node and the cutoff limit false discovery rate (FDR) value was set to 0.01. The selected spectra were used for the identification of histone proteins that were extracted and used for further analysis.

Verification of the distinctly expressed H1.3 by IHC

The formalin fixed paraffin embedded (FFPE) PDAC specimens corresponding to fresh frozen preserved tissue analyzed with LC-MS/MS and normal pancreatic tissue, were sectioned and stained for the presence of Histone H1.3 antigen. Tissue sections with the omitting of the primary antibody were used as negative control. 4 µm tissue sections attached on a respective slide were deparaffinized and epitope retrieved using PT Link -PT 11730 (Dako, Agilent Technologies, Santa Clara, CA, United States) for 20 min at 97 °C in 1× EnVision ™ Flex retrieval solution, low pH (Dako, Agilent Technologies). The slides were then rinsed with Tris-buffered saline (25 mM Tris-HCl, 75 mM NaCl, 0.025% Triton-X, [pH 7.4]) and pretreated with 5% normal goat serum in dilution buffer (Tris-buffered saline with 1% BSA) for 1 hour at RT. The sections were then incubated overnight at 4 °C with 5 µg/ml anti- histone H1.3 polyclonal IgG (Abcam, Cambridge, MA, USA) recognizing N-terminal amino acids 7–33 of human histone H1.3. The endogenous peroxidase was blocked for 15 min at RT using 0.3% hydrogen peroxide and 1% methanol dissolved in TBS. The primary antibody was labeled with horseradish peroxidase (HRP) conjugated secondary antibody (Sigma-Aldrich), diluted 1:200 in dilution buffer. Diaminobenzidine (DAB) kit (Vector Laboratories Inc., Burlingame, CA, USA) was used as the substrate for colored visualization of the antigen and the nuclear contrast was achieved with hematoxylin counterstaining. The sections were then dehydrated, cleared with xylene and mounted with Pertex. The distribution of H1.3 in the tissue, the immunoreactivity, the overall staining intensity as well as the subcellular location, was evaluated by a practicing pathologist specialized in pancreatic cancer diagnostics, blinded to the clinical data. The staining was scored according to Giaginis et al. reviewed in Table 1 [18]. Finally, score sum of 2 was classified as low H1.3 expression and the score sum of ≥ 3 as high H1.3 expression. Representative images were taken at 10 and 20 x magnification using Olympus BX53 microscope.

Analysis of H1.3 as a prognostic biomarker in PDAC
Clinical specimens
Clinical specimens were collected from patients with a suspected PDAC diagnosis, undergoing pancreaticoduodenectomy with a curative intent, at the department of Surgery, Skåne University Hospital in Lund, Sweden between 2000 and 2013. Resected tumors were histologically examined at the department of pathology, Skåne University Hospital in Lund to establish the diagnosis. Primary PDAC cases ($n = 62$) with a tumor located in caput pancreatis, were selected for the study and served as an external cohort for the evaluation of H1.3 as a prognostic biomarker. Pancreatic tissue obtained from patients with benign pancreatic disease ($n = 10$), were co-analyzed as a comparative control. The formalin fixed paraffin embedded (FFPE) specimens were acquired from the department of pathology, Skåne University Hospital in Lund for immunohistochemical analysis of H1.3, performed as reported above.

Statistical analysis
The findings regarding histone profile, analyzed by LC-MS/MS, were assessed as presence or absence of the respective histone protein variant and analyzed as categorical data using Fisher's exact test. In the analysis of H1.3 as a prognostic biomarker, the correlation between H1.3 expression and clinicopathological parameters was determined using the Mann-Whitney U test for continuous variables and Fisher's exact test or χ^2 for categorical variables. The Kaplan-Meier method was used to estimate the survival for patients with positive or negative H1.3 tumor expression. P-values estimating the differences between groups were calculated using the log-rank

Table 1 Evaluation of H1.3 immunohistochemistry [18]

Immunoreactivity	H1.3 + cells
0	0–4%
1	5–24%
2	25–49%
3	50–100%
Intensity	
0	negative
1	mild
2	intermediate
3	intense

test. Clinical relevant confounding variables were identified from previously published studies including age, gender, tumor diameter, grading, lymph node metastasis, margin status and adjuvant chemotherapy. Adjustment for these confounding variables was made using the Cox proportional hazard method. A value of $p < 0.05$ was considered as statistically significant. STATA MP statistical package version 14.1 (StataCorp LP, College Station, TX) was used for the statistical analyses.

Results
Analysis of the histone profile in PDAC using LC-MS/MS
Profile of histone variants and histone related PTMs
Overall, it was possible to classify between 1281 and 2767 protein identifications of which 11 to 16 different histone variants were detected in individual samples. The number of histone protein identification was independent of the total number of protein identifications. For each detected histone protein subtype, the number of unique peptides as well as the total yield of high confidence peptides resulting from both Glu-C and trypsin digestion, was comparable in both experimental groups. Even though the sequence coverage was substantially improved by using additional digestion enzyme, the sequence coverages for the reported histone variants varied between 12.45% and 73.02%.

In total, we identified 24 variants of histone proteins, represented by at least one unique peptide sequence alignment, classified to the linker histone H1 family or core families comprising H2A, H2B, H3 and H4. Fourteen histone subtypes (58%) distributed among the five main histone families displayed the same pattern of frequency in both pancreatic cancer tissue and normal pancreas. The comprehensive histone profile is summarized in Fig. 1.

Altogether, we have identified seven H1 histone subtypes including H1.1-H1–5, H1.0 and H1x, where H1.3 was found significantly more frequent ($p = 0.005$) in PDAC material as compared to healthy control. H1.1 was present in 20% of the PDAC material, while absent in normal tissue. H1.0, H1.2, H1.4, H1.5 as well as H1x, were distinguished in the majority of the analyzed material.

The H2A family comprised totally five diverse subtypes, H2A1-B/E, H2A2.B H2A.C, H2A.Z and H2A.V. The abundance of H2A1-B/E was significantly lower ($p = 0.005$) in PDAC material. H2A.V was absent in all patient samples and found exclusively in 10% of normal pancreatic tissue. The H2A2.B, H2A.C and H2A.Z were identified in more than 90% in all of the tissue specimens.

Concerning all measured samples, the H2B histone family was represented by eight subtypes, identified as H2B1.D, H2B1.C/E/F/G/I, H2B1.J- H2B1.N and H2B3.B.

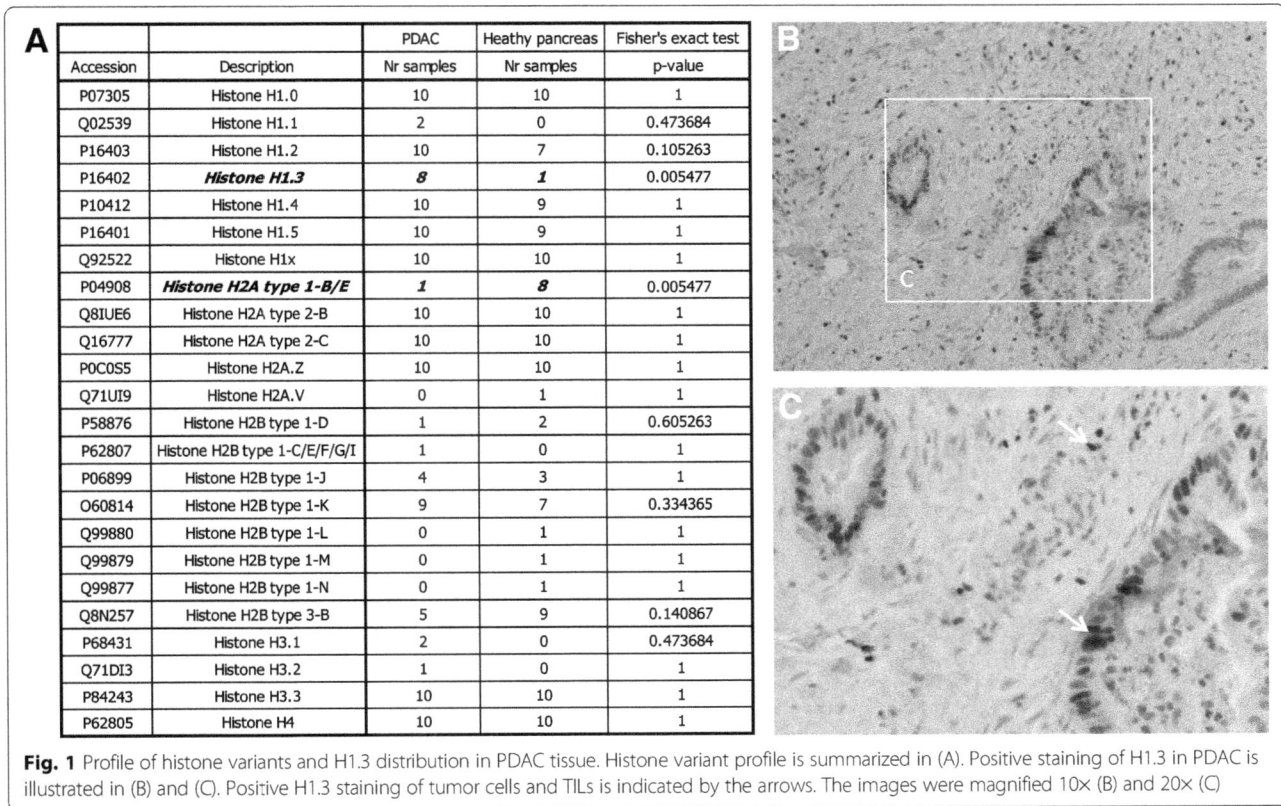

		PDAC	Heathy pancreas	Fisher's exact test
Accession	Description	Nr samples	Nr samples	p-value
P07305	Histone H1.0	10	10	1
Q02539	Histone H1.1	2	0	0.473684
P16403	Histone H1.2	10	7	0.105263
P16402	*Histone H1.3*	*8*	*1*	0.005477
P10412	Histone H1.4	10	9	1
P16401	Histone H1.5	10	9	1
Q92522	Histone H1x	10	10	1
P04908	*Histone H2A type 1-B/E*	*1*	*8*	0.005477
Q8IUE6	Histone H2A type 2-B	10	10	1
Q16777	Histone H2A type 2-C	10	10	1
P0C0S5	Histone H2A.Z	10	10	1
Q71UI9	Histone H2A.V	0	1	1
P58876	Histone H2B type 1-D	1	2	0.605263
P62807	Histone H2B type 1-C/E/F/G/I	1	0	1
P06899	Histone H2B type 1-J	4	3	1
O60814	Histone H2B type 1-K	9	7	0.334365
Q99880	Histone H2B type 1-L	0	1	1
Q99879	Histone H2B type 1-M	0	1	1
Q99877	Histone H2B type 1-N	0	1	1
Q8N257	Histone H2B type 3-B	5	9	0.140867
P68431	Histone H3.1	2	0	0.473684
Q71DI3	Histone H3.2	1	0	1
P84243	Histone H3.3	10	10	1
P62805	Histone H4	10	10	1

Fig. 1 Profile of histone variants and H1.3 distribution in PDAC tissue. Histone variant profile is summarized in (A). Positive staining of H1.3 in PDAC is illustrated in (B) and (C). Positive H1.3 staining of tumor cells and TILs is indicated by the arrows. The images were magnified 10× (B) and 20× (C)

H3.1 and H3.2 were present distinctly in 20% and 10% of PDAC samples, respectively. H3.3 and H4 were identified in all analyzed samples.

The detected peptides were investigated regarding possible dynamic PTMs. We have noted varied sporadic PTMs including acetylation (Ac), ubiquitination (Ub), methylation (Me), di- and trimethylation (Me2, Me3). The majority of the identified PTMs were annotated in a single sample within the respective group, showing a diffuse and inconsistent arrangement. PTMs presented in more than five samples in the individual groups (H2AR89Me, H2AK119Ub, H2AK120Ub, H2BR100Me, H2B109Ub, H3K80Me and H3K80Me2) revealed overlapping distribution pattern among the histone variants, resulting in a non-significant outcome. The complex array of the PTMs is summarized in Fig. 2.

Verification of the distinctly expressed H1.3
Immunohistochemistry was applied to verify the distinct expression pattern of linker histone variant H1.3 detected in PDAC tissue analyzed with LC-MS/MS ($n = 10$). Comprehensively, all investigated PDAC samples were positive for the H1.3 histone variant identified by a staining with the intensity ranging between mild and intense, assessed as a nuclear or membrane and cytoplasmic reaction. The H1.3 was identified in the 20–80% of tumor cells. H1.3 staining was also detected in tumor

infiltrating lymphocytes (TILs) situated throughout the inflammatory stroma. Normal pancreatic tissues ($n = 10$) stained negative for H1.3. The representative pattern of H1.3 intra-tumor distribution is illustrated in Fig. 1.

Analysis of H1.3 as a prognostic biomarker in an external PDAC cohort
Intratumor distribution of H1.3
The expression status of H1.3 in the PDAC specimens ($n = 62$) was evaluated using IHC. As presented in Fig. 3, 81% of the PDAC samples exhibited intratumor H1.3 expression, where nuclear reactivity was detected in the majority of the positively stained malignant cells (88%). In 34% of H1.3 positive cases, a nuclear, cytosolic and membrane reactivity was noted, while 12% of cases presented exclusively cytosolic and membrane reactivity. Lymphocytes infiltrating the tumor stroma stained positive for H1.3 in all PDAC specimens. Benign tissue stained negative for H1.3.

Expression of H1.3 correlates with poor prognosis in PDAC
As reported in Table 2, H1.3 expression was significantly associated with the age of the patient ($p = 0.012$). No significant correlations were shown between H1.3 expression and the additional clinicopathological factors including gender, tumor size, grade of differentiation,

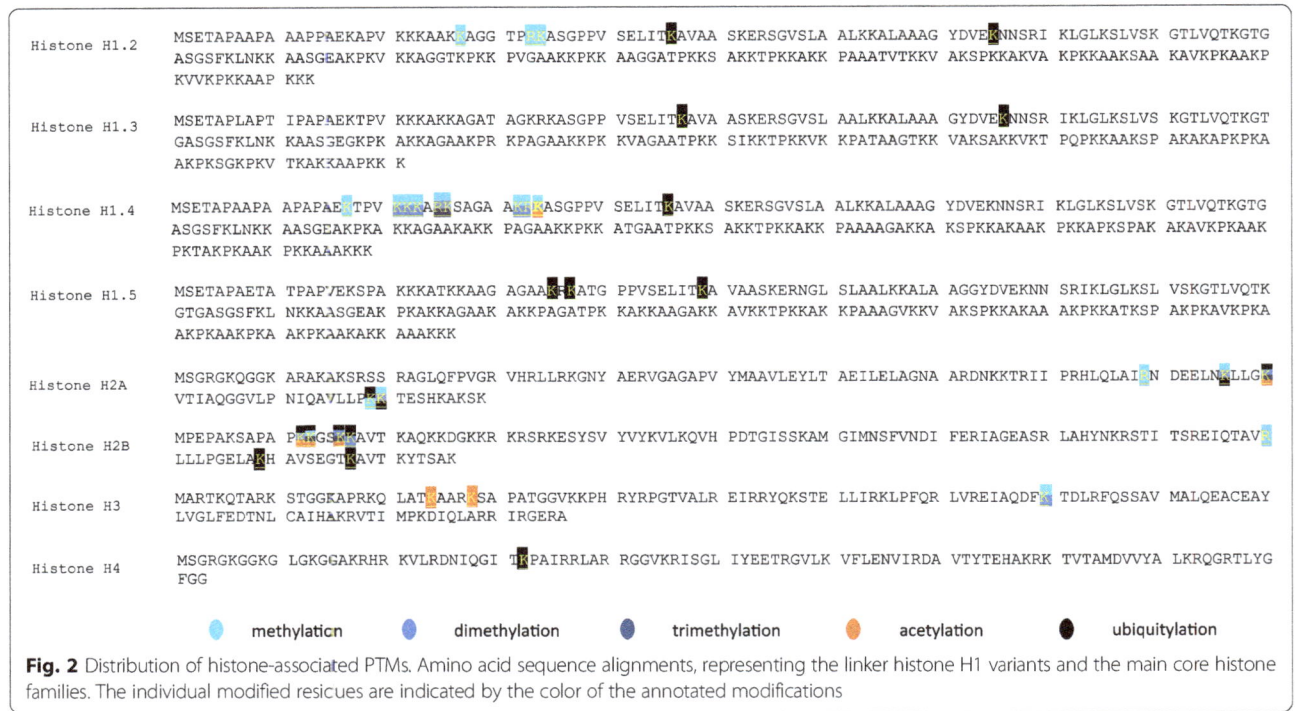

Fig. 2 Distribution of histone-associated PTMs. Amino acid sequence alignments, representing the linker histone H1 variants and the main core histone families. The individual modified resicues are indicated by the color of the annotated modifications

lymph node metastasis, resection margin status or adjuvant chemotherapy.

Kaplan-Meier analysis, reported in Fig. 4 revealed that H1.3 expression was associated with decreased median survival. The median survival of patients with negative H1.3 expression was estimated to 46 months with a 5-year survival of 42%. Patients with positive H1.3 expression showed a median survival of 28 months with a 5-year survival of 11% ($p = 0.010$).

Multivariate analysis indicated that the positive H1.3 expression was associated with a decreased survival, presented in Table 3.

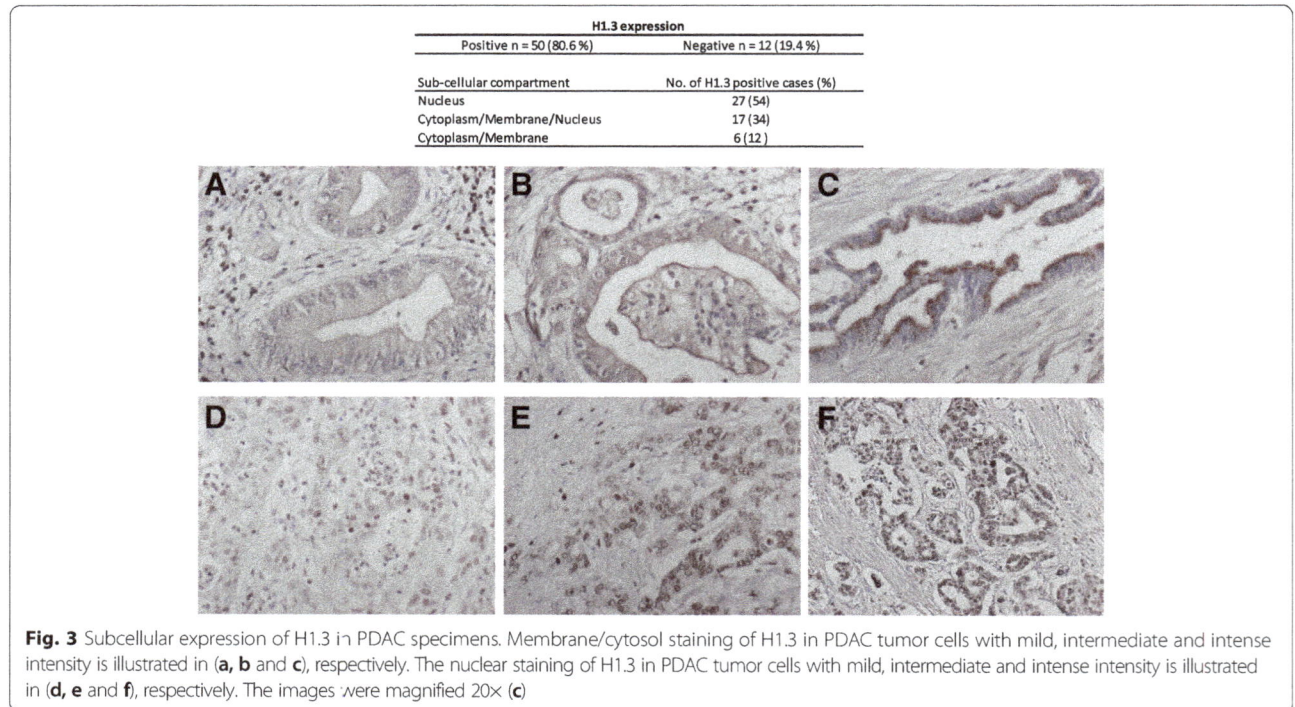

H1.3 expression	
Positive n = 50 (80.6 %)	Negative n = 12 (19.4 %)

Sub-cellular compartment	No. of H1.3 positive cases (%)
Nucleus	27 (54)
Cytoplasm/Membrane/Nucleus	17 (34)
Cytoplasm/Membrane	6 (12)

Fig. 3 Subcellular expression of H1.3 in PDAC specimens. Membrane/cytosol staining of H1.3 in PDAC tumor cells with mild, intermediate and intense intensity is illustrated in (**a, b** and **c**), respectively. The nuclear staining of H1.3 in PDAC tumor cells with mild, intermediate and intense intensity is illustrated in (**d, e** and **f**), respectively. The images were magnified 20× (**c**)

Table 2 The correlation between H1.3 expression and clinicopathological data in resected PDAC ($n = 62$)

| | No. of patients (%) | H1.3 expression | | |
		Positive $n = 50$	Negative $n = 12$	P-value
Age (years), median [IQR]	67 [43–76]	66 [43–78]	73 [58–76]	0.012
Male gender	29 (47)	25 (50)	4 (33)	0.173
Tumor size (cm), median [IQR]	3 [0.3–8.5]	3 [1–8.5]	3 [0.3–4]	0.285
Poor differentiation	36 (58)	31 (62)	5 (42)	0.173
Lymph node metastasis	38 (61)	31 (62)	7 (58)	0.815
Resection margin status (R1)	18 (29)	14 (28)	4 (33)	0.721
Adjuvant chemotherapy	46 (74)	36 (72)	10 (83)	0.420

IQR interquartile range

Discussion

Histone variants as chromatin remodeling proteins are emerging as important factors in cancer biology [9]. Thus the intratumor profiling of the distinct histone subtypes may lead to identification of interesting histone protein candidates, useful for the improvement of the disease management.

We performed a classical bottom-up MS analysis of PDAC tissues and normal pancreas biopsies to map the individual histone variants and histone related PTMs that could be correlated to chromatin dynamics in PDAC.

The profiling of histone variants revealed that H1.3, detected in the majority of patient samples and H2A1-B/E, primarily associated with the normal pancreatic tissue, displayed the opposite signatures of frequency with the overall accuracy of 95%. H1.3 expression in PDAC tissue was thereafter confirmed by IHC. H1.3 was thus considered as a possible PDAC specific histone variant candidate for further investigation. The immunohistochemical verification of H2A1-B/E was somewhat limited due to the high homology of the primary amino acid sequence of the H2A variants. However, MS based characterization of H2A histone family in ovarian cancer cells, revealed that the expression

of the canonical histone variant H2A1-B/E was associated with undetectable levels [19], which we estimated, supports our findings.

The H1 linker histone family represents the most heterogeneous and functionally divergent group of histones among the highly conserved histone protein families. In tumorigenesis, the most relevant functional differences between the individual H1 subtypes are related to chromatin dynamics and transcriptional regulation. [20]. H1 linker histones consist of a highly conserved globular domain, variable N-terminal region and C-terminal domain (CTD), rich in positively charged lysine and arginine residues, that mediates both chromatin condensation and protein-protein interactions [21]. H1.3 was defined as a histone H1 subtype with an intermediate chromatin affinity that is associated with more relaxed and accessible chromatin conformation [22]. The results of global habitation studies demonstrated that H1.3 binds chromatin with significantly higher dynamics compared to the main H1 variants, thus the effect of H1.3 nucleosomal incorporation may be more pronounced at the specific binding sites [23]. According to a recent report, the CTD of histone H1.3 possesses the ability to recruit and interact with DNA methyltransferases, DNMT1 and DNMT3B, leading to methylation of CpG sites and subsequent gene silencing [24]. In cancer, a hypermethylation of CpG islands in promotor regions was described to correlate with transcriptional silencing of tumor suppressor genes [25] or with genes critical for the sensitivity to chemotherapy [26]. H1 was also shown to inhibit acetylation of H3 as well as methylation of nucleosomal H3K4 by

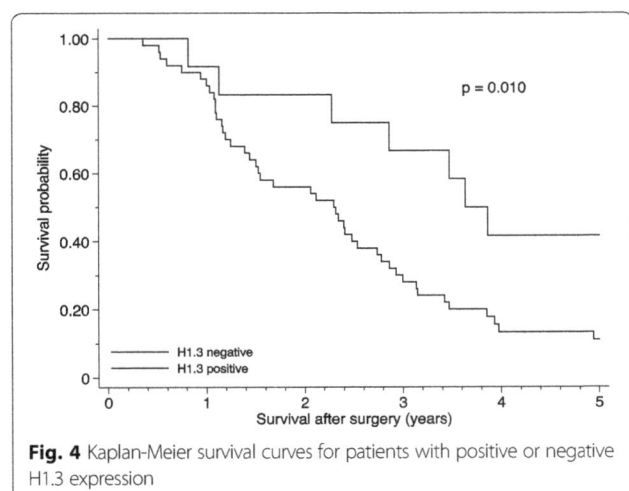

Fig. 4 Kaplan-Meier survival curves for patients with positive or negative H1.3 expression

Table 3 Multivariate Cox regression analysis ($n = 62$)

	Hazard ratio	95% CI	P-value
Unadjusted			
H1.3 expression (positive vs negative)	2.4	1.2–5.3	0.018
Adjusted[a]			
H1.3 expression (positive vs negative)	2.6	1.1–6.1	0.029

CI confidence interval. [a]Adjusted for age, gender, tumor size, differentiation, lymph node metastasis, margin status and adjuvant chemotherapy

interference with histone acetylase PCAF and histone-lysine N-methyltransferase SET7/9. Loss of histone acetylation as well as methylation of H3K4 represent events generally associated with a decreased transcriptional activity [24, 27, 28]. As recently reported, PTMs, H2AK119Ub and H2BK120Ub are involved in modulation of SET7/9 expression and regulation of H3K4Me2 and H3K9Me2 [29]. Moreover, methylation of individual CpG sites as well as low cellular levels of H3K4me2, H3K9Me2 and H3K18, were each reported as significant predictors of survival in PDAC [30, 31].

Our results indicate that H1.3 expression in PDAC tumors is associated with poor survival. Though, it remains possible that nucleosomal H1.3 may participate in the epigenetic regulation of gene repression in PDAC and by that contribute to the aggressiveness of the disease and poor prognosis.

The function of histone H1.3 subtype in pancreatic cancer is yet to be revealed and further investigations on this subject are necessary.

Interestingly, the positive H1.3 staining exhibited in tumor cells demonstrated, besides nuclear, also membrane and cytoplasmic distribution. Based on these results, we speculate that the biological role of H1.3 in PDAC may expand beyond the nuclear function. According to the findings from several reports, it appears that histones, in response to environmental stress, are frequently shuttled to the cell surface or cytoplasm where they act as signaling molecules [32]. Depending on the environmental conditions, histone proteins exposed to the extracellular matrix can function as basic ligands to negatively charged molecules, such as various proteoglycans, and regulate various cellular processes, including cell proliferation and matrix remodeling [33, 34]. The frequent cell proliferation associated with cancer development [35] may thus result in extensive transcription and synthesis of histone proteins. An overbalanced synthesis of nuclear proteins as histones may lead to cytoplasmic accumulation, as we observed in the IHC analysis of H1.3 in PDAC tissue.

Lymphocytes infiltrating the tumor and signaling pathways related to the immune system are frequently observed in the immunogenic subclass of pancreatic cancer [5]. Consistent with the findings of the present study, the infiltrating lymphocytes are found prevalently in the stromal compartment as a functional part of the tumor microenvironment [36]. Further investigation is however required to understand the possible contribution of TILs expressing high levels of H1.3 to the development and progression of pancreatic cancer.

Conclusions

We found that the expression of H1.3 in tumor cells provides prognostic information in patients with PDAC. Our results suggest that H1.3 may serve as a novel epigenetic biomarker for the prediction of clinical outcome after surgical resection. The intratumor histone profile, especially the distinct histone subtypes, may also contribute to the increased understanding of pancreatic tumor biology and should be considered for further investigation aiming to improve the clinical management of PDAC.

Acknowledgements
The authors would like to thank to the Lund University Diabetes Center (LUDC), a part of the national consortium Excellence of Diabetes Research in Sweden (EXODIAB), for providing us with the normal pancreatic tissue.

Funding
The study was supported by SWElife/Vinnova, the Royal Physiographic Society of Lund, the Magnus Bergvall Foundation, the Tore Nilsson Foundation and the Inga and John Hain Foundation for Medical Research. This work was also supported by grants from the National Research Foundation of Korea, funded by the Government of Republic of Korea.

Authors' contributions
MB made substantial contributions to conception and design; acquisition of data; analysis and interpretation of data; drafted the manuscript. TK made substantial contributions to MS analysis and interpretation of data. AS made substantial contributions to IHC analysis. BA made substantial contributions to analysis and interpretation of data. GMV made substantial contributions to MS analysis and interpretation of data. RA was involved in study design and revising the manuscript critically for important intellectual content. DA was involved in study design; collection of patient tissue and data; revising the manuscript critically for important intellectual content; gave final approval of the version to be published and agreed to be accountable for all aspects of the work in ensuring that questions related to the accuracy or integrity of any part of the work are appropriately investigated and resolved. All authors read and approved the final manuscript.

Competing interests
The authors have read the journal's authorship agreement and editorial policies on disclosure of potential conflicts of interest. The authors have no conflict of interest to declare.

Author details
[1]Department of Surgery, Clinical Sciences Lund, Lund University, Skåne University Hospital, SE-221 85 Lund, Sweden. [2]Clinical Protein Science & Imaging, Department of Biomedical Engineering, Lund University, Biomedical Center, Lund, Sweden. [3]Department of Pathology, Skåne University Hospital, Lund, Sweden.

References
1. Malvezzi M, Carioli G, Bertuccio P, Rosso T, Boffetta P, Levi F, La Vecchia C, Negri E. European cancer mortality predictions for the year 2016 with focus on leukaemias. Ann Oncol. 2016;27(4):725–31.
2. Siegel RL, Miller KD, Jemal A. Cancer statistics, 2016. CA Cancer J Clin. 2016; 66(1):7–30.
3. Ansari D, Tingstedt B, Andersson B, Holmquist F, Sturesson C, Williamsson C, Sasor A, Borg D, Bauden M, Andersson R. Pancreatic cancer: yesterday, today and tomorrow. Future Oncol. 2016;12(16):1929–46.
4. Parikh AA, Maiga A, Bentrem D, Squires MH 3rd, Kooby DA, Maithel SK, Weber SM, Cho CS, Katz M, Martin RC, et al. Adjuvant therapy in pancreas cancer: does it influence patterns of recurrence? J Am Coll Surg. 2016; 222(4):448–56.
5. Bailey P, Chang DK, Nones K, Johns AL, Patch AM, Gingras MC, Miller DK, Christ AN, Bruxner TJ, Quinn MC, et al. Genomic analyses identify molecular subtypes of pancreatic cancer. Nature. 2016;531(7592):47–52.

6. Guo M, Jia Y, Yu Z, House MG, Esteller M, Brock MV, Herman JG. Epigenetic changes associated with neoplasms of the exocrine and endocrine pancreas. Discov Med. 2014;17(92):67–73.

7. Omura N, Goggins M. Epigenetics and epigenetic alterations in pancreatic cancer. Int J Clin Exp Pathol. 2009;2(4):310–26.

8. Henikoff S, Smith MM. Histone variants and epigenetics. Cold Spring Harb Perspect Biol. 2015;7(1):a019364.

9. Vardabasso C, Hasson D, Ratnakumar K, Chung CY, Duarte LF, Bernstein E. Histone variants: emerging players in cancer biology. Cell Mol Life Sci. 2014; 71(3):379–404.

10. Luger K, Mader AW, Richmond RK, Sargent DF, Richmond TJ. Crystal structure of the nucleosome core particle at 2.8 a resolution. Nature. 1997; 389(6648):251–60.

11. Talbert PB, Henikoff S. Histone variants–ancient wrap artists of the epigenome. Nat Rev Mol Cell Biol. 2010;11(4):264–75.

12. Tessarz P, Kouzarides T. Histone core modifications regulating nucleosome structure and dynamics. Nat Rev Mol Cell Biol. 2014;15(11):703–8.

13. Weber CM, Henikoff S. Histone variants: dynamic punctuation in transcription. Genes Dev. 2014;28(7):672–82.

14. Cheema MS, Ausio J. The structural determinants behind the epigenetic role of Histone variants. Genes (Basel). 2015;6(3):685–713.

15. Ferraro A. Altered primary chromatin structures and their implications in cancer development. Cell Oncol (Dordr). 2016;39(3):195–210.

16. Kwak HG, Dohmae N. Proteomic characterization of histone variants in the mouse testis by mass spectrometry-based top-down analysis. Biosci Trends. 2016;

17. Bauden M, Kristl T, Andersson R, Marko-Varga G, Ansari D. Characterization of Histone-related PTMs and chemical modifications in FFPE and fresh frozen human pancreatic cancer Xenografts using LC-MS/MS. Lab Investig. 2017;97:279–88.

18. Giaginis C, Damaskos C, Koutsounas I, Zizi-Serbetzoglou A, Tsoukalas N, Patsouris E, Kouraklis G, Theocharis S. Histone deacetylase (HDAC)-1, −2, −4 and −6 expression in human pancreatic adenocarcinoma: associations with clinicopathological parameters, tumor proliferative capacity and patients' survival. BMC Gastroenterol. 2015;15:148.

19. Boyne MT 2nd, Pesavento JJ, Mizzen CA, Kelleher NL. Precise characterization of human histones in the H2A gene family by top down mass spectrometry. J Proteome Res. 2006;5(2):248–53.

20. Happel N, Warneboldt J, Hanecke K, Haller F, Doenecke D. H1 subtype expression during cell proliferation and growth arrest. Cell Cycle. 2009;8(14): 2226–32.

21. McBryant SJ, Lu X, Hansen JC. Multifunctionality of the linker histones: an emerging role for protein-protein interactions. Cell Res. 2010;20(5):519–28.

22. Clausell J, Happel N, Hale TK, Doenecke D, Beato M. Histone H1 subtypes differentially modulate chromatin condensation without preventing ATP-dependent remodeling by SWI/SNF or NURF. PLoS One. 2009;4(10): e0007243.

23. Rutowicz K, Puzio M, Halibart-Puzio J, Lirski M, Kotlinski M, Kroten MA, Knizewski L, Lange B, Muszewska A, Sniegowska-Swierk K, et al. A specialized Histone H1 variant is required for adaptive responses to complex Abiotic stress and related DNA Methylation in Arabidopsis. Plant Physiol. 2015;169(3):2080–101.

24. Yang SM, Kim BJ, Norwood Toro L, Skoultchi AI. H1 linker histone promotes epigenetic silencing by regulating both DNA methylation and histone H3 methylation. Proc Natl Acad Sci U S A. 2013;110(5):1708–13.

25. Herman JG, Baylin SB. Gene silencing in cancer in association with promoter hypermethylation. N Engl J Med. 2003;349(21):2042–54.

26. Tan AC, Jimeno A, Lin SH, Wheelhouse J, Chan F, Solomon A, Rajeshkumar NV, Rubio-Viqueira B, Hidalgo M. Characterizing DNA methylation patterns in pancreatic cancer genome. Mol Oncol. 2009;3(5–6):425–38.

27. Herrera JE, West KL, Schiltz RL, Nakatani Y, Bustin M. Histone H1 is a specific repressor of core histone acetylation in chromatin. Mol Cell Biol. 2000;20(2): 523–9.

28. Kouzarides T. Chromatin modifications and their function. Cell. 2007;128(4): 693–705.

29. Goru SK, Kadakol A, Pandey A, Malek V, Sharma N, Gaikwad AB. Histone H2AK119 and H2BK120 mono-ubiquitination modulate SET7/9 and SUV39H1 in type 1 diabetes-induced renal fibrosis. Biochem J. 2016;473(21): 3937–49.

30. Manuyakorn A, Paulus R, Farrell J, Dawson NA, Tze S, Cheung-Lau G, Hines OJ, Reber H, Seligson DB, Horvath S, et al. Cellular histone modification patterns predict prognosis and treatment response in resectable pancreatic adenocarcinoma: results from RTOG 9704. J Clin Oncol. 2010;28(8):1358–65.

31. Thompson MJ, Rubbi L, Dawson DW, Donahue TR, Pellegrini M. Pancreatic cancer patient survival correlates with DNA methylation of pancreas development genes. PLoS One. 2015;10(6):e0128814.

32. Chen R, Kang R, Fan XG, Tang D. Release and activity of histone in diseases. Cell Death Dis. 2014;5:e1370.

33. Hampton RY, Golenbock DT, Raetz CR, Lipid A. Binding sites in membranes of macrophage tumor cells. J Biol Chem. 1988;263(29):14802–7.

34. Henriquez JP, Casar JC, Fuentealba L, Carey DJ, Brandan E. Extracellular matrix histone H1 binds to perlecan, is present in regenerating skeletal muscle and stimulates myoblast proliferation. J Cell Sci. 2002;115(Pt 10): 2041–51.

35. Hanahan D, Weinberg RA. Hallmarks of cancer: the next generation. Cell. 2011;144(5):646–74.

36. Swartz MA, Iida N, Roberts EW, Sangaletti S, Wong MH, Yull FE, Coussens LM, DeClerck YA. Tumor microenvironment complexity: emerging roles in cancer therapy. Cancer Res. 2012;72(10):2473–80.

6

Basal metabolic state governs AIF-dependent growth support in pancreatic cancer cells

Andrew J. Scott, Amanda S. Wilkinson and John C. Wilkinson[*]

Abstract

Background: Apoptosis-inducing factor (AIF), named for its involvement in cell death pathways, is a mitochondrial protein that regulates metabolic homeostasis. In addition to supporting the survival of healthy cells, AIF also plays a contributory role to the development of cancer through its enzymatic activity, and we have previously shown that AIF preferentially supports advanced-stage prostate cancer cells. Here we further evaluated the role of AIF in tumorigenesis by exploring its function in pancreatic cancer, a disease setting that most often presents at an advanced stage by the time of diagnosis.

Methods: A bioinformatics approach was first employed to investigate AIF mRNA transcript levels in pancreatic tumor specimens vs. normal tissues AIF-deficient pancreatic cancer cell lines were then established via lentiviral infection. Immunoblot analysis was used to determine relative protein quantities within cells. Cell viability was measured by flow cytometry; in vitro and Matrigel™ growth/survival using Coulter™ counting and phase contrast microscopy; and glucose consumption in the absence and presence of Matrigel™ using spectrophotometric methods.

Results: Archival gene expression data revealed a modest elevation of AIF transcript levels in subsets of pancreatic tumor specimens, suggesting a possible role in disease progression. AIF expression was then suppressed in a panel of five pancreatic cancer cell lines that display diverse metabolic phenotypes. AIF ablation selectively crippled the growth of cells in vitro in a manner that directly correlated with the loss of mitochondrial respiratory chain subunits and altered glucose metabolism, and these effects were exacerbated in the presence of Matrigel™ substrate. This suggests a critical metabolic role for AIF to pancreatic tumorigenesis, while the spectrum of sensitivities to AIF ablation depends on basal cellular metabolic phenotypes.

Conclusions: Altogether these data indicate that AIF supports the growth and survival of metabolically defined pancreatic cancer cells and that this metabolic function may derive from a novel mechanism so far undocumented in other cancer types.

Keywords: Mitochondria, Cell death, Glycolysis, Oxidative phosphorylation

Background

Apoptosis-inducing factor (AIF) is a mitochondrial flavo-protein discovered and named for its involvement in caspase-independent cell death, and the mechanisms through which AIF mediates cellular toxicity have been largely defined [1–11]. Distinct from its death role, AIF also possesses an intrinsic NADH oxidase activity that is linked to control of mitochondrial structure and function [12, 13]. A complete picture of how AIF promotes mitochondrial homeostasis remains elusive, but it has become increasingly clear that through its enzymatic activity AIF has a primary role in maintaining cell survival. Inactivation of the AIF gene in mice causes embryonic lethality [14, 15], whereas the Harlequin mouse model exhibits severe and progressive neurodegeneration as a consequence of decreased AIF protein expression (>80 %) in all tissues [16]. Tissue-specific AIF deletion studies demonstrated a series of physiological defects including skeletal muscle atrophy and dilated cardiomyopathy resulting from severe

* Correspondence: john.wilkinson@ndsu.edu
Department of Chemistry and Biochemistry, North Dakota State University, Dept. 2710, P.O. Box 6050, Fargo, ND 58108-6050, USA

mitochondrial dysfunction and loss of cristae structure [17, 18]. More recent studies in humans have identified AIF mutations that lead to respiratory chain malfunction with a spectrum of clinical manifestations including mitochondrial encephalomyopathy [19], prenatal ventriculomegaly [20], and Cowchock syndrome [21]. The AIF-deficient phenotype is associated with concomitant depletions of mitochondrial respiratory chain subunits and subsequent impairment of oxidative phosphorylation [22], in part due to a resulting defective co-translational import system regulated by the AIF-interacting protein CHCHD4/MIA40 [23, 24]. It has been proposed that AIF functions in vivo as a metabolic sensor [25], supported by its contributory roles to disorders involving metabolic dysregulation including obesity, diabetes, and cancer [26–28]. While largely descriptive, these studies altogether illustrate a role for AIF as a critical regulator of cellular metabolism.

The pro-survival activity of AIF and its role in controlling metabolic homeostasis in healthy cells is well positioned to be exploited by cancer cells in order to promote growth, invasiveness, and chemoresistance [28, 29]. Indeed, increased AIF protein levels have been observed in esophageal, skin, colorectal, gastric, lymphatic, and prostate cancers [28, 30–35], and in colorectal cancer increased AIF levels elevate the general cellular oxidative state to protect cells from chemical stress [29]. Furthermore, we have shown that in prostate cancer the NADH oxidase activity of AIF promotes a metabolic state that supports growth and invasiveness in a manner specific to cells that have achieved advanced status [28]. Given our findings that AIF preferentially supports metabolism benefitting the aggressiveness of advanced-stage prostate cancer cells, we questioned whether AIF also contributes to pancreatic ductal adenocarcinoma (PDAC), a disease which almost always reaches an advanced stage before diagnosis [36]. Unfortunately for patient prognosis, late detection of PDAC makes it one of the most lethal cancers with a grim 5-year survival rate of 6 % [37]. As tumors progress and achieve advanced stages, reliance upon specific metabolic pathways for growth and survival increases substantially while cells become vulnerable to death by metabolic disruption, a trait known as metabolism addiction. As one of the most metabolically driven forms of cancer, mitochondrial function is frequently critical to pancreatic tumorigenesis [38, 39], leading us to hypothesize that AIF's metabolic function supports the growth and survival of PDAC cells.

In this study we identified AIF as a major contributor to the growth-promoting metabolic state of pancreatic tumor cells. The contribution of AIF to PDAC metabolism in our panel of cell lines was directly related to their basal metabolic preferences. While cells that use both glycolysis and mitochondrial energy metabolism rely on AIF for survival, those that rely only upon glycolysis cannot benefit from AIF's metabolic activity. Through a mechanism that appears distinct from its function in prostate cancer, we found that AIF facilitates a metabolic balance that maintains survival, a role that potentially extends to normal tissues and may explain the selective sensitivity to AIF suppression among cell types. Altogether our findings suggest that AIF is a significant support molecule to the development and progression of some pancreatic cancers and therefore represents a promising new target for therapeutic development.

Methods

Materials

MEM, DMEM, RPMI 1640, DMEM/F12, GlutaMAX, horse serum, insulin, transferrin, epidermal growth factor, trypsin, 4–12 % bis-tris polyacrylamide gels, and nitrocellulose membranes were obtained from Life Technologies; fetal bovine serum (FBS), phosphate buffered saline (PBS), and Pierce ECL 2 Western Blotting Substrate were from Thermo Scientific; QuantiChrom™ Glucose Assay Kit was from BioAssay Systems; Matrigel™ was from BD Biosciences; Matrigel Recovery Solution was from Corning; protease inhibitor tablets were from Roche Applied Science; all other materials were from Sigma. Antibodies were obtained as follows: anti-AIF (Santa Cruz Biotechnology, sc-13116), anti-complex I 39 kDa (Life Technologies, 459100), anti-complex I 20 kDa (Life Technologies, 459210), anti-complex I 17 kDa (Life Technologies, A21359), anti-COX IV (Life Technologies, A21347) anti-β-actin (Sigma, A5316), and peroxidase-conjugated anti-mouse (Amersham Biosciences, NA931V).

Oncomine data analysis

Data sets examining AIF mRNA expression in pancreatic tumors versus normal pancreatic tissue from 7 studies [40–46] were analyzed using Oncomine [47]. Statistical calculations and normalization techniques are given by the Oncomine website (http://www.oncomine.org).

Cell culture

PANC-1, BxPC-3, HPAF-II, HPAC, and MIA PaCa-2 cells were from ATCC (kind gift of Dr. Sanku Mallik, NDSU). HEK293T cells were as described [28]. Cells were grown in an atmosphere of 95 % air and 5 % CO_2 at 37 °C. All media was supplemented with 2 mM GlutaMAX. Cell lines were grown and cultured with the following media formulations: HEK293T and PANC-1 cells in DMEM supplemented with 10 % FBS; MIA PaCa-2 in DMEM supplemented with 10 % FBS and 2.5 % horse serum; BxPC-3 in RPMI 1640 supplemented with 10 % FBS; HPAF-II in MEM supplemented with 10 % FBS; and HPAC in a 1:1 mixture of DMEM and Ham's F12 medium supplemented with 5 % FBS, 2 µg/mL insulin, 5 µg/mL transferrin, 40 ng/mL hydrocortisone, and 10 ng/mL epidermal growth factor.

Lentivirus production and infection

FG12-derived plasmids for targeting of AIF and LacZ by RNA interference (RNAi) have been rigorously assessed and used as described [28, 48, 49]. Lentiviral packaging plasmids pRRE, pRSV-rev, and pHCMV-G are as described [50]. RNAi plasmids and equal amounts of lentiviral packaging plasmids were transfected into HEK293T cells using the calcium phosphate precipitation method [51]. Supernatants of transfected HEK293T cultures were then filtered through 0.45-μm PVDF Millex-HV filters (Millipore) and concentrated by centrifugation at 20,000 × g for 90 min at 4 °C. Viral pellets were resuspended in PBS and then incubated overnight at 4 °C prior to use. Cell lines were then infected as described [28]. PANC-1 and MIA PaCa-2 cells were infected with lentiviruses carrying shLacZ-GFP or shAIF-GFP, after which infection was verified by fluorescence microscopy and flow cytometry with an Accuri C6 flow cytometer. BxPC-3, HPAC, and HPAF-II cells were infected with lentiviruses carrying shLacZ-puro or shAIF-puro and then selected using 2 μg/mL puromycin.

Cell viability

Cells were seeded in replicate populations of 25,000-150,000 cells per well in 6-well plates and allowed to attach overnight. Cells were then left untreated or treated with 1 μg/mL actinomycin D, 1 μM gemcitabine, or 50 mM 2-deoxyglucose for 24–72 h. Cells were then harvested by trypsinization, washed, and resuspended in PBS containing 2 μg/mL propidium iodide. Cell viability was determined by flow cytometry.

SDS-PAGE and immunoblotting

Cells were harvested by trypsinization, washed, and resuspended in radioimmune precipitation assay lysis buffer (PBS containing 1 % Nonidet P-40, 0.5 % sodium deoxycholate, 0.1 % sodium dodecyl sulfate, 1 mM dithiothreitol, 1 mM phenylmethanesulfonyl fluoride, and 1 protease inhibitor mixture tablet per 10 mL). Lysates were then normalized for protein content, separated by SDS-PAGE, and transferred to nitrocellulose membranes. Membranes were blocked with 5 % milk in Tris-buffered saline with 0.1 % Tween-20 and incubated with primary antibodies for 1 h at room temperature. Membranes were then washed and incubated with peroxidase-conjugated anti-mouse IgG secondary antibody for 45 min at room temperature, followed by washing and visualization using enhanced chemiluminescence with a MyECL imaging system (Thermo Scientific).

Cell growth rate measurements

Cells were harvested by trypsinization, washed, resuspended in fresh medium, and seeded at equal densities in replicate 6-well plates. Cells were harvested and quantified by Coulter™ counting after 72 h. Fold change in growth was determined by dividing populations of AIF-deficient cells by corresponding control populations.

Scratch assay

Cells were harvested by trypsinization, washed, resuspended in fresh media, and seeded in replicate 6-well plates. Cells were allowed to attach for 12–36 h, and a single scratch was made through the middle of each well using a P200 pipette tip [52]. Cells were immediately washed, fresh media was added, and each scratch was imaged. Cells were then incubated for 6–48 h before final assessment of scratch width. All images were captured by phase contrast microscopy using the 10× objective of a Nikon TS100F microscope equipped with a Nikon DS-Fi1 digital camera detection system and NIS Elements 4.0 software.

Glucose consumption measurements

Cells were harvested by trypsinization, washed, resuspended in fresh medium, and seeded at equal densities in replicate 6-well plates. Cells were grown at 37 °C for 72 h. Media was then collected from each well, and total glucose was measured using the QuantiChrom™ Glucose Assay Kit (BioAssay Systems). Total cell number in each sample was determined by Coulter™ counting. To determine glucose consumed per cell, total glucose consumption per sample was divided by its corresponding cell count.

Matrigel™ experiments

Equal volumes of cold Matrigel™ were added to each well in 24-well plates and allowed to solidify at 37 °C for 1 h. Cells were harvested, washed, resuspended in fresh medium, and seeded in equal densities on solidified Matrigel™ layers. Cells were grown in Matrigel™ for up to 21 days with media replenished following each week of growth and imaged using phase contrast microscopy as described above. Cells were then extracted from substrate with the Matrigel Recovery Solution (Corning), and glucose consumption and growth measurements were performed as described above.

Results

Elevation of AIF mRNA transcripts in pancreatic cancer

To determine a potential involvement of AIF in pancreatic cancer, we began by analyzing archived expression data retrieved from the publically available cancer gene expression database Oncomine (oncomine.com). Archival data from a total of 7 data sets comparing relative AIF expression in pancreatic adenocarcinomas to normal pancreatic tissue are currently available [40–46]. When average AIF expression was compared between groups (cancer vs. normal) and for each data set, a trend towards elevated AIF transcripts in pancreatic cancer tissue was apparent (values ranging from essentially unchanged to an increase of 1.54 fold in cancer relative to normal). However, the observed increase in average expression was only statistically significant in one of the seven data sets, which indicated a 1.45-fold increase in AIF expression in pancreatic cancer tissue ([40], $p = 0.024$; for all other studies $p = 0.068–0.956$). Representative data are shown in Fig. 1a-d. At first glance these data suggested that altered AIF expression is not a global trend in pancreatic cancer, but that in a small fraction of tissue cohorts a modest (less than 2-fold) elevation of AIF expression can be observed.

To further explore AIF expression changes in these cohorts of cancer vs. normal tissues we compared individual expression data from each sample within each cohort (Figs. 1e-h). Interestingly, in 5 of the 7 data sets there appears a subtype within each cancer group that displays elevated AIF expression significantly beyond the 90 % confidence interval defined for normal tissues [40–43, 46]. This subtype represents ~36 % of the total among these five cohorts, and while elevated AIF is observed, the magnitude of this elevation remains modest (less than 3-fold relative to control tissue). These data are in close agreement with similar analyses examining AIF mRNA and protein expression in prostate cancer tissues [28]. Taken together these data suggest that while elevated AIF expression is not a global feature of pancreatic cancer, there exists a subtype of pancreatic tumors (approximately one-third of the total samples assessed) in which AIF expression is significantly elevated. That increased expression is modest likely reflects potential toxicity associated with AIF-mediated cell-killing when levels exceed a certain threshold [1].

Establishment of AIF-deficient cell lines

The above analysis of AIF gene expression data from clinically derived pancreatic cancer tissues suggested a connection between elevated AIF expression and subtypes of pancreatic tumors. In order to evaluate the role of AIF in the growth and survival of pancreatic cancer cells, we generated a panel of AIF-deficient PDAC cell lines. Given the metabolic activity of AIF in other systems, we targeted AIF in a panel of five cell types (PANC-1, BxPC-3, HPAC, HPAF-II, and MIA PaCa-2) that display diverse metabolic characteristics. Previously, metabolic phenotyping of PDAC cells was rigorously established by gene expression analysis, sensitivity to metabolic inhibitors, and metabolite profiling [53]. PANC-1 and BxPC-3 cells balance the metabolic requirements derived from glycolysis, pentose phosphate pathway, and mitochondrial energy metabolism, while HPAC cells display a pronounced bias towards lipogenic pathways; HPAF-II cells also require mitochondrial energy

pathways but are more reliant upon glycolysis than those previously described, and MIA PaCa-2 cells are highly glycolytic (Table 1). Within this panel of cell lines oncogene status varies slightly: all cells except BxPC-3 express mutant KRAS, and all cells except HPAC express mutant p53 [54–60]. Silencing of AIF expression by RNAi was achieved through infection with lentiviruses harboring short-hairpin RNA (shRNA) sequences targeting either AIF (shAIF) or LacZ (shLacZ) as a control. PANC-1 and MIA PaCa-2 cells were infected with lentiviruses that carried GFP expression cassettes which served to confirm stable integration and subsequent knockdown of targeted genes. Success of lentiviral infection was evaluated by observation of at least 95 % GFP positivity using fluorescence microscopy and flow cytometry (Fig. 2a, b). Due to lower infection efficiencies, BxPC-3, HPAC, and HPAF-II cells were infected with lentiviruses carrying the puromycin N-acetyl transferase gene as a selectable marker instead of GFP, and stably infected cells were derived by treatment with puromycin. To control for differences between lentiviruses bearing puromycin resistance vs. GFP, we additionally established PANC-1 cells via puromycin selection that were indistinguishable from GFP-infected cells in all assays performed (data not shown). To determine the extent of AIF protein ablation in our cell line panel, immunoblot analysis was employed, which demonstrated AIF knockdown levels greater than 95 % in all cases when compared to either uninfected cells or shLacZ negative controls (Fig. 2c).

AIF ablation does not affect chemical death induction in pancreatic cancer cells

In various cell types, AIF has been shown to promote both death induction and survival in response to toxic chemical triggers. To determine the role of AIF in regulating cell death in pancreatic cancer, we employed two death-inducing agents with distinct mechanisms of action: actinomycin D, an inhibitor of protein synthesis; and gemcitabine, a nucleoside analog and the first-line treatment for PDAC [61, 62]. Following treatment viability was measured by propidium iodide staining and flow cytometry. When compared to controls, AIF-deficient cell lines showed neither increased resistance (to actinomycin D) nor increased sensitivity (to gemcitabine) following treatment (Fig. 3). Similar results were obtained by treatment with etoposide, MNNG, arsenic trioxide, menadione, and hydrogen peroxide (data not shown). These data demonstrate that AIF does not play a significant regulatory role in the promotion of cell death in pancreatic cancer cells, and is consistent with previous studies evaluating AIF-mediated cell death in prostate cancer [28].

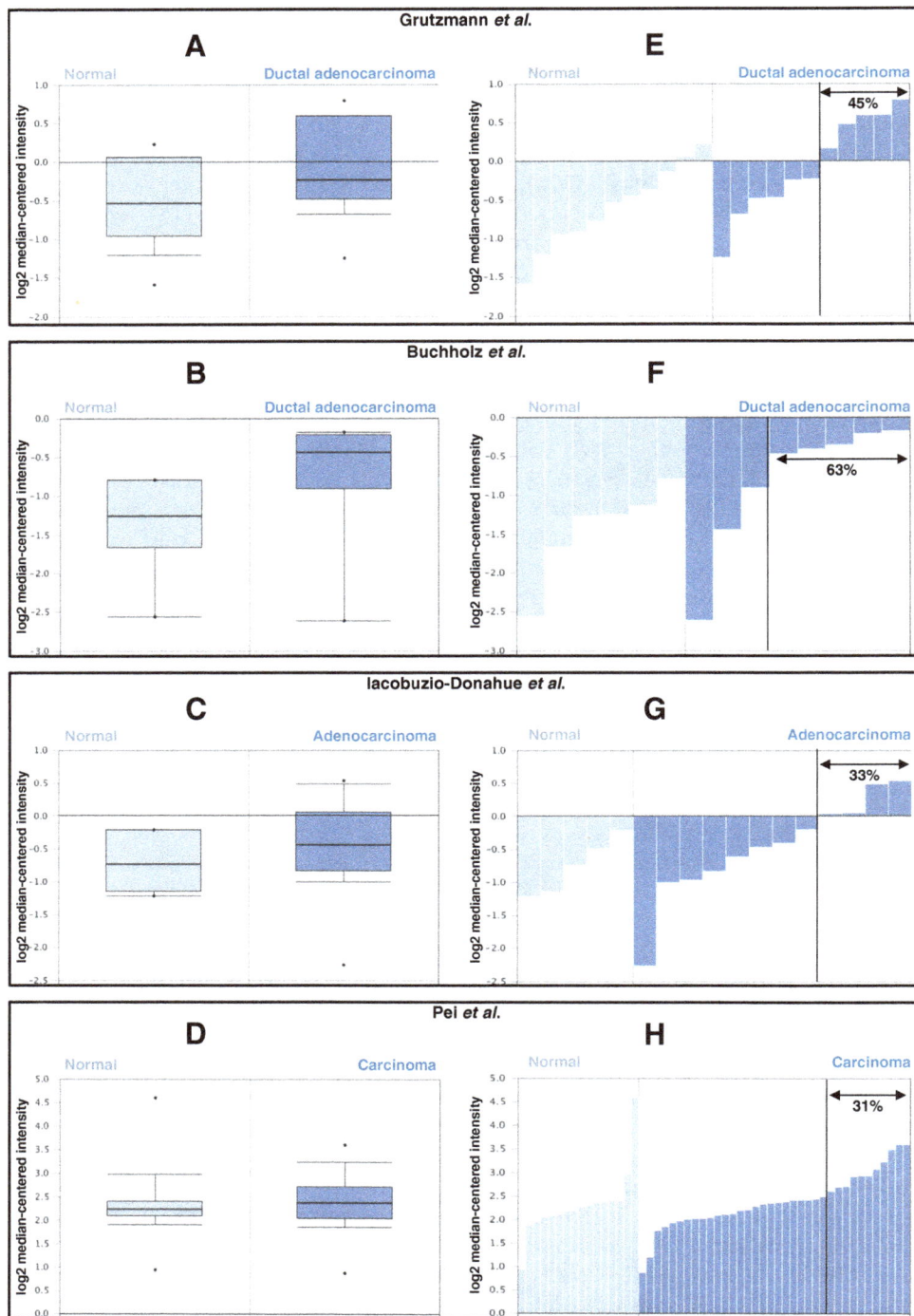

Fig. 1 AIF expression in pancreatic cancer. Data comparing AIF mRNA transcript expression in pancreatic tumors compared to normal pancreatic tissue was retrieved from the Oncomine database and assessed as shown in representative studies [40–42, 46]. Panels **a-d**: Average relative AIF mRNA expression in pancreatic tumors vs. normal pancreatic tissue. Panels **e-h**: Relative AIF mRNA levels within individual samples within each cohort. Fractions of tumor specimens within each cohort exhibiting statistically significant AIF expression changes relative to normal tissue are indicated in *red*

AIF selectively supports the growth and migration of pancreatic cancer cells

In order to determine whether AIF ablation impacts the rate of proliferation of pancreatic cancer cells, we measured the growth of AIF-deficient cells in vitro. Equal populations of cells were seeded in fresh media and allowed to proliferate for 72 h before quantification by Coulter™ counting. Notably, 4 of the 5 cell lines

Table 1 AIF dependence is related to metabolic phenotype [53] and sensitivity to glycolytic inhibition in pancreatic cancer cells

	Relative metabolic phenotype [53]		Sensitivity to glycolytic disruption	Sensitivity to AIF ablation
	Glycolysis/PPP	Fatty acid/ OXPHOS		
PANC-1	Moderate	Moderate	Insensitive	Sensitive
BxPC-3	Moderate	Moderate	Insensitive	Sensitive
HPAC	Low	High	Insensitive	Sensitive
HPAF-II	High	Moderate	Moderately sensitive	Moderately sensitive
MIA PaCa-2	High	Low	Sensitive	Insensitive

(PANC-1, BxPC-3, HPAC, and HPAF-II) showed a reduction in growth rate following ablation of AIF. After 3 days of proliferation, AIF-deficient PANC-1, BxPC-3, and HPAC cells exhibited only ~60 % of growth compared to shLacZ controls. AIF ablation resulted in a more modest reduction in proliferation rate in HPAF-II cells (~75 %), while growth was unaffected in MIA PaCa-2 cells (Fig. 4a). These results are distinct from our previous observations: in prostate cancer the growth rates of cells are largely unaffected by AIF ablation under nutrient-rich conditions in vitro, and it is not until exposure to Matrigel™ or growth stress in vivo that AIF-deficient prostate cancer cells exhibit substantial reductions in growth. This suggests that AIF is either more important in advanced PDAC vs. prostate cancer, and/or functions via alternative/additional mechanisms.

To further define the role of AIF in controlling the aggressiveness of pancreatic tumor cells, we next assessed the migration of AIF-deficient cells by scratch assay. High densities of cells were plated in replicate and allowed to attach for 12–36 h, and a scratch was made across the middle of each well with a P200 pipette tip. Scratch width was assessed immediately following cell displacement and 6–48 h later. AIF-deficient PANC-1, BxPC-3, and HPAC cells showed reduced migration while little change was observed in AIF-deficient HPAF-II or MIA PaCa-2 cells (Fig. 4b), in agreement with our proliferation rate data. It is notable that while MIA PaCa-2-shAIF cells displayed similar migration when compared to controls, when plated at the high densities used in the migration assay these cells took longer to adhere to plate surfaces. This suggests that AIF may be involved in cellular adhesion in this cell type; further studies are needed to define this function more clearly and determine the cancer specificity of this observation. Altogether, these data indicate that (1) the impact of AIF ablation upon pancreatic tumor cells is more severe than that observed in prostate cancer, (2) there is a spectrum of sensitivities to AIF ablation that is reflected by changes in cell growth patterns, and (3) AIF supports pancreatic tumorigenesis through a mechanism that appears different from that shown in prostate cancer.

Cellular energy phenotype determines the ability of AIF to promote growth and survival of pancreatic cancer cells

Having found that AIF selectively contributes to the rates of both cellular proliferation and migration in vitro, we sought to determine how AIF supports cell growth in pancreatic cancer and distinguish these effects based on cellular metabolic state. A common feature of cells that require AIF for basal metabolic activity is a loss of expression in protein subunits of complex I of the respiratory chain [22, 28]. To determine whether respiratory chain regulation is related to AIF-mediated cell growth, cells were lysed and probed for complex I subunits by immunoblot analysis. Following knockdown of AIF the concomitant changes in respiratory chain protein levels were diverse and directly correlated with both metabolic phenotype and changes in growth. AIF-deficient PANC-1, BxPC-3, and HPAC cells exhibited substantial reductions in 39-kDa, 20-kDa, and 17-kDa complex I subunits (Fig. 5). Interestingly, when AIF was suppressed in BxPC-3 cells, the expression of not only complex I subunits but also COX IV was reduced (Fig. 5), a change that has not been previously reported in cancer and may suggest a more global alteration in the mitochondrial proteome in this cell type. Changes in respiratory chain status were minimal when AIF was depleted from HPAF-II and MIA PaCa-2 cells (Fig. 5). These data indicate that loss of complex I in pancreatic cancer cells following AIF ablation is dependent on metabolic phenotype.

To further define the role of AIF in pancreatic cancer cells, we next evaluated the metabolic changes associated with AIF ablation by measuring glucose consumption rates within our cell line panel. Increased glucose consumption is a common adaptation following impairment of the mitochondrial respiratory chain, allowing cells to meet ATP demands directly through glycolysis. In agreement with the spectrum of respiratory deficiencies we observed, AIF-deficient PANC-1, BxPC-3, and HPAC cells consumed ~2–5-fold more glucose than their corresponding controls, while HPAF-II-shAIF and MIA PaCa-2-shAIF cells exhibited glucose consumption levels that were essentially unchanged when compared to controls (Fig. 6a). Notably, the magnitudes of altered glucose consumption in our panel of cell lines directly

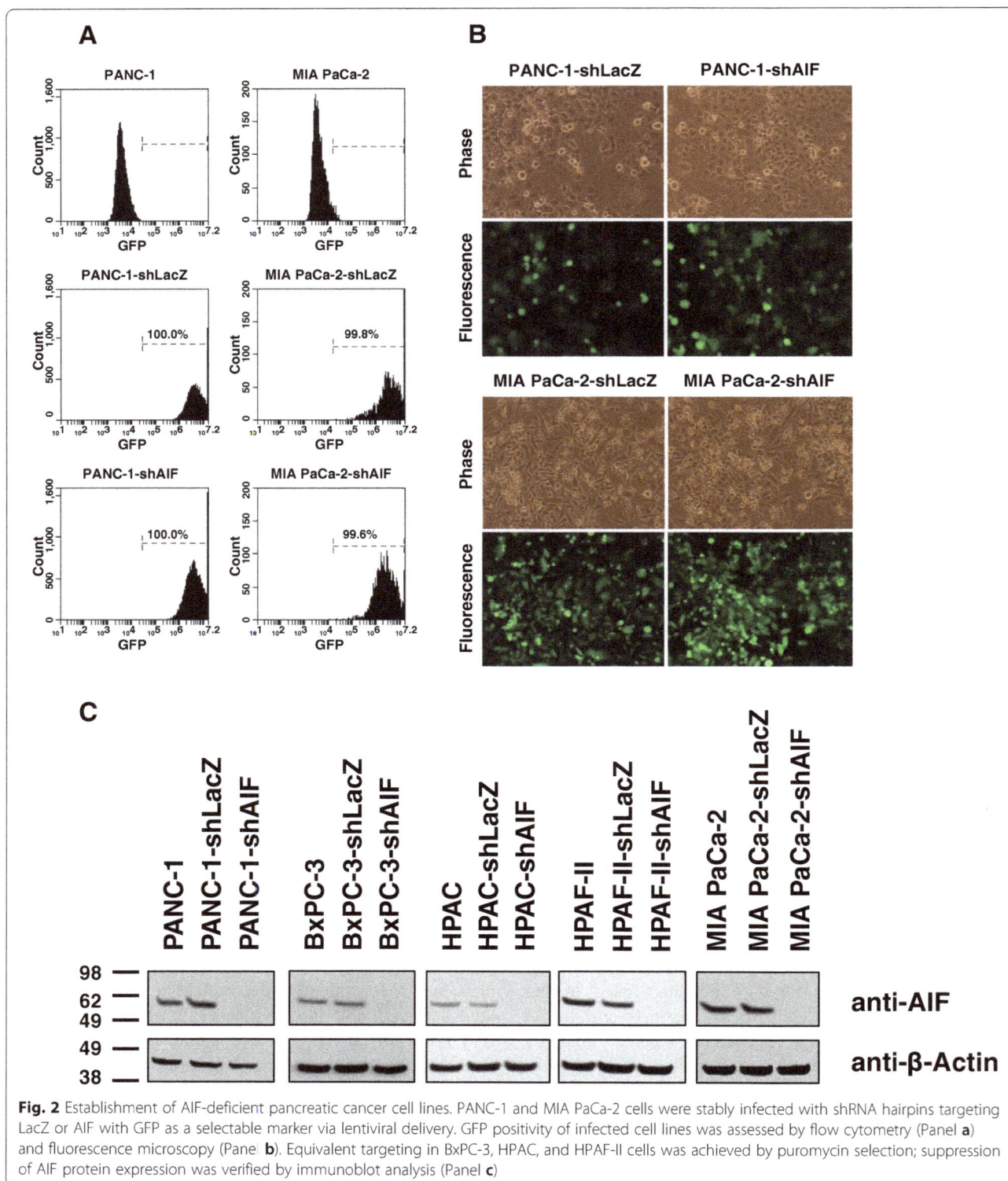

Fig. 2 Establishment of AIF-deficient pancreatic cancer cell lines. PANC-1 and MIA PaCa-2 cells were stably infected with shRNA hairpins targeting LacZ or AIF with GFP as a selectable marker via lentiviral delivery. GFP positivity of infected cell lines was assessed by flow cytometry (Panel **a**) and fluorescence microscopy (Panel **b**). Equivalent targeting in BxPC-3, HPAC, and HPAF-II cells was achieved by puromycin selection; suppression of AIF protein expression was verified by immunoblot analysis (Panel **c**)

correlated with the severity of respiratory chain deficiency that followed ablation of AIF (Fig. 5). This correlation suggests that differences in sensitivity to AIF ablation among cell types may stem from differential

metabolic requirements prior to AIF ablation. For example, due to a pre-existing decrease in respiratory chain activity [63], MIA PaCa-2 and HPAF-II cells have already adapted by upregulating glycolysis such that

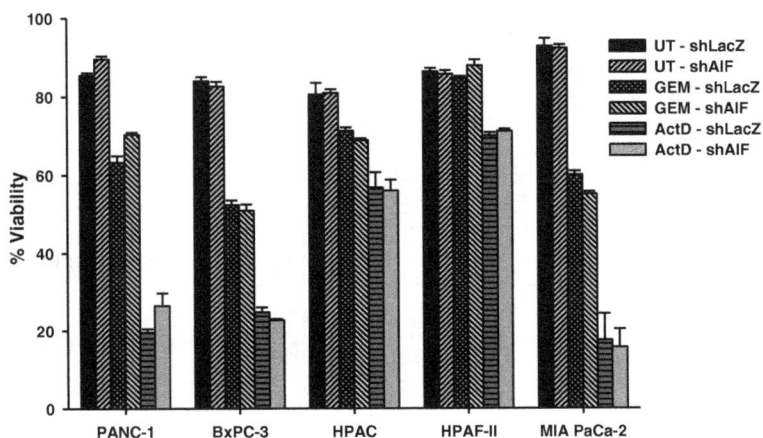

Fig. 3 AIF ablation does not impact chemical death induction in pancreatic cancer cells. Equal numbers of cells were harvested, washed, and allowed to attach overnight. Cells were then left untreated (UT) or treated with 1 μg/mL actinomycin D (ActD) for 24 h or 1 μM gemcitabine (GEM) for 48–72 h. Cell viability was then determined by propidium iodide staining and flow cytometry. Data are shown as average ± standard deviation

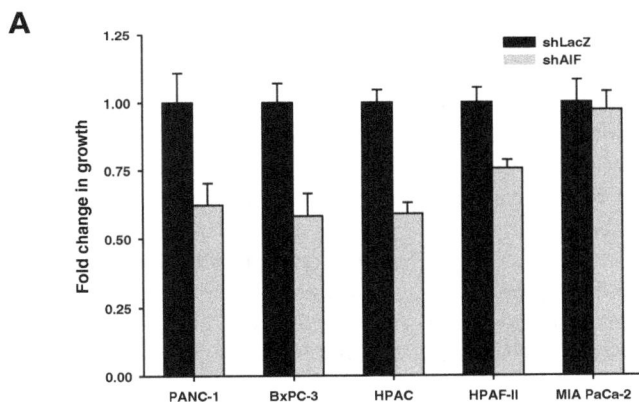

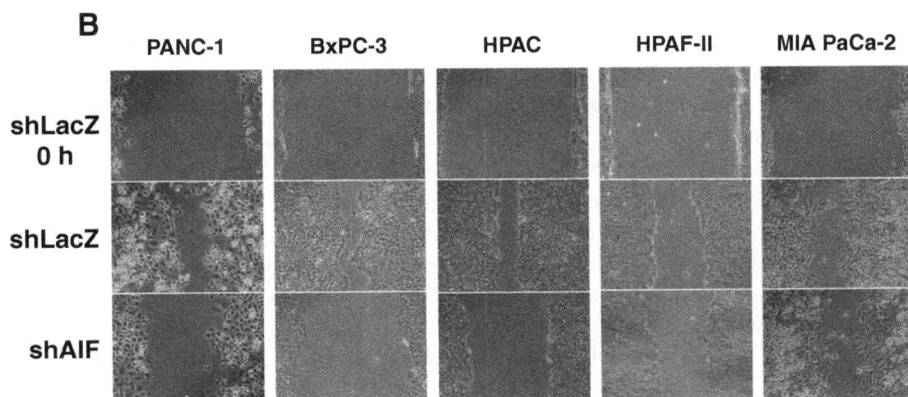

Fig. 4 Contribution of AIF to the growth and migration of pancreatic cancer cells in vitro. *Growth assay* (Panel **a**): cells were plated in equal densities in replicate, harvested, and quantified by Coulter™ counting after 72 h of growth. Data are shown as average ± standard deviation. *Scratch assay* (Panel **b**): high densities of cells were seeded in replicate wells and allowed to attach for 12–36 h. A single scratch was made through the middle of each well, and width was assessed at 0 h (all cell lines), 6 h (HPAC), 10 h (HPAF-II), 24 h (PANC-1), and 48 h (BxPC-3 and MIA PaCa-2). Representative images are shown (Panel **b**); all images were captured at 10× magnification

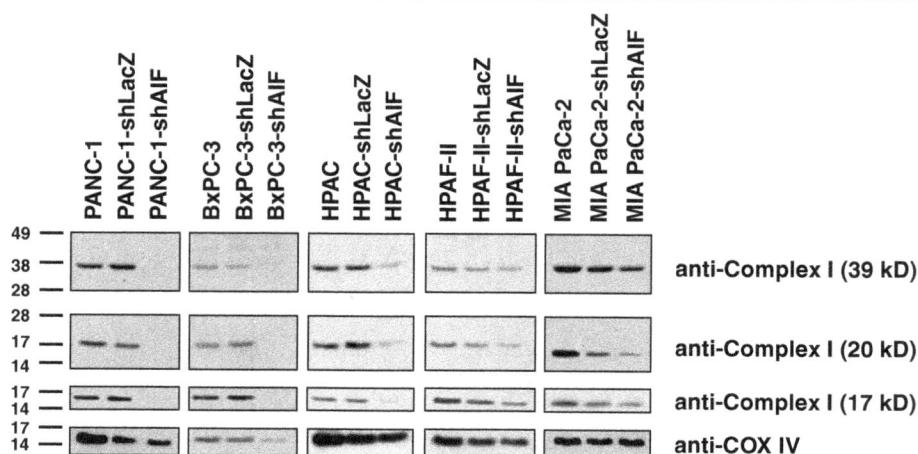

Fig. 5 AIF selectively controls respiratory chain protein expression in pancreatic cancer cells. Following suppression of AIF, respiratory chain status was assessed by immunoblot analysis of complex I (39-, 20-, and 17-kDa subunits) and COX IV

further impairment of the respiratory chain via AIF ablation has no additional effects upon glucose consumption.

To test this hypothesis and to determine the benefit of AIF-mediated glucose metabolism to cell survival, we next inhibited glycolysis in our panel of cell lines by treatment with 2-deoxyglucose. Glycolytic cell lines (*i.e.*, those that rely on glycolysis rather than oxidative phosphorylation as a primary source of energy production) will exhibit a higher sensitivity to treatment than those that remain capable of using other pathways (such as lipid catabolism or glutaminolysis) to compensate for this metabolic deficiency. To assess sensitivity, cell viability was measured using propidium iodide staining followed by flow cytometry. Our results revealed that while control PANC-1 and BxPC-3 cells are entirely resistant to 2-deoxyglucose, those that lack AIF exhibit substantial sensitivity with only ~40–50 % survival following treatment (Fig. 6b). Taken together with the corresponding respiratory statuses of these cell lines (Fig. 5), AIF is likely to regulate a balance between glycolysis and oxidative phosphorylation that is critical to the growth and survival of PANC-1 and BxPC-3 cells. In contrast, AIF ablation did not affect sensitivity to treatment in HPAC cells despite their complex I deficiency and elevated glucose consumption levels (Fig. 6b). This is not surprising given the lipogenic nature of the HPAC cell line [53], which allows cells to circumvent the metabolic requirement for AIF and complex I but at the expense of their proliferative capacity (Fig. 4). When compared to the resistant PANC-1, BxPC-3, and HPAC cell lines, control HPAF-II and MIA PaCa-2 cells both displayed a high basal sensitivity to 2-deoxyglucose, reflecting their dependence on glycolysis that is likely due to long-term adaptations to basal mitochondrial dysfunction. AIF ablation modestly increased sensitivity to glycolytic disruption in HPAF-II cells, but

MIA PaCa-2 cells displayed a pre-existing addiction to glycolysis [53, 64] that could not be amplified by AIF suppression. This sensitivity was comparable to PANC-1-shAIF and BxPC-3-shAIF cells following treatment (Fig. 6b) and is consistent with our glucose consumption data (Fig. 6a). In this context loss of AIF has little to no additional metabolic effect, an observation that further confirms the hypothesis that differences in glucose uptake among cell types following AIF ablation derive from differences in the intrinsic activities of their respiratory chains and/or glucose utilization.

Matrigel™ growth conditions amplify AIF dependence in pancreatic cancer cells

Following the observations that AIF supports metabolism benefiting the growth and survival of non-glycolytic pancreatic cancer cells in vitro, we next explored the metabolic function of AIF in an environment that more closely resembles conditions found in vivo. Matrigel™ is a cell growth substrate that consists of matrix protein polymers and proteoglycans found in natural extracellular environments and is often used as a model for studying tumorigenesis in a setting that approximates in vivo cell growth and survival. To assess the role of AIF in the growth and metabolism of pancreatic cancer cells under such conditions, glucose consumption and growth were measured following exposure to Matrigel™ substrate. These results were strikingly similar to those found in the absence of Matrigel™, except that the differences between control and AIF-deficient cells were amplified. When introduced into substrate, cells displayed a dependence on AIF expression for aggressive growth and normal glucose consumption. While control PANC-1, BxPC-3, and HPAC cells grew into spheroidal tumor-like structures, those without AIF exhibited substantial reductions in both size (Fig. 7a) and proliferation rate

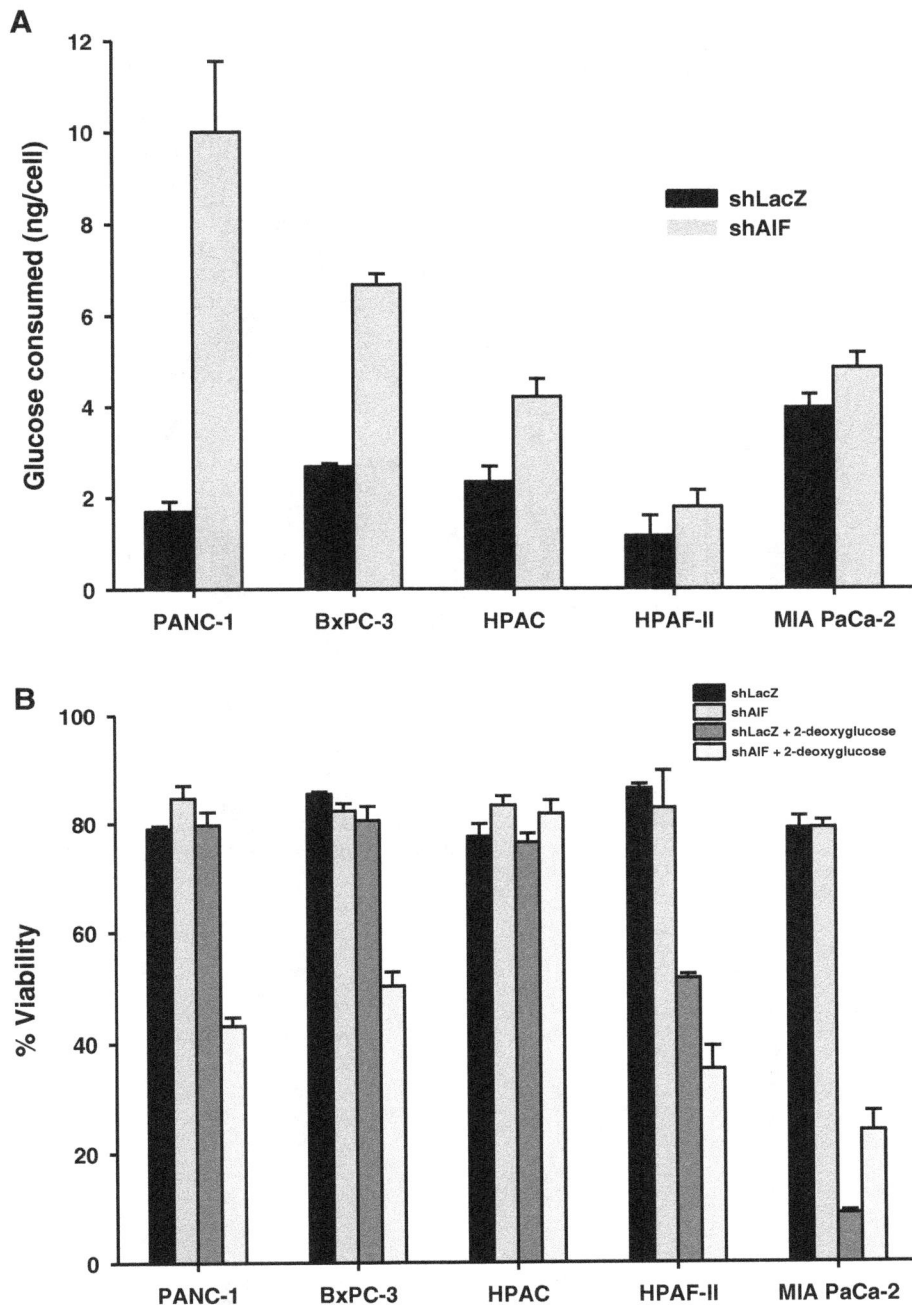

Fig. 6 Glycolytic dependence predicts metabolic sensitivity to AIF ablation. *Glucose consumption assay* (Panel **a**): equal densities of cells were plated in fresh media, and total glucose was measured using the QuantiChrom™ Glucose Assay Kit (BioAssay Systems) 72 h after seeding. Total numbers of cells in each well were used to determine glucose consumption per cell. *Sensitivity to glycolytic disruption* (Panel **b**): Cells were seeded in equal densities and allowed to attach overnight before treatment with 50 mM 2-deoxyglucose. After 48 h cells were collected, and viability was determined by propidium iodide staining and flow cytometry. Data are shown as average ± standard deviation

(Fig. 7b). Furthermore, AIF-deficient PANC-1, BxPC-3, and HPAC cells consumed ~3–7-fold more glucose than those with AIF (Fig. 7c), suggesting that glycolysis becomes critical for growth and survival under Matrigel™ growth conditions when AIF is depleted. In the HPAF-II

cell line, which exhibited modest changes in growth and metabolism following AIF ablation in vitro, both shLacZ controls and shAIF failed to invade the substrate to the extent of other cell lines, yet HPAF-II-shAIF cells showed a substantial reduction in growth rate and a 2-

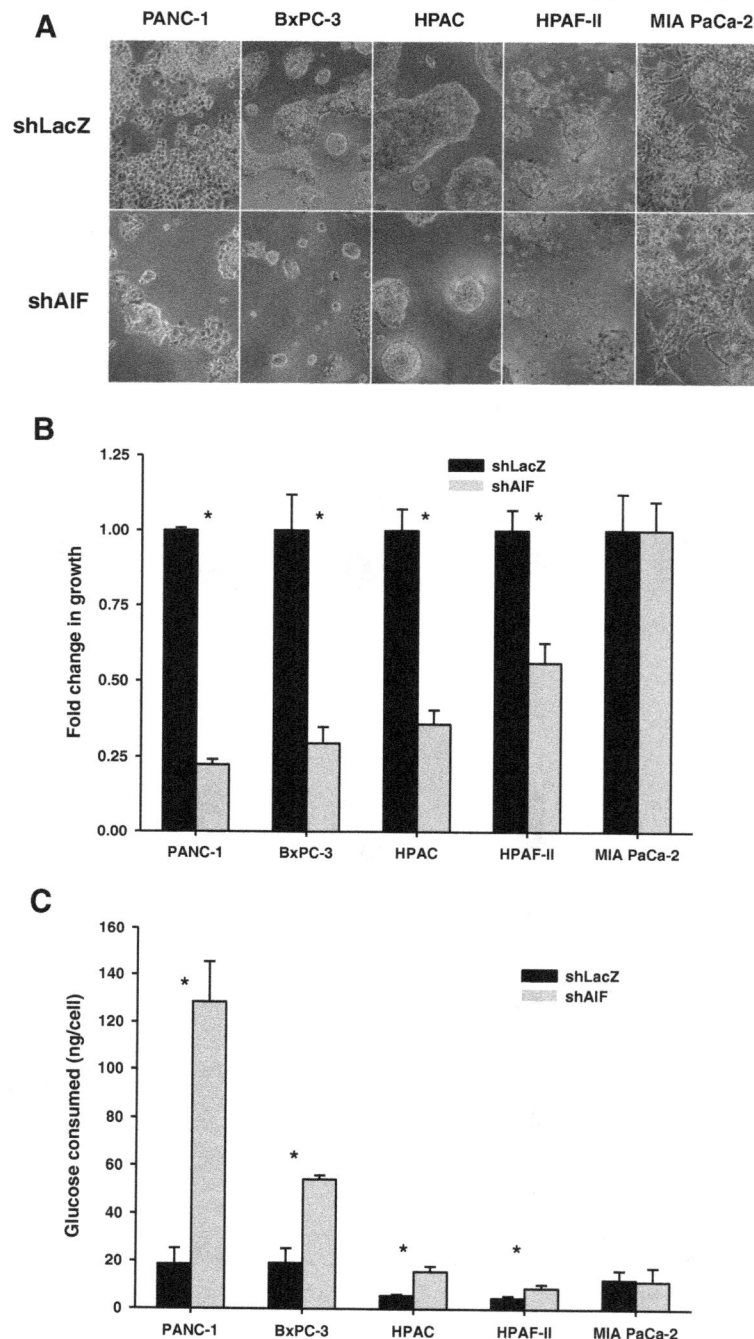

Fig. 7 Matrigel™ environment amplifies dependence upon AIF-mediated growth and metabolism. *Matrigel™ growth*: Cells were plated in replicate Matrigel™ layers and allowed to grow for up to 21 days. Representative images (captured at 10× magnification) are shown (Panel **a**). Cells were extracted from substrate and quantified by Coulter™ counting (Panel **b**). *Glucose consumption in Matrigel™ substrate* (Panel **c**): Cells were exposed to Matrigel™ conditions prior to media collection and total glucose measurements using the QuantiChrom™ Glucose Assay Kit (BioAssay Systems). Cells were extracted from substrate with the Matrigel Recovery Solution (Corning) and quantified by Coulter™ counting. Total numbers of cells in each well were used to determine glucose consumption per cell. Data are shown as average ± standard deviation. *$p < 0.05$

fold increase in glucose consumption. Taken together with previous data, this suggests that AIF plays a minor role in HPAF-II glucose metabolism under nutrient-rich conditions but that this role gains prominence upon exposure to Matrigel™. In contrast, MIA PaCa-2-derived cell lines did not display significant changes (Fig. 7), consistent with in vitro measurements. Following growth in Matrigel™ changes in both glucose uptake and growth in substrate were more severe but directly proportional to those found in vitro. Altogether, our data indicate that AIF supports the growth and survival of some pancreatic cancer cells by facilitating a metabolic balance, and this metabolic function is most beneficial to cell populations that do not rely fully on glycolysis for survival.

Discussion

When functioning in a pro-death role, AIF can undergo nuclear translocation followed by the induction of chromatin condensation and DNA degradation during various forms of cell death [65–69]. As a promoter of caspase-independent death, it is formally possible that AIF could act in a tumor-suppressive manner. Yet while AIF nuclear translocation has been observed in cancer [70, 71], this study and others [28, 29] show that loss of AIF suppresses tumorigenesis and that AIF's nuclear function is unlikely to make a significant contribution to death pathways despite overexpression in tumors [28, 30–35]. AIF elevation in cancer is modest (typically less than 3-fold), suggesting a threshold exists above which AIF expression is either no longer beneficial or actively disadvantageous. Despite this threshold, AIF elevation in cancer is both sufficient and necessary for AIF to promote survival through its enzymatic activity [28, 29].

Presently, AIF's enzymatic activity has been demonstrated to support tumorigenesis through at least two distinct mechanisms. In colorectal cancer cells, AIF elevates the cellular oxidative state to protect against chemical stress-induced apoptosis [29]. In prostate cancer, AIF promotes a metabolic state that selectively supports the growth and survival of cells that have achieved advanced status [28], suggesting that AIF addiction in cancer manifests as tumors become increasingly aggressive. Our current data agree with a similarly important contribution for AIF to pancreatic cancer progression, a disease setting that most often presents at an advanced stage by the time of diagnosis. However, in contrast to our observations in prostate cancer, the selectivity of AIF's support of different pancreatic cancer cell types was directly related to their cellular energy preferences.

PANC-1, BxPC-3, and HPAC cells, all of which display a metabolic phenotype not solely reliant upon glycolysis (Fig. 6b, Table 1, [53]), exhibited a remarkably similar reduced growth phenotype (~60 % of controls) following AIF ablation that also included respiratory chain depletion and elevated glucose consumption levels ranging from ~2–5-fold. When introduced into Matrigel™ substrate, we observed more drastic changes in both growth (20–30 % of controls) and glucose uptake (~3–7-fold increases). PANC-1 and BxPC-3 cell lines were also sensitized to glycolytic disruption, suggesting that glycolysis

becomes critical for survival following AIF ablation. This change was not observed in the HPAC cell line, likely due to a metabolic flexibility that derives from its lipogenic phenotype [53]; in this context AIF supports aggressive growth, yet cells remain capable of maintaining survival in the absence of AIF's metabolic activities.

HPAF-II cells, which exhibit a greater dependence on glycolysis than PANC-1, BxPC-3, or HPAC cells (Fig. 6b, Table 1, [53]), also showed changes following AIF ablation, although less severe. Cells did not lose complex I subunits, nor did they exhibit significantly increased glucose consumption in vitro. Despite this, AIF ablation further increased sensitivity to 2-deoxyglucose while modestly compromising in vitro growth. Moreover, introduction to Matrigel™ caused HPAF-II-shAIF cells to elevate glucose consumption by 2-fold while significantly reducing growth rate. No changes in either growth or glucose metabolism were identified in MIA PaCa-2 cells, which displayed a severe pre-existing addiction to glycolysis (Fig. 6b, Table 1, [53]) that could not be further exacerbated by AIF ablation.

While our data suggest that AIF is selectively beneficial to metabolically "flexible" PDAC cells that use both glycolysis and oxidative phosphorylation for energy production, the basis for the selective sensitivity of different cell types to AIF ablation has not been firmly established. It has been proposed that AIF functions as a metabolic sensor through binding and oxidizing NADH ligands [25]. In light of this hypothesis and extending our current data to other cell types, AIF may regulate respiratory chain expression and metabolic flux in response to NADH/NAD$^+$ availability (established by the overall metabolic state). By implication, AIF is consequently central to a self-regulating metabolic balance.

How might the presence of AIF impact metabolism addiction in pancreatic cancer? Otto Warburg first observed that cancer cells increase their glucose consumption levels relative to normal cells, hypothesizing that defective mitochondrial respiration contributes to tumorigenesis [72]. While elevated glucose consumption is a common characteristic of tumor cells, it is now well-established that many cancer cells rely on both glycolysis and mitochondrial energy metabolism to coordinate an efficient balance between glucose-derived macromolecule biosynthesis and energy production that permits aggressive growth and survival [73]. The supportive role of AIF in cancer derives from its ability to maintain efficient mitochondrial electron transport and oxidative phosphorylation, and this function becomes critical as cells become more aggressive and reliant on mitochondrial function. Indeed, several recent studies have identified paramount roles for oxidative phosphorylation in promoting the invasiveness of cancer cells [38, 74, 75].

When tumors undergoing aerobic glycolysis reach advanced stages, cancer cells often continue to rely on mitochondria as a source of energy production [76] and suffer a metabolic disadvantage when mitochondrial function is lost. In pancreatic cancer, this is especially true. Recently it has been shown that following ablation of the oncogene KRAS, mitochondrial function and oxidative phosphorylation become critical for survival in relapsing tumors [38]. Our data suggest that AIF expression is necessary to mediate a metabolic balance in certain pancreatic cancer cells (e.g., PANC-1, BxPC-3, and HPAC), and AIF ablation induces cellular adaptations that lead to a greater reliance upon glycolysis for survival in these cell types. Other cell types that exhibit a pre-existing addiction to glycolysis (e.g., HPAF-II and MIA PaCa-2) are therefore less sensitive to AIF ablation. This further emphasizes the impact of metabolic balance in support of pancreatic tumorigenesis, specifically through the expression of AIF.

In this study we established a pro-tumorigenic role for AIF in pancreatic cancer that derives from its metabolic activities. The selectivity of AIF dependence in tumorigenesis appears independent of oncogene/tumor suppressor status and instead stems from the overall cellular metabolic state, which results from the cumulative effect of genetic alterations. We found a direct relationship between basal metabolic state and dependence upon AIF expression (Table 1): as cells become aggressive such that they require a critical balance between mitochondrial energy metabolism and glycolysis, they become more dependent upon AIF. This correlation is in strong agreement with other studies. For example, PANC-1 cells (highly sensitive to AIF ablation) express higher levels of vascular endothelial growth factor than MIA PaCa-2 cells (insensitive to AIF ablation) [59, 77, 78]. This indicates a greater requirement for oxygen and mitochondrial function, and hence AIF activity, in the PANC-1 line. A recent report identified clear PDAC subtypes based upon metabolic requirements [53]. This extensive study characterized the metabolic states of all cell lines used in our study (Table 1) as well as numerous other cell lines, and their data strongly support our model. These data and our previous studies suggest that AIF's metabolic impact upon tumorigenesis increases with disease progression. Previously we showed that AIF promotes a metabolic state permitting progression to advanced stages. Based on our current data, we propose that in the most advanced tumor cells (such as in PDAC), which critically rely on metabolic reprogramming for growth and survival, AIF activity is maximally exploited and becomes entwined within the overall metabolic state, a situation in which the only limiting factor to AIF dependence is how the cell utilizes mitochondrial energy metabolism.

Altered AIF expression is not a general feature of cancerous tissues and AIF activity is not universally supportive to cancer development and progression. However, in studies presented here we have identified a subpopulation of pancreatic cancer samples in which AIF expression is elevated, and using a panel of cancer cell lines with defined metabolic phenotypes we have correlated AIF activity to basal metabolic state. At present the molecular mechanisms defining AIF sensitivity remain to be elucidated, yet the experiments presented outline a framework for determining those cells in which AIF activity is critical, based on criteria such as metabolic phenotype and fuel source preference/requirements. The promise of this framework is the potential for AIF-mediated therapy. Development of such therapy, either as a stand-alone approach or more likely in combination with other modalities, will depend on better understanding of AIF mechanism and accurate metabolic assessment, but offers significant potential for increasing our treatment arsenal for cancer patients suffering from advanced disease.

Conclusions

Altogether this study highlights the metabolic significance of AIF to PDAC and expands the range of AIF function in tumorigenesis. We found that the basal energetic requirements of PDAC cells determine the ability of AIF to support metabolic plasticity that benefits growth and survival. As a metabolic linchpin in cancer, AIF therefore represents a novel therapeutic target.

Ethics statement

All work performed in this study was carried out in accordance with the Declaration of Helsinki. Patient-derived gene expression data was obtained from the publically available database Oncomine, which requires written informed consent and institutional review board approval from all investigators prior to data deposition. All cell lines used in this study were obtained from commercial sources; no other clinical specimens or human subjects were employed.

Abbreviations
AIF: apoptosis-inducing factor; FBS: fetal bovine serum; PBS: phosphate buffered saline; RNAi: RNA interference; shRNA: short-hairpin RNA.

Competing interests
The authors declare that they have no competing interests.

Authors' contributions
AJS and ASW performed experiments. AJS and JCW wrote the manuscript. All authors read and approved the final manuscript.

Acknowledgements
The authors would like to thank Dr. Sanku Mallik for providing PANC-1, BxPC-3, HPAC, HPAF-II, and MIA PaCa-2 cell lines. This work was supported by

grant RSG-09-166-01-CCG (to JCW) from the American Cancer Society, and the State of North Dakota Experimental Program to Stimulate Competitive Research (ND-EPSCoR, project #FAR0022246, to JCW).

References

1. Susin SA, Lorenzo HK, Zamzami N, Marzo I, Snow BE, Brothers GM, Mangion J, Jacotot E, Costantini P, Loeffler M et al. Molecular characterization of mitochondrial apoptosis-inducing factor. Nature. 1999;397(6718):441–6.

2. Otera H, Ohsakaya S, Nagaura Z, Ishihara N, Mihara K. Export of mitochondrial AIF in response to proapoptotic stimuli depends on processing at the intermembrane space. Embo J. 2005;24(7):1375–86.

3. Polster BM, Basanez G, Etxebarria A, Hardwick JM, Nicholls DG. Calpain I induces cleavage and release of apoptosis-inducing factor from isolated mitochondria. J Biol Chem. 2005;280(8):6447–54.

4. Yuste VJ, Moubarak RS, Delettre C, Bras M, Sancho P, Robert N, d'Alayer J, Susin SA. Cysteine protease inhibition prevents mitochondrial apoptosis-inducing factor (AIF) release. Cell Death Differ. 2005;12(11):1445–8.

5. Bidere N, Lorenzo HK, Carmona S, Laforge M, Harper F, Dumont C, Senik A. Cathepsin D triggers Bax activation, resulting in selective apoptosis-inducing factor (AIF) relocation in T lymphocytes entering the early commitment phase to apoptosis. J Biol Chem. 2003;278(33):31401–11.

6. Cao G, Xing J, Xiao X, Liou AK, Gao Y, Yin XM, Clark RS, Graham SH, Chen J. Critical role of calpain I in mitochondrial release of apoptosis-inducing factor in ischemic neuronal injury. J Neurosci. 2007;27(35):9278–93.

7. Loeffler M, Daugas E, Susin SA, Zamzami N, Metivier D, Nieminen AL, Brothers G, Penninger JM, Kroemer G. Dominant cell death induction by extramitochondrially targeted apoptosis-inducing factor. Faseb J. 2001;15(3):758–67.

8. Cande C, Vahsen N, Kouranti I, Schmitt E, Daugas E, Spahr C, Luban J, Kroemer RT, Giordanetto F, Garrido C et al. AIF and cyclophilin A cooperate in apoptosis-associated chromatinolysis. Oncogene. 2004;23(8):1514–21.

9. Wang X, Yang C, Chai J, Shi Y, Xue D. Mechanisms of AIF-mediated apoptotic DNA degradation in Caenorhabditis elegans. Science. 2002; 298(5598):1587–92.

10. Zhu C, Wang X, Deinum J, Huang Z, Gao J, Modjtahedi N, Neagu MR, Nilsson M, Eriksson PS, Hagberg H et al. Cyclophilin A participates in the nuclear translocation of apoptosis-inducing factor in neurons after cerebral hypoxia-ischemia. J Exp Med. 2007;204(8):1741–8.

11. Artus C, Boujrad H, Bouharrour A, Brunelle MN, Hoos S, Yuste VJ, Lenormand P, Rousselle JC, Namane A, England P et al. AIF promotes chromatinolysis and caspase-independent programmed necrosis by interacting with histone H2AX. Embo J. 2010;29(9):1585–99.

12. Miramar MD, Costantini P, Ravagnan L, Saraiva LM, Haouzi D, Brothers G, Penninger JM, Peleato ML, Kroemer G, Susin SA et al. NADH oxidase activity of mitochondrial apoptosis-inducing factor. J Biol Chem. 2001;276(19):16391–8.

13. Churbanova IY, Sevrioukova IF. Redox-dependent changes in molecular properties of mitochondrial apoptosis-inducing factor. J Biol Chem. 2008; 283(9):5622–31.

14. Joza N, Susin SA, Daugas E, Stanford WL, Cho SK, Li CY, Sasaki T, Elia AJ, Cheng HY, Ravagnan L et al. Essential role of the mitochondrial apoptosis-inducing factor in programmed cell death. Nature. 2001;410(6828):549–54.

15. Brown D, Yu BD, Joza N, Benit P, Meneses J, Firpo M, Rustin P, Penninger JM, Martin GR. Loss of Aif function causes cell death in the mouse embryo, but the temporal progression of patterning is normal. Proc Natl Acad Sci U S A. 2006; 103(26):9918–23.

16. Klein JA, Longo-Guess CM, Rossmann MP, Seburn KL, Hurd RE, Frankel WN, Bronson RT, Ackerman SL. The harlequin mouse mutation downregulates apoptosis-inducing factor. Nature. 2002;419(6905):367–74.

17. Joza N, Oudit GY, Brown D, Benit P, Kassiri Z, Vahsen N, Benoit L, Patel MM, Nowikovsky K, Vassault A et al. Muscle-specific loss of apoptosis-inducing factor leads to mitochondrial dysfunction, skeletal muscle atrophy, and dilated cardiomyopathy. Mol Cell Biol. 2005;25(23):10261–72.

18. Cheung EC, Joza N, Steenaart NA, McClellan KA, Neuspiel M, McNamara S, MacLaurin JG, Rippstein P, Park DS, Shore GC et al. Dissociating the dual roles of apoptosis-inducing factor in maintaining mitochondrial structure and apoptosis. Embo J. 2006;25(17):4061–73.

19. Ghezzi D, Sevrioukova I, Invernizzi F, Lamperti C, Mora M, D'Adamo P, Novara F, Zuffardi O, Uziel G, Zeviani M. Severe X-linked mitochondrial encephalomyopathy associated with a mutation in apoptosis-inducing factor. Am J Hum Genet. 2010;86(4):639–49.

20. Berger I, Ben-Neriah Z, Dor-Wolman T, Shaag A, Saada A, Zenvirt S, Raas-Rothschild A, Nadjari M, Kaestner KH, Elpeleg O. Early prenatal ventriculomegaly due to an AIFM1 mutation identified by linkage analysis and whole exome sequencing. Mol Genet Metab. 2011;104(4):517–20.

21. Rinaldi C, Grunseich C, Sevrioukova IF, Schindler A, Horkayne-Szakaly I, Lamperti C, Landoure G, Kennerson ML, Burnett BG, Bonnemann C et al. Cowchock syndrome is associated with a mutation in apoptosis-inducing factor. Am J Hum Genet. 2012;91(6):1095–102.

22. Vahsen N, Cande C, Briere JJ, Benit P, Joza N, Larochette N, Mastroberardino PG, Pequignot MO, Casares N, Lazar V et al. AIF deficiency compromises oxidative phosphorylation. Embo J. 2004;23(23):4679–89.

23. Hangen E, Feraud O, Lachkar S, Mou H, Doti N, Fimia GM, Lam NV, Zhu C, Godin I, Muller K et al. Interaction between AIF and CHCHD4 Regulates Respiratory Chain Biogenesis. Mol Cell. 2015;58(6):1001–14.

24. Meyer K, Buettner S, Ghezzi D, Zeviani M, Bano D, Nicotera P. Loss of apoptosis-inducing factor critically affects MIA40 function. Cell Death Dis. 2015;6:e1814.

25. Ferreira P, Villanueva R, Martinez-Julvez M, Herguedas B, Marcuello C, Fernandez-Silva P, Cabon L, Hermoso JA, Lostao A, Susin SA et al. Structural insights into the coenzyme mediated monomer-dimer transition of the pro-apoptotic apoptosis inducing factor. Biochemistry. 2014;53(25):4204–15.

26. Pospisilik JA, Knauf C, Joza N, Benit P, Orthofer M, Cani PD, Ebersberger I, Nakashima T, Sarao R, Neely G et al. Targeted deletion of AIF decreases mitochondrial oxidative phosphorylation and protects from obesity and diabetes. Cell. 2007;131(3):476–91.

27. Modjtahedi N, Hangen E, Gonin P, Kroemer G. Metabolic epistasis among apoptosis-inducing factor and the mitochondrial import factor CHCHD4. Cell Cycle. 2015;14(17):2743–7.

28. Lewis EM, Wilkinson AS, Jackson JS, Mehra R, Varambally S, Chinnaiyan AM, Wilkinson JC. The Enzymatic Activity of Apoptosis Inducing Factor Supports Energy Metabolism Benefitting the Growth and Invasiveness of Advanced Prostate Cancer Cells. J Biol Chem. 2012;287(52):43862–75.

29. Urbano A, Lakshmanan U, Choo PH, Kwan JC, Ng PY, Guo K, Dhakshinamoorthy S, Porter A. AIF suppresses chemical stress-induced apoptosis and maintains the transformed state of tumor cells. Embo J. 2005; 24(15):2815–26.

30. Fan T, Tian F, Yi S, Ke Y, Han S, Zhang L, Liu H. Implications of Bit1 and AIF overexpressions in esophageal squamous cell carcinoma. Tumour Biol. 2014; 35(1):519–27.

31. Skyrlas A, Hantschke M, Passa V, Gaitanis G, Malamou-Mitsi V, Bassukas ID. Expression of apoptosis-inducing factor (AIF) in keratoacanthomas and squamous cell carcinomas of the skin. Exp Dermatol. 2011;20(8):674–6.

32. Jeong EG, Lee JW, Soung YH, Nam SW, Kim SH, Lee JY, Yoo NJ, Lee SH. Immunohistochemical and mutational analysis of apoptosis-inducing factor (AIF) in colorectal carcinomas. APMIS. 2006;114(12):867–73.

33. Millan A, Huerta S. Apoptosis-inducing factor and colon cancer. J Surg Res. 2009;151(1):163–70.

34. Lee JW, Jeong EG, Soung YH, Kim SY, Nam SW, Kim SH, Lee JY, Yoo NJ, Lee SH. Immunohistochemical analysis of apoptosis-inducing factor (AIF) expression in gastric carcinomas. Pathol Res Pract. 2006;202(7):497–501.

35. Li S, Wan M, Cao X, Ren Y. Expression of AIF and HtrA2/Omi in small lymphocytic lymphoma and diffuse large B-cell lymphoma. Arch Pathol Lab Med. 2011;135(7):903–8.

36. Cleary SP, Gryfe R, Guindi M, Greig P, Smith L, Mackenzie R, Strasberg S, Hanna S, Taylor B, Langer B et al. Prognostic factors in resected pancreatic adenocarcinoma: analysis of actual 5-year survivors. J Am Coll Surg. 2004; 198(5):722–31.

37. Siegel R, Ma J, Zou Z, Jemal A. Cancer statistics, 2014. CA Cancer J Clin. 2014;64(1):9–29.

38. Viale A, Pettazzoni P, Lyssiotis CA, Ying H, Sanchez N, Marchesini M, Carugo A, Green T, Seth S, Giuliani V et al. Oncogene ablation-resistant pancreatic cancer cells depend on mitochondrial function. Nature. 2014;514(7524):628–32.

39. Blum R, Kloog Y. Metabolism addiction in pancreatic cancer. Cell Death Dis. 2014;5:e1065.

40. Grutzmann R, Pilarsky C, Ammerpohl O, Luttges J, Bohme A, Sipos B, Foerder M, Alldinger I, Jahnke B, Schackert HK et al. Gene expression profiling of microdissected pancreatic ductal carcinomas using high-density DNA microarrays. Neoplasia. 2004;6(5):611–22.

41. Buchholz M, Braun M, Heidenblut A, Kestler HA, Kloppel G, Schmiegel W, Hahn SA, Luttges J, Gress TM. Transcriptome analysis of microdissected pancreatic intraepithelial neoplastic lesions. Oncogene. 2005;24(44):6626–36.

42. Iacobuzio-Donahue CA, Maitra A, O sen M, Lowe AW, van Heek NT, Rosty C, Walter K, Sato N, Parker A, Ashfaq R et al. Exploration of global gene expression patterns in pancreatic adenocarcinoma using cDNA microarrays. Am J Pathol. 2003;162(4):1151–62.

43. Segara D, Biankin AV, Kench JG, Langusch CC, Dawson AC, Skalicky DA, Gotley DC, Coleman MJ, Sutherland RL, Henshall SM. Expression of HOXB2, a retinoic acid signaling target in pancreatic cancer and pancreatic intraepithelial neoplasia. Clin Cancer Res. 2005;11(9):3587–96.

44. Ishikawa M, Yoshida K, Yamashita Y, Ota J, Takada S, Kisanuki H, Koinuma K, Choi YL, Kaneda R, Iwao T et al. Experimental trial for diagnosis of pancreatic ductal carcinoma based on gene expression profiles of pancreatic ductal cells. Cancer Sci. 2005;96(7):387–93.

45. Badea L, Herlea V, Dima SO, Dumitrascu T, Popescu I. Combined gene expression analysis of whole-tissue and microdissected pancreatic ductal adenocarcinoma identifies genes specifically overexpressed in tumor epithelia. Hepatogastroenterology. 2008;55(88):2016–27.

46. Pei H, Li L, Fridley BL, Jenkins GD, Kalari KR, Lingle W, Petersen G, Lou Z, Wang L. FKBP51 affects cancer cell response to chemotherapy by negatively regulating Akt. Cancer Cell. 2009;16(3):259–66.

47. Rhodes DR, Kalyana-Sundaram S, Mahavisno V, Varambally R, Yu J, Briggs BB, BB, Barrette TR, Anstet MJ, Kincead-Beal C, Kulkarni P et al. Oncomine 3.0: genes, pathways, and networks in a collection of 18,000 cancer gene expression profiles. Neoplasia. 2007;9(2):166–80.

48. Turner RL, Wilkinson JC, Ornelles DA. E1B and E4 oncoproteins of adenovirus antagonize the effect of apoptosis inducing factor. Virology. 2014;456–457:205–19.

49. Yu J, Wang P, Ming L, Wood MA, Zhang L. SMAC/Diablo mediates the proapoptotic function of PUMA by regulating PUMA-induced mitochondrial events. Oncogene. 2007;26(29):4189–98.

50. Qin XF, An DS, Chen IS, Baltimore D. Inhibiting HIV-1 infection in human T cells by lentiviral-mediated delivery of small interfering RNA against CCR5. Proc Natl Acad Sci U S A. 2003;100(1):183–8.

51. Galban S, Hwang C, Rumble JM, Oetjen KA, Wright CW, Boudreault A, Durkin J, Gillard JW, Jaquith JB, Morrs SJ et al. Cytoprotective effects of IAPs revealed by a small molecule antagonist. Biochem J. 2009;417(3):765–71.

52. Liang CC, Park AY, Guan JL. In vitro scratch assay: a convenient and inexpensive method for analysis of cell migration in vitro. Nat Protoc. 2007;2(2):329–33.

53. Daemen A, Peterson D, Sahu N, McCord R, Du X, Liu B, Kowanetz K, Hong R, Moffat J, Gao M et al. Metabolite profiling stratifies pancreatic ductal adenocarcinomas into subtypes with distinct sensitivities to metabolic inhibitors. Proc Natl Acad Sci U S A. 2015;112(32):E4410–4417.

54. Lieber M, Mazzetta J, Nelson-Rees W, Kaplan M, Todaro G. Establishment of a continuous tumor-cell line (panc-1) from a human carcinoma of the exocrine pancreas. Int J Cancer. 1975;15(5):741–7.

55. Tan MH, Nowak NJ, Loor R, Ochi H, Sandberg AA, Lopez C, Pickren JW, Berjian R, Douglass HO, Jr., Chu TM. Characterization of a new primary human pancreatic tumor line. Cancer Invest. 1986;4(1):15–23.

56. Gower Jr WR, Risch RM, Godellas CV, Fabri PJ. HPAC, a new human glucocorticoid-sensitive pancreatic ductal adenocarcinoma cell line. In Vitro Cell Dev Biol Anim. 1994;30A(3):151–61.

57. Yunis AA, Arimura GK, Russin DJ. Human pancreatic carcinoma (MIA PaCa-2) in continuous culture: sensitivity to asparaginase. Int J Cancer. 1977;19(1):128–35.

58. Metzgar RS, Gaillard MT, Levine SJ, Tuck FL, Bossen EH, Borowitz MJ. Antigens of human pancreatic adenocarcinoma cells defined by murine monoclonal antibodies. Cancer Res. 1982;42(2):601–8.

59. Deer EL, Gonzalez-Hernandez J, Coursen JD, Shea JE, Ngatia J, Scaife CL, Firpo MA, Mulvihill SJ. Phenotype and genotype of pancreatic cancer cell lines. Pancreas. 2010;39(4):425–35.

60. Moore PS, Sipos B, Orlandini S, Sorio C, Real FX, Lemoine NR, Gress T, Bassi C, Kloppel G, Kalthoff H et al. Genetic profile of 22 pancreatic carcinoma cell lines. Analysis of K-ras, p53, p16 and DPC4/Smad4. Virchows Arch. 2001;439(6):798–802.

61. Sobell HM. Actinomycin and DNA transcription. Proc Natl Acad Sci U S A. 1985;82(16):5328–31.

62. Burris 3rd HA, Moore MJ, Andersen J, Green MR, Rothenberg ML, Modiano MR, Cripps MC, Portenoy RK, Storniolo AM, Tarassoff P et al. Improvements in survival and clinical benefit with gemcitabine as first-line therapy for patients with advanced pancreas cancer: a randomized trial. J Clin Oncol. 1997;15(6):2403–13.

63. Palorini R, De Rasmo D, Gaviraghi M, Sala Danna L, Signorile A, Cirulli C, Chiaradonna F, Alberghina L, Papa S. Oncogenic K-ras expression is associated with derangement of the cAMP/PKA pathway and forskolin-

reversible alterations of mitochondrial dynamics and respiration. Oncogene. 2013;32(3):352–62.

64. Maher JC, Savaraj N, Priebe W, Liu H, Lampidis TJ. Differential sensitivity to 2-deoxy-D-glucose between two pancreatic cell lines correlates with GLUT-1 expression. Pancreas. 2005;30(2):e34–39.

65. Kim GT, Chun YS, Park JW, Kim MS. Role of apoptosis-inducing factor in myocardial cell death by ischemia-reperfusion. Biochem Biophys Res Commun. 2003;309(3):619–24.

66. Zhang X, Chen J, Graham SH, Du L, Kochanek PM, Draviam R, Guo F, Nathaniel PD, Szabo C, Watkins SC et al. Intranuclear localization of apoptosis-inducing factor (AIF) and large scale DNA fragmentation after traumatic brain injury in rats and in neuronal cultures exposed to peroxynitrite. J Neurochem. 2002;82(1):181–91.

67. Granville DJ, Cassidy BA, Ruehlmann DO, Choy JC, Brenner C, Kroemer G, van Breemen C, Margaron P, Hunt DW, McManus BM. Mitochondrial release of apoptosis-inducing factor and cytochrome c during smooth muscle cell apoptosis. Am J Pathol. 2001;159(1):305–11.

68. Cao G, Clark RS, Pei W, Yin W, Zhang F, Sun FY, Graham SH, Chen J. Translocation of apoptosis-inducing factor in vulnerable neurons after transient cerebral ischemia and in neuronal cultures after oxygen-glucose deprivation. J Cereb Blood Flow Metab. 2003;23(10):1137–50.

69. Zhu C, Qiu L, Wang X, Hallin U, Cande C, Kroemer G, Hagberg H, Blomgren K. Involvement of apoptosis-inducing factor in neuronal death after hypoxia-ischemia in the neonatal rat brain. J Neurochem. 2003;86(2):306–17.

70. Zhang W, Zhang C, Narayana N, Du C, Balaji KC. Nuclear translocation of apoptosis inducing factor is associated with cisplatin induced apoptosis in LNCaP prostate cancer cells. Cancer Lett. 2007;255(1):127–34.

71. Kang YH, Yi MJ, Kim MJ, Park MT, Bae S, Kang CM, Cho CK, Park IC, Park MJ, Rhee CH et al. Caspase-independent cell death by arsenic trioxide in human cervical cancer cells: reactive oxygen species-mediated poly(ADP-ribose) polymerase-1 activation signals apoptosis-inducing factor release from mitochondria. Cancer Res. 2004;64(24):8960–7.

72. Warburg O. On the origin of cancer cells. Science. 1956;123(3191):309–14.

73. Deberardinis RJ, Thompson CB. Cellular metabolism and disease: what do metabolic outliers teach us? Cell. 2012;148(6):1132–44.

74. Tan AS, Baty JW, Dong LF, Bezawork-Geleta A, Endaya B, Goodwin J, Bajzikova M, Kovarova J, Peterka M, Yan B et al. Mitochondrial Genome Acquisition Restores Respiratory Function and Tumorigenic Potential of Cancer Cells without Mitochondrial DNA. Cell Metab. 2015;21(1):81–94.

75. LeBleu VS, O'Connell JT, Gonzalez Herrera KN, Wikman H, Pantel K, Haigis MC, de Carvalho FM, Damascena A, Domingos Chinen LT, Rocha RM et al. PGC-1alpha mediates mitochondrial biogenesis and oxidative phosphorylation in cancer cells to promote metastasis. Nat Cell Biol. 2014; 16(10):992–1003–1001–1015.

76. Solaini G, Sgarbi G, Baracca A. Oxidative phosphorylation in cancer cells. Biochim Biophys Acta. 2011;1807(6):534–42.

77. Luo J, Guo P, Matsuda K, Truong N, Lee A, Chun C, Cheng SY, Korc M. Pancreatic cancer cell-derived vascular endothelial growth factor is biologically active in vitro and enhances tumorigenicity in vivo. Int J Cancer. 2001;92(3):361–9.

78. Holloway SE, Beck AW, Shivakumar L, Shih J, Fleming JB, Brekken RA. Selective blockade of vascular endothelial growth factor receptor 2 with an antibody against tumor-derived vascular endothelial growth factor controls the growth of human pancreatic adenocarcinoma xenografts. Ann Surg Oncol. 2006;13(8):1145–55.

7

Impact of RUNX2 on drug-resistant human pancreatic cancer cells with *p53* mutations

Toshinori Ozaki[1*†], Meng Yu[2†], Danjing Yin[3], Dan Sun[4], Yuyan Zhu[4], Youquan Bu[5] and Meixiang Sang[3]

Abstract

Background: Despite the remarkable advances in the early diagnosis and treatment, overall 5-year survival rate of patients with pancreatic cancer is less than 10%. Gemcitabine (GEM), a cytidine nucleoside analogue and ribonucleotide reductase inhibitor, is a primary option for patients with advanced pancreatic cancer; however, its clinical efficacy is extremely limited. This unfavorable clinical outcome of pancreatic cancer patients is at least in part attributable to their poor response to anti-cancer drugs such as GEM. Thus, it is urgent to understand the precise molecular basis behind the drug-resistant property of pancreatic cancer and also to develop a novel strategy to overcome this deadly disease.

Review: Accumulating evidence strongly suggests that *p53* mutations contribute to the acquisition and/or maintenance of drug-resistant property of pancreatic cancer. Indeed, certain p53 mutants render pancreatic cancer cells much more resistant to GEM, implying that *p53* mutation is one of the critical determinants of GEM sensitivity. Intriguingly, runt-related transcription factor 2 (RUNX2) is expressed at higher level in numerous human cancers such as pancreatic cancer and osteosarcoma, indicating that, in addition to its pro-osteogenic role, RUNX2 has a pro-oncogenic potential. Moreover, a growing body of evidence implies that a variety of miRNAs suppress malignant phenotypes of pancreatic cancer cells including drug resistance through the down-regulation of RUNX2. Recently, we have found for the first time that forced depletion of *RUNX2* significantly increases GEM sensitivity of *p53*-null as well as *p53*-mutated pancreatic cancer cells through the stimulation of p53 family TAp63/TAp73-dependent cell death pathway.

Conclusions: Together, it is likely that RUNX2 is one of the promising molecular targets for the treatment of the patients with pancreatic cancer regardless of their *p53* status. In this review article, we will discuss how to overcome the serious drug-resistant phenotype of pancreatic cancer.

Keywords: Gemcitabine, Mutant p53, p53 family, RUNX2

Background

Pancreatic cancer which is highly metastatic to lymph nodes, liver and the other distal sites, is one of the most lethal malignancies among human cancers with 5-year survival rate less than 10%, and its incidence is gradually increasing worldwide [1]. Although 20% of patients receive surgical resection at diagnosis, the remaining 80% of patients are identified as unresectable due to their late diagnosis [2]. Gemcitabine (GEM), a deoxycytidine analogue, has become a standard chemotherapeutic for the treatment of patients with advanced pancreatic cancer [3]. Unfortunately, its clinical efficacy is extremely limited and the extensive efforts to develop the combination regimes with GEM have resulted in only a minor improvement over the conventional therapies [4]. Therefore, it is urgent to develop novel treatment options against pancreatic cancer, and also to understand the precise molecular mechanisms how pancreatic cancer cells could acquire and maintain GEM-resistant phenotype.

As mentioned above, GEM resistance is a critical issue to be adequately addressed for the better treatment of pancreatic cancer patients. Accumulating evidence strongly suggests that the alterations within *KRAS*, *p53*, *CDKN2A* and *SMAD4* are frequently

* Correspondence: tozaki@chiba-cc.jp
†Equal contributors
[1]Laboratory of DNA Damage Signaling, Chiba Cancer Center Research Institute, Chiba 260-8717, Japan
Full list of author information is available at the end of the article

detected in pancreatic cancer tissues, and contribute to the genesis and/or maintenance of their advanced phenotypes including GEM resistance [5]. Among these genetic aberrations, *p53* mutations (around 75%) appear in the later stages of pancreatic cancer genesis and development [6, 7]. Since p53, which monitors and ensures the genomic integrity, is an essential molecular barrier against carcinogenesis [8, 9], it is possible that loss of function mutation of *p53* leads to the accumulation of genetic damage within pancreatic cancer cells, and thus they might acquire GEM-resistant property as well as metastatic potential.

RUNX2 (also called Osf2/Cbfa1, AML-3 or Peb-p2αA), a member of RUNX (runt-related transcription factor) family, has been shown to be one of the major determinants of osteoblast differentiation and bone formation [10]. As expected, RUNX2 transactivates number of pro-osteogenic target genes such as collagen type I, bone alkaline phosphatase, osteopontin and osteocalcin [11]. In addition to its pro-osteogenic role, a growing body of evidence strongly suggests that RUNX2 plays a vital role in tumor initiation, progression, invasion and metastasis. From the clinical point of view, the elevated expression level of RUNX2 has been shown to correlate to poor prognosis of patients with pancreatic cancer or with thyroid cancer [12, 13]. In support of these observations, it has been described that RUNX2 regulates numerous genes implicated in carcinogenesis including *MMP9* (matrixmetalloproteinase-9), *MMP13* (matrixmetalloproteinase-13), *VEGF* (vascular endothelial growth factor) and *survivin* [14–16]. Furthermore, Pratap et al. found that RUNX2 promotes invasion of bone metastatic cancer cells through the induction of MMP9, and also stimulates the early events of breast cancer progression [17, 18]. Recently, we have described for the first time that siRNA-mediated knockdown of *RUNX2* increases adriamycin (ADR) sensitivity of *p53*-wild-type osteosarcoma cells through the activation of p53 family-dependent cell death pathway [19, 20]. Our subsequent studies revealed that depletion of *RUNX2* improves GEM sensitivity of pancreatic cancer cells regardless of their *p53* status [21–23].

In this review article, we provide a brief overview of the molecular basis behind drug-resistant phenotype of pancreatic cancer cells, and also describe p53 family-dependent cell death pathway in response to DNA damage. Subsequently, we summarize the current understanding of oncogenic potential of RUNX2 and possible involvement of RUNX2 and various miRNAs in pancreatic cancer. Lastly, we discuss how to overcome the serious drug-resistant phenotype of pancreatic cancer.

Main text
Pancreatic cancer

Pancreatic cancer is ranked as the fourth leading cause of cancer-related death in the world (both in industrial countries as well as nonindustrial ones), and is known to exhibit the worst prognosis among cancers (5-year survival rate is less than 10%) [24, 25]. Its mortality rate is nearly equal to its incidence. Up to 80% of pancreatic cancer deaths take place within the first year of diagnosis. Although surgical resection is the only potentially curative approach against pancreatic cancer, greater than 80% of cases are judged as unresectable at the time of diagnosis due to its locally advanced property and/or metastasis. A highly invasive and metastatic nature of the advanced pancreatic cancer is often responsible for its extremely poor clinical outcome. Therefore, it is urgently required to identify the reliable diagnostic and/or prognostic markers. These biomarkers could be helpful to the accurate detection of pancreatic cancer in the early stage, and the prediction of its biological behavior.

Because of the low chance of successful surgery, chemotherapy is the most common approach to extend the survival time of pancreatic cancer patients. For advanced pancreatic cancer patients, a deoxycytidine analogue termed gemcitabine (GEM) (2′,2′-difluorodeoxycytidine) has been considered to be the first choice as a front-line chemotherapy based on the results of the Phase III trial [26, 27]. The cytotoxicity of GEM relies on its ability to promote cancer cell death. Similar to the related nucleoside analog termed cytarabine (Ara-C) [28], GEM is taken up within pancreatic cancer cells through equilibrative nucleoside transporter-1 (hENT1) [29], and subjected to deoxycytidine kinase (dCK)-mediated phosphorylation to become an active form (dFdCTP). dFdCTP is then incorporated at the end of the elongating DNA strand, terminates DNA replication process, and thereby inducing DNA fragmentation (cancer cell death) [30]. In addition to the advanced pancreatic cancer, GEM is also utilized to treat patients with the other serious diseases such as non-small-lung cell, breast, bladder, gastric and ovarian cancers. However, the response rate of GEM monotherapy is low and the improvement of 5-year survival rate is unsatisfied (less than 6 months) [31]. The efficacy of GEM is less than 20% of treated patients, and almost all the patients eventually become resistant to GEM [31].

Subsequently, the extensive studies to improve the unfavorable clinical outcome of the advanced pancreatic cancer patients by GEM-based combination therapies with the other anti-cancer drugs including fluorouracil, irinotecan, pemetrexed, oxaliplatin, exatecan, cisplatin and capecitabine, have been performed. Unfortunately, most of these combination therapies have failed to obtain much better results than GEM monotherapy [32–34]. Recently, it has been shown that the combination of GEM with erlotinib (Erlo) or GEM plus nab-paclitaxelm (nab-PTX) has marginal benefits in survival rate of patients with the advanced pancreatic cancer [35, 36]. In support of these observations, it is well known that pancreatic cancer is intrinsically resistant to GEM or acquires GEM resistance. To override GEM-resistant property of pancreatic cancer and improve clinical outcome of the patients, it is critical to understand the precise molecular mechanisms behind its GEM-resistance, and also to develop more efficient GEM-based treatment options for the patients.

Molecular basis underlying GEM-resistance of pancreatic cancer

As mentioned above, drug resistance is a hallmark of pancreatic cancer, and the poor clinical outcome of the patients is partly due to its drug-resistant phenotype. To date, various hypotheses explaining its drug resistance have been postulated. Firstly, it has been generally accepted that its drug resistance is generated by the aberrant overexpression of P-glycoprotein as well as the other transporters, and thereby reducing the accumulation of anti-cancer drugs inside cancer cells [37, 38]. For example, multidrug-resistance 1 (MDR1/ ABCB1/P-glycoprotein) is a transmembrane glycoprotein of 170 kDa and acts as an ATP-dependent drug-efflux pump. O'Driscoll et al. reported that MDR1 is expressed in the majority of pancreatic cancer tissues, indicative of its important contribution to their drug resistance [39]. Consistent with these observations, Song et al. demonstrated that depletion of *MDR1* sensitizes GEM-resistant pancreatic cancer Panc-1 cells to GEM [40]. Intriguingly, Zhang et al. found that Ser/Thr kinase PLK1 is expressed at higher level in pancreatic cancer tissues as compared to normal pancreatic ones, and a potent PLK1 inhibitor DMTC acts synergistically with GEM [41]. Recently, Li et al. demonstrated that PLK1 inhibitor GSK461364A enhances the efficacy of GEM [42]. As described [40], PLK1 augmented c-fos-mediated induction of MDR1, suggesting that PLK1 reduces GEM sensitivity of pancreatic cancer cells through up-regulation of MDR1. Another transporter responsible for drug resistance is MDR-related protein MRP1/2 (ABCC1/2). Lee et al. showed that MRP1 and MRP2 are expressed in 84 and 91% of pancreatic cancer cases [43]. Nath et al. found that a significantly higher expression level of *MRP1* is closely associated with GEM-resistant phenotype of pancreatic cancer cells [44].

Since the diffusion of hydrophilic GEM through the plasma membrane lipid bilayer is very slow, the efficient cellular uptake of GEM requires the specialized membrane nucleoside transporter protein(s) [45]. Among the nucleoside transporters, it has been shown that human equilibrative nucleoside transporter 1 (hENT1) plays a major role to facilitate the intracellular uptake of GEM across the plasma membrane [46]. Indeed, *ENT1*-deficient cells were highly resistant to GEM [45], and forced expression of hENT1 enhanced GEM response of pancreatic cancer cells [47]. In accordance with these results, hENT-positive pancreatic cancer patients had a prolonged survival rate after GEM treatment relative to the patients without detectable hENT [48]. Similarly, Nordh et al. described that the expression level of hENT is a reliable predictive indicator for pancreatic cancer patients treated with GEM [49]. Therefore, it is likely that the defect(s) in hENT-mediated intracellular uptake of GEM renders pancreatic cancer cells resistant to GEM.

Meanwhile, it has been well documented that tumor suppressor *p53* is frequently mutated in pancreatic cancer tissues (around 75%) [50], indicating that mutant p53 contributes to the development of GEM-resistant nature of pancreatic cancer. Notably, Florini et al. detected GEM-mediated stabilization of mutant p53 at protein level in pancreatic cancer cells [51]. We have also observed the similar phenomenon [22]. In the next chapter, we would like to describe p53 and its family members.

p53-dependent cell death pathway

p53 is one of the well-studied tumor suppressor genes. Since p53 is able to protect cells from serious DNA damage and thus prevent carcinogenesis, p53 is called "guardian of the genome" [52]. Under the normal conditions, p53 is kept at an extremely low level. Upon cellular stresses such as DNA damage, oncogene activation, hypoxia and telomere shortening, p53 becomes stabilized at protein level, activated through the sequential post-translational modifications and then triggers a cascade of the molecular events which determines cell fate such as cell cycle arrest, cellular senescence and/or cell death [53]. These chemical modifications including phosphorylation and acetylation, which attenuate MDM2 (murine double minute 2 homolog)-mediated degradation of p53, extend the half-life of p53, and thereby increasing the intracellular p53 level. MDM2 with an E3 ubiquitin protein ligase enzymatic activity, catalyzes poly-ubiquitination of p53 and facilitates its rapid degradation through proteasome [54, 55]. Once activated, p53 functions as a sequence-specific transcription factor to transactivate a large number of its downstream target genes implicated in the regulation of the above-mentioned cellular processes. For example, p21^{WAF1} and 14-3-3σ are involved in the induction of p53-dependent G1/S and G2/M cell cycle arrest (cell survival), respectively. While, p53-mediated transcriptional activation of BAX, PUMA, NOXA and/or p53AIP1 participates in the proper cell death response. Therefore, p53 stands at the crossroad between cell survival and death, which might rely on the intensity of stress signal and/or extent of cellular damage (Fig. 1).

p53 is frequently mutated in around 50% of human cancers [56]. The majority of mutations occur within its central core sequence-specific DNA-binding domain with 6 hot spots at codons such as R175, G245, R248, R249, R273 and R282, and result in the production of conformationally aberrant p53 proteins (mutant p53). *p53* hot spot mutations account for 30% of all reported ones. These observations indicate that mutant p53 lacks the sequence-specific transactivation capability. Since pro-apoptotic function of wild-type p53 is tightly linked to its sequence-specific transcriptional activity, mutant p53 fails to suppress tumor initiation as well as progression. Of note, most common *p53* mutations not only impair its tumor-suppressor function (loss of function) but also confer novel pro-oncogenic potential on p53 (gain of function), which markedly enhances tumor progression and drug resistance [57]. Knock-in mice expressing mutant p53 (R175H and R273H) displayed an accelerated tumor growth, which was more invasive and metastatic relative to that of *p53*-deficient mice [58]. In addition to R175H and R273H mutants, Hanel et al. found that R248 mutant mice show gain of function in carcinogenesis [59]. These findings strongly suggest that at least certain p53 mutants exhibit gain of function. In

support of this notion, it has been demonstrated that mutant p53 has an ability to transactivate various pro-oncogenic genes such as *MYC*, *PDGFR*, *HGFR*, *EGFR* and *MDR1* [60]. Recently, Zhao et al. described that Pontin with an ATPase activity interacts with mutant p53 and facilitates its transcriptional activity [61]. Intriguingly, overexpression of Pontin is detectable in a variety of cancer tissues, and strongly associated with poor prognosis of the patients [62]. In addition to Pontin, PML and Pin1 have been shown to enhance the transcriptional capability of mutant p53 through the direct interaction [63, 64].

In a sharp contrast to wild-type p53 with an extremely short half-life (around 20 min), mutant p53, which escapes from ubiquitin/proteasome-dependent degradation pathway mediated by MDM2, has an extended half-life. It has been shown that molecular chaperone Hsp90 is associated with mutant p53, prevents its degradation, and thus facilitates its accumulation in cancer cells [65]. The strong immunohistochemical positivity for p53 has been employed as a diagnostic indicator for the presence of a *p53* mutation [57]. Since the vast majority of *p53* mutations occur within its central core sequence-specific DNA-binding domain, mutant p53 retains an intact COOH-terminal oligomerization domain. Therefore, a large amount of mutant p53 forms a hetero-oligomer with wild-type p53 *via* its oligomerization domain through which mutant p53 displays a dominant-negative

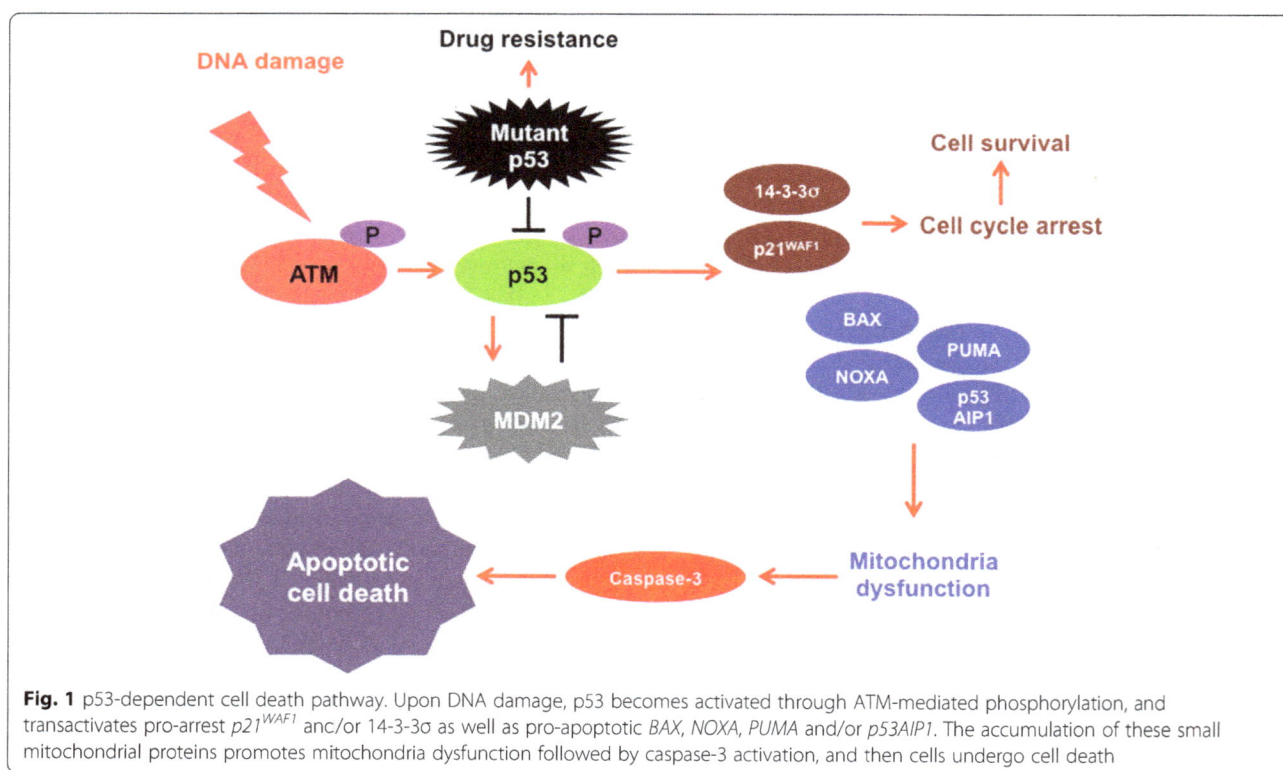

Fig. 1 p53-dependent cell death pathway. Upon DNA damage, p53 becomes activated through ATM-mediated phosphorylation, and transactivates pro-arrest *p21^{WAF1}* anc/or 14-3-3σ as well as pro-apoptotic *BAX*, *NOXA*, *PUMA* and/or *p53AIP1*. The accumulation of these small mitochondrial proteins promotes mitochondria dysfunction followed by caspase-3 activation, and then cells undergo cell death

behavior against wild-type p53 [66]. This hetero-oligomerization diminishes the tumor-suppressive function of wild-type p53. Emerging evidence suggests that *p53* status of cancer cells is closely associated with their sensitivity to anti-cancer drugs [67–69]. Together, the gain of function (GOF) and/or loss of function (LOF) mutations of *p53* might be one of the possible molecular mechanisms of the serious drug resistance of cancer cells. Considering that one half of cancer cells express wild-type p53 but not mutant p53, the presence of *p53* mutation-independent mechanisms, which could disrupt p53-dependent cell death pathway, should also be kept in mind.

MDM2, a negative regulator of p53

As described above, around half of cancer patients carry wild-type *p53*, raising a question why the patients harboring wild-type *p53* sometimes do not respond to the standard chemotherapy. A number of evidence indicates that, apart from mutant p53, the other cellular factors might directly prohibit wild-type p53 and/or disrupt the upstream or downstream p53-dependent cell death pathway. Among them, MDM2 is one of the major negative regulators of p53. MDM2 deficiency promoted p53-dependent cell death in a variety of cells [70]. *p53* is infrequently mutated in glioblastoma; however, wild-type p53 remains dysfunctional due to the overexpression of MDM2 [71]. In addition to the stimulation of proteasomal degradation of p53, MDM2 binds to NH_2-terminal transactivation domain I (TD1) of p53, strongly prohibits it from serving as a transcriptional activator, and thereby attenuates p53-mediated cell death in response to DNA damage. Alternatively, MDM2 interacts with p53 and drives its sequestration in the cytoplasm. Subcellular localization of p53 is regulated through its ubiquitination status. It has been shown that MDM2-mediated monoubiquitination of p53 induces its nuclear export and polyubiquitination facilitates its proteasomal degradation [72].

Since *MDM2* is one of the downstream target genes of p53, its expression is tightly regulated in a p53-dependent manner. Thus, p53 modulates the intracellular expression level of its own negative regulator MDM2 *via* a feedback loop [73]. As a result of this regulatory system, the amounts of p53 and MDM2 are maintained at extremely low level under the healthy conditions. In contrast to normal cells, *MDM2* gene is sometimes amplified and/or aberrantly overexpressed in number of cancers including pancreatic cancer [74, 75]. The overall frequency of *MDM2* gene amplification in human cancers is around 7%; however, cancer tissues such as osteosarcoma (16%), soft tissue tumors (31%), hepatocellular carcinoma (44%) and Hodgkin disease (67%) have the

higher frequencies of *MDM2* gene amplification [76]. It is worth noting that the elevated level of *MDM2* expression is significantly associated with poor clinical outcome of the patients with pancreatic cancer [77, 78]. In a good agreement with these observations, the abnormal overexpression of MDM2 caused by its gene amplification and/or transcriptional activation mediated by p53, disrupts the balance between the intracellular amounts of p53 and MDM2, and then promotes tumor development [79]. Wade et al. described that a 2-fold increase in MDM2 expression level is enough to prohibit p53 activation [80]. As expected, shRNA-mediated knockdown of *MDM2* suppressed proliferation rate and tumor growth potential of highly metastatic pancreatic cancer cells [81]. Under their experimental conditions, depletion of *MDM2* caused an up- and down-regulation of *p53* and *MMP9*, respectively.

Consistent with those results, Kondo et al. have described that MDM2 plays a vital role in the development of resistance to CDDP (cisplatin) in human glioblastoma cells [82]. Suzuki et al. demonstrated that forced expression of MDM2 overrides wild-type p53 and confers ADR (adriamycin) resistance on breast cancer cells [83]. Meijer et al. reported that a small chemical compound termed Nutlin-3, which binds to MDM2 and inhibits its interaction with p53, preferentially enhances drug-sensitivity of wild-type *p53*-expressing ovarian cancer cells through the accumulation of wild-type p53 [84]. Collectively, MDM2-mediated dysfunction of p53 is one of the primary molecular mechanisms underlying *p53* mutation-independent acquisition of chemo-resistance.

p53 family

Following the identification of p53, two independent p53-related nuclear transcription factors such as p73 and p63 have been discovered (p53 family members) [85, 86]. These p53 family members have a similar exon/intron organization and display a remarkable amino acid sequence similarity especially in their central DNA-binding domains (around 63%). Subsequent studies revealed that both *p73* and *p63* genes encode multiple variants, which are basically divided into two groups such as transcription-competent TA (TAp73 and TAp63) and transcription-deficient ΔN (ΔNp73 and ΔNp63) isoforms. The alternative splicing events produce various TA isoforms with the distinct COOH-terminal portions as well as the different tranactivation potential. While, the alternative promoter usage gives rise to NH_2-terminaly truncated ΔN isoforms, which lack the first TA (transactivation) domain. As expected from their differential transactivation potentials, TA and ΔN isoforms have their own physiological functions. As described [87, 88], *TAp73-* or *TAp63*-null mice developed spontaneous tumors, indicating that, like p53, TAp73 and TAp63 act as tumor suppressors. On the other hand, *ΔNp73-* or *ΔNp63*-deficient mice displayed complex developmental defects in the nervous system or in the epidermis and limbs, respectively [89, 90].

Like p53, TAp73/TAp63 are induced following genotoxic insults, recruited onto p53-responsive elements within the promoter regions of the overlapping set of p53-target pro-apoptotic genes including *BAX*, *PUMA*, *NOXA* and/or *p53AIP1*, and then efficiently promote cell death [91]. The expression of TAp73 is regulated at both mRNA and protein levels. Lissy et al. revealed that *TAp73* is transactivated by E2F-1 in response to cell death stimulus [91]. Basically similar results were also reported from several independent groups, suggesting that E2F-1 triggers cell death through the activation of TAp73-dependent cell death pathway [92–94]. Alternatively, several lines of evidence suggest that Sp1 (specificity protein 1) and Nrf-2 (nuclear factor erythroid 2-related factor 2) stimulate *TAp73* transcription [95, 96]. By contrast, Fontemaggi et al. found that *TAp73* expression is down-regulated by the transcriptional repressor ZEB-1 during differentiation [97]. While, Rossi et al. found that HECT domain-containing Nedd4-like E3 ubiquitin ligase Itch binds to TAp73/TAp63 and promotes their proteolytic degradation through proteasome [98, 99]. According to their results, the expression level of Itch was significantly reduced in response to DNA damage caused by ADR, VP16 or ADR, implying that DNA damage-mediated reduction of Itch contributes at least in part to the increased stability of TAp73/TAp63. Consistent with these observations, Hansen et al. described that silencing of *Itch* increases drug sensitivity of cancer cells even in the absence of functional p53 [100]. Notably, it has been shown that TAp73/TAp63 are required for p53-dependent cell death in response to DNA damage, whereas TAp73/TAp63 induce DNA damage-mediated cell death without functional p53 [101]. Since *p73/p63* are rarely mutated in human cancer tissues [102], TAp73/TAp63 are expressed as the functional wild-type forms, raising a possibility that, instead of wild-type p53, TAp73/TAp63 might trigger DNA damage-mediated cell death in *p53*-null and/or *p53*-mutated cancer cells.

Unlike TAp73/TAp63, ΔNp73/ΔNp63 lack the acidic NH$_2$-terminal transactivation domain. As expected, ΔNp73/ΔNp63 fail to specifically transactivate p53-target gene promoters, although they are capable to bind to p53-responsve elements within them. Intriguingly, it has been described that ΔNp73/ΔNp63 exert their own transcriptional activities, which is dependent on two additional transactivation domains located between their COOH-terminal oligomerization domain and SAM domain, and close to the Pro-rich domain [103]. Therefore, ΔNp73/ΔNp63 have an ability to activate their own downstream target gene promoters [104]. For example, Wu et al. found that ΔNp63 activates pro-metastatic *Hsp70* gene transcription [105]. Soldevilla et al. reported that *ABCB1* and *HMGB1* are the putative downstream target genes of ΔNp73 [106]. In addition to the transactivation of pro-oncogenic genes, ΔNp73/ΔNp63 act as the dominant-negative inhibitors against TAp73/TAp63 and wild-type p53 through the formation of the inactive complexes with them or the competition for promoter binding sites [107]. Indeed, ΔNp73 is overexpressed in a variety of cancers including lung, breast, brain, thymus, colon, ovary, skin and prostate cancers [108, 109], and this up-regulation of ΔNp73 has been shown to tightly link to poor prognosis of cancer patients [110]. Leung et al. demonstrated that ΔNp73 contributes to the development of CDDP resistance of ovarian cancer cells through the activation of pro-oncogenic AKT signaling pathway [111]. For ΔNp63, its overexpression was detectable in head and neck, lung, esophagus, bladder, liver and tongue cancers [112, 113], and the increased expression of ΔNp63 has been considered to be unfavorable clinical indicator of patients with melanoma [114]. Rocco et al. found that ΔNp63 attenuates TAp73-dependent cell death pathway, and acts as the major determinant of CDDP sensitivity of head and neck cancer [115]. Together, it is likely that, although mutant p53 and ΔNp73/ΔNp63 have a strong dominant-negative potential against TAp73/TAp63, the response to anti-cancer drugs of cancer cells lacking wild-type p53 might be determined at least in part by functional TAp73/TAp63 (Fig. 2). With these in mind, we have to discuss especially how to override the negative effect of mutant p53 on TAp73/TAp63.

Pro-oncogenic RUNX2

Runt-domain containing transcription factor 2 (also called Osf2/Cbfa1, AML-3 or Pebp2αA) is a member of RUNX family, which is identified by an evolutionary conserved DNA-binding/protein-protein interaction domain called runt-homology domain. In contrast to the other RUNX family members such as RUNX1 and RUNX3 whose mutations are tightly linked to the promotion of leukemia and gastric cancer, respectively [116, 117], the initial studies strongly suggest that RUNX2 acts as a master regulator of osteoblast differentiation and bone development. In support of this notion, *RUNX2*-deficient mice died shortly after birth due to a complete lack of bone formation with arrest of osteoblast differentiation [118, 119]. During bone development, RUNX2 facilitates the differentiation of mesenchymal stem cells into the osteoblast lineage [120]. As expected, RUNX2 transactivates its downstream target gene promoters implicated in these cellular and

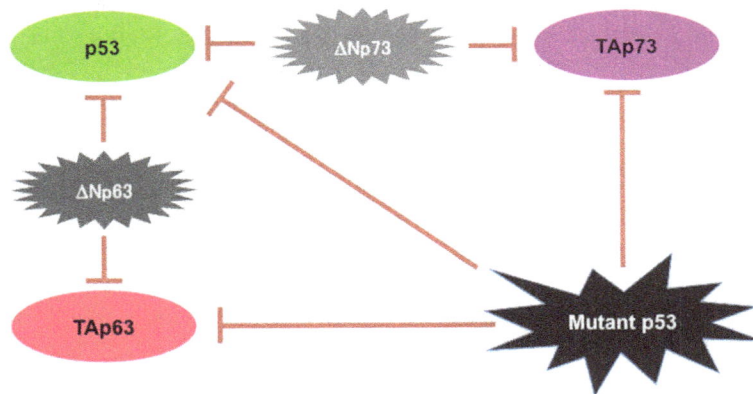

Fig. 2 Functional interplay among p53 family members. Mutant p53 inhibits pro-apoptotic wild-type p53, TAp73 and TAp63 through the direct interaction, and thus contributes to the acquisition and/or maintenance of the serious drug-resistant phenotype of malignant tumors

developmental processes including collagen type I, bone alkaline phosphatase, osteopontin and osteocalcin. Of note, Liu et al. demonstrated that RUNX2 is a prerequisite for the early stage of osteoblast differentiation, whereas its overexpression attenuates the subsequent osteoblast maturation [121]. Thus, it is indicative that *RUNX2* is under the strict transcriptional and/or post-translational regulation during the cellular differentiation as well as development.

Recently, the possible involvement of RUNX2 in tumor initiation/progression has been increasingly recognized depending on the cellular context. In addition to osteogenesis-related genes, RUNX2 has an ability to transactivate its downstream target genes involved in tumor progression, invasion and metastasis such as *MMP9*, *MMP13*, *VEGF*, *survivin*, *IL-8* and *TGFβR* [14–16, 122–124]. The extensive expression studies demonstrated that the expression level of RUNX2 is aberrantly elevated in numerous cancer tissues as compared to their corresponding normal ones including pancreatic cancer, breast cancer, prostate cancer and osteosarcoma [125]. Of note, overexpression of RUNX2 has been shown to cause a poor response to chemotherapy of certain cancer cells. For example, *RUNX2* gene is sometimes amplified, overexpressed in osteosarcomas and thus has been employed as a reliable marker for the estimation of their chemo-resistance [126, 127]. Roos et al. have revealed that loss of RUNX2 expression increases ADR sensitivity of osteosarcoma cells [128]. Similarly, RUNX2 was aberrantly overexpressed in breast cancer cells and promoted their progression [17, 18, 129]. Consistent with these observations, El-Gendi and Mostafa have described that the expression level of RUNX2 is a potential prognostic indicator for breast cancer [130]. As expected, targeting of *RUNX2* suppressed breast cancer progression and bone metastasis

[131]. Additionally, it has been shown that the abnormally higher RUNX2 expression level in prostate cancer tissues is positively associated with their stage and aggressiveness [132]. For pancreatic cancer, Kayed et al. found that the increased expression level of *RUNX2* correlates to unfavorable prognosis of the patients with this serious disease [12]. Given those findings, it is suggestive that RUNX2 is a potential diagnostic marker and/or therapeutic target of the advanced tumors such as pancreatic cancer.

Growth of solid tumors including pancreatic cancer often depends on angiogenesis with the continuous blood vessel formation, and thus the inhibition of tumor angiogenesis is a potential strategy for cancer treatment [133]. Indeed, numerous studies have shown that the attenuation of tumor angiogenesis prohibits pancreatic cancer growth and metastasis [134–136]. Among RUNX2-target gene products as described above, VEGF is the most potent angiogenic cytokine [137]. Through the binding to its receptors (VEGFR-1 and VEGFR-2) whose expression is predominantly restricted to endothelial cells in blood vessels, VEGF triggers a variety of downstream survival and migration pathways, and then induces angiogenesis. For transcriptional regulation of *VEGF*, a large body of evidence suggests that *VEGF* is transcriptionally activated by hypoxia-inducible factor (HIF). Hypoxia is a major stimulator of angiogenesis. HIF is a heterodimeric transcription factor composed of an oxygen-sensitive alpha subunit (HIF-1α or HIF-2α) and a constitutively expressed beta subunit (HIF-1β). Under normoxic conditions, HIF-1α and HIF-2α are subjected to a rapid hydroxylation at their proline residues, followed by proteasomal degradation mediated by an E3 ubiquitin ligase VHL (von Hippel-Lindau). By contrast, HIF-1α as well as HIF-2α is stabilized at protein level due to the strong inhibition of its hydroxylation and ubiquitination under hypoxic conditions, forms an active HIF transcriptional complex with its binding partner HIF-1β in cell nucleus and regulates its downstream target gene expression. Since HIF-1β is not affected by oxygen concentration and is expressed in excess, the protein levels of HIF-1α and HIF-2α are responsible for HIF transcriptional activity [138, 139]. As expected from those observations, HIF-1α was highly expressed in several solid tumors, and forced suppression of HIF-1α impaired tumor angiogenesis, growth and metastasis [140, 141].

In addition to HIF transcription complex, Zelzer et al. demonstrated for the first time that RUNX2 directly binds to *VEGF* promoter region, and stimulates its transcription [142]. According to their results, targeting *RUNX2* resulted in a significant loss of VEGF expression in mice, and overexpression of RUNX2 in cultured murine fibroblasts caused an obvious increase in *VEGF* mRNA level. Alternatively, Lee et al. found that RUNX2 has an ability to increase the protein stability and transcriptional activity of HIF-1α by competing with VHL to block its ubiquitination [143]. From their results, ectopic expression of RUNX2 promoted the nuclear access of HIF-1α, elevated the secretion of VEGF, and augmented the *in vitro* and *in vivo* angiogenesis, indicative that RUNX2 acts as a potent inducer of angiogenesis through the enhancement of HIF-1α-dependent transactivation of *VEGF*. Intriguingly, Rhaman et al have reported that VEGF enhances the protein stability of RUNX2 by blocking its degradation, indicating the presence of a positive feedback loop between VEGF and RUNX2, which might synergistically modulate angiogenesis [144]. In a sharp contrast to RUNX2, it has been shown that RUNX3 is recruited onto the putative RUNX3-binding sites of *VEGF* promoter, trans-represses its transcription, and suppresses gastric cancer angiogenesis [145]. Peng et al. described that RUNX1 physically interacts with HIF-1α and prohibits its transcriptional activity [146]. Under their experimental conditions, forced expression of RUNX1 resulted in a marked decrease in *VEGF* mRNA level. These observations raise a possibility that RUNX family members might differentially regulate angiogenesis. Since, among RUNX family proteins, RUNX2 strongly stimulates VEGF-dependent angiogenesis, RUNX2 might be an attractive molecular target for therapies, which seek to repress malignant progression of solid tumors such as pancreatic cancer.

Functional interplay between p53 family and RUNX2

Previously, we have found that tumor-suppressive RUNX3 enhances pro-apoptotic activity of p53 in osteosarcoma-derived U2OS cells exposed to ADR through the stimulation of ATM-dependent phosphorylation of p53 at Ser-15 [147]. Subsequent studies revealed that another RUNX family member RUNX1 facilitates

p300-mediated acetylation of p53 at Lys-373/382 and thus augments p53-induced cell death of U2OS cells in response to ADR [148]. We then asked whether there could exist a functional interaction between p53 and the remaining RUNX family member RUNX2. In a sharp contrast to RUNX1 and RUNX3, we have found for the first time that RUNX2 strongly prohibits p53/TAp73-mediated cell death of U2OS cells following ADR exposure. Based on our prior results, RUNX2 was associated with histone deacetylase HDAC6 as well as p53 and impaired its transcriptional and pro-apoptotic activities. In addition to p53, RUNX2 repressed *TAp73* transcription and also bound to TAp73 to diminish its pro-apoptotic activity. These observations were in accordance with the recent findings of Roos et al. showing that shRNA-mediated knockdown of *RUNX2* increases ADR sensitivity of osteosarcoma cells [128].

As described above, U2OS cells bearing wild-type *p53* undergo cell death following DNA damage primarily in a p53-dependent manner. Therefore, it is of interest to ask whether RUNX2 could be also involved in poor drug response of *p53*-null or *p53*-mutated cancer cells. To this end, we have employed pancreatic cancer cells in which *p53* is frequently mutated. Firstly, Sugimoto et al. revealed that depletion of *RUNX2* improves GEM sensitivity of *p53*-negative pancreatic cancer AsPC-1 cells through the stimulation of TAp63-dependent cell death pathway [21]. Secondary, Nakamura et al. demonstrated that GEM sensitivity of *p53*-mutated pancreatic cancer MiaPaCa-2 cells is increased by *RUNX2* depletion-mediated up-regulation of TAp73 [22]. Recently, we have found that RUNX2 suppresses TAp63 expression and also impairs its pro-apoptotic activity in *p53*-mutated pancreatic cancer Panc-1 cells [23]. These observations imply that RUNX2 is implicated in poor response to GEM of pancreatic cancer cells lacking functional p53, and TAp73/TAp63 might potentiate GEM-induced cell death of *RUNX2*-knocked down pancreatic cancer cells instead of wild-type p53 (Fig. 3). Previously, Flores et al. described that p53 requires TAp73 and/or TAp63 for DNA damage-induced cell death, whereas TAp73 or TAp63 is capable to promote cell death in response to DNA damage without functional p53 [101]. Thus, it is possible that *RUNX2* gene silencing-mediated up-regulation of TAp63 augments GEM-induced cell death of *p53*-null AsPC-1 cells. For *p53*-mutated MiaPaCa-2 and Panc-1 cells, it has been shown that mutant p53 acts as a strong dominant-negative inhibitor against TAp73 and TAp63 [149].

The question is how *RUNX2* depletion could partially override the negative effect of mutant p53 on TAp73/TAp63. Recently, Wang et al. reported that, in contrast to *RUNX2*, low ATF3 (activating transcription factor 3) expression level is significantly associated with poor

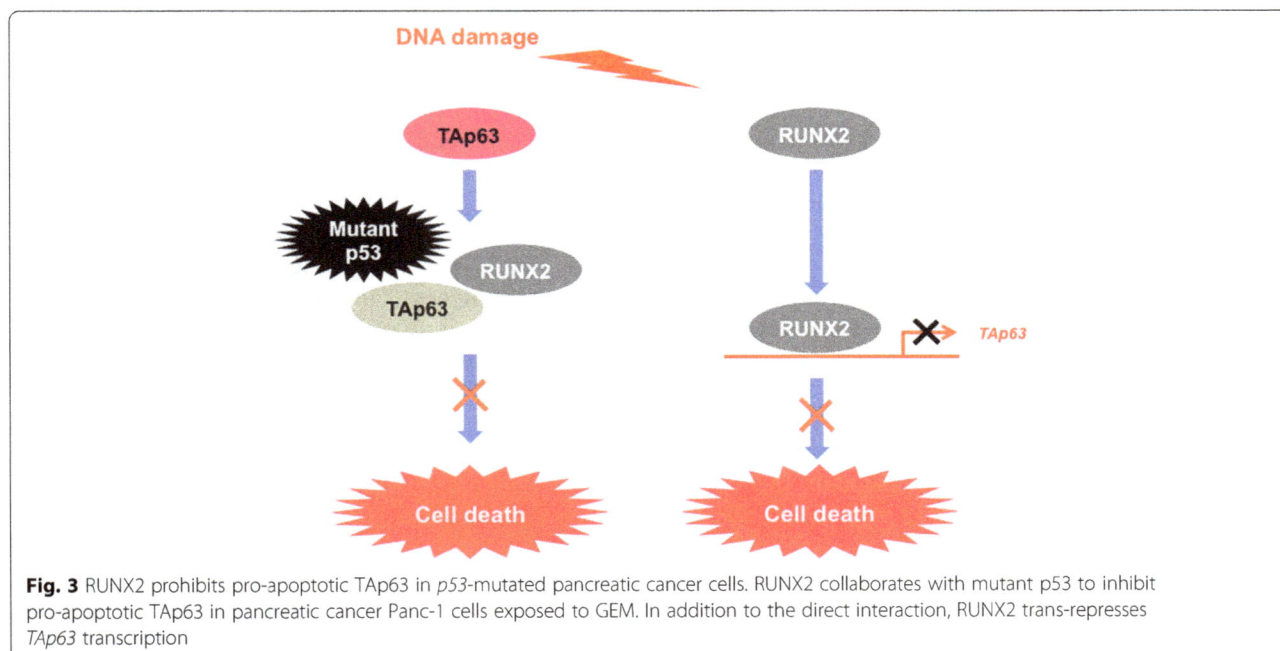

Fig. 3 RUNX2 prohibits pro-apoptotic TAp63 in *p53*-mutated pancreatic cancer cells. RUNX2 collaborates with mutant p53 to inhibit pro-apoptotic TAp63 in pancreatic cancer Panc-1 cells exposed to GEM. In addition to the direct interaction, RUNX2 trans-represses *TAp63* transcription

survival of prostate cancer patients, indicating that ATF3 might serve as a tumor suppressor against prostate cancer [150]. In line with these findings, *ATF3* deficiency promoted prostate cancer development in *PTEN*-knockout mice [151]. Of note, Wei et al. found that ATF3 binds to COOH-terminal portion of mutant p53 and diminishes its pro-oncogenic activity [152]. Forced expression of ATF3 sensitized mutant p53-expressing cancer cells to CDDP or VP16. Further analysis demonstrated that ATF3 disrupts the physical interaction between mutant p53 and TAp63, and thereby facilitates the reactivation of TAp63. In addition to TAp63 reactivation, ATF3 impaired pro-oncogenic activity of mutant p53 through the direct binding. Therefore, it is suggestive that *RUNX2* depletion might enhance ATF3 expression and/or activity and thereby augment TAp63-mediated cell death even in the presence of a large amount of mutant p53. However, Gokulnath et al. described that ATF3 is efficiently recruited onto *RUNX2* promoter and stimulates its transcription in bone metastatic breast cancer cells, indicating that *RUNX2* is a direct downstream target gene of ATF3 [153]. Further studies should be necessary to verify the functional significance of the interaction among RUNX2, ATF3, mutant p53 and TAp63 in the acquisition and/or maintenance of drug-resistant phenotype of pancreatic cancer cells.

Implication of microRNA-mediated down-regulation of *RUNX2* in pancreatic cancer

MicroRNAs (miRNAs) are a family of small (20-25 nucleotides in length) and single-stranded non-coding RNAs, which bind to the 3'-untranslated region of their target mRNAs in a sequence-specific manner, and repress their expressions through mRNA degradation and/or translation inhibition [154, 155]. An individual miRNA has a capability to regulate numerous distinct mRNAs. Intriguingly, miRNAs act as either oncogenes or tumor suppressor genes, which might be dependent on their target genes. It has been described that the dysregulated expression of certain miRNAs is closely associated with proliferation rate, invasion potential and chemo-sensitivity of pancreatic cancer cells [156]. For example, Lu et al. found that miR-301a whose expression level is specifically elevated in pancreatic cancer tissues, contributes to the persistent activation of NF-κB-mediated pro-oncogenic signaling pathway [157]. By contrast, Liang et al. demonstrated that miR-33a is capable to increase the sensitivity of pancreatic cancer cells to GEM through the down-regulation of pro-oncogenic AKT/Gsk-3β/β-catenin signaling pathway [158]. Ji et al. reported that miR-34 family members have tumor-suppressive function downstream of p53, and their restoration renders *p53*-mutated pancreatic cancer cells 2-3-fold more sensitive to GEM [159].

Meanwhile, Huang et al. found the inverse relationship between the expression levels of miR-204/miR-211 and RUNX2 during adipocyte differentiation, and also demonstrated for the first time that miR-204/miR-211 bind to the 3'-untranslated region of *RUNX2*, and attenuate its expression, indicating that miR-204/miR-211 act as the negative regulators of *RUNX2* [160]. In support of their observations, Wu et al. described that miR-30 family members prohibit BMP-2-induced osteoblast differentiation by targeting *RUNX2* [161]. It has been shown that the additional miRNAs (miR-23a, miR-34c, miR-133a, miR-135a, miR-205 and miR-217) also attenuate osteogenesis by targeting *RUNX2* [162, 163]. In addition to adipocyte and osteoblast differentiation, Saini et al. revealed that ectopic expression of miR-203 impairs the development of metastasis originated from prostate cancer in association with the down-regulation of pro-metastatic genes such as *ZEB2*, *survivin* and *RUNX2* [164]. van der Deen et al. described that p53-mediated stimulation of miR-34c expression causes a massive decrease in RUNX2 and reduces the metastatic potential of osteosarcoma cells [165]. Considering that the aberrant overexpression of RUNX2 correlates to resistance to chemotherapy [166], it is indicative that miR-34c contributes to the improvement of chemo-sensitivity of drug-resistant osteosarcoma cells through the down-regulation of RUNX2. Moreover, Li et al. found that the lower expression level of miR-23b is associated with worse prognosis of ovarian cancer patients, and miR-23b-induced repression of RUNX2 slow downs ovarian cancer cell proliferation [167]. Recently, Taipaleenmäki et al. showed that malignant phenotypes of breast cancer cells are significantly suppressed by miR-135/miR-203-caused direct reduction of RUNX2. Together, these observations suggest that *RUNX2*-targeting miRNAs effectively suppress the progression and/or metastasis of various types of aggressive tumors including pancreatic cancer.

Notably, miR-203, which prohibits prostate cancer cell metastasis, has also been shown to reduce migration/

invasion capacity of pancreatic cancer cells [168]. Chen et al. reported that miR-204 is highly expressed in normal pancreatic ductal tissues relative to pancreatic cancer tissues, and promotes pancreatic cancer cell death [169]. miRNA profiling studies revealed that miR-205 is down-regulated in GEM-resistant pancreatic cancer cells and metastatic pancreatic cancer tissues [170]. Zhao et al. found that the expression level of miR-217 is significantly lower in pancreatic cancer tissues as compared to that in normal ones, and exogenous miR-217 reduces tumor growth in mouse xenograft models [171]. As mentioned above, these miRNAs such as miR-203, miR-204, miR-205 and miR-217 negatively regulate RUNX2 expression, raising a possibility that miRNA-induced down-regulation of RUNX2 contributes to the suppression of malignant properties of pancreatic cancer cells such as drug resistance (Fig. 4).

Conclusions

Since the patients with pancreatic cancer show the worst prognosis despite the extensive therapy, it is urgent to develop a novel strategy to enable its early detection and increase its drug sensitivity. For this purpose, the precise understanding of the biology of pancreatic cancer and also molecular mechanisms how pancreatic cancer cells could acquire and maintain this serious drug-resistant phenotype should be required. An increasing body of evidence has demonstrated that RUNX2 is aberrantly overexpressed in numerous cancer tissues including pancreatic cancer relative to their corresponding normal

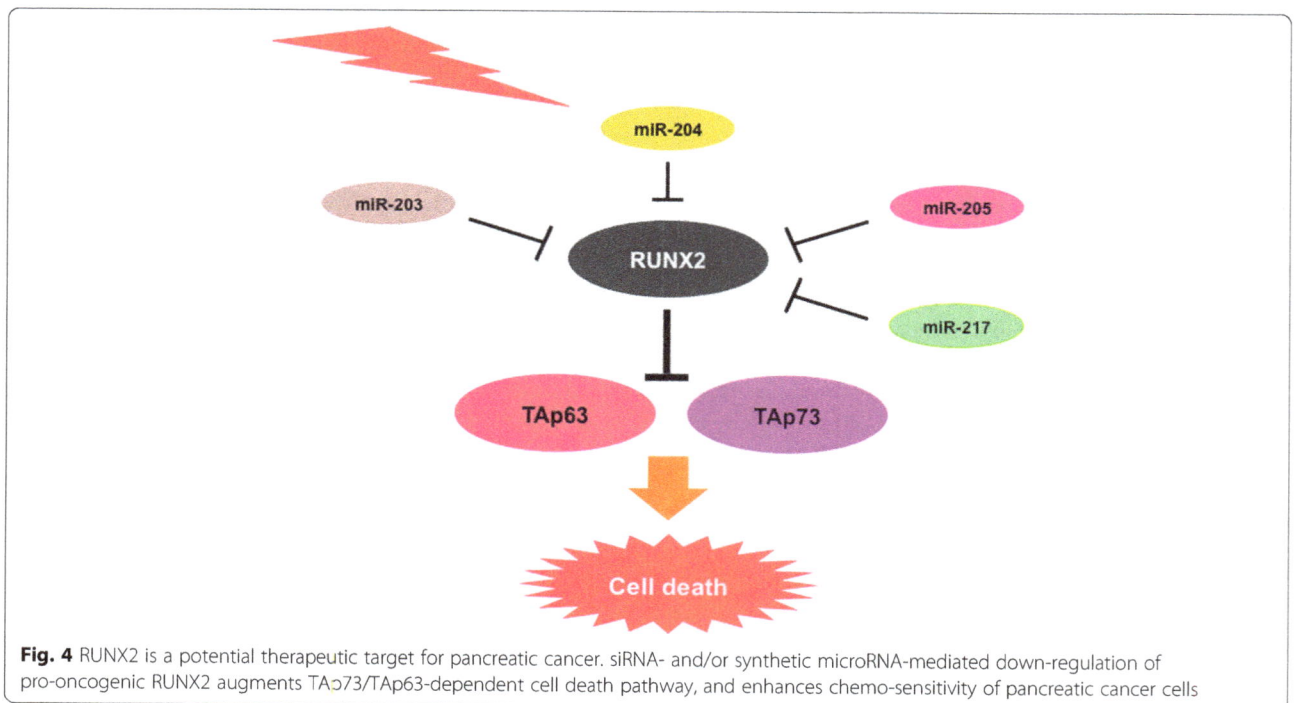

Fig. 4 RUNX2 is a potential therapeutic target for pancreatic cancer. siRNA- and/or synthetic microRNA-mediated down-regulation of pro-oncogenic RUNX2 augments TAp73/TAp63-dependent cell death pathway, and enhances chemo-sensitivity of pancreatic cancer cells

ones, and its depletion suppresses their malignant phenotypes such as migration, invasion, metastasis and drug resistance. Consistent with these observations, we have demonstrated that siRNA-mediated knockdown of *RUNX2* improves GEM sensitivity of various pancreatic cancer cells regardless of their *p53* status. According to our results, *RUNX2* gene silencing increased GEM sensitivity of *p53*-null pancreatic cancer AsPC-1 cells [21] as well as *p53*-mutated pancreatic cancer MiaPaCa-2 and Panc-1 cells [22, 23], raising a possibility that *RUNX2* depletion improves GEM sensitivity of pancreatic cancer cells without functional p53. In a sharp contrast to *p53*, *TAp73/TAp63* is rarely mutated in cancer tissues. Of note, it has been shown that pro-apoptotic p53 family TAp73/TAp63 has an ability to promote DNA damage-mediated cell death in the absence of functional p53. Mutant p53 acts as a strong dominant-negative inhibitor against p53 family members; however, *RUNX2* depletion-mediated up-regulation of TAp73 and/or TAp63 resulted in an increase in GEM sensitivity of *p53*-mutated pancreatic cancer cells, which might be at least in part due to the disruption of the intracellular balance between the amounts of mutant p53 and TAp73/TAp63. Furthermore, miRNAs targeting *RUNX2* suppress malignant phenotypes of pancreatic cancer cells, suggesting that the delivery of chemically stable synthetic miRNAs to pancreatic cancer tissues is an attractive strategy to treat advanced pancreatic cancer patients. Although it is unknown whether miRNA-mediated down-regulation of RUNX2 could lead to the potentiation of TAp73/TAp63-dependent cell death pathway, *RUNX2* silencing-mediated restoration of TAp73/TAp63 and down-regulation of its pro-oncogenic downstream target genes might represent a promising approach to override the serious drug-resistant phenotype of pancreatic cancer with *p53* mutation.

Abbreviations
ADR: Adriamycin; ATF3: Activating transcription factor 3; ATM: Ataxia telangiectasia mutated; GEM: Gemcitabine; HDAC: Histone deacetylase; hENT1: Equilibrative nucleoside transporter-1; HIF: Hypoxia-inducible factor; MDM2: Murine double minute 2; MDR1: Multidrug-resistance 1; miRNA: microRNA; MMP9: Matrixmetalloproteinase-9; MMP13: Matrixmetalloproteinase-13; Nrf-2: Nuclear factor erythroid 2-related factor 2; PLK1: Polo-like kinase 1; RUNX2: Runt-related transcription factor 2; siRNA: Small interfering RNA; shRNA: Small hairpin RNA; TA: Transactivation; TD1: Transactivation domain I; VEGF: Vascular endothelial growth factor; VHL: Von Hippel-Lindau

Acknowledgements
We thank Dr. Hiroki Nagase (Laboratory of Cancer Genetics, Chiba Cancer Center Research Institute) for his valuable discussion.

Funding
This work was supported in part by JSPS (MEXT) KAKENHI Grant Number 23501278. The funding body was not involved in the study design, data collection, analysis and interpretation of data, or in writing of this review article.

Authors' contributions
TO provided direction throughout the preparation of this manuscript. TO, DY and MY wrote the manuscript. DS, YZ, YB and MS reviewed and made significant revisions on the manuscript. All authors approved the final manuscript.

Competing interests
The authors declare that they have no competing interests.

Author details
[1]Laboratory of DNA Damage Signaling, Chiba Cancer Center Research Institute, Chiba 260-8717, Japan. [2]Department of Laboratory Animal of China Medical University, Shenyang 110001, People's Republic of China. [3]Research Center, Fourth Hospital of Hebei Medical University, Shijiazhuang, Hebei 050017, People's Republic of China. [4]Department of Urology, First Hospital of China Medical University, Shenyang 110001, People's Republic of China. [5]Department of Biochemistry and Molecular Biology, Chongqing Medical University, Chongqing 400016, People's Republic of China.

References
1. Vincent A, Herman J, Schulick R, Hruban RH, Goggins M. Pancreatic cancer. Lancet. 2011;378:607–20.
2. Li D, Xie K, Wolff R, Abbruzzese JL. Pancreatic cancer. Lancet. 2004;363: 1049–57.
3. Abbruzzese JL. New applications of gemcitabine and future directions in the management of pancreatic cancer. Cancer. 2002;15:941–5.
4. Van CE, Verslype C, Grusenmeyer PA. Lessons learned in the management of advanced pancreatic cancer. J Clin Oncol. 2007;25:1949–52.
5. Hezel AF, Kimmelman AC, Stanger BZ, Bardeesy N, Depinho RA. Genetics and biology of pancreatic ductal adenocarcinoma. Genes Dev. 2006;15: 1218–49.
6. Boschman CR, Stryker S, Reddy JK, Rao MS. Expression of p53 protein in precursor lesions and adenocarcinoma of human pancreas. Am J Pathol. 1994;145:1291–5.
7. Maitra A, Adsay NV, Argani P, Iacobuzio-Donahue C, De Marzo A, Cameron JL, Yeo CJ, Hruban RH. Multicomponent analysis of the pancreatic adenocarcinoma progression model using a pancreatic intraepithelial neoplasia tissue microarray. Mod Pathol. 2003;16:902–12.
8. Vousden KH, Lu X. Live or let die: the cell's response to p53. Nat Rev Cancer. 2002;2:594–604.
9. Muller PA, Vousden KH. p53 mutations in cancer. Nat Cell Biol. 2013;15:2–8.
10. Karsenty G, Kronenberg HM, Settembre C. Genetic control of bone formation. Annu Rev Cell Dev Biol. 2009;25:629–48.
11. Cohen MM Jr. Perspectives on RUNX genes: an update. Am J Med Genet Part A. 2009. 149A: 2629-2646.
12. Kayed H, Jiang X, Keleg S, Jesnowski R, Giese T, Berger MR, Esposito I, Löhr M, Friess H, Kleeff J. Regulation and functional role of the Runt-related transcription factor-2 in pancreatic cancer. Br J Cancer. 2007;97:1106–15.
13. Endo T, Ohta K, Kobayashi T. Expression and function of Cbfa-1/Runx2 in thyroid papillary carcinoma cells. J Clin Endocr Metab. 2008;93:2409–12.
14. Akech J, Wixted JJ, Bedard K, van der Deen M, Hussain S, Guise TA, van Wijnen AJ, Stein JL, Languino LR, Altieri DC, Pratap J, Keller E, Stein GS, Lian JB. Oncogene. 2010;29:811–21.

15. Mendoza-Villanueva D, Deng W, Lopez-Camacho C, Shore P. The Runx transcriptional co-activator, CBFbeta, is essential for invasion of breast cancer cells. Mol Cancer. 2010;9:171.

16. Lim M, Zhong C, Yang S, Bell AM, Cohen MB, Roy-Burman P. RUNX2 regulates survivin expression in prostate cancer cells. Lab Invest. 2010;90:222–33.

17. Pratap J, Javed A, Languino LR, van Wijnen AJ, Stein JL, Stein GS, Lian JB. The RUNX2 osteogenic transcription factor regulates matrix metalloproteinase 9 in bone metastatic cancer cells and controls cell invasion. Mol Cell Biol. 2005;25:8581–91.

18. Pratap J, Imbalzano KM, Underwood JM, Cohet N, Gokul K, Akech J, van Wijnen AJ, Stein JL, Imbalzano AN, Nickerson JA, Lian JB, Stein GS. Ectopic RUNX2 expression in mammary epithelial cells disrupts formation of normal acini structure: implications for breast cancer progression. Cancer Res. 2009;69:6307–14.

19. Ozaki T, Wu D, Sugimoto H, Nagase H, Nakagawara A. Runt-related transcription factor 2 (RUNX2) inhibits p53-dependent apoptosis through the collaboration with HDAC6 in response to DNA damage. Cell Death Dis. 2013;4:e610.

20. Ozaki T, Sugimoto H, Nakamura M, Hiraoka K, Yoda H, Sang M, Fujiwara K, Nagase H. Runt-related transcription factor 2 attenuates the transcriptional activity as well as DNA damage-mediated induction of pro-apoptotic TAp73 to regulate chemosensitivity. FEBS J. 2015;282:114–28.

21. Sugimoto H, Nakamura M, Yoda H, Hiraoka K, Shinohara K, Sang M, Fujiwara K, Shimozato O, Nagase H, Ozaki T. Silencing of RUNX2 enhances gemcitabine sensitivity of p53-deficient human pancreatic cancer AsPC-1 cells through the stimulation of TAp63-mediated cell death. Cell Death Discov. 2015;1:15010.

22. Nakamura M, Sugimoto H, Ogata T, Hiraoka K, Yoda H, Sang M, Sang M, Zhu Y, Yu M, Shimozato O, Ozaki T. Improvement of gemcitabine sensitivity of p53-mutated pancreatic cancer MiaPaCa-2 cells by RUNX2 depletion-mediated augmentation of TAp73-dependent cell death. Oncogenesis. 2016;5:e233.

23. Ozaki T, Nakamura M, Ogata T, Sang M, Yoda H, Hiraoka K, Sang M, Shimozato O. Depletion of pro-oncogenic RUNX2 enhances gemcitabine (GEM) sensitivity of p53-mutated pancreatic cancer Panc1 cells through the induction of pro-apoptotic TAp63. Oncotarget. 2016;7:71937–50.

24. Sporn MB. The war on cancer. Lancet. 1996;347:1377–81.

25. Wan L, Pantel K, Kang Y. Tumor metastasis: moving new biological insights into the clinic. Nat Med. 2013;19:1450–64.

26. Burris HA 3rd, Moore MJ, Andersen J, Green MR, Rothenberg ML, Modiano MR, Cripps MC, Portenoy RK, Storniolo AM, Tarassoff P, Nelson R, Dorr FA, Stephens CD, Von Hoff DD. Improvements in survival and clinical benefit with gemcitabine as first-line therapy for patients with advanced pancreas cancer: a randomized trial. J Clin Oncol. 1997;15:2403–13.

27. Louvet C, Labianca R, Hammel P, Lledo G, Zampino MG, Andre T, Zaniboni A, Ducreux M, Aitini E, Taieb J, Faroux R, Lepere C, de GA. Gemcitabine in combination with oxaliplatin compared with gemcitabine alone in locally advanced or metastatic pancreatic cancer: results of a GERCOR and GISCAD phase III trial. J Clin Oncol. 2005;23:3509–16.

28. Li ZR, Campbell J, Rustum YM. Effect of 3-deazauridine on the metabolism, toxicity, and antitumor activity of azacitidine in mice bearing L1210 leukemia sensitive and resistant to cytarabine. Cancer Treat Rep. 1983;67:547–54.

29. Farrell JJ, Elsaleh H, Garcia M, Lai R, Ammar A, Regine WF, Abrams R, Benson AB, Macdonald J, Cass CE, Dicker AP, Mackey JR. Human equilibrative nucleoside transporter 1 levels predict response to gemcitabine in patients with pancreatic cancer. Gastroenterol. 2009;136:187–95.

30. Plunkett W, Huang P, Xu YZ, Heinemann V, Grunewald R, Gandhi V. Gemcitabine: metabolism, mechanisms of action, and self-potentiation. Sem. Oncol. 1995;22:3–10.

31. Oettle H, Post S, Neuhaus P, Gellert K, Langrehr J, Ridwelski K, Schramm H, Fahlke J, Zuelke C, Burkart C, Gutberlet K, Kettner E, Schmalenberg H, Weigang-Koehler K, Bechstein WO, Niedergethmann M, Schmidt-Wolf I, Roll L, Doerken B, Riess H. Adjuvant chemotherapy with gemcitabine vs observation in patients undergoing curative-intent resection of pancreatic cancer: a randomized controlled trial. JAMA. 2007;297:267–77.

32. Berlin JD, Catalano P, Thomas JP, Kugler JW, Haller DG, Benson AB 3rd. Phase III study of gemcitabine in combination with fluorouracil versus gemcitabine alone in patients with advanced pancreatic carcinoma: Eastern Cooperative Oncology Group Trial E2297. J Clin Oncol. 2002;20:3270–5.

33. Rocha Lima CM, Green MR, Rotche R, Miller WH Jr, Jeffrey GM, Cisar LA, Morganti A, Orlando N, Gruia G, Miller LL. Irinotecan plus gemcitabine results in no survival advantage compared with gemcitabine monotherapy in patients with locally advanced or metastatic pancreatic cancer despite increased tumor response rate. J Clin Oncol. 2004;22:3776–83.

34. Heinemann V, Quietzsch D, Gieseler F, Gonnermann M, Schönekäs H, Rost A, Neuhaus H, Haag C, Clemens M, Heinrich B, Vehling-Kaiser U, Fuchs M, Fleckenstein D, Gesierich W, Uthgenannt D, Einsele H, Holstege A, Hinke A, Schalhorn A, Wilkowski R. Randomized phase III trial of gemcitabine plus cisplatin compared with gemcitabine alone in advanced pancreatic cancer. J Clin Oncol. 2006;24:3946–52.

35. Wang Y, Hu GF, Zhang QQ, Tang N, Guo J, Liu LY, Han X, Wang X, Wang ZH. Efficacy and safety of gemcitabine plus erlotinib for locally advanced or metastatic pancreatic cancer: a systematic review and meta-analysis. Drug Des Dev Ther. 2016;10:1961–72.

36. Von Hoff DD, Ervin T, Arena FP, Chiorean EG, Infante J, Moore M, Seay T, Tjulandin SA, Ma WW, Saleh MN, Harris M, Reni M, Dowden S, Laheru D, Bahary N, Ramanathan RK, Tabernero J, Hidalgo M, Goldstein D, Van Cutsem E, Wei X, Iglesias J, Renschler MF. Increased survival in pancreatic cancer with nab-paclitaxel plus gemcitabine. New Engl J Med. 2013;369:1691–703.

37. Gottesman MM, Fojo T, Bates SE. Multidrug resistance in cancer: role of ATP-dependent transporters. Nat Rev Cancer. 2002;2:48–58.

38. Fletcher JI, Haber M, Henderson MJ, Norris MD. ABC transporters in cancer: more than just drug efflux pumps. Nat Rev Cancer. 2010;10:147–56.

39. O'Driscoll L, Walsh N, Larkin A, Ballot J, Ooi WS, Gullo G, O'Connor R, Clynes M, Crown J, Kennedy S. MDR1/P-glycoprotein and MRP-1 drug efflux pumps in pancreatic carcinoma. Anticancer Res. 2007;27:2115–20.

40. Song B, Liu XS, Rice SJ, Kuang S, Elzey BD, Konieczny SF, Ratliff TL, Hazbun T, Chiorean EG, Liu X. Plk1 phosphorylation of orc2 and hbo1 contributes to gemcitabine resistance in pancreatic cancer. Mol Cancer Ther. 2013;12:58–68.

41. Zhang C, Sun X, Ren Y, Lou Y, Zhou J, Liu M, Li D. Validation of Polo-like kinase 1 as a therapeutic target in pancreatic cancer cells. Cancer Biol Ther. 2012;13:1214–20.

42. Li J, Wang R, Schweickert PG, Karki A, Yang Y, Kong Y, Ahmad N, Konieczny SF, Liu X. Plk1 inhibition enhances the efficacy of gemcitabine in human pancreatic cancer. Cell Cycle. 2016;15:711–9.

43. Lee SH, Kim H, Hwang JH, Lee HS, Cho JY, Yoon YS, Han HS. Breast cancer resistance protein expression is associated with early recurrence and decreased survival in resectable pancreatic cancer patients. Pathol Int. 2012; 62:167–75.

44. Nath S, Daneshvar K, Roy LD, Grover P, Kidiyoor A, Mosley L, Sahraei M, Mukherjee P. MUC1 induces drug resistance in pancreatic cancer cells via upregulation of multidrug resistance genes. Oncogenesis. 2013;2:e51.

45. Mackey JR, Mani RS, Selner M, Mowles D, Young JD, Belt JA, Crawford CR, Cass CE. Functional nucleoside transporters are required for gemcitabine influx and manifestation of toxicity in cancer cell lines. Cancer Res. 1998;58:4349–57.

46. Mackey JR, Yao SY, Smith KM, Karpinski E, Baldwin SA, Cass CE, Young JD. Gemcitabine transport in xenopus oocytes expressing recombinant plasma membrane mammalian nucleoside transporters. J Nat Cancer Inst. 1999;91: 1876–81.

47. Pérez-Torras S, García-Manteiga J, Mercadé E, Casado FJ, Carbó N, Pastor-Anglada M, Mazo A. Adenoviral-mediated overexpression of human equilibrative nucleoside transporter 1 (hENT1) enhances gemcitabine response in human pancreatic cancer. Biochem Pharm. 2008;76:322–9.

48. Spratlin J, Sangha R, Glubrecht D, Dabbagh L, Young JD, Dumontet C, Cass C, Lai R, Mackey JR. The absence of human equilibrative nucleoside transporter 1 is associated with reduced survival in patients with gemcitabine-treated pancreas adenocarcinoma. Clin Cancer Res. 2004;10:6956–61.

49. Nordh S, Ansari D, Andersson R. hENT1 expression is predictive of gemcitabine outcome in pancreatic cancer: A systematic review. World J Gastroenterol. 2014;20:8482–90.

50. Nigro JM, Baker SJ, Preisinger AC, Jessup JM, Hostetter R, Cleary K, Bigner SH, Davidson N, Baylin S, Devilee P, Glover T, Collins FS, Weston A, Modali R, Harris CC, Vogelstein B. Mutations in the p53 gene occur in diverse human tumour types. Nature. 1989;342:705–8.

51. Fiorini C, Cordani M, Padroni C, Blandino G, Di Agostino S, Donadelli M. Mutant p53 stimulates chemoresistance of pancreatic adenocarcinoma cells to gemcitabine. Biochim Biophys Acta. 2015;1853:89–100.

52. Lane DP. Cancer p53 guardian of the genome. Nature. 1992;358:15–6.
53. Vogelstein B, Lane DP, Levine AJ. Surfing the p53 network. Nature. 2000;408: 307–10.
54. Kubbutat MH, Jones SN, Vousden KH. Regulation of p53 stability by Mdm2. Nature. 1997;387:299–303.
55. Haupt Y, Maya R, Kazaz A, Oren M. Mdm2 promotes the rapid degradation of p53. Nature. 1997;387:296–9.
56. Hollstein M, Sidransky D, Vogelstein B, Harris CC. p53 mutations in human cancers. Science. 1991;253:49–53.
57. Brosh R, Rotter V. When mutants gain new powers: news from the mutant p53 field. Nat Rev Cancer. 2009;9:701–13.
58. Liu DP, Song H, Xu Y. A common gain of function of p53 cancer mutants in inducing genetic instability. Oncogene. 2010;29:949–56.
59. Hanel W, Marchenko N, Xu S, Yu SX, Weng W, Moll U. Two hot spot mutant p53 mouse models display differential gain of function in tumorigenesis. Cell Death Differ. 2013;20:898–909.
60. Strano S, Dell'Orso S, Di Agostino S, Fontemaggi G, Sacchi A, Blandino G. Mutant p53: an oncogenic transcription factor. Oncogene. 2007;26:2212–9.
61. Zhao Y, Zhang C, Yue X, Li X. Liu J, Yu H, Belyi VA, Yang Q, Feng Z, Hu W. Pontin, a new mutant p53-binding protein, promotes gain-of-function of mutant p53. Cell Death Differ. 2015;22:1824–36.
62. Lauscher JC, Elezkurtaj S, Dullat S, Lipka S, Gröne J, Buhr HJ, Huber O, Kruschewski M. Increased Pontin expression is a potential predictor for outcome in sporadic colorectal carcinoma. Oncol Rep. 2012;28:1619–24.
63. Haupt S, di Agostino S, Mizrahi I, Alsheich-Bartok O, Voorhoeve M, Damalas A, Blandino G, Haupt Y. Promyelocytic leukemia protein is required for gain of function by mutant p53. Cancer Res. 2009;69:4818–26.
64. Girardini JE, Napoli M, Piazza S, Rustighi A, Marotta C, Radaelli E, Capaci V, Jordan L, Quinlan P, Thompson A, Mano M, Rosato A, Crook T, Scanziani E, Means AR, Lozano G, Schneider C, Del Sal GA. Pin1/mutant p53 axis promotes aggressiveness in breast cancer. Cancer Cell. 2011;20:79–91.
65. Muller P, Hrstka R, Coomber D, Lane DP, Vojtesek B. Chaperone-dependent stabilization and degradation of p53 mutants. Oncogene. 2008;27:3371–83.
66. Blagosklonny MV. p53 from complexity to simplicity: mutant p53 stabilization, gain-of-function, and dominant-negative effect. FASEB J. 2000; 14:1901–7.
67. Fan S, el-Deiry WS, Bae I, Freeman J, Jondle D, Bhatia K, Fornace AJ Jr, Magrath I, Kohn KW, O'Connor PM. p53 gene mutations are associated with decreased sensitivity of human lymphoma cells to DNA damaging agents. Cancer Res. 1994;54:5824–30.
68. Lai SL, Perng RP, Hwang J. p53 gene status modulates the chemosensitivity of non-small cell lung cancer cells. J Biomed Sci. 2000;7:64–70.
69. Huang Y, Sadee W. Membrane transporters and channels in chemoresistance and -sensitivity of tumor cells. Cancer Lett. 2006;239:168–82.
70. Montes de Oca Luna R, Wagner DS, Lozano G. Rescue of early embryonic lethality in mdm2-deficient mice by deletion of p53. Nature. 1995;378:203–6.
71. Ohgaki H, Kleihues P. Genetic alterations and signaling pathways in the evolution of gliomas. Cancer Sci. 2009;100:2235–41.
72. Li M, Brooks CL, Wu-Baer F, Chen D, Baer R, Gu W. Mono- versus polyubiquitination: differential control of p53 fate by Mdm2. Science. 2003;302:1972–5.
73. Meek DW, Hupp TR. The regulation of MDM2 by multisite phosphorylation—opportunities for molecular-based intervention to target tumours? Sem Cancer Biol. 2010;20(1):9–28.
74. Rayburn E, Zhang R, He J, Wang H. MDM2 and human malignancies: expression, clinical pathology, prognostic markers, and implications for chemotherapy. Curr Cancer Drug Targets. 2005;5:27–41.
75. Rayburn ER, Ezell SJ, Zhang R. Recent advances in validating MDM2 as a cancer target. Anticancer Agents Med Chem. 2009;9:882–903.
76. Toledo F, Wahl GM. Regulating the p53 pathway: in vitro hypotheses, in vivo veritas. Nat Rev Cancer. 2006;6:909–23.
77. Grochola LF, Taubert H, Greither T, Bhanot U, Udelnow A, Würl P. Elevated transcript levels from the MDM2 P1 promoter and low p53 transcript levels are associated with poor prognosis in human pancreatic ductal adenocarcinoma. Pancreas. 2011;40:265–70.
78. Sheng W, Dong M, Chen C, Wang Z, Li Y, Wang K, Li Y, Zhou J. Cooperation of Musashi-2, Numb, MDM2, and P53 in drug resistance and malignant biology of pancreatic cancer. FASEB J. in press
79. Onel K, Cordon-Cardo C. MDM2 and prognosis. Mol Cancer Res. 2004;2:1–8.
80. Wade M, Wang YV, Wahl GM. The p53 orchestra: Mdm2 and Mdmx set the tone. Trends Cell Biol. 2010;20:299–309.

81. Shi W, Meng Z, Chen Z, Hua Y, Gao H, Wang P, Lin J, Zhou Z, Luo J, Liu L. RNA interference against MDM2 suppresses tumor growth and metastasis in pancreatic carcinoma SW1990HM cells. Mol Cell Biochem. 2014;387:1–8.
82. Kondo S, Barnett GH, Hara H, Morimura T, Takeuchi J. MDM2 protein confers the resistance of a human glioblastoma cell line to cisplatin-induced apoptosis. Oncogene. 1995;10:2001–6.
83. Suzuki A, Toi M, Yamamoto Y, Saji S, Muta M, Tominaga T. Role of MDM2 overexpression in doxorubicin resistance of breast carcinoma. Jpn J Cancer Res. 1998;89:221–7.
84. Meijer A, Kruyt FA, van der Zee AG, Hollema H, Le P, ten Hoor KA, Groothuis GM, Quax WJ, de Vries EG, de Jong S. Nutlin-3 preferentially sensitises wild-type p53-expressing cancer cells to DR5-selective TRAIL over rhTRAIL. Br J Cancer. 2013;109:2685–95.
85. Kaghad M, Bonnet H, Yang A, Creancier L, Biscan JC, Valent A, Minty A, Chalon P, Lelias JM, Dumont X, Ferrara P, McKeon F, Caput D. Monoallelically expressed gene related to p53 at 1p36, a region frequently deleted in neuroblastoma and other human cancers. Cell. 1997;90:809–19.
86. Yang A, Kaghad M, Wang Y, Gillett E, Fleming MD, Dötsch V, Andrews NC, Caput D, McKeon F. p63, a p53 homolog at 3q27-29, encodes multiple products with transactivating, death-inducing, and dominant-negative activities. Mol Cell. 1998;2:305–16.
87. Tomasini R, Tsuchihara K, Wilhelm M, Fujitani M, Rufini A, Cheung CC, Khan F, Itie-Youten A, Wakeham A, Tsao MS, Iovanna JL, Squire J, Jurisica I, Kaplan D, Melino G, Jurisicova A, Mak TW. TAp73 knockout shows genomic instability with infertility and tumor suppressor functions. Genes Dev. 2008;22:2677–91.
88. Su X, Chakravarti D, Cho MS, Liu L, Gi YJ, Lin YL, Leung ML, El-Naggar A, Creighton CJ, Suraokar MB, Wistuba I, Flores ER. TAp63 suppresses metastasis through coordinate regulation of Dicer and miRNAs. Nature. 2010;467:986–90.
89. Wilhelm MT, Rufini A, Wetzel MK, Tsuchihara K, Inoue S, Tomasini R, Itie-Youten A, Wakeham A, Arsenian-Henriksson M, Melino G, Kaplan DR, Miller FD, Mak TW. Isoform-specific p73 knockout mice reveal a novel role for delta Np73 in the DNA damage response pathway. Genes Dev. 2010;24:549–60.
90. Chakravarti D, Su X, Cho MS, Bui NH, Coarfa C, Venkatanarayan A, Benham AL, Flores González RE, Alana J, Xiao W, Leung ML, Vin H, Chan IL, Aquino A, Müller N, Wang H, Cooney AJ, Parker-Thornburg J, Tsai KY, Gunaratne PH, Flores ER. Induced multipotency in adult keratinocytes through down-regulation of ΔNp63 or DGCR8. Proc Natl Acad Sci USA. 2014;111:E572–1.
91. Lissy NA, Davis PK, Irwin M, Kaelin WG, Dowdy SFA. common E2F-1 and p73 pathway mediates cell death induced by TCR activation. Nature. 2000;407: 642–5.
92. Irwin M, Marin MC, Phillips AC, Seelan RS, Smith DI, Liu W, Flores ER, Tsai KY, Jacks T, Vousden KH, Kaelin WG Jr. Role for the p53 homologue p73 in E2F-1-induced apoptosis. Nature. 2000;407:645–8.
93. Stiewe T, Pützer BM. Role of the p53-homologue p73 in E2F1-induced apoptosis. Nat Genet. 2000;26:464–9.
94. Zaika A, Irwin M, Sansome C, Moll UM. Oncogenes induce and activate endogenous p73 protein. J Biol Chem. 2001;276:11310–6.
95. Logotheti S, Michalopoulos I, Sideridou M, Daskalos A, Kossida S, Spandidos DA, Field JK, Vojtesek B, Liloglou T, Gorgoulis V, Zoumpourlis V. Sp1 binds to the external promoter of the p73 gene and induces the expression of TAp73gamma in lung cancer. FEBS J. 2010;277:3014–27.
96. Lai J, Nie W, Zhang W, Wang Y, Xie R, Wang Y, Gu J, Xu J, Song W, Yang F, Huang G, Cao P, Guan X. Transcriptional regulation of the p73 gene by Nrf-2 and promoter CpG methylation in human breast cancer. Oncotarget. 2014;5:6909–22.
97. Fontemaggi G, Gurtner A, Strano S, Higashi Y, Sacchi A, Piaggio G, Blandino G. The transcriptional repressor ZEB regulates p73 expression at the crossroad between proliferation and differentiation. Mol Cell Biol. 2001;21:8461–70.
98. Rossi M, De Laurenzi V, Munarriz E, Green DR, Liu YC, Vousden KH, Cesareni G, Melino G. The ubiquitin-protein ligase Itch regulates p73 stability. EMBO J. 2005;24:836–48.
99. Rossi M, Aqeilan RI, Neale M, Candi E, Salomoni P, Knight RA, Croce CM, Melino G. The E3 ubiquitin ligase Itch controls the protein stability of p63. Proc Natl Acad Sci U S A. 2006;103:12753–8.
100. Hansen TM, Rossi M, Roperch JP, Ansell K, Simpson K, Taylor D, Mathon N, Knight RA, Melino G. Itch inhibition regulates chemosensitivity in vitro. Biochem Biophys Res Commun. 2007;361:33–6.
101. Flores ER, Tsai KY, Crowley D, Sengupta S, Yang A, McKeon F, Jacks T. p63 and p73 are required for p53-dependent apoptosis in response to DNA damage. Nature. 2002;416:560–4.

102. Melino G, Lu X, Gasco M, Crook T, Knight RA. Functional regulation of p73 and p63: development and cancer. Trends Biochem Sci. 2003;28:663–70.

103. Helton ES, Zhu J, Chen X. The unique NH_2-terminally deleted (DeltaN) residues, the PXXP motif, and the PPXY motif are required for the transcriptional activity of the DeltaN variant of p63. J Biol Chem. 2006;281: 2533–42.

104. Ghioni P, Bolognese F, Duijf PH, Van Bokhoven H, Mantovani R, Guerrini L. Complex transcriptional effects of p63 isoforms: identification of novel activation and repression domains. Mol Cell Biol. 2002;22:8659–68.

105. Wu G, Osada M, Guo Z, Fomenkov A, Begum S, Zhao M, Upadhyay S, Xing M, Wu F, Moon C, Westra WH, Koch WM, Mantovani R, Califano JA, Ratovitski E, Sidransky D, Trink B. DeltaNp63alpha up-regulates the Hsp70 gene in human cancer. Cancer Res. 2005;65:758–66.

106. Soldevilla B, Díaz R, Silva J, Campos-Martín Y, Muñoz C, García V, García JM, Peña C, Herrera M, Rodriguez M, Gómez I, Mohamed N, Marques MM, Bonilla F, Domínguez G. Prognostic impact of ΔTAp73 isoform levels and their target genes in colon cancer patients. Clin Cancer Res. 2011;17:6029–39.

107. Melino G, De Laurenzi V, Vousden KH. p73: Friend or foe in tumorigenesis. Nat Rev Cancer. 2002;2:605–15.

108. Oswald C, Stiewe T. In good times and bad: p73 in cancer. Cell Cycle. 2008; 7:1726–31.

109. Vilgelm AE, Hong SM, Washington MK, Wei J, Chen H, El-Rifai W, Zaika A. Characterization of DeltaNp73 expression and regulation in gastric and esophageal tumors. Oncogene. 2010;29:5861–8.

110. Müller M, Schleithoff ES, Stremmel W, Melino G, Krammer PH, Schilling T. One, two, three–p53, p63, p73 and chemosensitivity. Drug Resist Updat. 2006;9:288–306.

111. Leung TH, Wong SC, Chan KK, Chan DW, Cheung AN, Ngan HY. The interaction between C35 and ΔNp73 promotes chemo-resistance in ovarian cancer cells. Br J Cancer. 2013;109:965–75.

112. Ramsey MR, Wilson C, Ory B, Rothenberg SM, Faquin W, Mills AA, Ellisen LW. FGFR2 signaling underlies p63 oncogenic function in squamous cell carcinoma. J Clin Invest. 2013;123:3525–38.

113. Ram Kumar RM, Betz MM, Robl B, Born W, Fuchs B. ΔNp63α enhances the oncogenic phenotype of osteosarcoma cells by inducing the expression of GLI2. BMC Cancer. 2014;14:559.

114. Matin RN, Chikh A, Chong SL, Mesher D, Graf M, Sanza' P, Senatore V, Scatolini M, Moretti F, Leigh IM, Proby CM, Costanzo A, Chiorino G, Cerio R, Harwood CA, Bergamaschi D. p63 is an alternative p53 repressor in melanoma that confers chemoresistance and a poor prognosis. J Exp Med. 2013;210:581–603.

115. Rocco JW, Leong CO, Kuperwasser N, DeYoung MP, Ellisen LW. p63 mediates survival in squamous cell carcinoma by suppression of p73-dependent apoptosis. Cancer Cell. 2006;9:45–56.

116. Song WJ, Sullivan MG, Legare RD, Hutchings S, Tan X, Kufrin D, Ratajczak J, Resende IC, Haworth C, Hock R, Loh M, Felix C, Roy DC, Busque L, Kurnit D, Willman C, Gewirtz AM, Speck NA, Bushweller JH, Li FP, Gardiner K, Poncz M, Maris JM, Gilliland DG. Haploinsufficiency of CBFA2 causes familial thrombocytopenia with propensity to develop acute myelogenous leukaemia. Nat Genet. 1999;23:166–75.

117. Li QL, Ito K, Sakakura C, Fukamachi H, Ki I, Chi XZ, Lee KY, Nomura S, Lee CW, Han SB, Kim HM, Kim WJ, Yamamoto H, Yamashita N, Yano T, Ikeda T, Itohara S, Inazawa J, Abe T, Hagiwara A, Yamagishi H, Ooe A, Kaneda A, Sugimura T, Ushijima T, Bae SC, Ito Y. Causal relationship between the loss of RUNX3 expression and gastric cancer. Cell. 2002;109:113–24.

118. Komori T, Yagi H, Nomura S, Yamaguchi A, Sasaki K, Deguchi K, Shimizu Y, Bronson RT, Gao YH, Inada M, Sato M, Okamoto R, Kitamura Y, Yoshiki S, Kishimoto T. Cell. 1997;89:755–64.

119. Otto F, Thornell AP, Crompton T, Denzel A, Gilmour KC, Rosewell IR, Stamp GW, Beddington RS, Mundlos S, Olsen BR, Selby PB, Owen MJ. Cbfa1, a candidate gene for cleidocranial dysplasia syndrome, is essential for osteoblast differentiation and bone development. Cell. 1997;89:765–71.

120. Komori T. Regulation of bone development and extracellular matrix protein genes by RUNX2. Cell Tissue Res. 2010;339:189–95.

121. Liu W, Toyosawa S, Furuichi T, Kanatani N, Yoshida C, Liu Y, Himeno M, Narai S, Yamaguchi A, Komori T. Overexpression of Cbfa1 in osteoblasts inhibits osteoblast maturation and causes osteopenia with multiple fractures. J Cell Biol. 2001;155:157–66.

122. Blyth K, Cameron ER, Neil JC. The RUNX genes: gain or loss of function in cancer. Nat Rev. 2005;5:376–87.

123. Pratap J, Lian JB, Javed A, Barnes GL, van Wijnen AJ, Stein JL, Stein GS. Regulatory roles of Runx2 in metastatic tumor and cancer cell interactions with bone. Cancer Metastasis Rev. 2006;25:589–600.

124. Chua CW, Chiu YT, Yuen HF, Chan KW, Man K, Wang X, Ling MT, Wong YC. Suppression of androgen-independent prostate cancer cell aggressiveness by FTY720: validating Runx2 as a potential antimetastatic drug screening platform. Clin Cancer Res. 2009;15:4322–35.

125. Ito Y, Bae SC, Chuang LS. The RUNX family: developmental regulators in cancer. Nat Rev Cancer. 2015;15:81–95.

126. Man TK, Lu XY, Jaeweon K, Perlaky L, Harris CP, Shah S, Ladanyi M, Gorlick R, Lau CC, Rao PH. Genome-wide array comparative genomic hybridization analysis reveals distinct amplifications in osteosarcoma. BMC Cancer. 2004;4:45.

127. Sadikovic B, Thorner P, Chilton-Macneill S, Martin JW, Cervigne NK, Squire J, Zielenska M. Expression analysis of genes associated with human osteosarcoma tumors shows correlation of RUNX2 overexpression with poor response to chemotherapy. BMC Cancer. 2010;10:202.

128. Roos A, Satterfield L, Zhao S, Fuja D, Shuck R, Hicks MJ, Donehower LA, Yustein JT. Loss of Runx2 sensitises osteosarcoma to chemotherapy-induced apoptosis. Br J Cancer. 2015;113:1289–97.

129. Pratap J, Wixted JJ, Gaur T, Zaidi SK, Dobson J, Gokul KD, Hussain S, van Wijnen AJ, Stein JL, Stein GS, Lian JB. Runx2 transcriptional activation of Indian Hedgehog and a downstream bone metastatic pathway in breast cancer cells. Cancer Res. 2008;68:7795–802.

130. El-Gendi SM, Mostafa MF. Runx2 Expression as a Potential Prognostic Marker in Invasive Ductal Breast Carcinoma. Pathol Oncol Res. 2016;22:461–70.

131. Taipaleenmäki H, Browne G, Akech J, Zustin J, van Wijnen AJ, Stein JL, Hesse E, Stein GS, Lian JB. Targeting of Runx2 by miRNA-135 and miRNA-203 impairs progression of breast cancer and metastatic bone disease. Cancer Res. 2015;75:1433–44.

132. Dutta A, Li J, Lu H, Akech J, Pratap J, Wang T, Zerlanko BJ, TJ FG, Jiang Z, Birbe R, Wixted J, Violette SM, Stein JL, Stein GS, Lian JB, Languino LR. Integrin $\alpha v \beta 6$ promotes an osteolytic program in cancer cells by upregulating MMP2. Cancer Res. 2014;74:1598–608.

133. Hanahan D, Weinberg RA. The hallmarks of cancer. Cell. 2000;100:57–70.

134. Ishikawa T, Chen J, Wang J, Okada F, Sugiyama T, Kobayashi T, Shindo M, Higashino F, Katoh H, Asaka M, Kondo T, Hosokawa M, Kobayashi M. Adrenomedullin antagonist suppresses in vivo growth of human pancreatic cancer cells in SCID mice by suppressing angiogenesis. Oncogene. 2003;22: 1238–42.

135. Wei D, Wang L, He Y, Xiong HQ, Abbruzzese JL, Xie K. Celecoxib inhibits vascular endothelial growth factor expression in and reduces angiogenesis and metastasis of human pancreatic cancer via suppression of Sp1 transcription factor activity. Cancer Res. 2004;64:2030–8.

136. Maruyama Y, Ono M, Kawahara A, Yokoyama T, Basaki Y, Kage M, Aoyagi S, Kinoshita H, Kuwano M. Tumor growth suppression in pancreatic cancer by a putative metastasis suppressor gene Cap43/NDRG1/Drg-1 through modulation of angiogenesis. Cancer Res. 2006;66:6233–42.

137. Holash J, Maisonpierre PC, Compton D, Boland P, Alexander CR, Zagzag D, Yancopoulos GD, Wiegand SJ. Vessel cooption, regression, and growth in tumors mediated by angiopoietins and VEGF. Science. 1999;284:1994–8.

138. Wang GL, Jiang BH, Rue EA, Semenza GL. Hypoxia-inducible factor 1 is a basic-helix-loop-helix-PAS heterodimer regulated by cellular O2 tension. Proc Natl Acad Sci USA. 1995;92:5510–4.

139. Kaelin WG Jr, Ratcliffe PJ. Oxygen sensing by metazoans: the central role of the HIF hydroxylase pathway. Mol Cell. 2008;30:393–402.

140. Maxwell PH, Dachs GU, Gleadle JM, Nicholls LG, Harris AL, Stratford IJ, Hankinson O, Pugh CW, Ratcliffe PJ. Hypoxia-inducible factor-1 modulates gene expression in solid tumors and influences both angiogenesis and tumor growth. Proc Natl Acad Sci USA. 1997;94:8104–9.

141. Zhong H, De Marzo AM, Laughner E, Lim M, Hilton DA, Zagzag D, Buechler P, Isaacs WB, Semenza GL, Simons JW. Overexpression of hypoxia-inducible factor 1alpha in common human cancers and their metastases. Cancer Res. 1999;59:5830–5.

142. Zelzer E, Glotzer DJ, Hartmann C, Thomas D, Fukai N, Soker S, Olsen BR. Tissue specific regulation of VEGF expression during bone development requires Cbfa1/Runx2. Mech Dev. 2001;106:97–106.

143. Lee SH, Che X, Jeong JH, Choi JY, Lee YJ, Lee YH, Bae SC, Lee YM. Runx2 protein stabilizes hypoxia-inducible factor-1α through competition with von Hippel-Lindau protein (pVHL) and stimulates angiogenesis in growth plate hypertrophic chondrocytes. J Biol Chem. 2012;287:14760–71.

144. Rahman SU, Lee MS, Baek JH, Ryoo HM, Woo KM. The prolyl hydroxylase inhibitor dimethyloxalylglycine enhances dentin sialophoshoprotein expression through VEGF-induced Runx2 stabilization. PLoS One. 2014;9:e112078.

145. Peng Z, Wei D, Wang L, Tang H, Zhang J, Le X, Jia Z, Li Q, Xie K. RUNX3 inhibits the expression of vascular endothelial growth factor and reduces the angiogenesis, growth, and metastasis of human gastric cancer. Clin Cancer Res. 2006;12:6386–94.

146. Peng ZG, Zhou MY, Huang Y, Qiu JH, Wang LS, Liao SH, Dong S, Chen GQ. Physical and functional interaction of Runt-related protein 1 with hypoxia-inducible factor-1alpha. Oncogene. 2008;27:839–47.

147. Yamada C, Ozaki T, Ando K, Suenaga Y, Inoue K, Ito Y, Okoshi R, Kageyama H, Kimura H, Miyazaki M, Nakagawara A. RUNX3 modulates DNA damage-mediated phosphorylation of tumor suppressor p53 at Ser-15 and acts as a co-activator for p53. J Biol Chem. 2010;285:16693–703.

148. Wu D, Ozaki T, Yoshihara Y, Kubo N, Nakagawara A. Runt-related transcription factor 1 (RUNX1) stimulates tumor suppressor p53 protein in response to DNA damage through complex formation and acetylation. J Biol Chem. 2013;288:1353–64.

149. Gaiddon C, Lokshin M, Ahn J, Zhang T, Prives C. A subset of tumor-derived mutant forms of p53 down-regulate p63 and p73 through a direct interaction with the p53 core domain. Mol Cell Biol. 2001;21:1874–87.

150. Wang Z, Kim J, Teng Y, Ding HF, Zhang J, Hai T, Cowell JK, Yan C. Loss of ATF3 promotes hormone-induced prostate carcinogenesis and the emergence of CK5+CK8+ epithelial cells. Oncogene. 2016;35:3555–64.

151. Wang Z, Xu D, Ding HF, Kim J, Zhang J, Hai T, Yan C. Loss of ATF3 promotes Akt activation and prostate cancer development in a Pten knockout mouse model. Oncogene. 2016;34:4975–84.

152. Wei S, Wang H, Lu C, Malmut S, Zhang J, Ren S, Yu G, Wang W, Tang DD, Yan C. The activating transcription factor 3 protein suppresses the oncogenic function of mutant p53 proteins. J Biol Chem. 2014;289:8947–59.

153. Gokulnath M, Partridge NC, Selvamurugan N. Runx2, a target gene for activating transcription factor-3 in human breast cancer cells. Tumour Biol. 2015;36:1923–31.

154. Chitwood DH, Timmermans MC. Small RNAs are on the move. Nature. 2010; 467:415–9.

155. Kosik KS. MicroRNAs and cellular phenotype. Cell. 2010;143:21–6.

156. Sun T, Kong X, Du Y, Li Z. Aberrant microRNAs in pancreatic cancer: Researches and clinical implications. Gastroenterol Res Pract. 2014;2014:386561.

157. Lu Z, Li Y, Takwi A, Li B, Zhang J, Conklin DJ, Young KH, Martin R, Li Y. miR-301a as an NF-κB activator in pancreatic cancer cells. EMBO J. 2011; 30:57–67.

158. Liang C, Yu XJ, Guo XZ, Sun MH, Wang Z, Song Y, Ni QX, Li HY, Mukaida N, Li YY. MicroRNA-33a-mediated downregulation of Pim-3 kinase expression renders human pancreatic cancer cells sensitivity to gemcitabine. Oncotarget. 2015;6:14440–55.

159. Ji Q, Hao X, Zhang M, Tang W, Yang M, Li L, Xiang D, Desano JT, Bommer GT, Fan D, Fearon ER, Lawrence TS, Xu L. MicroRNA miR-34 inhibits human pancreatic cancer tumor-initiating cells. PLoS One. 2009;4:e6816.

160. Huang J, Zhao L, Xing L, Chen D. MicroRNA-204 regulates Runx2 protein expression and mesenchymal progenitor cell differentiation. Stem Cells. 2010;28:357–64.

161. Wu T, Zhou H, Hong Y, Li J, Jiang X, Huang H. miR-30 family members negatively regulate osteoblast differentiation. J Biol Chem. 2012;287:7503–11.

162. Li Z, Hassan MQ, Volinia S, van Wijnen AJ, Stein JL, Croce CM, Lian JB, Stein GS. A microRNA signature for a BMP2-induced osteoblast lineage commitment program. Proc Natl Acad Sci USA. 2008;105:13906–11.

163. Zhang Y, Xie RL, Croce CM, Stein JL, Lian JB, van Wijnen AJ, Stein GS. A program of microRNAs controls osteogenic lineage progression by targeting transcription factor Runx2. Proc Natl Acad Sci USA. 2011; 108: 9863–9868.

164. Saini S, Majid S, Yamamura S, Tabatabai L, Suh SO, Shahryari V, Chen Y, Deng G, Tanaka Y, Dahiya R. Regulatory Role of mir-203 in Prostate Cancer Progression and Metastasis. Clin Cancer Res. 2011;17:5287–98.

165. van der Deen M, Taipaleenmäki H, Zhang Y, Teplyuk NM, Gupta A, Cinghu S, Shogren K, Maran A, Yaszemski MJ, Ling L, Cool SM, Leong DT, Dierkes C, Zustin J, Salto-Tellez M, Ito Y, Bae SC, Zielenska M, Squire JA, Lian JB, Stein JL, Zambetti GP, Jones SN, Galindo M, Hesse E, Stein GS, van Wijnen AJ. MicroRNA-34c inversely couples the biological functions of the runt-related transcription factor RUNX2 and the tumor suppressor p53 in osteosarcoma. J Biol Chem. 2013;288:21307–19.

166. Martin JW, Zielenska M, Stein GS, van Wijnen AJ, Squire JA. The role of RUNX2 in osteosarcoma oncogenesis. Sarcoma. 2011;2011:282745.

167. Li W, Liu Z, Chen L, Zhou L, Yao Y. MicroRNA-23b is an independent prognostic marker and suppresses ovarian cancer progression by targeting runt-related transcription factor-2. FEBS Lett. 2014;588:1608–15.

168. Miao L, Xiong X, Lin Y, Cheng Y, Lu J, Zhang J, Cheng N. miR-203 inhibits tumor cell migration and invasion via caveolin-1 in pancreatic cancer cells. Oncol Lett. 2014;7:658–62.

169. Chen Z, Sangwan V, Banerjee S, Mackenzie T, Dudeja V, Li X, Wang H, Vickers SM, Saluja AK. miR-204 mediated loss of Myeloid cell leukemia-1 results in pancreatic cancer cell death. Mol Cancer. 2013;12:105.

170. Singh S, Chitkara D, Kumar V, Behrman SW, Mahato RI. miRNA profiling in pancreatic cancer and restoration of chemosensitivity. Cancer Lett. 2013;334:211–20.

171. Zhao WG, Yu SN, Lu ZH, Ma YH, Gu YM, Chen J. The miR-217 microRNA functions as a potential tumor suppressor in pancreatic ductal adenocarcinoma by targeting KRAS. Carcinogenesis. 2010;31:1726–33.

8

Non-invasively predicting differentiation of pancreatic cancer through comparative serum metabonomic profiling

Shi Wen[1], Bohan Zhan[2], Jianghua Feng[2*], Weize Hu[1], Xianchao Lin[1], Jianxi Bai[1] and Heguang Huang[1*] (iD)

Abstract

Background: The differentiation of pancreatic ductal adenocarcinoma (PDAC) could be associated with prognosis and may influence the choices of clinical management. No applicable methods could reliably predict the tumor differentiation preoperatively. Thus, the aim of this study was to compare the metabonomic profiling of pancreatic ductal adenocarcinoma with different differentiations and assess the feasibility of predicting tumor differentiations through metabonomic strategy based on nuclear magnetic resonance spectroscopy.

Methods: By implanting pancreatic cancer cell strains Panc-1, Bxpc-3 and SW1990 in nude mice in situ, we successfully established the orthotopic xenograft models of PDAC with different differentiations. The metabonomic profiling of serum from different PDAC was achieved and analyzed by using ^{1}H nuclear magnetic resonance (NMR) spectroscopy combined with the multivariate statistical analysis. Then, the differential metabolites acquired were used for enrichment analysis of metabolic pathways to get a deep insight.

Results: An obvious metabonomic difference was demonstrated between all groups and the pattern recognition models were established successfully. The higher concentrations of amino acids, glycolytic and glutaminolytic participators in SW1990 and choline-contain metabolites in Panc-1 relative to other PDAC cells were demonstrated, which may be served as potential indicators for tumor differentiation. The metabolic pathways and differential metabolites identified in current study may be associated with specific pathways such as serine-glycine-one-carbon and glutaminolytic pathways, which can regulate tumorous proliferation and epigenetic regulation.

Conclusion: The NMR-based metabonomic strategy may be served as a non-invasive detection method for predicting tumor differentiation preoperatively.

Keywords: Pancreatic ductal adenocarcinoma, Nuclear magnetic resonance, Metabonomics, Tumor differentiation

Background

Pancreatic ductal adenocarcinoma (PDAC) is one of the most malignant tumors with an extremely poor prognosis. Only about 7% of patients can be survived in 5 years, making PDAC the fourth leading cause of death among tumors [1]. Many risk factors have been correlated with prognosis, including tumor size [2, 3], lymph node metastasis [3, 4], nerve plexus invasion [5, 6], vascular invasion [6, 7], tumor differentiation [2, 3, 8], surgical margin status [3, 9] and specific molecular prognostic factors [10, 11]. Thereinto, poorly differentiated/high grade tumors are closely associated with poor outcome of the patients [12]. Furthermore, previous researches also linked tumor histological grading to an increased risk of early death within 1 year [13, 14]. As an important component of early mortality risk score, tumor differentiation can help to assessing short-term tumor-related mortality [14, 15]. Given the important role of tumor differentiation in PDAC management, increased interest in preoperative tumor differentiation assessment were emerged in order to identify high-risk patients, which can benefit the most from neoadjuvant treatment [13, 16–19], even over than upfront surgery [20, 21].

* Correspondence: jianghua.feng@xmu.edu.cn; heguanghuang2@163.com; hhuang2@aliyun.com
[2]Department of Electronic Science, Fujian Provincial Key Laboratory of Plasma and Magnetic Resonance, Xiamen University, Xiamen 361005, China
[1]Department of General Surgery, Fujian Medical University Union Hospital, Fuzhou 350001, China

Thus, notarizing differentiation of tumors preoperatively can provide constructive information for prognostic evaluation and management of PDAC [22].

Conventionally, the preoperative assessments of tumor differentiation were conducted by tissue histological observations derived from fine needle aspiration. This method has been realized to be an effective way to grade the pancreatic neuroendocrine tumors and intraductal papillary mucinous neoplasms [23, 24]. However, this technique is highly invasive for many patients and the achievable samples are too limited to give a reliable histological grading, making this technique still being far away from application in clinical PDAC differentiation assessment [19]. Thus, it would be of great importance to develop an easily acceptable and reliable method to assess the differentiation of PDAC preoperatively.

Nuclear magnetic resonance (NMR) spectroscopy-based metabonomic technique is a promising diagnostic tool with the advantages of high sensitivity, non-invasion and high throughput. This technique can analyze the disease-related metabonomic differences occurred in various types of biosamples (etc. tissues, body fluids and cells) to identify differential metabolites and further biomarkers contributed to establishment of recognition models for diagnosis. At present, NMR-based diagnostic strategy has demonstrated a favorable clinical performance in many diseases [25–31]. Particularly noticeable, magnetic resonance spectroscopy have also been recommended for diagnosis of brain, prostate and breast cancer in European cancer conference [29]. In addition, by using NMR-based methods, many reports on detecting PDAC *in vivo* or *in vitro* have showed an encouraging result to distinguish PDAC from not only the normal but also other benign lesions [32–35]. Therefore, in present study, we used ^{1}H NMR spectroscopy to analyze serum metabonomes from PDAC mice models established by implantations of Panc-1, BxPC-3 and SW1990 (being poor, poor to moderate and moderate to well differentiated [36–39], respectively) cell strains on pancreas, thus, to assess the feasibility of this strategy in predicting the differentiation of tumor.

Methods

Cell culture and animals feeding

PDAC cell strains (Panc-1, BxPC-3 and SW1990, Catalog NO. SCSP-535, TCHu 12 and TCHu 201) were obtained from Shanghai Institute of Cell Biology, Chinese Academy of Sciences (Shanghai, China) authenticated with short tandem repeat test and mycoplasma culture. At the circumstance of 5% CO_2 and 37 °C, these strains were incubated in dulbecco's modified eagle medium (DMEM, Gibco, Thermo Fisher Scientific Inc., USA) added with 10% fetal bovine serum (Gibco) in cell incubator (3110, Thermo Scientific). Then, cells were

digested by 0.125% trypsinogen (Life Technologies, Grand Island, NY, USA) for the passage with the ratio of 1:2-4 every 2-3 days. BALB/c nude mice (male, 4 weeks, weighing 18-20 g), purchased from Shanghai Slac laboratory animals Co., Ltd. (NO: SCXK (HU) 2012-0002), were bred in Fujian Medical University Animals Centre (Fuzhou, china) with a standard SPF-grade laboratory conditions.

Establishment of animal models

This experimental protocol was in accordance with the principles of National Institutes of Health guide for the care and use of laboratory animals and approved by Ethical Committee of Fujian Medical University. Three PDAC cell strains in the exponential phase were digested with 0.125% trypsinogen, washed by phosphate buffered saline (PBS) for three times, then collected and resuspended in PBS (1×10^7 cells per milliliter). After skin degerming, the cell suspension liquids were subcutaneously injected into the axilla of mice (one cell strain each mouse), followed by a month of normal feeding. The tumors with a size of 5 to 10 mm in diameter generated in the injected positions of mice. Consequently, the mice were executed by a mercy killing, and the tumor tissues of Panc-1, BxPC-3 and SW1990 were carefully collected and divided into pieces of 1 mm^3 for implantation *in situ*.

Forty-five mice were randomly divided into 3 groups using random number table. Before surgery, all mice have a 12-h fasting without drink-deprivation. A 2-cm horizontal incision was made on the middle of abdominal wall to expose the pancreas. One piece of tumors was placed on the body or tail of pancreas and fixed with biogum (BaiYun medical glue Co., Ltd., Guangzhou, China), followed by carefully organ restoration and suture. Three groups were dealt with tumor tissues of Panc-1, BxPC-3 and SW1990, respectively ($n = 15$ for each).

Tissues samples collection and preparation

Thirty days after surgeries, 1 mL of blood from each group was collected by aortic puncture under continuous airway anesthesia of isoflurane (Jiupai pharmaceutical Co., Ltd., Shijiazhuang, China) and stored in clear 1.5-mL Eppendorf tubes. After standing for 30 min, the blood went through a 10-min centrifugation at 10,000 g and 4 °C. The supernate was collected and immediately frozen by liquid nitrogen and stored at –80 °C. For the detection of ^{1}H NMR spectroscopy, 400 μL of serum were melted on the surface of ice, and then mixed with 200 μL of 90 mM deuterated phosphate buffer (NaH_2PO_4 and K_2HPO_4, pH 7.4). The mixture of serum and buffer were centrifuged again, and finally, 550 μL of the supernate was moved into 5-mm NMR tubes (ST500, NORELL, Inc., Morganton, North Carolina, USA).

Detection of 1H NMR spectroscopy and preprocessing

The ^{1}H NMR spectroscopy of serum samples were performed on a Varian NMR system (Agilent Technologies Co, Palo Alto, California, USA) with a 500.13 MHz of proton frequency at the temperature of 298 K. For each sample, a water-suppressed CPMG (Carr-Purcell-Meiboom-Gill) spin-echo pulse sequence (RD-90°-(τ-180°-τ)$_n$-ACQ) was used to acquire the NMR spectrum. Herein, a total of 64 scans with a spectral width of 6 KHz and a data point of 12 K were accumulated for all spectra. Spin-echo loop time (2nτ) of 70 ms was applied with a relaxation delay of 2.0 s. The NMR spectra were processed by using MestReNova (V9.0.1, Mestrelab Research S. L., Spain). In order to increase the signal-to-noise ratio, all free induction decays were multiplied by an exponential weighting function equivalent to a 1 Hz linebroadening and subsequently disposed with Fourier transformation. To make the spectra more comparable, the manual phase rectifications and baseline corrections were conducted by using MestReNova. The chemical shifts were referenced to the double-peak of endogenic lactate at δ1.33 for metabolites identification. Automatically, the spectral regions δ9.0-0.5 of the processed NMR spectra were segmented into scatter integral regions of 0.002 ppm with a removal of spectral region δ6.40-5.50 and δ5.19-4.36 to eliminate the impacts of residual water signal and urea signal, respectively. Finally, for each spectrum, the integrated data were normalized to the total sum of the spectrum in favour of multivariate statistical analysis.

Multivariate statistical analysis

The multivariate statistical analysis, including principal component analysis (PCA), partial least squares discriminant analysis (PLS-DA) and orthogonal partial least squares discriminant analysis (OPLS-DA), were performed in SIMCA-P$^+$ (V14.0 Umetrics, Sweden) to analyze the metabonomic differences between three PDAC groups. PCA, performed in the approach of mean-centered scaling, could simplify the normalized date into several components, which can roughly evaluate the clusters distributions and identify the existence of outlines. PLS-DA and OPLS-DA, which can be classified as supervised multivariate statistical analysis, were conducted in the approach of parato-scaling approach for better extraction and maximization of the metabonomic differences between PDAC groups. Furthermore, the OPLS-DA models coefficients, which were back-calculated from the coefficients, incorporated with the weight of the variables, and then to be plotted with color-coded coefficients to enhance interpretability of the models. As a result, the metabolites responsible for the metabonomic differences between groups can be extracted from the corresponding color-coded loading plots and displayed visually. By assistance of MATLAB (V7.1, the Mathworks Inc., Natick, USA), the color-coded coefficient loading plots were drew and color-coded according to the absolute value of coefficient. That meant, in the loading plots, a warm-toned color (i.e. red) represents for the metabolites being positive or negative significant in distinguishing different groups while a cool-toned

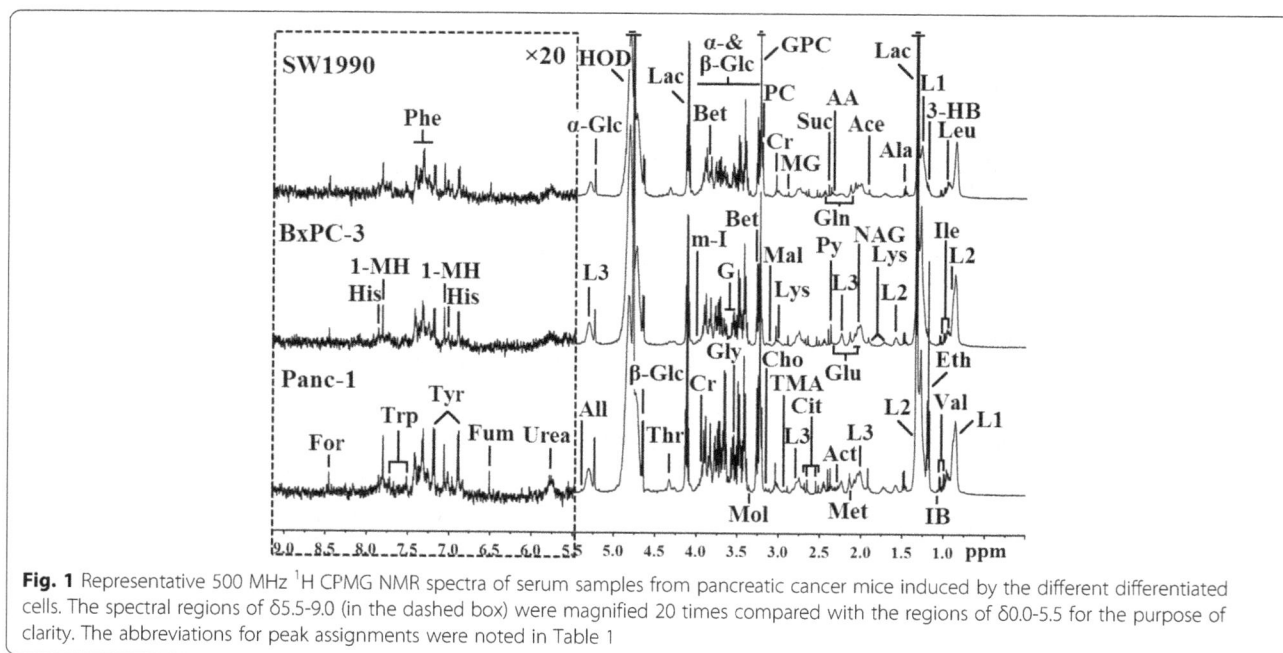

Fig. 1 Representative 500 MHz ^{1}H CPMG NMR spectra of serum samples from pancreatic cancer mice induced by the different differentiated cells. The spectral regions of δ5.5-9.0 (in the dashed box) were magnified 20 times compared with the regions of δ0.0-5.5 for the purpose of clarity. The abbreviations for peak assignments were noted in Table 1

Table 1 The metabolites assignments from NMR spectra of serum from PDAC mice[a]

Abbreviation	Metabolites	^{1}H chemical shift(multiplicity)[b]
1-MH	1-Methylhistidine	7.06(s), 7.78(s)
3-HB	3-Hydroxybutyrate	1.20(d), 2.31(dd), 2.40(m), 4.16(m)
Ace	Acetate	1.92(s)
AA	Acetoacetate	2.28(s)
Act	Acetone	2.24(s)
Ala	Alanine	1.48(d)
All	Allantoin	5.39(s)
Bet	Betaine	3.27(s), 3.90(s)
Cho	Choline	3.20(s)
Cit	Citrate	2.53(d), 2.67(d)
Cr	Creatine	3.04(s), 3.93(s)
Eth	Ethanol	1.18(t), 3.61(q)
For	Formate	8.46(s)
Fum	Fumarate	6.52(s)
Glu	Glutamate	2.08(m), 2.11(m), 2.35(m), 3.75(t)
Gln	Glutamine	2.14(m), 2.45(m), 3.75(t)
G	Glycerol	3.55(m), 3.66(dd), 3.78(m)
GPC	Glycerolphosphocholine	3.23(s), 4.33(m)
Gly	Glycine	3.56(s)
His	Histidine	7.08(s), 7.82(s)
HOD	Residual water signal	4.76(br)
IB	Isobutyrate	1.07(d)
Ile	Isoleucine	0.94(t), 1.01(d)
L1	LDL	0.86(br), 1.28(br)
L2	VLDL	0.89(br), 1.30(br), 1.58(br)
L3	Unsaturated fatty acid	2.04(br), 2.24(br), 2.76(br), 5.31(br)
Lac	Lactate	1.33(d), 4.11(q)
Leu	Leucine	0.96(d)
Lys	Lysine	1.46(m), 1.73(m), 1.91(m), 3.03(m), 3.76(t)
Mal	Malonate	3.11(s)
Met	Methionine	2.14(s), 2.63(t)
MG	Methylguanidine	2.83(s), 3.36(s)
Mol	Methanol	3.36(s)
m-I	myo-Inositol	3.52(dd), 3.61(dd), 4.07(m)
NAG	N-acetyl glycoprotein	2.03(s)
Phe	Phenylalanine	7.32(d), 7.37(t), 7.42(dd)
PC	Phosphocholine	3.21(s)
Py	Pyruvate	2.37(s)
Suc	Succinate	2.40(s)
Thr	Threonine	1.33(d), 4.26(m)
TMA	Trimethylamine	2.89(s)
Trp	Tryptophan	7.27(m), 7.30(s), 7.54(d), 7.73(d)
Tyr	Tyrosine	6.90(d), 7.19(d)

Table 1 The metabolites assignments from NMR spectra of serum from PDAC mice[a] *(Continued)*

Abbreviation	Metabolites	^{1}H chemical shift(multiplicity)[b]
Urea	Urea	5.80(br)
Val	Valine	0.99(d), 1.04(d)
α-Glc	α-Glucose	3.42(t), 3.54(dd), 3.71(t), 3.73(m), 3.84(m), 5.24(d)
β-Glc	β-Glucose	3.24(ddb), 3.41(t), 3.46(m), 3.49(t), 3.90(dd), 4.65(d)

[a]PDAC pancreatic ductal adenocarcinoma
[b]multiplicity:s, singlet; d, doublet; t, triplet; q, quartet; dd, doublets; m, multiplet; br, broad resonance

color (i.e. blue) corresponds to the metabolites not being significant in discriminations. Moreover, to screen out differential metabolites, the cutoff value of correlation coefficients ($|r| > 0.576$) was determined according to the statistical significance of the Pearson correlation coefficient test at the level of $P < 0.05$ and *df* (degree of freedom) =10. In order to assess the quality and validity of models, the 10-fold cross validation and response permutation testing ($n = 200$) were performed and the corresponding parameters R^2 and Q^2 in the permutated plots presented the degree of model fitting and the potentially predictive ability of models, respectively.

The metabolic pathways and interactions analysis

The differential metabolites derived from multivariate statistical analysis were further analyzed for the metabolic pathways by using KEGG (www.genome.jp/kegg) and MBROLE 1.0 (http://csbg.cnb.csic.es/mbrole/) [40, 41].

Results

NMR spectral profiles of serum samples from Panc-1, BxPC-3, SW1990 groups

After visual confirmation for tumorgenesis, 12, 13, and 11 serum samples from Panc-1, BxPC-3 and SW1990 groups were included for the detections with ^{1}H NMR spectroscopy, respectively. Typical one-dimensional 500-MHz ^{1}H NMR spectra of serum samples from models induced by the different differentiated PDAC cells are presented in Fig. 1, which provided an integrated overview of all metabolites. Forty-seven metabolites were identified from the NMR spectra (Table 1) based on the relative literatures and public databases [42, 43]. A certain degree of metabolic differences could be noticed between different PDAC groups visually such as ethanol and phosphocholine. But considering the high similarity of spectra, the metabonomic information acquired was quite limited and the multivariate statistic analysis will help to extract the detailed information.

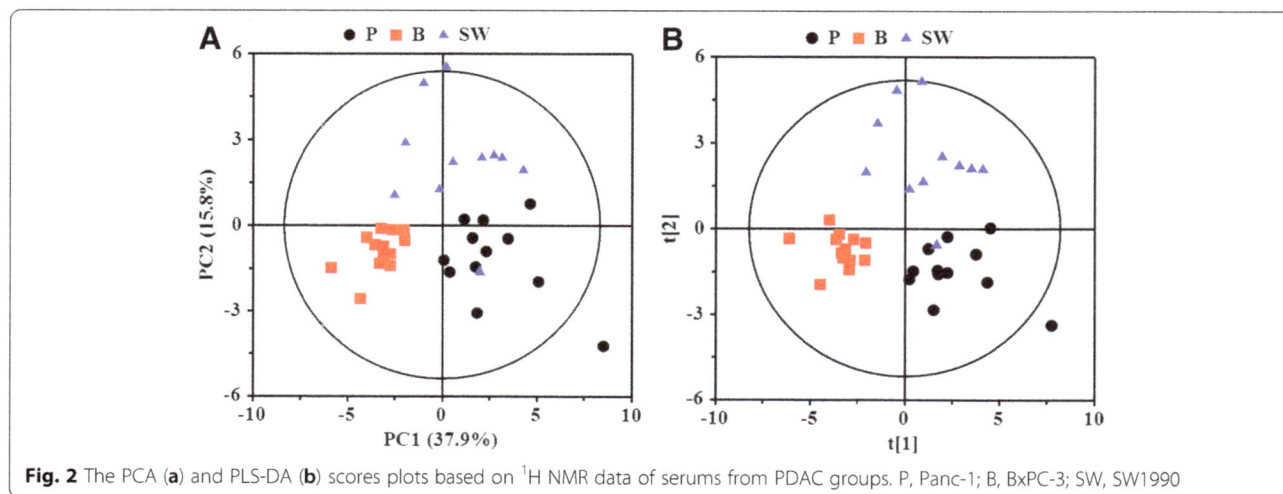

Fig. 2 The PCA (a) and PLS-DA (b) scores plots based on ^{1}H NMR data of serums from PDAC groups. P, Panc-1; B, BxPC-3; SW, SW1990

Metabonomic characteristics of serum from the PDAC groups

To show an overview of ^{1}H NMR data collected from the serum of Panc-1, BxPC-3, and SW1990 groups, the PCA and PLS-DA were performed. The PCA scores plot showed a certain degree of separated trends between the three PDAC groups (Fig. 2a) though a little overlap or dispersity was demonstrated, indicating their obvious metabonomic differences. In further, a greater discrimination in cluster distributions of Panc-1, Bxpc-3 and SW1990 could be observed visually in PLS-DA scores plot (Fig. 2b), demonstrating a significant differences with each other.

To get deep insight into the metabolites responsible for the metabonomic alterations occurred in three PDAC groups, pair-wise comparisons were conducted by using the PLS-DA combined with orthogonal projection (OPLS-DA). The pronounced separations were demonstrated in OPLS-DA scores plots (Fig. 3 upper left panels) and the metabolites corresponding to the metabolic difference were marked in loading plots (Fig. 3 bottom panels). The summarized dominant metabolites, based on the cutoff value of correlation coefficient ($|r| > 0.576$), and the correlation coefficients were listed in detail based on their biochemical types (Table 2). Overall, the levels of metabolites belonged to glycolysis and glutaminolysis, alcohols and amino acids were lower in SW1990 group while the high concentrations of choline and its derivatives were noticeable in Panc-1 group. The favorable fit and prediction parameters (R^2 and Q^2) of the OPLS-DA models and the corresponding permutation test and probability (p-value) via CV-ANOVA also confirmed the strong predictive ability of the models to guarantee a reliable identification of characteristic metabolites.

The biochemical pathways related with the metabonomic difference between PDAC groups

For better understanding of the bioinformation contained in discriminatory metabolites, the biochemical

pathways were identified based on the differential metabolites derived from OPLS-DA of pair-comparisons and those with p-value less than 0.01 were demonstrated on Fig. 4. The p-value for pathway identification were calculated automatically by the MBROLE [40].

In the analysis to compare SW1990 with Bxpc-3, the numerous amino acid-related pathways were noticeable, including metabolism of essential and non-essential amino acids, the biosynthesis of aminoacyl-tRNA and ABC transporters. In addition, the pathways related with glycolysis involving pyruvate, galactose, glutamine and glutamate were also identified as differential features to distinguish the Bxpc-3 from the SW1990. Meanwhile, except the pathways of lysine, histidine and thiamine metabolisms, most pathways involved in Bxpc-3 vs SW1990 were also identified in the comparison between Panc-1 and Sw1990. In addition, the pathways of glycerophospholipid metabolism and the degradation of valine, leucine and isoleucine were also identified to be a signature contributed to distinguish Panc-1 from SW1990. In term of metabolic diversity between Panc-1 and BxPC-3, the metabolic discrimination seems to be quite limited where only a few pathways related with amino acids and glycerophospholipid metabolism were identified.

Discussion

In this study, we tried to evaluate the potential value of non-targeted NMR strategy to predict the tumor differentiation. Since many factors (e.g., drugs, operations) could influence the metabonomic characteristics of serum from patients. We chose three PDAC strains, Panc-1, BxPC-3 and SW1990 which can form tumors *in vivo* with typical histopathologic characters from poor, poor to moderate and moderate to well differentiation respectively [36–39] to establish PDAC models for research. By using animal models, the interference factors can be furthest eliminated. It is beneficial to purify

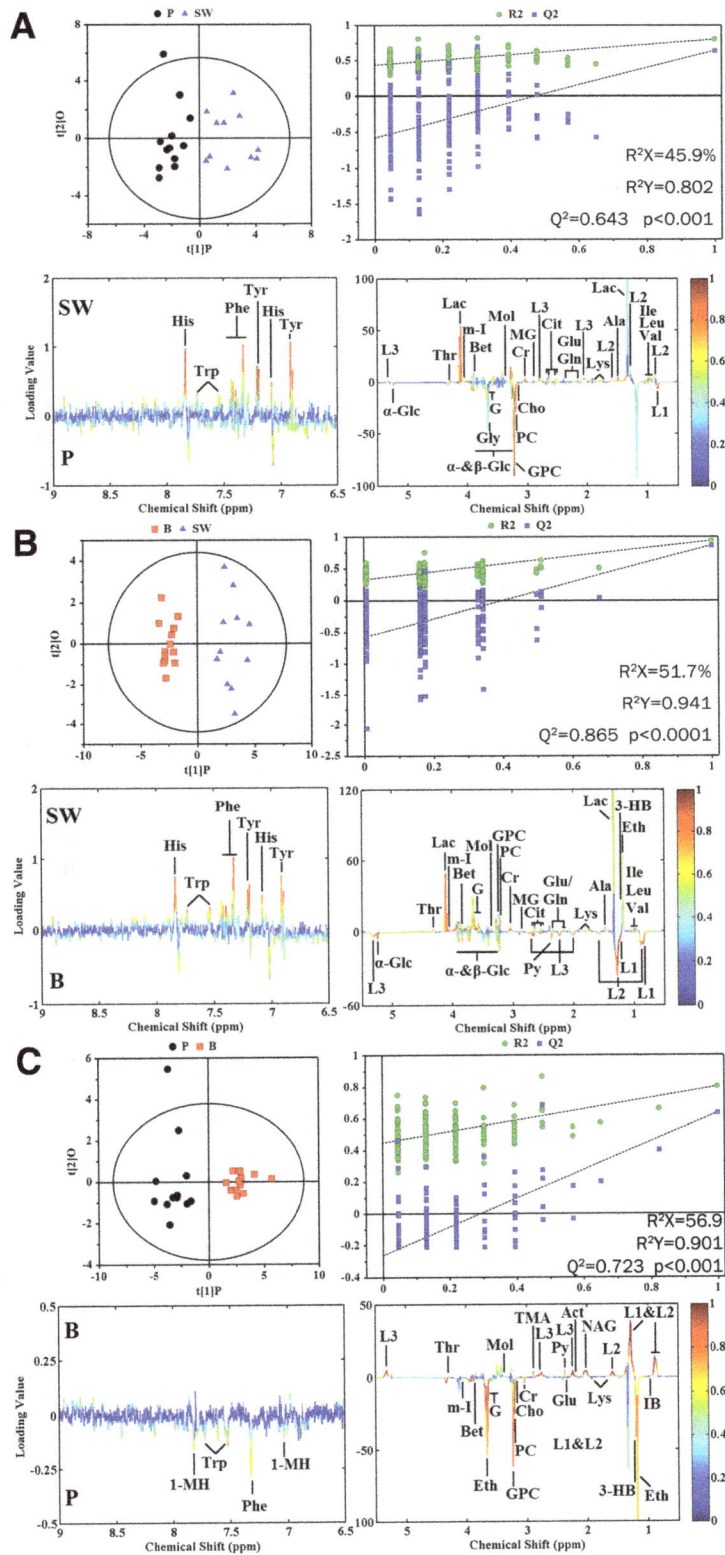

Fig. 3 (See legend on next page.)

(See figure on previous page.)
Fig. 3 OPLS-DA scores plots (upper left panels) and plots of permutation tests ($n = 200$) (upper right panels) derived from ^{1}H NMR spectra of serum samples and corresponding coefficient loading plots (bottom panels) from the pair-wise comparisons between Panc-1, Bxpc-3 and SW1990 groups. **a**. Panc-1 vs SW1990, **b**. BxPC-3 vs SW1990, **c**. Panc-1 vs BxPC-3. The color map shows the significance of metabolites variations between the two classes. Keys of the assignments were shown in Table 1. P, Panc-1; B, BxPC-3; SW, SW1990

serum metabonomic alteration caused by tumor with different differentiation and also specify the association between tumor differentiation and serum metabonomes. To amplify the metabolic difference between the tumors in different differentiations, all groups were compared directly. Given most of clinical patients were diagnosed with moderately differentiated PDAC and the significant clinical value for the identification of tumors in poor differentiation, we focus on the metabonomic difference between SW1990 and other two strains.

Comparative low levels of lactate, glutamate and glutamine indicate a poor differentiation

In present study, we found that the high concentration of citrate, lactate, glutamate and glutamine can help to distinguish the SW1990 from Panc-1 and Bxpc-3. Being well known, the tumor metabolic reprogramming has been validated to be the cornerstone for malignant transformation and one common composition in this process is the aerobic glycolysis (Warburg effect). Through the aerobic glycolysis, rather than tricarboxylic acid (TCA) cycle, the tumor cells derive the predominant ATP/energy and generate extensive lactate from pyruvate to result in environmental acidosis which promote the spreading of the tumor cells [44]. Meanwhile, the lactate generated from hypoxic PDAC can be taken up by normoxic PDAC cells nearby as fuel to maintain proliferation, creating a phenomenon called tumor symbiosis [45]. Thus, the tumor metabolic impact upon the level of lactate in peripheral circulation may be determined by the dynamic balance of release and uptake of lactate around tumor microenvironment. Our outcome indicates that the tumor with a poorer differentiation could induce a lower concentration of lactate in serum relative to that with a better differentiation, which may be due to a stronger ability of lactate recirculation. It's also implied by inconsistent variation trends of lactate in serum reported by previous studies [46, 47]. In addition, due to the breakdown of TCA cycle, glutaminolysis is enhanced in PDAC cells to generate TCA intermediates (e.g. malate, oxaloacetate and citrate) which is called anaplerosis reaction, and subsequently served as building blocks for synthesis of lipid and non-essential amino acids [48]. Besides, glutamine can also act as fuel to support energy metabolism through aspartate, oxaloacetate and pyruvate transformation process, thus promoting growth of pancreatic cancer via *Kras*-regulated metabolic pathway [49]. Therefore, the significantly low levels

of glutamine, glutamate and citrate may indicate that the tumor with poorer differentiation may provide a more dramatic glutaminolysis and deprive more glutamine and glutamate from peripheral circulation.

Comparative low levels of amino acids in serum imply poor differentiation

Likewise, the higher concentrations of amino acids could also contribute to the distinguishing of the SW1990 from Panc-1 and Bxpc-3, which could serve as key participants in the cancer metabolism reprogramming. Under the influence of the abnormal expression of oncogenes and tumor suppress genes, the anabolic metabolism and transport of amino acid were tremendously enhanced for rapid proliferation of cancer cells. To provide required nutrients for cancer growth, the catabolic metabolism of whole-body tissue would be enhanced, leading to an increased circulating amino acids at the early stage of PDAC [50]. But the catabolic metabolism cannot maintain in a high level for a long time and end in a severe nutritional imbalance called cachexia, thus creating a decrease of amino acids in serum at last. In this process, L-type amino-acid transporter 1 (LAT-1), the most important transporter of neutral amino acids, plays a key role in internalized transportation of essential amino acids (EAAs) in PDAC. As previous reports demonstrated, the overexpression of LAT-1 can promote cancer growth via mammalian target-of-rapamycin (mTOR) and serve as a prognostic factor in PDAC [51, 52]. Thus, the higher concentration of EAAs in SW1990 group than in Panc-1 and BxPC-3 group indicates that the tumors with poor differentiation may have a higher expression of LAT1 and nutritional stress from rapid proliferation, which can associated with poor prognosis.

With regard to the non-essential amino acids (NEAAs), several pathways were involved to enhance their biosynthesis and utilization for cell proliferation. As noted above, the accumulated glycolysis intermediates could also promote the biosynthesis of glycine, serine and threonine through 3-phospho-D-glycerate pathway. In addition, the increased glutaminolysis provides numerous substrates (e.g. isocitrate, malate, alpha-ketoglutaric acid) not only to supply the lipids synthesis but also to promote the biosynthesis of alanine and aspartate. Besides being used as building blocks and fuels for cell proliferation, NEAAs have been indicated to bridge the interplay metabolism and epigenetics, thus

Table 2 OPLS-DA coefficients of metabolites in different pair-comparisons derived from NMR-data

Metabolites	r[a]		
	BxPC-3 vs SW1990	Panc-1 vs SW1990	Panc-1 vs BxPC-3
Glycolysis and glutaminolysis			
α-Glucose	−0.788	−0.631	−
β-Glucose	−0.735	−0.842	−
Citrate	0.817	0.921	−
Glutamate	0.808	0.747	−0.789
Glutamine	0.767	0.856	−
Lactate	0.906	0.905	−
pyruvate	−0.880	−	0.793
Succinate	−	−	−
Carboxylic acids and derivatives			
Acetate	−	−	−
Formate	−	−	−
Fumarate	−	−	−
Isobutyrate	−	−	−0.709
Malonate	−	−	−0.648
Alcohols			
Ethanol	0.879	−	−0.804
Methanol	0.702	0.760	0.667
myo-Inositol	0.889	0.817	−0.877
Glycerol	0.935	0.784	−0.916
Lipid			
LDL	−0.899	−0.847	0.912
VLDL	−0.774	0.720	0.921
Unsaturated fatty acid	−0.899	−0.847	0.912
ketone body			
3-Hydroxybutyrate	0.747	−	−0.636
Acetoacetate	−	−	−
Acetone	−0.760	−	0.912
Choline and derivatives			
Choline	−	−0.836	−0.841
Glycerolphosphocholine	0.671	−0.912	−0.894
Phosphocholine	0.736	−0.832	−0.892
Amino acid			
Non-essential amino acid			
1-methylhistidine	−	−	−0.651
Alanine	0.750	0.778	−
Betaine	0.812	0.834	−0.769
Creatine	0.930	0.826	−0.849
Glycine	0.871	0.674	−
Histidine	0.776	0.602	−
Tyrosine	0.832	0.859	−

Table 2 OPLS-DA coefficients of metabolites in different pair-comparisons derived from NMR-data (Continued)

Metabolites	r[a]		
	BxPC-3 vs SW1990	Panc-1 vs SW1990	Panc-1 vs BxPC-3
Essential amino acid			
Isoleucine	0.749	0.795	−
Leucine	0.707	0.775	−
Lysine	0.886	0.822	−0.780
Methionine	−	0.645	−
Phenylalanine	0.878	0.813	−0.642
Threonine	0.630	0.794	0.730
Tryptophan	0.846	0.847	−0.673
Valine	0.839	0.858	−
Others			
Methylguanidine	0.650	0.732	−
Allantoin	−0.687	−	−
N-acetyl glycoprotein	−	0.661	0.914
Trimethylamine	−0.855	0.750	0.782

[a]Correlation coefficients, positive and negative signs indicate positive and negative correlation in the concentrations. $|r| > 0.576$ was the cutoff value for significance based on discrimination significance of $p = 0.05$ and df = 10. "-" means $|r| < 0.576$

serve as programmed switch for cell differentiation [53]. For instance, several NEAAs including glycine could be associated with gene signatures of cell proliferation and *Myc* target activation through the serine-glycine-one-carbon pathway (SGOC pathway), which contribute significantly to energy generation and biosynthesis of NADPH and purine [54]. In addition, the mTOR-dependent induction of SGOC pathways can also lead to DNA methylation and tumorigenesis under the cooperatively oncogenic function of the loss of liver kinase B1 and activation of Kras, which highly involved in epigenetics [55]. Thus, NEAAs are highly associated with genesis, progression and epigenetics, and their relative concentration in serum may be indicators for the differentiation of PDAC.

Relative high concentration metabolites of choline metabolism may imply a poor differentiation

Impressively, the high correlation coefficient of choline groups in the pair-comparison of Panc-1 vs BxPC-3 and Panc-1 vs SW1990 implied that relatively high concentration of choline-like metabolites including phosphocholine (PC) and glycerolphosphocholine (GPC) may be significant metabolic features for poor differentiation of PDAC. According to previous study, the tumor-associated choline metabolism plays a key role in cell malignant transformation, tumor migration and metastasis [56, 57], characterized by elevated level of PC and total choline in tissue [45, 46]. Thereinto, the

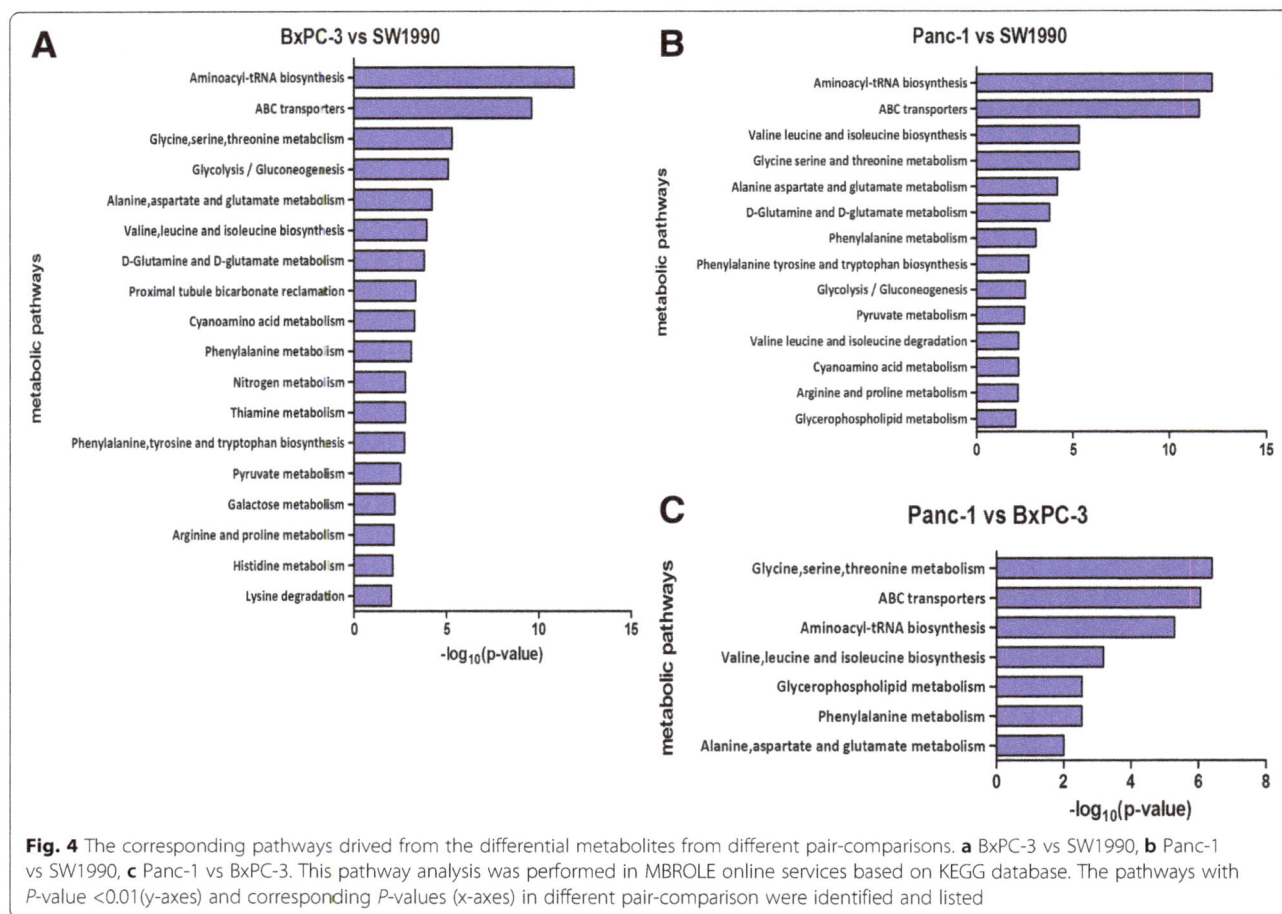

Fig. 4 The corresponding pathways drived from the differential metabolites from different pair-comparisons. **a** BxPC-3 vs SW1990, **b** Panc-1 vs SW1990, **c** Panc-1 vs BxPC-3. This pathway analysis was performed in MBROLE online services based on KEGG database. The pathways with P-value <0.01(y-axes) and corresponding P-values (x-axes) in different pair-comparison were identified and listed

overexpression of choline kinase-α (Chk-a) induced by hypoxia-inducible factor (HIF) accounts for the increase of cellular PC and total choline [58], generating excessive phosphatidylcholine for biosynthesis of cell membrane. In addition, the EDI3-intermediated choline metabolism, a pathways verified in other solid tumor, can not only cleave GPC to form choline to supplement Kennedy pathway, but also generate glycerol-3-phosphate and its sequentially downstream intermediators for cellular signaling to regulate migration, invasion, proliferation and differentiation [57]. Other research detecting serum from PDAC patients also indicated that the choline metabolism were obviously altered and could potentially serve as biomarkers to detect PDAC in early stage. Thus, the difference of choline metabolism in PDAC could reflect and create a handful of regulatory functions on tumor progression and differentiation.

There are some pitfalls in this study. The PDAC models were established by using three PDAC cell lines which could only represent a part of metabonome landscape of pancreatic cancer, which inevitably lower the level of evidence provided from our study. The heterogeneity of pancreatic cancer in patients may compromise the directly clinical transformation application of our results. Thus, the further validation based on a large patient cohort will be performed in the future.

Conclusions
In this study, we compared the serum metabonomic profiling between PDAC with different differentiations and successfully established pattern recognition models to distinguish with each other. The lower concentration of amino acids, glycolytic and glutaminolytic participators may serve as the predictors for poor differentiation of tumor. Thus, NMR-based metabonomic strategy can be a promising non-invasive approach to predict tumor differentiation preoperatively.

Abbreviations
1-MH: 1-Methylhistidine; 3-HB: 3-Hydroxybutyrate; AA: Acetoacetate; Ace: Acetate; Act: Acetone; Ala: Alanine; All: Allantoin; Bet: Betaine; Cho: Choline; Cit: Citrate; CPMG: Carr-Purcell-Meiboom-Gill; Cr: Creatine; EAAs: Essential amino acids; Eth: Ethanol; For: Formate; Fum: Fumarate; G: Glycerol; Gln: Glutamine; Glu: Glutamate; Gly: Glycine; GPC: Glycerolphosphocholine; His: Histidine; HOD: Residual water signal; IB: Isobutyrate; Ile: Isoleucine; L1: LDL; L2: VLDL; Lac: Lactate; LAT-1: L-type amino-acid transporter 1; Leu: Leucine; Lys: Lysine; Mal: Malonate; Met: Methionine; MG: Methylguanidine; m-I: myo-Inositol; Mol: Methanol; mTOR: Mammalian target-of-rapamycin; NAG: N-acetyl glycoprotein;

NEAAs: Non-essential amino acids; NMR: Nuclear magnetic resonance; OPLS-DA: Orthogonal partial least squares discriminant analysis; PC: Phosphocholine; PCA: Principal component analysis; PDAC: Pancreatic ductal adenocarcinoma; Phe: Phenylalanine; PLS-DA: Partial least squares discriminant analysis; Py: Pyruvate; SGOC pathway: Serine-glycine-one-carbon pathway; Suc: Succinate; TCA: Tricarboxylic acid; Thr: Threonine; TMA: Trimethylamine; Trp: Tryptophan; Tyr: Tyrosine; Val: Valine; α-Glc: α-Glucose; β-Glc: β-Glucose

Acknowledgements

No applicable

Funding

This work is sponsored by a. the National Natural Science Foundation of China (No. 81272581, 31671920); b. the United Fujian Provincial Health and Education Project for Tackling the Key Research (No.WKJ-FJ-10); c. National Key Clinical Specialty Discipline Construction Program of China and Key Clinical Specialty Discipline Construction Program of Fujian.

Authors' contributions

SW established the animal models, interpreted the metabonomic data regarding PDAC and was the main writer for this manuscript. BZ was in charge of NMR detection of samples and the disposition of spectrum. JF designed the protocol of NMR detection, check the whole experimental data and was a major contributor in writing the manuscript. WH, XL and JB were major contributors to animal models and the preparation of samples. HH was the initiator of this study, design the whole experimental protocol and as the ultimate checker for this manuscript. All authors have read and approved the final version of this manuscript.

Competing interests

The authors declare that they have no competing interests.

References

1. Siegel RL, Miller KD, Jemal A. Cancer statistics, 2015. CA Cancer J Clin. 2015; 65(1):5–29.
2. Sohn T, Yeo C, Lillemoe K, Koniaris L, Kaushal S, Sauter P, Coleman J, Hruban R, Cameron J. Resected adenocarcinoma of the pancreas - 616 patients: results, outcome and prognostic indicators. Gastroenterology. 2000;118(4):A1059.
3. Winter J, Cameron J, Campbell K, Chang D, Coleman J, Hodgin M, Sauter P, Hruban R, Riall T, Schulick R. 1423 Pancreaticoduodenectomies for pancreatic cancer: a single-institution experience. J Gastrointest Surg. 2006; 10(9):1199–211.
4. Makowiec F, Riediger H, Fischer E, Keck T, Opitz OG, Adam U, Hopt UT. M1547 the lymph node-ratio is the strongest factor predicting survival after resection of pancreatic cancer. Gastroenterology. 2008;134(4):A-870.
5. Nagai S, Fujii T, Kodera Y, Kanda M, Sahin TT, Kanzaki A, Yamada S, Sugimoto H, Nomoto S, Takeda S. Impact of operative blood loss on survival in invasive Ductal Adenocarcinoma of the pancreas. Pancreas. 2010;40(1):3–9.
6. Shimada K, Sano T, Sakamoto Y, Kosuge T. Clinical implications of combined portal vein resection as a palliative procedure in patients undergoing pancreaticoduodenectomy for pancreatic head carcinoma. Ann Surg Oncol. 2006;13(12):1569–78.
7. Mitsuro K, Tsutomu F, Sahin TT, Akiyuki K, Shunji N, Suguru Y, Hiroyuki S, Shuji N, Shin T, Yasuhiro K. Invasion of the splenic artery is a crucial prognostic factor in carcinoma of the body and tail of the pancreas. Ann Surg. 2010;251(3):483–7.
8. Sugiura T, Uesaka K, Mihara K, Sasaki K, Kanemoto H, Mizuno T, Okamura Y. Margin status, recurrence pattern, and prognosis after resection of pancreatic cancer. Surgery. 2013;154(5):1078–86.
9. Neoptolemos JP, Stocken DD, Dunn JA, Almond J, Beger HG, Pederzoli P, Bassi C, Dervenis C, Fernandez-Cruz L, Lacaine F, et al. Influence of resection margins on survival for patients with pancreatic cancer treated by adjuvant chemoradiation and/or chemotherapy in the ESPAC-1 randomized controlled trial. Ann Surg. 2001;234(6):758–68.
10. Saukkonen K, Hagstrom J, Mustonen H, Juuti A, Nordling S, Kallio P, Alitalo K, Seppanen H, Haglund C. PROX1 and beta-catenin are prognostic markers in pancreatic ductal adenocarcinoma. BMC Cancer. 2016;16:472.
11. Reiser-Erkan C, Erkan M, Pan Z, Bekasi S, Giese NA, Streit S, Michalski CW, Friess H, Kleeff J. Hypoxia-inducible proto-oncogene Pim-1 is a prognostic marker in pancreatic ductal adenocarcinoma. Cancer Biol Ther. 2008;7(9):1352–9.
12. Neoptolemos JP, Stocken DD, Friess H, Bassi C, Dunn JA, Hickey H, Beger H, Fernandez-Cruz L, Dervenis C, Lacaine F, et al. A randomized trial of chemoradiotherapy and chemotherapy after resection of pancreatic cancer. N Engl J Med. 2004;350(12):1200–10.
13. Barugola G, Partelli S, Marcucci S, Sartori N, Capelli P, Bassi C, Pederzoli P, Falconi M. Resectable pancreatic cancer: who really benefits from resection? Ann Surg Oncol. 2009;16(12):3316–22.
14. Hsu CC, Wolfgang CL, Laheru DA, Pawlik TM, Swartz MJ, Winter JM, Robinson R, Edil BH, Narang AK, Choti MA, et al. Early mortality risk score: identification of poor outcomes following upfront surgery for resectable pancreatic cancer. J Gastrointest Surg. 2012;16(4):753–61.
15. Joliat GR, Petermann D, Demartines N, Schafer M. External assessment of the early mortality risk score in patients with adenocarcinoma undergoing pancreaticoduodenectomy. HPB (Oxford). 2015;17(7):605–10.
16. Mornex F, Girard N, Delpero JR, Partensky C. Radiochemotherapy in the management of pancreatic cancer–part I: neoadjuvant treatment. Semin Radiat Oncol. 2005;15(4):226–34.
17. Quiros RM, Brown KM, Hoffman JP. Neoadjuvant therapy in pancreatic cancer. Cancer Investig. 2007;25(4):267–73.
18. Varadhachary GR, Tamm EP, Abbruzzese JL, Xiong HQ, Crane CH, Wang H, Lee JE, Pisters PW, Evans DB, Wolff RA. Borderline resectable pancreatic cancer: definitions, management, and role of preoperative therapy. Ann Surg Oncol. 2006;13(8):1035–46.
19. Larghi A, Correale L, Ricci R, Abdulkader I, Monges G, Iglesias-Garcia J, Giovannini M, Attili F, Vitale G, Hassan C, et al. Interobserver agreement and accuracy of preoperative endoscopic ultrasound-guided biopsy for histological grading of pancreatic cancer. Endoscopy. 2015;47(4):308–14.
20. Nurmi A, Haglund C, Mustonen H, Seppänen H. Neoadjuvant therapy offers longer survival for pancreatic cancer patients over upfront surgery. Pancreatology. 2017;17(3):S73.
21. Mokdad AA, Minter RM, Zhu H, Augustine MM, Porembka MR, Wang SC, Yopp AC, Mansour JC, Choti MA, Polanco PM. Neoadjuvant therapy followed by resection versus upfront resection for Resectable pancreatic cancer: a propensity score matched analysis. J Clin Oncol. 2016;35(4):515-22.
22. Network NCC. NCCN clinical practice guidelines in oncology: pancreatic Adenocarcinoma(version 2.2014). Fort Washington: National Comprehensive Cancer Network; 2014. http://www.nccn.org/professionals/physician_gls/pdf/pancreatic.pdf
23. Farrell JM, Pang JC, Kim GE, Tabatabai ZL. Pancreatic neuroendocrine tumors: accurate grading with Ki-67 index on fine-needle aspiration specimens using the WHO 2010/ENETS criteria. Cancer Cytopathol. 2014;122(10):770–8.
24. Pitman MB, Centeno BA, Genevay M, Fonseca R, Mino-Kenudson M. Grading epithelial atypia in endoscopic ultrasound-guided fine-needle aspiration of intraductal papillary mucinous neoplasms: an international interobserver concordance study. Cancer Cytopathol. 2013;121(12):729–36.
25. Brindle JT, Antti H, Holmes E, Tranter G, Nicholson JK, Bethell HWL, Clarke S, Schofield PM, Mckilligin E, Mosedale DE. Rapid and noninvasive diagnosis of the presence and severity of coronary heart disease using 1H-NMR-based metabonomics. Nat Med. 2002;8(12):1439–44.
26. Bartella L, Morris EA, Dershaw DD, Liberman L, Thakur SB, Moskowitz C, Guido J, Huang W. Proton MR spectroscopy with choline peak as malignancy marker improves positive predictive value for breast cancer diagnosis: preliminary study. Radiology. 2006;239(3):686–92.
27. Huzjan R, Sala E, Hricak H. Magnetic resonance imaging and magnetic resonance spectroscopic imaging of prostate cancer. Nat Clin Pract Urol. 2005;2(9):434–42.
28. Khan SA, Cox IJ, Thillainayagam AV, Bansi DS, Thomas HC, Taylor-Robinson SD. Proton and phosphorus-31 nuclear magnetic resonance spectroscopy of human bile in hepatopancreaticobiliary cancer. Eur J Gastroenterol Hepatol. 2005;17(7):733–8.
29. Kwock L, Smith JK, Castillo M, Ewend MG, Collichio F, Morris DE, Bouldin TW, Cush S. Clinical role of proton magnetic resonance spectroscopy in oncology: brain, breast, and prostate cancer. Lancet Oncol. 2006;7(10):859–68.

30. Rehman L, Rehman UL, Azmat SK, Mohammad Hashim AS. Magnetic resonance spectroscopy: novel non-invasive technique for diagnosing brain tumors. J Coll Physicians Surg Pak. 2015;25(12):863–6.

31. Thomas MA, Wyckoff N, Yue K, Binesh N, Banakar S, Chung HK, Sayre J, DeBruhl N. Two-dimensional MR spectroscopic characterization of breast cancer in vivo. Technol Cancer Res Treat. 2005;4(1):99–106.

32. Kaplan O, Kushnir T, Askenazy N, Knubovets T, Navon G. Role of nuclear magnetic resonance spectroscopy (MRS) in cancer diagnosis and treatment: 31P, 23Na, and 1H MRS studies of three models of pancreatic cancer. Cancer Res. 1997;57(8):1452–9.

33. Bathe OF, Shaykhutdinov R, Kopciuk K, Weljie AM, McKay A, Sutherland FR, Dixon E, Dunse N, Sotiropoulos D, Vogel HJ. Feasibility of identifying pancreatic cancer based on serum metabolomics. Cancer Epidemiol Biomarkers Prev. 2011;20(1):140–7.

34. Zhang L, Jin H, Guo X, Yang Z, Zhao L, Tang S, Mo P, Wu K, Nie Y, Pan Y, et al. Distinguishing pancreatic cancer from chronic pancreatitis and healthy individuals by (1)H nuclear magnetic resonance-based metabonomic profiles. Clin Biochem. 2012;45(13-14):1064–9.

35. Fang F, He X, Deng H, Chen Q, Lu J, Spraul M, Yu Y. Discrimination of metabolic profiles of pancreatic cancer from chronic pancreatitis by high-resolution magic angle spinning 1H nuclear magnetic resonance and principal components analysis. Cancer Sci. 2007;98(11):1678–82.

36. Tan MH, Nowak NJ, Loor R, ., Ochi H, ., Sandberg AA, Lopez C, ., Pickren JW, Berjian R, ., Douglass HO, Chu TM. Characterization of a new primary human pancreatic tumor line. Cancer Investig 1986, 4(1):15-23.

37. Kyriazis AP, Sandberg AA, Kyriazis AA, Sloane NH, Lepera R. Establishment and characterization of human pancreatic adenocarcinoma cell line SW-1990 in tissue culture and the nude mouse. Cancer Res. 1983;43(9):4393–401.

38. Lieber M, ., Mazzetta J, ., Nelson-Rees W, ., Kaplan M, ., Todaro G,. Establishment of a continuous tumor-cell line (panc-1) from a human carcinoma of the exocrine pancreas. Int J Cancer 1975, 15(5):741-747.

39. Deer EL, Jessica GH, Coursen JD, Shea JE, Josephat N, Scaife CL, Firpo MA, Mulvihill SJ. Phenotype and genotype of pancreatic cancer cell lines. Pancreas. 2010;39(4):425–35.

40. Chagoyen M, Pazos F. MBRole: enrichment analysis of metabolomic data. Bioinformatics. 2011;27(5):730–1.

41. Kanehisa M, Goto S, Sato Y, Kawashima M, Furumichi M, Tanabe M. Data, information, knowledge and princple: back to metabolism in KEGG. Nucleic Acids Res. 2014;42(Database issue):D199–205.

42. Wishart DS, Knox C, Guo AC, Eisner R, Young N, Gautam B, Hau DD, Psychogios N, Dong E, Bouatra S, et al. HMDB: a knowledgebase for the human metabolome. Nucleic Acids Res. 2009;37(Database issue): D603–10.

43. Cui Q, Lewis IA, Hegeman AD, Anderson ME, Li J, Schulte CF, Westler WM, Eghbalnia HR, Sussman MR, Markley JL. Metabolite identification via the Madison Metabolomics consortium database. Nat Biotechnol. 2008;26(2):162–4.

44. Hirschhaeuser F, Sattler UG, Mueller-Klieser W. Lactate: a metabolic key player in cancer. Cancer Res. 2011;71(22):6921–5.

45. Guillaumond F, Leca J, Olivares O, Lavaut MN, Vidal N, Berthezene P, Dusetti NJ, Loncle C, Calvo E, Turrini O, et al. Strengthened glycolysis under hypoxia supports tumor symbiosis and hexosamine biosynthesis in pancreatic adenocarcinoma. Proc Natl Acad Sc U S A. 2013;110(10):3919–24.

46. OuYang D, Xu J, Huang H, Chen Z. Metabolomic profiling of serum from human pancreatic cancer patients using 1H NMR spectroscopy and principal component analysis. Appl Biochem Biotechnol. 2011;165(1):148–54.

47. Kobayashi T, Nishiumi S, Ikeda A, Yoshie T, Sakai A, Matsubara A, Izumi Y, Tsumura H, Tsuda M, Nishisaki H, et al. A novel serum metabolomics-based diagnostic approach to pancreatic cancer. Cancer Epidemiol Biomarkers Prev. 2013;22(4):571–9.

48. Soga T. Cancer metabolism: key players in metabolic reprogramming. Cancer Sci. 2013;104(3):275–81.

49. Son J, Lyssiotis CA, Ying H, Wang X, Hua S, Ligorio M, Perera RM, Ferrone CR, Mullarky E, Shyh-Chang N, et al. Glutamine supports pancreatic cancer growth through a KRAS-regulated metabolic pathway. Nature. 2013; 496(7443):101–5.

50. Mayers JR, Wu C, Clish CB, Kraft P, Torrence ME, Fiske BP, Yuan C, Bao Y, Townsend MK, Tworoger SS, et al. Elevation of circulating branched-chain amino acids is an early event in human pancreatic adenocarcinoma development. Nat Med. 2014;20(10):1193–8.

51. Fuchs BC, Bode BP. Amino acid transporters ASCT2 and LAT1 in cancer: partners in crime? Semin Cancer Biol. 2005;15(4):254–66.

52. Kaira K, Sunose Y, Arakawa K, Ogawa T, Sunaga N, Shimizu K, Tominaga H, Oriuchi N, Itoh H, Nagamori S, et al. Prognostic significance of L-type amino-acid transporter 1 expression in surgically resected pancreatic cancer. Br J Cancer. 2012;107(4):632–8.

53. Phang JM, Liu W, Hancock C. Bridging epigenetics and metabolism: role of non-essential amino acids. Epigenetics. 2013;8(3):231–6.

54. Tedeschi PM, Markert EK, Gounder M, Lin H, Dvorzhinski D, Dolfi SC, Chan LL, Qiu J, DiPaola RS, Hirshfield KM, et al. Contribution of serine, folate and glycine metabolism to the ATP, NADPH and purine requirements of cancer cells. Cell Death Dis. 2013;4:e877.

55. Kottakis F, Nicolay BN, Roumane A, Karnik R, Gu H, Nagle JM, Boukhali M, Hayward MC, Li YY, Chen T, et al. LKB1 loss links serine metabolism to DNA methylation and tumorigenesis. Nature. 2016;539(7629):390-95.

56. Glunde K, Bhujwalla ZM, Ronen SM. Choline metabolism in malignant transformation. Nat Rev Cancer. 2011;11(12):835–48.

57. Stewart JD, Marchan R, Lesjak MS, Lambert J, Hergenroeder R, Ellis JK, Lau CH, Keun HC, Schmitz G, Schiller J, et al. Choline-releasing glycerophosphodiesterase EDI3 drives tumor cell migration and metastasis. Proc Natl Acad Sci U S A. 2012;109(21):8155–60.

58. Penet MF, Shah T, Bharti S, Krishnamachary B, Artemov D, Mironchik Y, Wildes F, Maitra A, Bhujwalla ZM. Metabolic imaging of pancreatic ductal adenocarcinoma detects altered choline metabolism. Clin Cancer Res. 2015; 21(2):386–95.

9

Nomograms predict long-term survival for patients with periampullary adenocarcinoma after pancreatoduodenectomy

Chaobin He[†], Yize Mao[†], Jun Wang, Fangting Duan, Xiaojun Lin and Shengping Li[*]

Abstract

Background: The prognosis of patients with periampullary adenocarcinoma after pancreatoduodenectomy is diverse and not yet clearly illustrated. The aim of this study was to develop a nomogram to predict individual risk of overall survival (OS) and progression-free survival (PFS) in patients with periampullary adenocarcinoma after pancreatoduodenectomy.

Methods: A total of 205 patients with periampullary adenocarcinoma after pancreatoduodenectomy were retrospectively included. OS and PFS were evaluated by the Kaplan-Meier method. Two nomograms for predicting OS and PFS were established, and the predictive accuracy was measured by the concordance index (Cindex) and calibration plots.

Results: Lymph node ratio (LNR), carbohydrate antigen 19–9 (CA19–9) and anatomical location were incorporated into the nomogram for OS prediction and LNR, CA19–9; anatomical location and tumor differentiation were incorporated into the nomogram for PFS prediction. All calibration plots for the probability of OS and PFS fit well. The Cindexes of the nomograms for OS and PFS prediction were 0.678 and 0.68, respectively. The OS and PFS survival times were stratified significantly using the nomogram-predicted survival probabilities.

Conclusions: The present nomograms for OS and PFS prediction can provide valuable information for tailored decision-making for patients with periampullary adenocarcinoma after pancreatoduodenectomy.

Keywords: Periampullary adenocarcinoma, Pancreatoduodenectomy, Nomogram, Prediction, Prognosis

Background

The periampullary region is a complex region that is composed of distinct anatomical structures: the head of the pancreas, the distal common bile duct (CBD), the second portion of the duodenum, and the ampulla of Vater. Periampullary adenocarcinoma is now classified by the anatomic location of origin according to the 8th edition of American Joint Committee on Cancer (AJCC) staging [1]. Although periampullary adenocarcinoma accounts for approximately 0.2% of all gastrointestinal tract tumors [2]

and is a relatively uncommon neoplasm, there has been an increasing trend of occurrence in recent years [3]. Periampullary adenocarcinoma is a common malignancy for which patients receive pancreaticoduodenectomy (PD), especially in Asia [4, 5]. The resectability is often limited by early local invasion of the surrounding anatomical structures, such as the superior mesenteric vein and superior mesenteric artery. The periampullary adenocarcinomas, including pancreatic head carcinoma, have a relatively low resectable rate of only 15–20% at diagnosis due to the absence of early detection methods [6, 7]. Patient survival after radical resection of adenocarcinomas of the pancreas, CBD, duodenum, and ampulla of Vater greatly varies [2, 8, 9], although some studies have reported that there is a comparatively favorable prognosis among periampullary

* Correspondence: lishp@sysucc.org.cn
[†]Equal contributors
Department of Hepatobiliary and Pancreatic Surgery, State Key Laboratory of Oncology in South China, Collaborative Innovation Center for Cancer Medicine, Sun Yat-sen University Cancer Center, Guangzhou, Guangdong 510060, People's Republic of China

adenocarcinomas, with 5-year overall survival (OS) rates of 30–70% after radical resection [10, 11].

Some reports have shown survival differences among different kinds of periampullary adenocarcinomas [2, 12]. Howe et al. reported that there was a higher resection rate, a lower recurrence rate, and a better OS rate for ampullary carcinomas compared with other periampullary adenocarcinomas [13]. However, pancreatic head carcinoma has been reported to have a poor prognosis even after curative therapy [14]. Anatomic location seems to provide some prognostic information in resected periampullary adenocarcinomas. Additionally, whether the ratio of lymph node (LN) with metastasis is or is not a predictor of OS in patients with periampullary adenocarcinomas has been controversial in recent years. Some studies [15, 16] suggested that the ratio of LN with metastasis was a strong predictor of OS in patients with periampullary adenocarcinomas while some reports [17, 18] failed to show that. Currently, the predictive value of variables is still uncertain. There is a lack of a staging system and consensus regarding specific risk profiles for OS and progression-free survival (PFS) in patients with periampullary adenocarcinomas; this lack makes appropriate risk stratification and physician-patient communication challenging. Risk equations and risk functions are widely applied in patient management, especially for predicting survival outcomes. Given these risk analyses and the current interest in precision medicine, it is necessary to establish prognostic tools to identify patients at risk of long-term survival and optimize patients' selection for appropriate treatment therapy.

A nomogram, which has been developed for various cancers [19–21], is a simple graphical presentation of a multivariate predictive model showing the impact of each included variable on an outcome of interest that provides a numerical probability of the outcome [22]. Some reports have demonstrated some prognostic factors for the survival of patients with periampullary adenocarcinomas, although these prognostic factors were analyzed separately in different cohorts [12, 23]. Further, nomograms, which are capable of utilizing multiple prognostic variables, can provide a single numerical estimate of survival and an individualized prediction of survival. Unfortunately, nomograms have only been available for pancreatic carcinoma [24, 25], and few studies [12, 26] have reported nomograms for ampullary carcinoma; these studies were based on a small cohorts or without relative high concordance indexes (C-index), indicating that these nomograms were not better choices compared with the tumor-node-metastasis (TNM) stage system. Additionally, there is a lack of specific nomograms that can predict long-term survival outcomes for patients with periampullary adenocarcinomas. In the present study, we constructed nomograms from a cohort study of patients with periampullary adenocarcinoma after pancreaticoduodenectomy to predict OS and PFS.

Methods

Patients

Consecutive patients with newly pathologically proven periampullary adenocarcinoma after pancreatoduodenectomy carried out between February 2009 and September 2016 at the Department of Hepatobiliary and Pancreatic Surgery of Sun Yat-sen University Cancer Center were enrolled into this study. Exclusion criteria are as follows: (1) patients with major vascular invasion (superior mesenteric vein, superior mesenteric artery, or inferior vena cava) (n = 28); (2) patients who underwent limited surgery (e.g. ampullectomy) (n = 5); (3) microscopic or macroscopic incomplete resection (n = 2); (4) patients diagnosed with distant metastasis with or without palliative therapy (n = 25); (5) pathologic cell types was not adenocarcinoma (n = 65); (6) patients diagnosed with other concurrent primary tumors (n = 12); (7) lost to follow-up (n = 18). All patients were followed up for at least 1 year after treatment. A total of 205 patients were included for this study.

Clinical data collection

All clinical and pathological data for diagnosis were retrieved from medical records archived at Sun Yat-sen University Cancer Center. The following clinical and pathological data were collected and analyzed: age, gender, white blood cell (WBC) count, C-reactive protein (CRP), alanine transaminase (ALT), aspartate aminotransferase (AST), albumin (ALB), total bilirubin (TBIL), alkaline phosphatase (ALP), serum levels of Carbohydrate antigen 19–9 (CA19–9), anatomical location, tumor differentiation, tumor diameter, lymph node ratio (LNR), LN metastasis and LN total number. LNR was defined as the number of LNs with metastases divided by the total number of excised LNs. The tumor stage was categorized according to the pathological TNM staging system issued by 8th edition of AJCC [1].

Treatment procedure

Resection was performed when there was no evidence of metastasis and no arterial involvement. A classical Whipple operation was the standard resection, which was performed for all the included patients. Regional lymphadenectomy included dissection of the LNs in the hepatoduodenal ligament along the superior mesenteric vessels, and on the surface of the pancreas. After resection, a pancreaticojejunostomy, hepaticojejunostomy and gastrojejunostomy were performed. After anastomotic reconstruction, two or three silicone abdominal drains were left posterior to the pancreaticojejunostomy and hepaticojejunostomy.

Follow-up

Patients were followed up at least every 2 months during the first year and every 3 months thereafter. CA19–9 test, liver ultrasonography, CT, and MRI were selectively performed as needed. Progression was defined as identification of suspicious imaging finding or biopsy-proven tumor in the tumor bed, regional LN area or distant area. OS was defined as the duration from the date of operation until death or the last follow-up. PFS was defined as the duration from the date of operation until the date when tumor progression was diagnosed or the last follow-up. The last follow-up was completed on August 31, 2017.

Statistical analysis

SPSS version 22 software (SPSS Inc., Chicago, IL, USA) was used to analyze the data. The optimal cutoff value for LNR was determined using time-dependent receiver operating characteristic (ROC) analysis, which was performed using the package "survivalROC" in R version 3. 2.5. The laboratory threshold was used as a cutoff value for other clinical data. Categorical variables were compared using the chi-square test and Fisher's exact test. Continuous variables were compared using the two-tailed unpaired t-test or Mann–Whitney U-test.

Survival times were estimated using the Kaplan–Meier method and compared using the log-rank test. Analyses for survival curves were performed using MedCalc software version 11.4.2.0 (MedCalc, Ostend, Belgium). Univariate analysis was performed to assess significance of clinical and pathological characteristics. Multivariate analysis was performed using the Cox regression model for variables that were significantly associated with OS or PFS in the univariate analysis, and the corresponding 95% confidence intervals (CI) were calculated. Two-tailed P values less than 0.05 were considered statistically significant.

A nomogram was developed based on the independent risk factors identified in the multivariate analysis. A final model selection for the nomogram was performed by a backward step-down selection process using a threshold P-value of 0.05. The performance of the nomogram was measured by C-index and assessed by calibration curves. The C-index reflected the probability that a randomly selected patient with a lower probability of survival predicted via the nomogram died earlier than another randomly selected patient with a higher predicted probability. The calibration curves were used to compare the predicted probability with the observed probability in the study cohort. Bootstraps with 1000 resamples were used for the development of the nomogram and calibration curve to reduce the overfit bias. All statistical analyses were conducted using R software version 3.2.5 (R Development Core Team; http://www.r-project.org) and the "rms" package developed by Harrell (Harrell et al.).

Results

Patient characteristics

Of the 205 patients with periampullary adenocarcinoma who underwent pancreatoduodenectomy, ampullary adenocarcinoma was the most common diagnosis (123 patients, 60%), followed by pancreatic adenocarcinoma (67 patients, 32.7%) and duodenal adenocarcinoma (15 patients, 7.3%). Baseline characteristics of patients are shown in Table 1. The median age of all patients was 56.2 years (range 25–84 years). Most of the patients (128 patients, 62.4%) were men in the whole study cohort. Jaundice (TBIL ≥20.5 mmol/L) was reported most frequently in patients with ampullary adenocarcinoma ($P = 0.045$). These patients were more likely to have elevated values of CRP ($P = 0.027$), AST ($P = 0.035$), ALP ($P = 0.010$) and GGT ($P < 0.001$). The proportion of patients with large tumors was higher in the duodenal adenocarcinoma group than that in the ampullary adenocarcinoma group or pancreatic adenocarcinoma group ($P = 0.002$). All three groups were similar with respect to age, gender, WBC, ALT, ALB, tumor differentiation, LNR, LN metastasis and chemotherapy treatment. With the cutoff value of 0.17, LNR was associated with the optimal Youden index for OS and PFS prediction.

OS analysis

The median OS time was 533 days and the 1-year, 3-year and 5-year OS rates were 88.2%, 66% and 53%, respectively. In the univariate analysis, age, gender, WBC, CRP, ALT, AST, ALB, TBIL, ALP, GGT, tumor differentiation, tumor diameter, LN metastasis, LN total number and chemotherapy treatment were not related to OS ($P > 0.05$). However, LNR, CA19–9 and anatomical location were significantly associated with OS (Table 2). These three risk factors were entered into the multivariate Cox regression analysis. After a stepwise removal of variables, LNR (HR = 1.788, 95% CI = 1.103–3.155, $P = 0.045$), CA19–9 (HR = 2.090, 95% CI = 1.082–4.037, $P = 0.028$) and anatomical location (HR = 1.892, 95% CI = 1.083–3. 306, $P = 0.025$) remained significant predictors for OS (Table 3). All the included patients were further stratified by LNR ($P = 0.015$, Fig. 1a), CA19–9 ($P = 0.007$, Fig. 1b) and anatomical location ($P = 0.006$, Fig. 1c) for OS analysis. The differences of OS rates were all significant.

PFS analysis

Tumor progression was observed in 60 (29.3%) patients in the study cohort. The median progression time was 418 days. The 1-year, 3-year and 4-year OS rates were 77.2%, 62.6% and 57.1%, respectively. The univariate analysis revealed that LNR, CA19–9, tumor differentiation, LN metastasis and anatomical location were all associated with PFS ($P < 0.05$, Table 2). Multivariate analysis was then performed to delineate various prognostic indicators. Variables that were significantly associated with survival status in the univariate Cox analyses were included in the multivariate analysis. To avoid multicollinearity, the LN metastasis

Table 1 The relationship between clinicolpathological factors and periampullary adenocarcinoma

Characteristic		N	Periampullary adenocarcinoma			P
			Panceatic head adenocarcinoma	Duodenal adenocarcinoma	Ampullary adenocarcinoma	
Total		205	67	15	123	
Age	< 60	127	38	10	79	0.551
	≥ 60	78	29	5	44	
Gender	Male	128	41	12	75	0.345
	Female	77	26	3	48	
WBC (× 10^9/L)	< 10	172	58	13	101	0.695
	≥ 10	33	9	2	22	
CRP (mg/L)	< 8	58	27	4	27	0.027
	≥ 8	147	40	11	96	
ALT (U/L)	< 40	79	48	5	26	0.455
	≥ 40	156	49	10	97	
AST (U/L)	< 45	47	20	6	21	0.035
	≥ 45	158	47	9	102	
ALB (g/L)	< 35	52	11	3	38	0.080
	≥ 35	153	56	12	85	
TBIL (mmol/L)	< 20.5	38	18	4	16	0.045
	≥ 20.5	167	49	11	107	
ALP (U/L)	< 100	31	16	4	11	0.010
	≥ 100	174	51	11	112	
GGT (U/L)	< 50	25	15	4	6	< 0.001
	≥ 50	180	52	11	117	
Tumor differentiation	W	5	0	1	4	0.463
	W-M	8	4	0	4	
	M	108	31	7	70	
	M-P	63	23	6	34	
	P	21	9	1	11	
Tumor diameter (cm)	< 2	69	14	2	53	0.002
	≥ 2	136	53	13	70	
LNR	< 0.17	151	50	12	89	0.798
	≥ 0.17	54	17	3	34	
LN metastasis	Absent	116	36	9	71	0.836
	Present	89	31	6	52	
Chemotherapy	No	87	28	7	52	0.941
	Yes	118	39	8	71	

WBC white blood cell count, *CRP* C-reactive protein, *ALT* alanine transaminase, *AST* aspartate aminotransferase, *ALB* albumin, *TBIL* total bilirubin, *ALP* alkaline phosphatase, *GGT* gamma-glutamyl transpeptidase, *W* well, *M* moderate, *P* poor, *W-M* well-moderate, *M-P* moderate-poor, *LN* lymph node

was not included in the multivariate analysis, as the LNR accounted for the absence or presence of LN metastasis. After adjusting for other risk factors the multivariate analysis showed that LNR (HR = 1.883, 95% CI = 1.094–3.242, *P* = 0.022), CA19–9 (HR = 1.863, 95% CI = 1.010–3.436, *P* = 0.046), tumor differentiation (HR = 1.031, 95% CI = 1.005–1.058, *P* = 0.019) and anatomical location (HR = 1.545, 95% CI = 1.172–2.036, *P* = 0.002) all remained independently associated with PFS. Additionally, LNR, CA19–9 and anatomical location were all independent predictive factors for both OS and PFS (Table 3). All the included patients were further stratified by LNR (*P* = 0.019, Fig. 2a), CA19–9 (*P* = 0.014, Fig. 2b), tumor

Table 2 Univariate of OS and PFS in the study cohort

Characteristic		OS		PFS	
		HR (95% CI)	P	HR (95% CI)	P
Age	< 60/ 60	1.496 (0.867–2.582)	0.148	0.643 (0.362–1.141)	0.131
Gender	male/ female	1.478 (0.857–2.547)	0.160	0.738 (0.425–1.283)	0.2821
WBC (×10⁹/L)	< 10/ ≥ 10	0.951 (0.429–2.109)	0.902	1.181 (0.598–2.330)	0.632
CRP (mg/L)	< 8/ ≥ 8	0.914 (0.508–1.645)	0.765	1.096 (0.618–1.943)	0.753
ALT (U/L)	< 40/ ≥ 40	0.869 (0.478–1.580)	0.645	1.929 (0.949–3.919)	0.069
AST (U/L)	< 45/ ≥ 45	0.670 (0.376–1.193)	0.174	1.397(0.727–2.688)	0.316
ALB (g/L)	< 35/ ≥ 35	0.987 (0.535–1.819)	0.966	0.747(0.430–1.299)	0.302
TBIL (mmol/L)	< 20.5/ ≥20.5	0.772 (0.419–1.422)	0.406	2.106 (0.957–4.634)	0.064
ALP (U/L)	< 100/ ≥ 100	0.761 (0.382–1.156)	0.438	1.73(0.744–4.023)	0.203
GGT (U/L)	< 50/ ≥ 50	0.571 (0.294–1.109)	0.098	0.906(0.430–1.909)	0.796
CA19-9 (U/ml)	< 35/ ≥ 35	2.362 (1.235–4.159)	0.009	2.095(1.147–3.829)	0.016
Tumor differrntiation	W/W-M/M/M-H/H	1.005 (0.976–1.035)	0.74	1.030(1.005–1.057)	0.020
Tumor diameter (cm)	< 2/≥ 2	0.991 (0.557–1.765)	0.976	1.486(0.828–2.666)	0.184
LNR	< 0.17/≥ 0.17	1.982 (1.13–3.479)	0.017	1.880(1.098–3.220)	0.021
LN metastasis	Absent / Present	1.408 (0.819–2.423)	0.216	2.328 (1.391–3.895)	0.001
LN total numbers	< 12/≥ 12	0.755 (0.430–1.324)	0.327	0.802 (0.478–1.344)	0.402
Anatomical location	Pancreatic/Duodenal/ Ampullary	2.287(1.325–3.948)	0.003	2.542 (1.517–4.262)	< 0.001
Chemotherapy	No/Yes	1.176(0.682–2.027)	0.559	1.713(1.006–2.915)	0.051

HR hazard ratio, *CI* confidence interval
Other abbreviations as in Table 1

differentiation (*P* = 0.001, Fig. 2c) and anatomical location (*P* = 0.001, Fig. 2d), respectively for PFS analysis. The differences of PFS rates were all significant.

Construction and validation of nomograms

All of the independent predictors of OS and PFS of patients in the study cohort were integrated into the nomogram (OS, Fig. 3; PFS, Fig. 4). The nomogram demonstrated good accuracy for OS prediction, with a C-index of 0.678 (95% CI = 0.612–0.744). Calibration plots for the probabilities of 1-, 2-, and 3-year OS showed fair agreement between the nomogram-predicted survival and the observed survival (Fig. 5a, b, c). The nomogram for PFS (Fig. 4) prediction was generated via the Cox proportional hazards model including the above-mentioned variables that were independently associated with PFS. The C-index for PFS prediction

was 0.680 (95% CI = 0.617–0.743). Calibration plots for the probabilities of 1-, 2-, and 3-years PFS showed an optimal agreement between prediction by the nomogram and the actual observation (Fig. 5d, e, f, respectively). Additionally, the bias-corrected C-indexes of the established nomograms were higher than those of the TNM 8th stage system for both OS and PFS analyses: OS = 0.678 (95% CI = 0.612–0.744) vs OS = 0.510 (95% CI = 0.429–0.591; *P* < 0.001); PFS = 0.680 (95% CI = 0.617–0.743) vs PFS = 0.634 (95% CI = 0.566–0.702; *P* = 0.042).

Survival analysis according to the risk stratification based on the nomogram

All the patients in this study were categorized into several risk groups according to the probability score calculated by the nomogram. Patients with the probability

Table 3 Multivariate of OS and PFS in the study cohort

Characteristic		OS		PFS	
		HR (95% CI)	P	HR (95% CI)	P
CA19-9 (U/ml)	< 35/ ≥ 35	2.090 (1.082–4.037)	0.028	1.863(1.010–3.436)	0.046
Tumor differrntiation	W/W-M/M/M-H/H		NI	1.031(1.005–1.058)	0.019
LNR	< 0.17/≥ 0.17	1.788 (1.103–3.155)	0.045	1.883(1.094–3.242)	0.022
Anatomical location	Pancreatic/Duodenal/ Ampullary	1.892(1.083–3.306)	0.025	1.545 (1.172–2.036)	0.002

NI not include
Other abbreviations as in Table 1

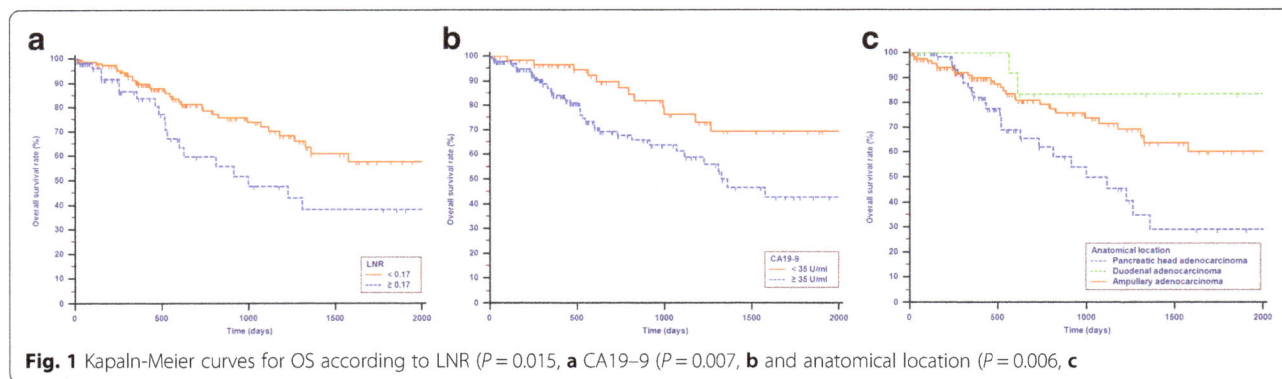

Fig. 1 Kapaln-Meier curves for OS according to LNR (*P* = 0.015, **a** CA19–9 (*P* = 0.007, **b** and anatomical location (*P* = 0.006, **c**

score of < 10, 10–15 and ≥ 15 were assigned into the low risk group, middle risk group and high risk group, respectively. Figure 6 shows the Kaplan-Meier survival curves separated by nomogram-based grouping. The OS rates and PFS rates of patients in the low risk group were significantly higher than those of patients in the high risk group (*P* < 0.001).

Discussion

The annual incidence of periampullary adenocarcinoma is steadily on the rise [3]. The only curative therapy for periampullary adenocarcinoma is surgical resection, usually performed as PD; the curative resectable rate is only 20% [27]. The long-term survival rate of periampullary adenocarcinoma is low and varies in a wide range among

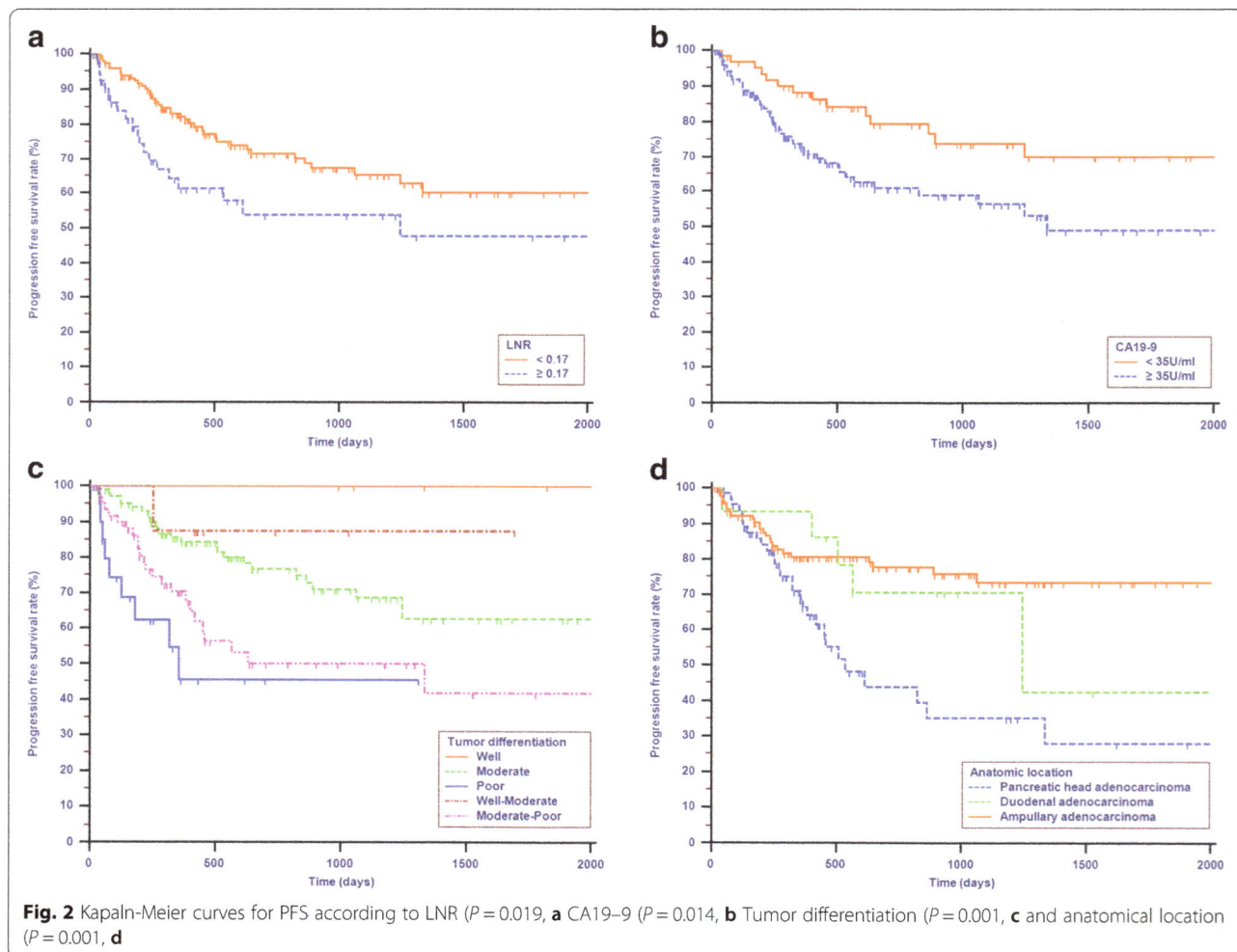

Fig. 2 Kapaln-Meier curves for PFS according to LNR (*P* = 0.019, **a** CA19–9 (*P* = 0.014, **b** Tumor differentiation (*P* = 0.001, **c** and anatomical location (*P* = 0.001, **d**

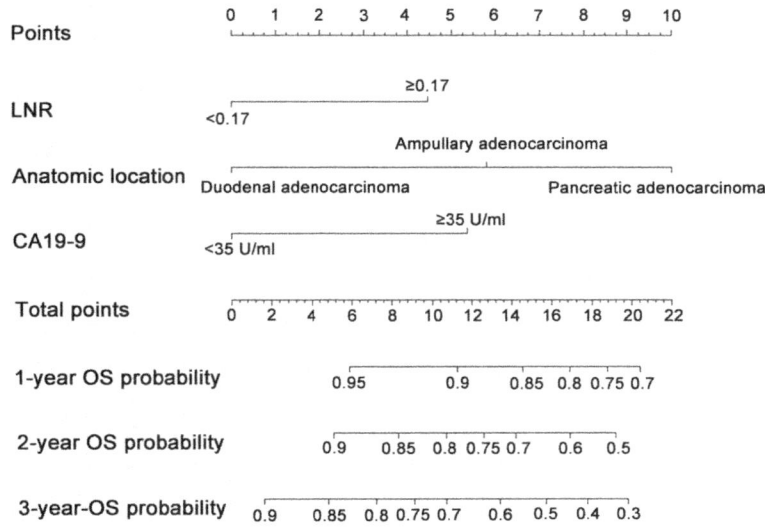

Fig. 3 Nomogram-predicted probabilities of 1-, 2-, and 3-years OS of patients with periampullary adenocarcinoma after pancreatoduodenectomy. The nomogram is used by adding up the points identified on the scale for three or four variables. The sum is located on the "Total points" scale, and a line is drawn downward to the survival axes to determine the probability of 1-, 2-, and 3-years OS

adenocarcinomas of different anatomical locations in the periampullary region [8]. Additionally, the long-term survival rate is greatly influenced by the rate of early progression [28, 29]. In this study, we identified 205 patients who underwent pancreatoduodenectomy for periampullary adenocarcinoma and grouped them by different anatomical locations. We found that ampullary adenocarcinoma constituted a relatively large proportion (60%) of all adenocarcinomas of the periampullary region, which was equivalent to the results from other studies [4, 13]. It is possible that the higher rate of resectability of ampullary adenocarcinoma at diagnosis, specified in the literature as up to 80%, which is significantly higher than that for pancreatic adenocarcinoma (20%) [2, 30], contributes to this situation. Jaundice,

which is caused by the exophytic growth pattern of the tumor, was more frequently occurring in patients with ampullary adenocarcinoma in this study. This result may also partly explain the higher resectability rate of ampullary adenocarcinoma [31]. The low probability of jaundice could also lead to the late detection of patients with duodenal adenocarcinoma, along with relatively larger tumors. Further, inflammation-based markers, such as AST, ALP, GGT and CRP, are more likely to be elevated in patients with jaundice [32], similarly to our study.

The prognostic factors of patients with pancreatic adenocarcinoma [15, 33], ampullary adenocarcinoma [17], or duodenal adenocarcinoma [34] have been reported in several studies. There are few reports that focus on the prognostic factors and survival predictive

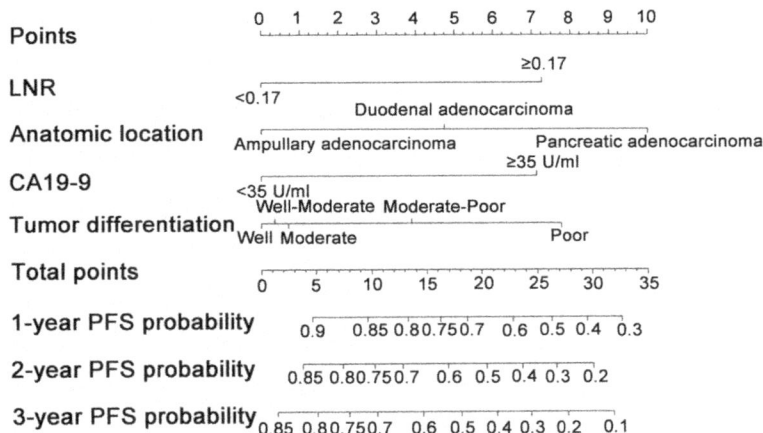

Fig. 4 Nomogram-predicted probabilities of 1-, 2-, and 3-years PFS of patients with periampullary adenocarcinoma after pancreatoduodenectomy

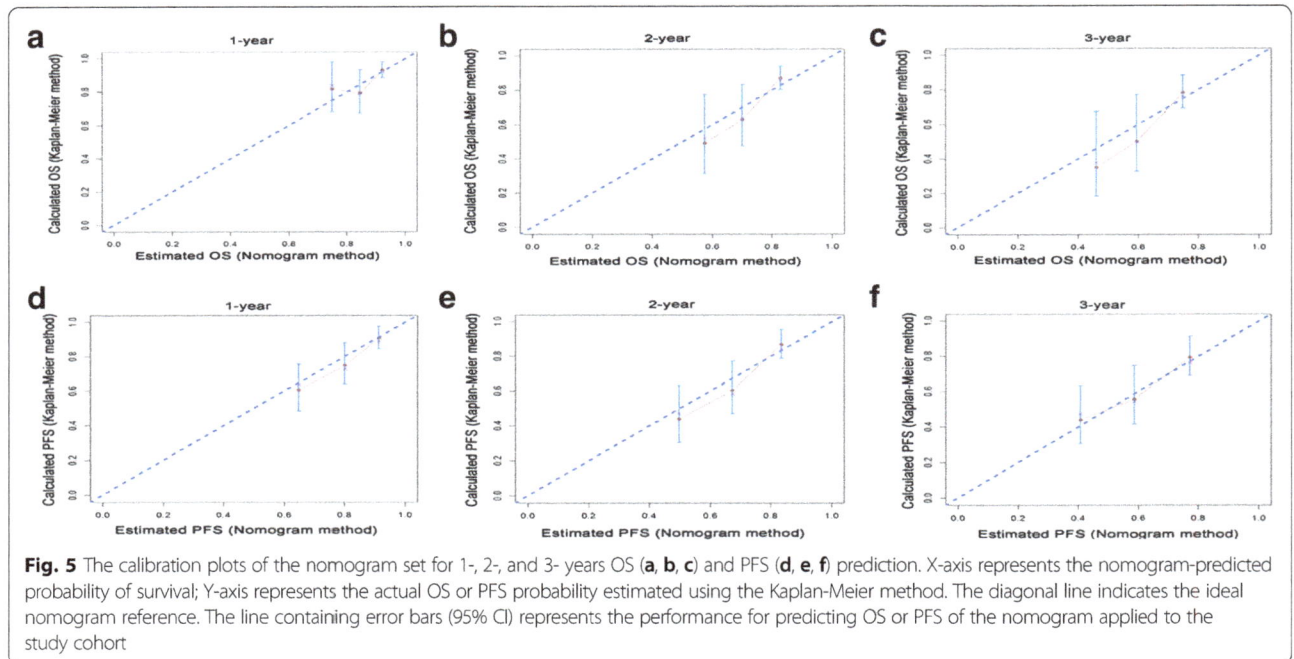

Fig. 5 The calibration plots of the nomogram set for 1-, 2-, and 3- years OS (**a, b, c**) and PFS (**d, e, f**) prediction. X-axis represents the nomogram-predicted probability of survival; Y-axis represents the actual OS or PFS probability estimated using the Kaplan-Meier method. The diagonal line indicates the ideal nomogram reference. The line containing error bars (95% CI) represents the performance for predicting OS or PFS of the nomogram applied to the study cohort

systems for patients with periampullary adenocarcinoma. By using a relative large patient cohort, we found that LNR, CA19–9 and anatomical location were independently predictive factors for both OS and PFS. Lower tumor differentiation was also associated with poorer PFS. Compared with pancreatic adenocarcinoma and ampullary adenocarcinoma, patients with duodenal adenocarcinoma had higher OS rates. The PFS rates were the highest for patients with ampullary adenocarcinoma in the study cohort, which is similar to the results of other studies [13, 31]. However, chemotherapy was not an independent predictor for either OS or PFS. The need for chemotherapy after surgery was

determined by a surgeon in cases with poor prognostic factors, such as LN metastasis. It is possible that the independent significance of chemotherapy was affected by the selective administration in this study. In addition, we developed a nomogram as an easy-to-apply model to predict the individual survival risk of patients with periampullary adenocarcinoma after pancreatoduodenectomy in the current study. For these patients, the nomogram internally showed that the prognosis would be better in terms of OS for patients with duodenal adenocarcinoma after pancreatoduodenectomy compared with the other two adenocarcinomas. For patients with a specific kind of

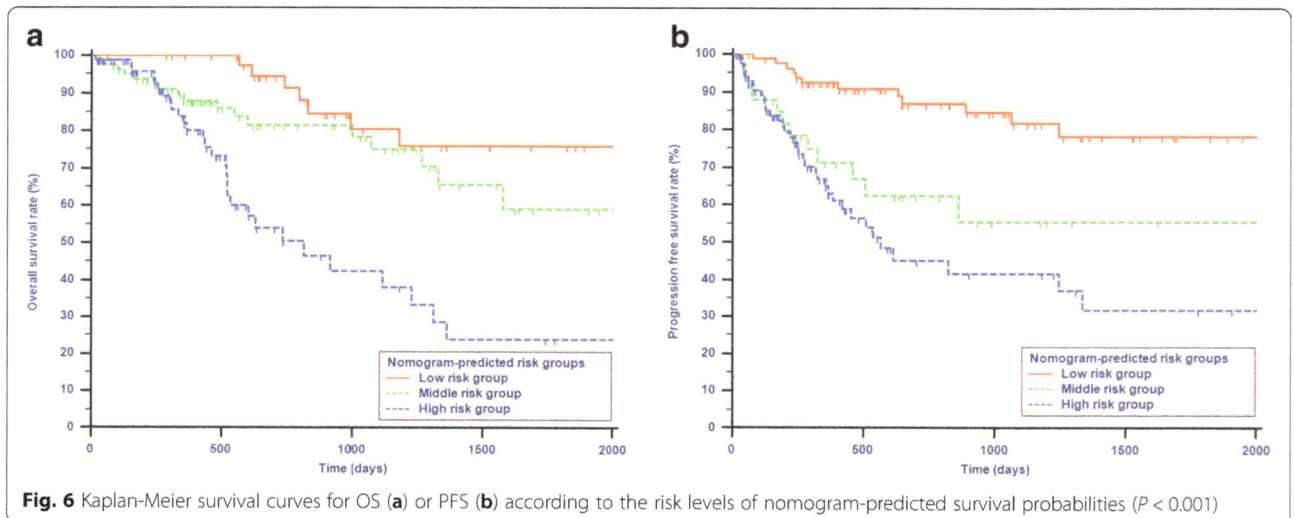

Fig. 6 Kaplan-Meier survival curves for OS (**a**) or PFS (**b**) according to the risk levels of nomogram-predicted survival probabilities (*P* < 0.001)

periampullary adenocarcinoma, the nomogram can serve as a quantitative scoring system to estimate OS and PFS.

All variables in the nomogram were clinical or pathological characteristics. By treating continuous variables, including CA19–9 and LNR, as binary predictors, this nomogram provided a simple and visual friendly method for prognosis estimation. Further, current nomograms allow the visual tracing of the estimated risk and impact on risk when various modifiable risk factors are added or removed. Of all variables included in the nomagram, CA199–9 was previously accepted as a prognostic factor for OS and PFS of patients with ampullary adenocarcinoma [23, 35, 36]. With the cutoff value of 35 U/ml, patients can be easily separated into groups with elevated values or normal values of CA19–9. Previous reports have shown that patients with higher preoperative CA19–9 levels were more likely to have higher tumor burdens and reduced chances of survival [37]. In the current study, we found that patients with elevated CA19–9 levels were more likely to have reduced OS and PFS. Our results are similar to the study by Cristina et al. [23], which showed that a lower preoperative CA19–9 level correlated not only with a lower pathologic stage but also with an increased postoperative survival.

LNR was demonstrated as a predictor of survival by many reports [12, 26]. The present study showed that a higher LNR was significantly associated with poorer OS and PFS. Our study did not show an association between the total number of resected nodes and OS or PFS in patients with periampullary adenocarcinoma. This result was similar to other reports [38, 39] in which the total number of nodes examined was not a predictive factor for survival. Furthermore, as demonstrated in the present study [16, 40], it was found that LNR was a superior predictor of survival compared with the total number of resected LNs. AJCC recommends at least 12 harvested nodes for accurate staging because insufficient LNs may lead to understage the N category in many kinds of tumors, such as gastric carcinoma or pancreatic carcinoma [1, 41, 42]. A patient with fewer resected LNs may have a decreased survival. The elevated LNR was a sign that showed the tendency of metastasis or progression and was associated with the poorer OS and PFS in this study. Our study demonstrated results similar to previous research [43] conducted by the MD Anderson Cancer Center, in which the strong association between high LNR (> 0.15) and low distant metastasis-free survival was detected.

OS and PFS of patients with adenocarcinoma from different anatomical locations in the periampullary region were analyzed and compared. Some studies [2, 44, 45] reported the 5-year OS rates of duodenal adenocarcinoma, ampullary adenocarcinoma and pancreatic carcinoma were 59%, 39% and 15%, respectively. As in the previous studies, our study showed that patients with duodenal adenocarcinoma had a better long-term OS. Interestingly, patients with ampullary adenocarcinoma kept an even higher long-term PFS rate compared with duodenal adenocarcinoma and pancreatic adenocarcinoma. Bucher et al. [31] also reported that ampullary carcinomas had a lower recurrence rate, which was in contrast with other carcinomas of the periampullary region. It is possible that the adenoma-to-carcinoma sequence of ampullary carcinoma, which is similar to colon carcinoma, contributed to this phenomenon [46]. In addition to the anatomical location, other pathological characteristics, such as tumor differentiation, have been reported to be associated with the progression of periampullary carcinoma [47, 48]. Park et al. [49] revealed that tumor differentiation was a significant influencing factor of early progression in patients with periampullary carcinoma. In our multivariate analysis, we also found that poor tumor differentiation was a poor prognostic factor for PFS. In general, it should seem that OS rate would be reduced in patients with poor tumor differentiation [50, 51], and our data showed such a tendency, but failed to show statistical significance, possibly due to the small total number of patients in the study. Tumor differentiation as a prognostic factor for PFS needs to be further elucidated by future prospective randomized controlled studies.

All the variables included in the nomograms were significant predictive factors for OS and FPS in this study. Our nomograms showed good C-indexes in the study cohort. The C-indexes of the nomograms for OS and PFS prediction were 0.678 and 0.680, respectively. This means that if two patients with different nomogram points are selected, the probabilities that the patient with the higher nomogram score would die earlier and of which the disease would progress earlier are both over 67%. Further, the comparison of C-indexes showed that the established nomogram displayed more powerful efficiency of discrimination for both OS and CSS prediction compared with the TNM 8th edition stage system. Calibration plots show how accurate the results are as predicted by the nomogram model compared with the results estimated by the Kaplan-Meier method. The calibration plots of internal validation demonstrated good fitness for OS and PFS prediction, as the predicted survival probabilities at 1-, 2-, and 3-years estimated via the nomogram were closely aligned with the actual survival times. Additionally, a clear risk stratification of survival times using nomogram-predicted survival probabilities was demonstrated by survival curves. Therefore, a user-friendly nomogram can help physicians to predict the prognosis of patients and provide individualized treatment.

There were several limitations in this study. First, it was a retrospective study that relied on a single-institutional dataset. Geographic and institutional heterogeneity of patients may affect these results. Second, some of the potential predictive variables could not be included into the nomograms. Third, an external validation for predictive accuracy of the nomograms was not conducted in our study, which decreased the applicability of the nomograms to an external cohort. Large prospective studies are needed to further validate the accuracy of these prognostic nomograms.

Conclusions

The predictive power of variables for survival prediction in patients was analyzed in this study. This was the first study that included LNR and anatomical location to nomograms for predicting OS and PFS in patients with periampullary adenocarcinoma after pancreatoduodenectomy, potentially facilitating highly tailored patient management.

Abbreviations

ALB: Albumin; ALP: Alkaline phosphatase; ALT: Alanine transaminase; AST: Aspartate aminotransferase; CA19–9: Carbohydrate antigen 19–9; CBD: Distal common bile duct; CI: Confidence interval; C-index: Concordance index; CRP: C-reactive protein; GGT: Gamma-glutamyl transpeptidase; LN: Lymph node; LNR: Lymph node ratio; OS: Overall survival; PD: Pancreaticoduodenectomy; PFS: Progression free survival; ROC: Receiver operating characteristic; TBIL: Total bilirubin; TNM: Tumor-node-metastasis; WBC: White blood cell

Acknowledgements

We acknowledged the Medical Records Department for collecting the survival data of patients.

Funding

This work was supported by grants from the National Natural Science Foundation of China (81171890; 81672390), and the Major National Scientific Research Projects of China (No. 2013CB910304).

Authors' contributions

CBH and YZM collected and analyzed data, drafted and revised the manuscript. JW collected and analyzed data. FTD and XJL collected data. SPL designed this study, revised the manuscript and finally approved of the manuscript. All authors read and approved the final manuscript.

Competing interests

The authors declare that they have no competing interests.

References

1. Amin MBES, Greene F. AJCC Cancer staging manual. 8th ed. Chicago: Springer; 2017.
2. Yeo CJ, Sohn TA, Cameron JL, Hruban RH, Lillemoe KD, Pitt HA. Periampullary adenocarcinoma: analysis of 5-year survivors. Ann Surg. 1998; 227(6):821–31.
3. Siegel RL, Miller KD, Jemal A. Cancer statistics, 2016. CA Cancer J Clin. 2016; 66(1):7–30.
4. Nakase A, Matsumoto Y, Uchida K, Honjo I. Surgical treatment of cancer of the pancreas and the periampullary region: cumulative results in 57 institutions in Japan. Ann Surg. 1977;185(1):52–7.

5. Petrova E, Ruckert F, Zach S, Shen Y, Weitz J, Grutzmann R, Wittel UA, Makowiec F, Hopt UT, Bronsert P, et al. Survival outcome and prognostic factors after pancreatoduodenectomy for distal bile duct carcinoma: a retrospective multicenter study. Langenbeck's Arch Surg. 2017;402(5):831–40.
6. Westgaard A, Tafjord S, Farstad IN, Cvancarova M, Eide TJ, Mathisen O, Clausen OP, Gladhaug IP. Pancreatobiliary versus intestinal histologic type of differentiation is an independent prognostic factor in resected periampullary adenocarcinoma. BMC Cancer. 2008;8:170.
7. Herreros-Villanueva M, Hijona E, Cosme A, Bujanda L. Adjuvant and neoadjuvant treatment in pancreatic cancer. World J Gastroenterol. 2012; 18(14):1565–72.
8. van Geenen RC, van Gulik TM, Offerhaus GJ, de Wit LT, Busch OR, Obertop H, Gouma DJ. Survival after pancreaticoduodenectomy for periampullary adenocarcinoma: an update. Eur J Surg Oncol. 2001;27(6):549–57.
9. Jang JY, Kim SW, Park DJ, Ahn YJ, Yoon YS, Choi MG, Suh KS, Lee KU, Park YH. Actual long-term outcome of extrahepatic bile duct cancer after surgical resection. Ann Surg. 2005;241(1):77–84.
10. Narang AK, Miller RC, Hsu CC, Bhatia S, Pawlik TM, Laheru D, Hruban RH, Zhou J, Winter JM, Haddock MG, et al. Evaluation of adjuvant chemoradiation therapy for ampullary adenocarcinoma: the Johns Hopkins Hospital-Mayo Clinic collaborative study. Radiat Oncol. 2011;6:126.
11. Kim K, Chie EK, Jang JY, Kim SW, Oh DY, Im SA, Kim TY, Bang YJ, Ha SW. Role of adjuvant chemoradiotherapy for ampulla of Vater cancer. Int J Radiat Oncol Biol Phys. 2009;75(2):436–41.
12. Tol JA, Brosens LA, van Dieren S, van Gulik TM, Busch OR, Besselink MG, Gouma DJ. Impact of lymph node ratio on survival in patients with pancreatic and periampullary cancer. Br J Surg. 2015;102(3):237–45.
13. Howe JR, Klimstra DS, Moccia RD, Conlon KC, Brennan MF. Factors predictive of survival in ampullary carcinoma. Ann Surg. 1998;228(1):87–94.
14. Seppanen H, Juuti A, Mustonen H, Haapamaki C, Nordling S, Carpelan-Holmstrom M, Siren J, Luettges J, Haglund C, Kiviluoto T. The results of pancreatic resections and long-term survival for pancreatic ductal adenocarcinoma: a single-institution experience. Scand J Surg. 2017;106(1):54–61.
15. House MG, Gonen M, Jarnagin WR, D'Angelica M, DeMatteo RP, Fong Y, Brennan MF, Allen PJ. Prognostic significance of pathologic nodal status in patients with resected pancreatic cancer. J Gastrointest Surg. 2007;11(11):1549–55.
16. Pawlik TM, Gleisner AL, Cameron JL, Winter JM, Assumpcao L, Lillemoe KD, Wolfgang C, Hruban RH, Schulick RD, Yeo CJ, et al. Prognostic relevance of lymph node ratio following pancreaticoduodenectomy for pancreatic cancer. Surgery. 2007;141(5):610–8.
17. Pomianowska E, Westgaard A, Mathisen O, Clausen OP, Gladhaug IP. Prognostic relevance of number and ratio of metastatic lymph nodes in resected pancreatic, ampullary, and distal bile duct carcinomas. Ann Surg Oncol. 2013;20(1):233–41.
18. Hurtuk MG, Hughes C, Shoup M, Aranha GV. Does lymph node ratio impact survival in resected periampullary malignancies? Am J Surg. 2009;197(3):348–52.
19. He CB, Lao XM, Lin XJ. Transarterial chemoembolization combined with recombinant human adenovirus type 5 H101 prolongs overall survival of patients with intermediate to advanced hepatocellular carcinoma: a prognostic nomogram study. Chin J Cancer. 2017;36(1):59.
20. Kattan MW, Karpeh MS, Mazumdar M, Brennan MF. Postoperative nomogram for disease-specific survival after an R0 resection for gastric carcinoma. J Clin Oncol. 2003;21(19):3647–50.
21. Kawai K, Ishihara S, Yamaguchi H, Sunami E, Kitayama J, Miyata H, Watanabe T. Nomogram prediction of metachronous colorectal neoplasms in patients with colorectal cancer. Ann Surg. 2015;261(5):926–32.
22. Fu YP, Ni XC, Yi Y, Cai XY, He HW, Wang JX, Lu ZF, Han X, Cao Y, Zhou J, et al. A novel and validated inflammation-based score (IBS) predicts survival in patients with hepatocellular carcinoma following curative surgical resection: a STROBE-compliant article. Medicine. 2016;95(7):e2784.
23. Ferrone CR, Finkelstein DM, Thayer SP, Muzikansky A, Fernandez-delCastillo C, Warshaw AL. Perioperative CA19-9 levels can predict stage and survival in patients with resectable pancreatic adenocarcinoma. J Clin Oncol. 2006;24(18):2897–902.
24. Deng QL, Dong S, Wang L, Zhang CY, Ying HF, Li ZS, Shen XH, Guo YB, Meng ZQ, Yu JM, et al. Development and validation of a nomogram for predicting survival in patients with advanced pancreatic ductal adenocarcinoma. Sci Rep. 2017;7(1):11524.
25. Song W, Miao DL, Chen L. Nomogram for predicting survival in patients with pancreatic cancer. OncoTargets and therapy. 2018;11:539–45.

26. Kwon J, Kim K, Chie EK, Kim BH, Jang JY, Kim SW, Oh DY, Bang YJ. Prognostic relevance of lymph node status for patients with ampullary adenocarcinoma after radical resection followed by adjuvant treatment. Eur J Surg Oncol. 2017;43(9):1690–6.

27. Kamisawa T, Wood LD, Itoi T, Takaori K. Pancreatic cancer. Lancet (London, England). 2016;388(10039):73–85.

28. Fischer R, Breidert M, Keck T, Makowiec F, Lohrmann C, Harder J. Early recurrence of pancreatic cancer after resection and during adjuvant chemotherapy. Saudi J Gastroenterol. 2012;18(2):118–21.

29. Shimada K, Sakamoto Y, Sano T, Kosuge T. The role of paraaortic lymph node involvement on early recurrence and survival after macroscopic curative resection with extended lymphadenectomy for pancreatic carcinoma. J Am Coll Surg. 2006;203(3):345–52.

30. Kim RD, Kundhal PS, McGilvray ID, Cattral MS, Taylor B, Langer B, Grant DR, Zogopoulos G, Shah SA, Greig PD, et al. Predictors of failure after pancreaticoduodenectomy for ampullary carcinoma. J Am Coll Surg. 2006; 202(1):112–9.

31. Bucher P, Chassot G, Durmishi Y, Ris F, Morel P. Long-term results of surgical treatment of Vater's ampulla neoplasms. Hepato-Gastroenterology. 2007; 54(76):1239–42.

32. Jin H, Pang Q, Liu H, Li Z, Wang Y, Lu Y, Zhou L, Pan H, Huang W. Prognostic value of inflammation-based markers in patients with recurrent malignant obstructive jaundice treated by reimplantation of biliary metal stents: a retrospective observational study. Medicine. 2017;96(3):e5895.

33. Bhatti I, Peacock O, Awan AK, Semeraro D, Larvin M, Hall RI. Lymph node ratio versus number of affected lymph nodes as predictors of survival for resected pancreatic adenocarcinoma. World J Surg. 2010;34(4):768–75.

34. Ecker BL, McMillan MT, Datta J, Lee MK, Karakousis GC, Vollmer CM Jr, Drebin JA, Fraker DL, Roses RE. Adjuvant chemotherapy versus chemoradiotherapy in the management of patients with surgically resected duodenal adenocarcinoma: a propensity score-matched analysis of a nationwide clinical oncology database. Cancer. 2017;123(6):967–76.

35. Okano K, Oshima M, Yachida S, Kushida Y, Kato K, Kamada H, Wato M, Nishihira T, Fukuda Y, Maeba T, et al. Factors predicting survival and pathological subtype in patients with ampullary adenocarcinoma. J Surg Oncol. 2014;110(2):156–62.

36. Kurihara C, Yoshimi F, Sasaki K, Iijima T, Kawasaki H, Nagai H. Clinical value of serum CA19-9 as a prognostic factor for the ampulla of Vater carcinoma. Hepato-Gastroenterology. 2013;60(127):1588–91.

37. Nakao A, Oshima K, Nomoto S, Takeda S, Kaneko T, Ichihara T, Kurokawa T, Nonami T, Takagi H. Clinical usefulness of CA-19-9 in pancreatic carcinoma. Semin Surg Oncol. 1998;15(1):15–22.

38. Sierzega M, Popiela T, Kulig J, Nowak K. The ratio of metastatic/resected lymph nodes is an independent prognostic factor in patients with node-positive pancreatic head cancer. Pancreas. 2006;33(3):240–5.

39. Hartwig W, Hackert T, Hinz U, Gluth A, Bergmann F, Strobel O, Buchler MW, Werner J. Pancreatic cancer surgery in the new millennium: better prediction of outcome. Ann Surg. 2011;254(2):311–9.

40. John BJ, Naik P, Ironside A, Davidson BR, Fusai G, Gillmore R, Watkins J, Rahman SH. Redefining the R1 resection for pancreatic ductal adenocarcinoma: tumour lymph nodal burden and lymph node ratio are the only prognostic factors associated with survival. HPB. 2013;15(9):674–80.

41. Datta J, Lewis RS Jr, Mamtani R, Stripp D, Kelz RR, Drebin JA, Fraker DL, Karakousis GC, Roses RE. Implications of inadequate lymph node staging in resectable gastric cancer: a contemporary analysis using the National Cancer Data Base. Cancer. 2014;120(18):2855–65.

42. Slidell MB, Chang DC, Cameron JL, Wolfgang C, Herman JM, Schulick RD, Choti MA, Pawlik TM. Impact of total lymph node count and lymph node ratio on staging and survival after pancreatectomy for pancreatic adenocarcinoma: a large, population-based analysis. Ann Surg Oncol. 2008; 15(1):165–74.

43. Roland CL, Katz MH, Gonzalez GM, Pisters PW, Vauthey JN, Wolff RA, Crane CH, Lee JE, Fleming JB. A high positive lymph node ratio is associated with distant recurrence after surgical resection of ampullary carcinoma. J Gastrointest Surg. 2012;16(11):2056–63.

44. Warren KW, Choe DS, Plaza J, Relihan M. Results of radical resection for periampullary cancer. Ann Surg. 1975;181(5):534–40.

45. Michelassi F, Erroi F, Dawson PJ, Pietrabissa A, Noda S, Handcock M, Block GE. Experience with 647 consecutive tumors of the duodenum, ampulla, head of the pancreas, and distal common bile duct. Ann Surg. 1989;210(4): 544–54. discussion 554-546

46. Klein F, Jacob D, Bahra M, Pelzer U, Puhl G, Krannich A, Andreou A, Gul S, Guckelberger O. Prognostic factors for long-term survival in patients with ampullary carcinoma: the results of a 15-year observation period after pancreaticoduodenectomy. HPB Surg. 2014;2014:970234.

47. Moriya T, Kimura W, Hirai I, Mizutani M, Ma J, Kamiga M, Fuse A. Nodal involvement as an indicator of postoperative liver metastasis in carcinoma of the papilla of Vater. J Hepato-Biliary-Pancreat Surg. 2006;13(6):549–55.

48. Talamini MA, Moesinger RC, Pitt HA, Sohn TA, Hruban RH, Lillemoe KD, Yeo CJ, Cameron JL. Adenocarcinoma of the ampulla of Vater. A 28-year experience. Ann Surg. 1997;225(5):590–9. discussion 599-600

49. Park JS, Yoon DS, Kim KS, Choi JS, Lee WJ, Chi HS, Kim BR. Factors influencing recurrence after curative resection for ampulla of Vater carcinoma. J Surg Oncol. 2007;95(4):286–90.

50. Hornick JR, Johnston FM, Simon PO, Younkin M, Chamberlin M, Mitchem JB, Azar RR, Linehan DC, Strasberg SM, Edmundowicz SA, et al. A single-institution review of 157 patients presenting with benign and malignant tumors of the ampulla of Vater: management and outcomes. Surgery. 2011;150(2):169–76.

51. Winter JM, Cameron JL, Olino K, Herman JM, de Jong MC, Hruban RH, Wolfgang CL, Eckhauser F, Edil BH, Choti MA, et al. Clinicopathologic analysis of ampullary neoplasms in 450 patients: implications for surgical strategy and long-term prognosis. J Gastrointest Surg. 2010;14(2):379–87.

10

Switch in *KRAS* mutational status during an unusual course of disease in a patient with advanced pancreatic adenocarcinoma: implications for translational research

Sibylle Baechmann[1†], Steffen Ormanns[1†] iD, Michael Haas[2], Stephan Kruger[2], Anna Remold[1,2], Dominik Paul Modest[2], Thomas Kirchner[1,4], Andreas Jung[1,4], Jens Werner[3], Volker Heinemann[2,4†] and Stefan Boeck[2*†]

Abstract

Background: Despite the introduction of novel effective treatment regimens like gemcitabine plus nab-paclitaxel and FOLFIRINOX, pancreatic ductal adenocarcinoma (PDAC) remains one of the most aggressive epithelial tumors. Among the genetic alterations frequently found in PDAC, mutations in the *KRAS* gene might play a prognostic role regarding overall survival and may also have the potential to predict the efficacy of anti-EGFR treatment.

Case presentation: We report the clinical case of a 69 year old Caucasian female that was diagnosed with histologically confirmed locally advanced PDAC with lymph node involvement in August 2010. At the time of first diagnosis, tumor tissue obtained from an open regional lymph node biopsy showed a poorly differentiated adenocarcinoma with a wild type sequence within exon 2 (codon 12/13) of the *KRAS* gene. The patient initially received single-agent gemcitabine and a subsequent 5-FU-based chemoradiotherapy with a sequential maintenance chemotherapy with oral capecitabine resulting in a long term disease control. Local disease progression occurred in May 2014 and the patient underwent pancreaticoduodenectomy in September 2014. A novel *KRAS* gene mutation (c.35G > T, p.G12 V) in exon 2 (codon 12) was detected within the surgical specimen. As of January 2016 the patient is still alive and without evidence of the underlying disease.

Conclusions: Specifically in the context of clinical trials and translational research in PDAC a re-assessment of molecular biomarkers, i. e. *KRAS*, at defined time points (e. g. relapse, disease progression, unusual clinical course) may be indicated in order to detect a potential switch in biomarker status during the course of disease.

Keywords: Pancreatic ductal adenocarcinoma (PDAC), *KRAS* mutation, Tumor heterogeneity

Background

Pancreatic ductal adenocarcinoma (PDAC) is one of the most aggressive epithelial tumors worldwide. In most patients it represents a deadly disease [1] due to an advanced stage at the time of diagnosis and the difficulties in therapeutic treatment, but also due to genetic heterogeneity [2]. Surgical resection remains the only curative treatment option for localized PDAC. During the last decade, systemic treatment with single-agent gemcitabine has evolved as standard chemotherapy for the adjuvant and palliative treatment setting [3, 4]. Gemcitabine offers a median survival of about 5 to 7 months in patients with advanced disease and shows comparatively good tolerability [5]; more recently, gemcitabine-based combination regimens with the oral epidermal growth factor receptor (EGFR) inhibitor erlotinib or together with nab-paclitaxel [6] showed a statistically significant improvement in overall survival (OS). The development and progression of PDAC

* Correspondence: stefan.boeck@med.uni-muenchen.de
†Equal contributors
[2]Department of Internal Medicine III and Comprehensive Cancer Center, Klinikum Grosshadern, Ludwig-Maximilans University of Munich, Marchioninistr. 15, 81377 Munich, Germany
Full list of author information is available at the end of the article

include different genetic alterations in oncogenic activation, loss of tumor-suppressor gene function and overexpression of receptor-ligand systems [7, 8]. Among these genetic alterations, mutations in the *KRAS* gene, which often are already present in precursor lesions, play an important role in tumor development and progression [8]. Gain of function mutations in the *KRAS* gene are detected in about 70 to 90% of PDAC cases [9], commonly as point mutations in exon 2 (codon 12/13), most frequently as p.G12D (c.35G > A) or p.G12 V (p.35G > T). Several studies showed that constitutively activating *KRAS* mutations are associated with worse OS, whereas *KRAS* wildtype status is associated with improved OS in PDAC [7, 10, 11]. Thus, in PDAC, *KRAS* mutations may be regarded as prognostic biomarker. The role of *KRAS* mutational status as predictive biomarker regarding the use of EGFR-targeting agents like erlotinib in advanced PDAC still remains a matter of debate to date [12–14].

Here, we report the case of a PDAC patient with an unusual clinical course: the tumor of the patient harbored a wildtype *KRAS* gene at the time of initial PDAC diagnosis; however, upon disease progression 4 years later, a mutation within exon 2 of the *KRAS* gene was detectable.

Case presentation

A currently 75-year-old woman was diagnosed with locally advanced PDAC at our comprehensive cancer center (CCC) in 2010. An explorative laparotomy in August 2010 showed metastatic disease spread extensively to regional lymph nodes and thus the primary tumor in the pancreatic head was not resected. By CT imaging criteria no other distant metastatic disease was evident. Lymph nodes were sampled surgically from the right gastric artery, the hepatic artery, the coeliac trunc and from the interaortocaval region; in all samples, tumor infiltration by a poorly differentiated adenocarcinoma was confirmed by histology. Immunohistochemical staining was positive for CK7, CK20 and CA 19–9 (with CDX-2 being negative). At that time point an additional analysis for *KRAS* mutational status and EGFR protein expression (which were conducted within a translational research project) detected a wildtype sequence of *KRAS* exon 2 by pyrosequencing and a moderately positive immunohistochemical staining for membranous EGFR expression in about 80% of the tumor cells.

The patient initially received systemic chemotherapy with three cycles of standard dose (1000 mg/m^2) gemcitabine between September and December 2010. Imaging studies in January 2011 confirmed stable disease and the CA 19–9 levels decreased from 3700 U/ml at first diagnosis to 180 U/ml. In February 2011 5-FU-based chemoradiotherapy (30 Gy) was applied at an external hospital.

During re-exploration performed in May 2011 surgical biopsies from the peritoneum histologically confirmed metastatic disease of PDAC; thus, no attempt to resect the primary tumor in the pancreas was performed. We then decided, also based on the wish of the patient, to re-start systemic chemotherapy and treatment with oral capecitabine was initiated in July 2011 and given until April 2012. During this chemotherapy, a further decline of CA 19–9 values was observed (nadir: 30 U/ml) and repeated CT imaging did not show any signs of local disease progression or metastatic disease (as assessed by imaging criteria). After a treatment rest for two years (beginning in May 2012), local tumor progression of the pancreatic primary was observed within a CT scan in May 2014. Again, no radiographic signs of distant metastasis were observed. Systemic chemotherapy with single-agent gemcitabine was re-introduced in June 2014 resulting in a CA 19–9 decrease from 690 U/ml at disease progression to 380 U/ml after three gemcitabine applications. Due to a progressive duodenal infiltration with clinical and endoscopic signs of gastrointestinal obstruction, a surgical re-exploration was performed in September 2014. Intraoperatively, no signs of peritoneal carcinomatosis were apparent and a liver biopsy showed no signs of malignancy. Thus, the pancreatic primary was removed by a pylorus preserving pancreaticoduodenectomy (modified Whipple-Kausch procedure). The tumor was classified as ypT3 ypN0 (0/15) L0 V0 Pn0, ductal adenocarcinoma G3, R0 resection (according to UICC criteria, TNM classification 7th edition, 2010). An additionally executed *KRAS* mutational analysis at this time point revealed a new point mutation p.G12 V (c.35G > T) in exon 2, codon 12. After surgery, CA 19–9 values decreased to levels of 20 U/ml. The patient was offered adjuvant chemotherapy with S-1 (tegafur, gimeracil, oteracil) after pancreaticoduodenectomy and started this treatment December 2014; however, S-1 was tolerated poorly due to gastrointestinal toxicity (diarrhea grade 4 and accompanying renal insufficiency) and was therefore terminated in March 2015. As of January 2016 the patient is still alive and without clear evidence of the underlying disease. An overview of this unusual disease course is shown within Fig. 1.

Discussion

Up to now, no prognostic or predictive tissue biomarker is available for PDAC [12]. In contrast to other diseases like breast, lung or colorectal cancer no specific biomarker has been validated for clinical use in pancreatic cancer and several clinical and translational trials are ongoing in order to better define the molecular basis of this disease and to search specifically for predictive markers for treatment efficacy. Thus, only limited data is available on the clinical role of biomarkers in PDAC

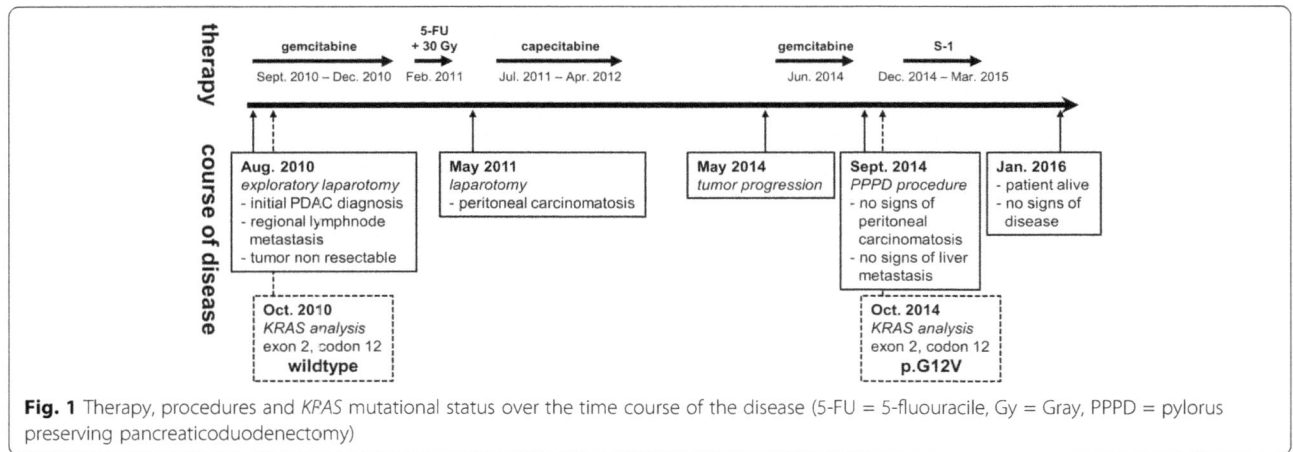

Fig. 1 Therapy, procedures and *KRAS* mutational status over the time course of the disease (5-FU = 5-fluouracile, Gy = Gray, PPPD = pylorus preserving pancreaticoduodenectomy)

[12]; specifically, there are no clear recommendations at which time points biomarkers should be assessed. In CRC for example, a good correlation between biomarker results from the primary tumor and from (metachronous) CRC metastases has been reported, resulting in the acceptance of e. g. *RAS* status of primary tumor tissue in patients with a metachronous relapse [15]. In contrast, in other diseases like breast cancer a switch in e. g. Her2/neu (ERBB2) status is well known resulting in the recommendation of repeated tumor biopsies at relapse or disease progression [16]. At least to our knowledge, studies investigating this issue have not yet been performed in PDAC.

Within this manuscript we report a rather unusual clinical course of a PADC patient, with a corresponding switch in *KRAS* mutational status during the course of disease. Of note, we detected the new *KRAS* mutation upon disease progression in September 2014; furthermore, it may be important to highlight the fact that this patient did not receive previous anti-EGFR treatment (e.g. with erlotinib) before the detection of the new *KRAS* mutation.

Several possible explanations may be hypothesized for the observation of a *KRAS* switch during the course of disease in our PDAC patient:

1. Appearance of a truly new tumor KRAS mutation upon disease progression in September 2014 without previous application of agents targeting the EGFR pathway:
   The reason for tumor progression could be caused by an evolved new mutation event in the *KRAS* gene, specifically in the light of selection pressure during previous treatment with chemotherapy and radiotherapy. In colorectal cancer, increasing evidence exists that the appearance of new *KRAS* mutations during treatment with agents targeting the EGFR (like cetuximab or panitumumab) may

be linked to an acquired resistance to anti-EGFR therapy [17, 18]. Of note, our patient did not receive anti-EGFR treatment for example with erlotinib before the detection of the new *KRAS* mutation. If other treatments like cytotoxic chemotherapy (gemcitabine, fluoropyrimidines) or radiotherapy to the pancreatic primary may also induce a "selection pressure" for the development of new genetic events remains unknown.

2. Tumor heterogeneity with distinct results in KRAS analysis at initial diagnosis (lymph node metastasis analyzed) and at progression (primary tumor analyzed):
   There is increasing evidence for intratumoral heterogeneity in different types of cancer that could be determined by multiregion sequencing [19]. In non-small cell lung cancer it was shown that ALK rearrangements (that were previously thought to be mutually exclusive with activating *EGFR* and *KRAS* mutations) can be found together with EGFR mutations in rare cases [20]. Moreover, it was shown that spatially separated subclones of the same tumor harbor different oncogenic drivers [21]. If these observations are transferable to PDAC, this might explain the differences in *KRAS* mutational status observed in our patient reported here. However, the scarce currently available data comparing pancreatic primary tumors and corresponding metastases, showed the same *KRAS* mutational status in the primary tumor and each metastatic site examined, thus supporting the idea of a newly apparent KRAS mutation [22, 23].

3. Technical aspects of the discrepant KRAS sequencing results (see Fig. 2):
   Potentially, the initial *KRAS* wildtype status detected in 2010 could be the effect of a false negative sequencing result. Both *KRAS* analyses in the tumor tissue of the patient reported here were performed

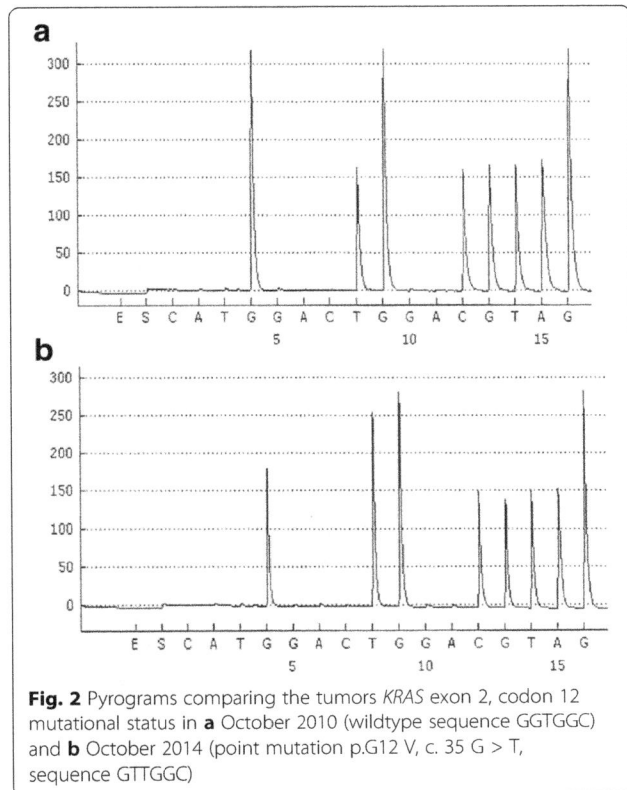

Fig. 2 Pyrograms comparing the tumors *KRAS* exon 2, codon 12 mutational status in **a** October 2010 (wildtype sequence GGTGGC) and **b** October 2014 (point mutation p.G12 V, c. 35 G > T, sequence GTTGGC)

in the same specialized and certified laboratory for molecular pathology. For both analyses, formalin fixed paraffin embedded (FFPE) tumor tissue was microdissected under visual control using a microscope to reduce contamination by adjacent normal tissue. In both situations, sufficient tumor tissue was available: In 2010 a subtotally infiltrated lymph node metastasis, 22 mm in diameter, containing insignificant residual lymphatic tissue and in 2014 whole tumor resection tissue was used for analysis. Moreover, the pyrosequencing assay employed here is highly sensitive and requires only 10% of tumor DNA in the whole DNA extracted to reliably detect the *KRAS* mutational status [24]. Thus, a false negative sequencing result is a very unlikely event to explain the discrepancy in the present case.

Conclusions

KRAS mutational status may change during the course of disease in PDAC. Thus, in well-defined clinical scenarios (e. g. relapse after surgery in curative intent, disease progression during/after chemotherapy, unusual clinical course) a re-assessment of the *KRAS* status should be discussed, specifically within the setting of controlled clinical and translational trials. As *KRAS* is not yet established as a clinically relevant biomarker in

PDAC, future translational trials in pancreatic cancer that evaluate a broad range of novel biomarkers should, at least to our opinion, include a repeated biomarker assessment during the course of disease within their prospective study protocols. Novel promising techniques like liquid biopsy approaches may thereby help to overcome the limitations of obtaining tumor tissue safely in PDAC [25]. As it may be difficult to obtain sufficient tumor tissue in PDAC by percutaneous- or endosonography-guided biopsy techniques, a sampling error may occur specifically in the light of tumor heterogeneity. In that context, liquid biopsy techniques may also eventually help to overcome these limitations.

Abbreviations
5-FU: 5-fluorouracil; ALK: Anaplastic lymphoma kinase; CA19–9: Carbohydrate antigen 19–9; CDX2: Caudal type homeo-box transcription factor 2; CK: Cytokeratin; CRC: Colorectal cancer; CT: Computed tomography; EGFR: Epidermal growth factor receptor; ERBB2: Human epidermal growth factor receptor 2; FFPE: Formalin fixed paraffin embedded; FOLFIRINOX: Folinic acid, 5-FU, irinotecan, oxaliplatin; Gy: Gray; KRAS: Kirsten rat sarcoma viral oncogene homologue; nab-paclitaxel: Nanoparticle albumin-bound paclitaxel; OS: Overall survival; PDAC: Pancreatic ductal adenocarcinoma; UICC: International union against cancer

Acknowledgments
We thank all the lab technicians at the Institute of Pathology for their excellent technical support.

Funding
SO is supported by grants from the Friedrich-Baur-Stiftung, Munich and the association for the promotion of research and science at the medical faculty LMU (wifomed), Munich.

Authors' contributions
SB, SO, AR, TK and AJ did the pathological investigations and the molecular-pathological analyses of the reported case. MH, SK, DPM, VH and SB were the treating oncologists. JW was the surgeon who performed the pancreaticoduodenectomy. SB, SO, VH, AJ and SB designed the study, collected the clinical data and drafted the manuscript. All authors have read and approved the manuscript of this case report.

Authors' information
The authors are experienced pathologists, oncologists or surgeons involved in the multidisciplinary management of pancreatic cancer patients at the comprehensive cancer center of a large tertiary care university hospital.

Competing interests
The authors declare that they have no competing interests.

Author details
[1]Institute of Pathology, Ludwig-Maximilians University of Munich, Munich, Germany. [2]Department of Internal Medicine III and Comprehensive Cancer Center, Klinikum Grosshadern, Ludwig-Maximilians University of Munich, Marchioninistr. 15, 81377 Munich, Germany. [3]Department of General, Visceral, Vascular and Transplantation Surgery, Klinikum Grosshadern, Ludwig-Maximilians-University of Munich, Munich, Germany. [4]DKTK, German Cancer Consortium, German Cancer Research Center (DKFZ), Heidelberg, Germany.

References

1. Siegel RL, Miller KD, Jemal A. Cancer statistics, 2016. CA: A cancer journal for clinicians; 2015.
2. Eser S, et al. Oncogenic KRAS signalling in pancreatic cancer. Br J Cancer. 2014;111(5):817–22.
3. Burris HA 3rd, et al. Improvements in survival and clinical benefit with gemcitabine as first-line therapy for patients with advanced pancreas cancer: a randomized trial. J Clin Oncol. 1997;15(6):2403–13.
4. Heinemann V, et al. Randomized phase III trial of gemcitabine plus cisplatin compared with gemcitabine alone in advanced pancreatic cancer. J Clin Oncol. 2006;24(24):3946–52.
5. Heinemann V, Haas M, Boeck S. Systemic treatment of advanced pancreatic cancer. Cancer Treat Rev. 2012;38(7):843–53.
6. Goldstein, D., et al., nab-Paclitaxel plus gemcitabine for metastatic pancreatic cancer: long-term survival from a phase III trial. Journal of the National Cancer Institute, 2015. 107(2): p. dju413.
7. Shin SH, et al. Genetic alterations of K-ras, p53, c-erbB-2, and DPC4 in pancreatic ductal adenocarcinoma and their correlation with patient survival. Pancreas. 2013;42(2):216–22.
8. Sinn BV, et al. KRAS mutations in codon 12 or 13 are associated with worse prognosis in pancreatic ductal adenocarcinoma. Pancreas. 2014;43(4):578–83.
9. Miglio U, et al. KRAS mutational analysis in ductal adenocarcinoma of the pancreas and its clinical significance. Pathology-Research and Practice. 2014; 210(5):307–11.
10. Lee J, et al. Impact of epidermal growth factor receptor (EGFR) kinase mutations, EGFR gene amplifications, and KRAS mutations on survival of pancreatic adenocarcinoma. Cancer. 2007;109(8):1561–9.
11. Boeck S, et al. EGFR pathway biomarkers in erlotinib-treated patients with advanced pancreatic cancer: translational results from the randomised, crossover phase 3 trial AIO-PK0104. Br J Cancer. 2013;108(2):469–76.
12. Kruger S, et al. Translational research in pancreatic ductal adenocarcinoma: current evidence and future concepts. World J Gastroenterol: WJG. 2014; 20(31):10769.
13. Kim ST, et al. Impact of KRAS mutations on clinical outcomes in pancreatic cancer patients treated with first-line gemcitabine-based chemotherapy. Mol Cancer Ther. 2011;10(10):1993–9
14. Boeck S, et al. KRAS mutation status is not predictive for objective response to anti-EGFR treatment with erlotinib in patients with advanced pancreatic cancer. J Gastroenterol. 2013;48(4):544–8.
15. Allegra, C.J., et al., Extended RAS gene mutation testing in metastatic colorectal carcinoma to predict response to anti–epidermal growth factor receptor monoclonal antibody therapy: American Society of Clinical Oncology provisional clinical opinion update 2015. Journal of clinical Oncology, 2015: p. JCO 2015.63. 9674.
16. Wolff AC, et al. Recommendations for human epidermal growth factor receptor 2 testing in breast cancer: American Society of Clinical Oncology/ College of American Pathologists clinical practice guideline update. Arch Pathol Lab Med. 2013;138(2):241–56.
17. Misale S, et al. Emergence of KRAS mutations and acquired resistance to anti-EGFR therapy in colorectal cancer. Nature. 2012;486(7404):532–6.
18. Diaz LA Jr, et al. The molecular evolution of acquired resistance to targeted EGFR blockade in colorectal cancers. Nature. 2012;486(7404):537–40.
19. Gerlinger M, et al. Intratumor heterogeneity and branched evolution revealed by multiregion sequencing. N Engl J Med. 2012;366(10):883–92.
20. Birkbak NJ, Hiley CT, Swanton C. Evolutionary precision medicine: a role for repeat epidermal growth factor receptor analysis in ALK-rearranged lung adenocarcinoma? J Clin Oncol. 2015;33(32):3681–3.
21. Cai, W., et al., Intratumoral heterogeneity of ALK-rearranged and ALK/EGFR coaltered lung adenocarcinoma. Journal of Clinical Oncology, 2015: p. JCO. 2014.58. 8293.
22. Embuscado EE, et al. Immortalizing the complexity of cancer metastasis: genetic features of lethal metastatic pancreatic cancer obtained from rapid autopsy. Cancer biology & therapy. 2005;4(5):548–54.
23. Yachida S, et al. Distant metastasis occurs late during the genetic evolution of pancreatic cancer. Nature. 2010;467(7319):1114–7.
24. Ogino S, et al. Sensitive sequencing method for KRAS mutation detecting by pyrosequencing. The Journal of Molecular Diagnostics. 2005;7(3):413–21.
25. Kinugasa H, et al. Detection of K-ras gene mutation by liquid biopsy in patients with pancreatic cancer. Cancer. 2015;121(13):2271–80.

Association between alcohol intake and the risk of pancreatic cancer: a dose–response meta-analysis of cohort studies

Ye-Tao Wang, Ya-Wen Gou, Wen-Wen Jin, Mei Xiao and Hua-Ying Fang[*]

Abstract

Background: Studies examining the association between alcohol intake and the risk of pancreatic cancer have given inconsistent results. The purpose of this study was to summarize and examine the evidence regarding the association between alcohol intake and pancreatic cancer risk based on results from prospective cohort studies.

Methods: We searched electronic databases consisting of PubMed, Ovid, Embase, and the Cochrane Library identifying studies published up to Aug 2015. Only prospective studies that reported effect estimates with 95 % confidence intervals (CIs) for the risk of pancreatic cancer, examining different alcohol intake categories compared with a low alcohol intake category were included. Results of individual studies were pooled using a random-effects model.

Results: We included 19 prospective studies (21 cohorts) reporting data from 4,211,129 individuals. Low-to-moderate alcohol intake had little or no effect on the risk of pancreatic cancer. High alcohol intake was associated with an increased risk of pancreatic cancer (risk ratio [RR], 1.15; 95 % CI: 1.06–1.25). Pooled analysis also showed that high liquor intake was associated with an increased risk of pancreatic cancer (RR, 1.43; 95 % CI: 1.17–1.74). Subgroup analyses suggested that high alcohol intake was associated with an increased risk of pancreatic cancer in North America, when the duration of follow-up was greater than 10 years, in studies scored as high quality, and in studies with adjustments for smoking status, body mass index, diabetes mellitus, and energy intake..

Conclusions: Low-to-moderate alcohol intake was not significantly associated with the risk of pancreatic cancer, whereas high alcohol intake was associated with an increased risk of pancreatic cancer. Furthermore, liquor intake in particular was associated with an increased risk of pancreatic cancer.

Keywords: Alcohol, Pancreatic cancer, Meta-analysis

Background

Pancreatic cancer is the fourth leading cause of cancer-related death for both men and women worldwide, with approximately 338,000 new cases diagnosed each year [1]. Over the past few decades, studies have shown that cigarette smoking, diabetes mellitus, and obesity are associated with an increased risk of pancreatic cancer [2–4]. Therefore, lifestyle changes are suggested as a preventative measure to reduce the incidence of pancreatic cancer. Changes in alcohol consumption may be an additional lifestyle change that might reduce the risk of pancreatic cancer. However, the association between alcohol intake and subsequent pancreatic cancer development is still under investigation, and more concrete results may be of great public health value given the prevalence of alcohol intake in many populations [5].

Several studies using pooled analyses [6–8] have investigated the association between alcohol intake and pancreatic cancer risk, and have demonstrated that moderate alcohol intake has no significant effect, while high alcohol intake has been shown to be associated with an increased risk of pancreatic cancer. In contrast, previous cohort studies have shown no association between alcohol intake and pancreatic cancer risk [9–11]. Importantly, cigarette smoking, diabetes mellitus, and

* Correspondence: fanghuayinganhui@126.com
Department of gastroenterology, Anhui provincial hospital, NO.17, Lujiang Road, Hefei City, Anhui Province 230001, China

obesity are established risk factors for pancreatic cancer and should be adjusted for in analyses examining alcohol use [12]. Furthermore, inclusion of retrospective case–control studies in analyses serves as a potential drawback as these studies are sensitive to confounding factors and biases, especially recall bias. Thus, the association between alcohol intake and pancreatic cancer risk remains unclear due to a lack of supporting evidence.

Recently, additional large-scale prospective cohort studies investigating the association between alcohol intake and subsequent pancreatic cancer morbidity have been completed [13–16]. To better understand any effect of alcohol intake on subsequent pancreatic cancer development, data from these recent studies need to be re-evaluated and combined with data from the existing literature. Therefore, we conducted a systematic review and meta-analysis of pooled data from prospective cohort studies to assess the possible association between alcohol intake and pancreatic cancer risk.

Methods
Data sources, search strategy, and selection criteria
This review was conducted and reported according to the criteria for conducting and reporting meta-analysis of observational studies in epidemiology (Additional file 1) [17]. Any prospective study that examined the association between alcohol intake and subsequent pancreatic cancer risk was eligible for inclusion in this study, with no restrictions placed on language or publication status.

Relevant studies were identified using the following procedures. We searched electronic databases including PubMed, Embase, Ovid, and the Cochrane Library for articles published up to Aug 2015. Search terms examining both medical subject headings and free-language searches for "ethanol" OR "alcohol" OR "alcoholic beverages" OR "drinking behavior" OR "alcohol drinking" OR "drink" OR "liquor" OR "ethanol intake" OR "alcohol drink" OR "ethanol drink" AND ("pancreas" OR "pancreatic") AND ("cancer" OR "carcinoma" OR "neoplasm") AND ("cohort" OR "cohort studies") were used. Other sources included meeting abstracts, meta-analyses, or reviews already published on related topics. Authors were contacted for essential information from publications that were not available in full. The medical subject heading, methods, population, study design, exposure, and outcome variables of these articles were used to identify the relevant studies.

The literature search was independently undertaken by two investigators using a standardized approach. Any inconsistencies between these investigators were identified by the principal investigator and resolved by consensus. We restricted our meta-analysis to prospective cohort studies that were less likely to be subject to confounding variables and bias than traditional case control studies. A study was eligible for inclusion if the study had a prospective cohort design, the study investigated the association between alcohol intake and the risk of pancreatic cancer, and the authors reported effect estimates (risk ratio [RR] or hazard ratio [HR]) and 95 % confidence intervals (CIs) comparing different alcohol intake categories with the lowest alcohol intake category.

Data collection and quality assessment
The information collected included the study group's name, country, study design, sample size, age at baseline, follow-up duration, effect estimate, and covariates, all of which were included in the fully adjusted model. We also extracted the number of cases, persons, person-years, the effect of different exposure categories, and their 95 % CIs. For studies that reported several multivariable adjusted RRs, we selected the effect estimate that was maximally adjusted for potential confounders. The Newcastle-Ottawa Scale (NOS), which is comprehensive and has been partially validated for evaluating the quality of observational studies in meta-analyses, was used to evaluate methodological quality [18, 19]. The NOS is based on three subscales, selection consisting of four items, comparability consisting of one item, and outcome consisting of three items. A "star system" (range, 0–9) has been developed for assessment [18]. Data extraction and quality assessment were independently conducted by two authors. The data was then independently examined and adjudicated by an additional author, while referring to the original studies.

Statistical analysis
We examined the relationship between alcohol intake and risk of pancreatic cancer based on the effect estimate (RR or HR) and its 95 % CI as published in each study. We used a fixed-effect model to calculate summary RRs and 95 % CIs for different alcohol intake levels compared with the lowest alcohol intake level or no alcohol intake [20, 21]. We then used a random-effects model to calculate summary RRs and 95 % CIs for different alcohol intake levels compared with the lowest alcohol intake level or no alcohol intake [22, 23]. We converted all measurements into grams per day and defined one drink as 12 g of alcohol intake. Using a semi-parametric method, we evaluated the association between light (0–12 g per day), moderate (≥12-24 g per day), or heavy alcohol (≥24 g per day) intake and the risk of pancreatic cancer. The value assigned to each alcohol intake category was the mid-point for closed categories and the median for open categories. Furthermore, we constructed a dose response curve based on the correlated natural log of RRs or HRs across alcohol intake categories, and modeled alcohol intake by using restricted cubic splines with three knots at fixed percentiles of 10 %, 50 %, and 90 % of the distribution [24, 25]. Heterogeneity between studies was investigated using the I^2 statistic as a measure

of the proportion of total variation between studies that is attributable to heterogeneity, where I^2 values of 25 %, 50 %, and 75 % were assigned as cut-off points for low, moderate, and high degrees of heterogeneity [26–28]. Subgroup analyses were conducted based on country, duration of follow-up, adjustment of covariates (including smoking status, body mass index [BMI], diabetes mellitus, and energy intake [EI]), and study quality. We also performed a sensitivity analysis by eliminating individual studies from the meta-analysis [29]. Several methods were used to check for potential publication bias, including visually inspecting the Funnel plots for pancreatic cancer, and using the Egger [30] and Begg [31] tests for a statistical bias assessment. All reported P values are 2-sided, and P values <0.05 were considered statistically significant for all included studies. Statistical analyses were performed using STATA software (version 12.0; Stata Corporation, College Station, TX, USA).

Results

Literature search

The study-selection process is illustrated in Fig. 1. We identified 469 articles during our initial electronic search, of which, 425 were excluded as duplicates or irrelevant, leaving 44 potentially eligible studies to be selected. After detailed evaluations, 19 prospective studies consisting of 21 cohorts were selected for the final meta-analysis [9–11, 13–16, 32–43]. A manual search of the reference lists from these studies did not yield any additional eligible studies. The general characteristics of the included studies are presented in Table 1.

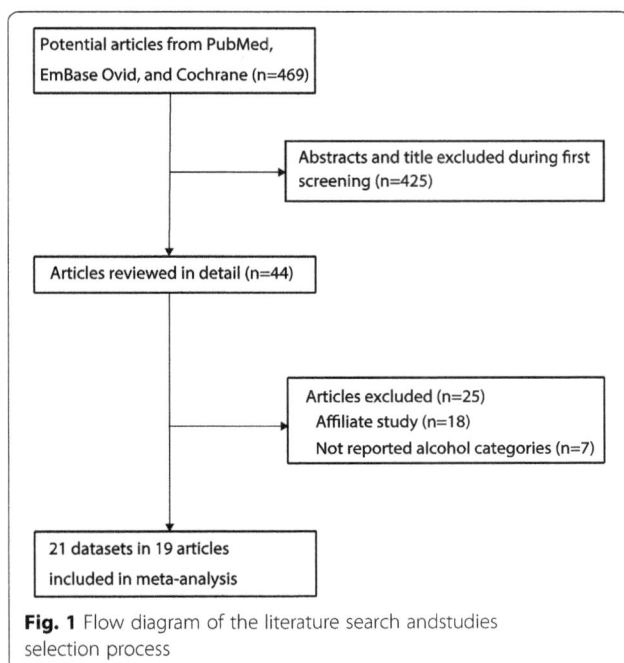

Fig. 1 Flow diagram of the literature search andstudies selection process

Study characteristics

In the included studies, follow-up periods for participants ranged from six to 30 years, and had from 7132 to 1,290,000 individuals included. Nine studies (ten cohorts) were conducted in the United States [11, 16, 32, 35, 36, 38–40, 42], six (seven cohorts) in Europe [9, 13, 33, 34, 37, 43], and four in other countries [10, 14, 15, 41]. In total, the meta-analysis included 11,846 incident cases and more than 4,211,129 individuals. Study quality was assessed using the NOS, with studies receiving a score ≥8 considered to be high quality (Table 1). Overall, four cohorts had a score of 9 [14, 16, 33, 34], eight cohorts (six studies) had a score of 8 [9, 11, 13, 38, 39, 43], five cohorts had a score of 7 [10, 15, 35, 37, 41], and the remaining four cohorts had a score of 6 [32, 36, 40, 42].

Alcohol intake and pancreatic cancer risk

In the pooled analysis (Fig. 2), low (RR, 0.97; 95 % CI, 0.89–1.05; $P = 0.389$; Additional file 2: Figure S1), moderate (RR, 0.98; 95 % CI: 0.93–1.03; $P = 0.513$; Additional file 3: Figure S2), and total alcohol intake (RR, 1.02; 95 % CI: 0.95–1.08; $P = 0.634$; Additional file 4: Figure S3) were not associated with pancreatic cancer risk, compared with the lowest alcohol intake level. However, high alcohol intake was associated with an increased risk of pancreatic cancer (RR, 1.15; 95 % CI: 1.06–1.25; $P = 0.001$; Additional file 5: Figure S4). Between-study heterogeneity was moderate for total alcohol intake ($I^2 = 39.4$ %) and low for low ($I^2 = 0.0$ %), moderate ($I^2 = 0.0$ %), and high alcohol intake ($I^2 = 14.5$ %). Analysis using the summary RR showed that low (RR, 0.98; 95 % CI, 0.84–1.15; $P = 0.836$), moderate (RR, 0.93; 95 % CI, 0.80–1.09; $P = 0.372$), and total alcohol intake (RR, 1.03; 95 % CI, 0.91–1.17; $P = 0.664$) were not associated with pancreatic cancer risk in men, compared with the lowest alcohol intake level. However, high alcohol intake was associated with an increased risk of pancreatic cancer in men (RR, 1.18; 95 % CI: 1.00–1.39; $P = 0.045$). Results from men exhibited substantial heterogeneity for total alcohol intake ($I^2 = 48.7$ %), moderate heterogeneity for low alcohol intake ($I^2 = 21.2$ %), and low heterogeneity for moderate ($I^2 = 0.0$ %) or high alcohol intake ($I^2 = 12.9$ %). No significant association was found between low, moderate, high, or total alcohol intake and pancreatic cancer risk in women, and there was no evidence of heterogeneity across studies in this population (low: $I^2 = 0.0$ %; moderate: $I^2 = 0.0$ %; high: $I^2 = 0.0$ %).

Types of alcohol intake and pancreatic cancer risk

Analysis based on the type of alcohol showed that, high liquor intake was associated with an increased risk of pancreatic cancer in men (RR, 1.66; 95 % CI: 1.24–2.23; Fig. 3) and in the total cohort (RR, 1.43; 95 % CI: 1.17–1.74; Fig. 3). However, there was no significant association between any other types of alcohol intake and risk of pancreatic cancer.

Table 1 Baseline characteristic of studies included

Study	Country	Sex	Study design	Sample size	Cases	Age at baseline	Effect estimate	Follow-up (year)	Covariates in fully adjusted model	NOS score
JACC [10]	Japan	Men	Cohort	46,465	94	40–79	RR	8.1	Age and smoking status	7
		Women	Cohort	64,327	97	40–79	RR	8.1		
KIRS and MIHDPs [13]	Lithuania	Men	Cohort	7,132	77	45–59	HR	30.0	Age, smoking status, education, BMI.	8
LWLH [32]	US	Both	Cohort	13,979	65	75.0	RR	9.0	Sex, age and smoking status	6
ATBC [33]	Finland	Men	Cohort	27,101	157	50–69	HR	13.0	Age and intervention	9
NLCS [34]	Netherland	Men	Cohort	58,279	144	55–69	HR	13.3	Age, sex, smoking status, EI, BMI, vegetable intake, and fruit intake	9
		Women	Cohort	62,573	115	55–69	HR	13.3		
NIH-AARP [35]	US	Men	Cohort	280,084	748	50–71	RR	7.3	Sex, smoking status, EI, energy-adjusted saturated fat, red meat, and total folate intake, BMI, PA, and DM	7
		Women	Cohort	190,597	401	50–71	RR	7.3		
IWHS [36]	US	Women	Cohort	33,976	66	55–69	RR	8.0	Age, smoking status	6
HPFS [11]	US	Men	Cohort	51,529	130	40–75	RR	12.0	Age, smoking status, BMI, history of DM, history of cholecysectomy, and EI	8
NHS [11]	US	Women	Cohort	121,700	158	30–55	RR	16.0	Age, smoking status, BMI, history of DM, history of cholecysectomy, and EI	8
CPS II [16]	US	Men	Cohort	453,770	3443	>30	RR	24.0	Age, sex, race/ethnicity, education, marital status, BMI, FHPC, and history of gallstones, DM, or smoking status	9
		Women	Cohort	576,697	3404	>30	RR	24.0		
TGP [15]	Japan	Men	Cohort	14,241	33	>35	HR	7.0	Age, smoking, BMI, history of DM	7
		Women	Cohort	16,585	18	>35	HR	7.0		
EPIC [9]	Europe	Both	Cohort	478,400	555	52.2	RR	8.9	Age, sex, centre, smoking status, height and weight, and history of DM	8
MWS [37]	UK	Women	Cohort	1,290,000	1338	55.9	RR	7.2	Age, region, socioeconomic status, smoking status, BMI and height	7
NYSC [38]	US	Men	Cohort	30,363	90	>15	RR	7.0	Smoking status, DM, BMI, and EI	8
		Women	Cohort	22,550	48	>15	RR	7.0		
BCDDP [39]	US	Women	Cohort	43,162	102	40–93	RR	11.0	Smoking status, DM, BMI, and EI	8
CTS [40]	US	Women	Cohort	100,030	116	>22	RR	8.1	Smoking status, DM, BMI, and EI	6
CNBSS [41]	Canada	Women	Cohort	49,654	105	40–59	RR	16.5	Smoking status, DM, BMI, and EI	7
PLCO [42]	US	Men	Cohort	29,914	90	55–74	RR	6.0	Smoking status, DM, BMI, and EI	6
		Women	Cohort	28,315	60	55–74	RR	6.0		
SMC [43]	Swedish	Women	Cohort	36,630	54	49–83	RR	6.8	Smoking status, DM, BMI, and EI	8
COSM [43]	Swedish	Men	Cohort	45,338	75	45–79	RR	6.8	Smoking status, DM, BMI, and EI	8
MCCS [14]	Australia	Men	Cohort	14,908	28	40–69	RR	15.0	Smoking status, DM, BMI, and EI	9
		Women	Cohort	22,830	35	40–69	RR	15.0		

*BMI body mass index, DM diabetes mellitus, EI energy intake, PA physical activity, FHPC family history of pancreatic cancer

Dose–response restricted cubic splines

A total of 13 cohorts (12 studies) were included in the restricted cubic splines analysis examining the association between alcohol intake and the incidence of pancreatic cancer. As shown in Fig. 4, we found no evidence for a potential nonlinear relationship between alcohol intake and the risk of pancreatic cancer ($P = 0.0874$), although alcohol intake greater than 15 g/day seemed to be associated with an increased risk of pancreatic cancer. A dose–response analysis examining the association

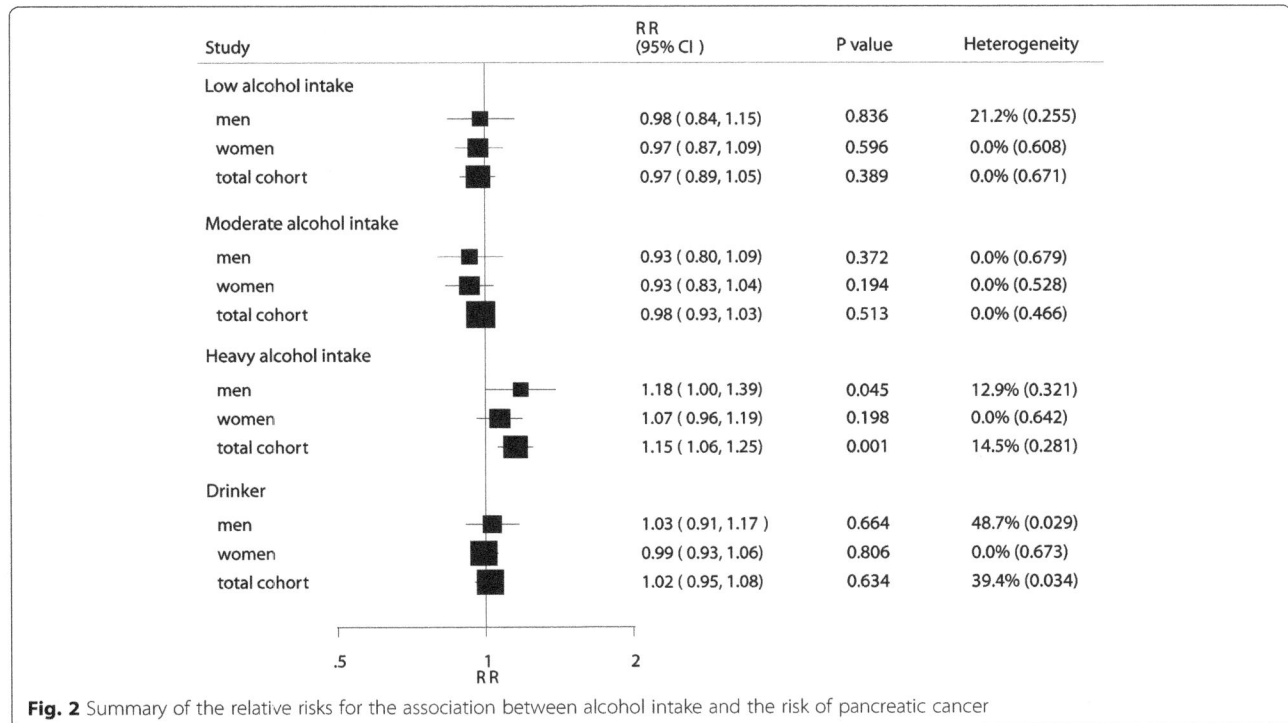

Study		RR (95% CI)	P value	Heterogeneity
Low alcohol intake				
men		0.98 (0.84, 1.15)	0.836	21.2% (0.255)
women		0.97 (0.87, 1.09)	0.596	0.0% (0.608)
total cohort		0.97 (0.89, 1.05)	0.389	0.0% (0.671)
Moderate alcohol intake				
men		0.93 (0.80, 1.09)	0.372	0.0% (0.679)
women		0.93 (0.83, 1.04)	0.194	0.0% (0.528)
total cohort		0.98 (0.93, 1.03)	0.513	0.0% (0.466)
Heavy alcohol intake				
men		1.18 (1.00, 1.39)	0.045	12.9% (0.321)
women		1.07 (0.96, 1.19)	0.198	0.0% (0.642)
total cohort		1.15 (1.06, 1.25)	0.001	14.5% (0.281)
Drinker				
men		1.03 (0.91, 1.17)	0.664	48.7% (0.029)
women		0.99 (0.93, 1.06)	0.806	0.0% (0.673)
total cohort		1.02 (0.95, 1.08)	0.634	39.4% (0.034)

Fig. 2 Summary of the relative risks for the association between alcohol intake and the risk of pancreatic cancer

between alcohol intake and pancreatic cancer risk in men was performed with seven cohorts, and found no significant relationship between alcohol intake and the risk of pancreatic cancer ($P = 0.8450$; Additional file 6: Figure S5A). Alcohol intake rates of 25.0–55.0 g/day seemed to be associated with an increased risk of pancreatic cancer, but alcohol intake rates greater than 55.0 g/day were not associated with the risk of pancreatic cancer. This analysis performed on data from women, as shown in Additional file 6: Figure S5B, found no evidence of a nonlinear relationship between alcohol intake and the risk of pancreatic cancer based on the P value for nonlinearity ($P = 0.0524$).

Subgroup analysis

We conducted subgroup analyses to minimize heterogeneity among the included studies and evaluated the association between alcohol intake and risk of pancreatic cancer in specific subpopulations (Table 2). First, we noted that high alcohol intake was associated with an increased risk of pancreatic cancer in North America; when the duration of follow-up was greater than 10 years; in studies with adjustments for smoking status, BMI, diabetes mellitus, and EI; and in studies scored as high quality. Second, high alcohol intake was associated with an increased risk of pancreatic cancer in men if the duration of the follow-up was less than 10 years. Third, high alcohol intake was associated with an increased risk of pancreatic cancer in women if the follow-up duration

was greater than 10 years and if the study adjusted for EI. Lastly, alcohol intake was associated with an increased risk of pancreatic cancer in men in studies scored as low quality.

Publication bias

After review of the funnel plots, we could not rule out the potential for publication bias (Fig. 5). However, the Egger [30] and Begg [31] tests showed no evidence of publication bias (Egger test, $P = 0.199$; Begg test, $P = 0.928$).

Discussion

Our meta-analysis drew exclusively from prospective studies and explored all possible correlations between alcohol intake and the risk of pancreatic cancer. This large quantitative analysis included 4,211,129 individuals from 19 prospective studies (21 cohorts) with a broad population range. The findings of this meta-analysis suggest that high alcohol intake is associated with an increased risk of pancreatic cancer, but other levels of alcohol intake have no significant effect on this risk. The results suggest a potential J-shaped correlation between increasing alcohol intake and the risk of pancreatic cancer. Our findings support the results of a previous pooled analysis and provide evidence that associations might differ in analysis of differently stratified groups. The magnitude of association between alcohol intake and the risk of pancreatic cancer was similar between sexes and after adjustment for most factors. These findings need to be

Study	RR (95% CI)
Beer	
Men	
light alcohol intake	1.06 (0.84, 1.34)
moderate alcohol intake	1.14 (0.94, 1.39)
Women	
light alcohol intake	1.00 (0.76, 1.30)
moderate alcohol intake	0.94 (0.56, 1.57)
Total cohort	
light alcohol intake	0.98 (0.86, 1.11)
moderate alcohol intake	1.05 (0.93, 1.19)
heavy alcohol intake	1.08 (0.90, 1.30)
Wine	
Men	
light alcohol intake	1.00 (0.85, 1.18)
moderate alcohol intake	1.00 (0.84, 1.18)
Women	
light alcohol intake	1.00 (0.86, 1.15)
moderate alcohol intake	0.95 (0.74, 1.23)
Total cohort	
light alcohol intake	0.97 (0.87, 1.07)
moderate alcohol intake	0.95 (0.85, 1.07)
heavy alcohol intake	1.09 (0.79, 1.49)
Liquor	
Men	
light alcohol intake	0.97 (0.73, 1.28)
moderate alcohol intake	1.01 (0.84, 1.18)
heavy alcohol intake	1.66 (1.24, 2.23)
Women	
light alcohol intake	1.06 (0.90, 1.26)
moderate alcohol intake	1.08 (0.90, 1.31)
heavy alcohol intake	1.46 (0.80, 2.67)
Total cohort	
light alcohol intake	1.02 (0.90, 1.16)
moderate alcohol intake	1.09 (0.99, 1.19)
heavy alcohol intake	1.43 (1.17, 1.74)

RR

.5   1   2

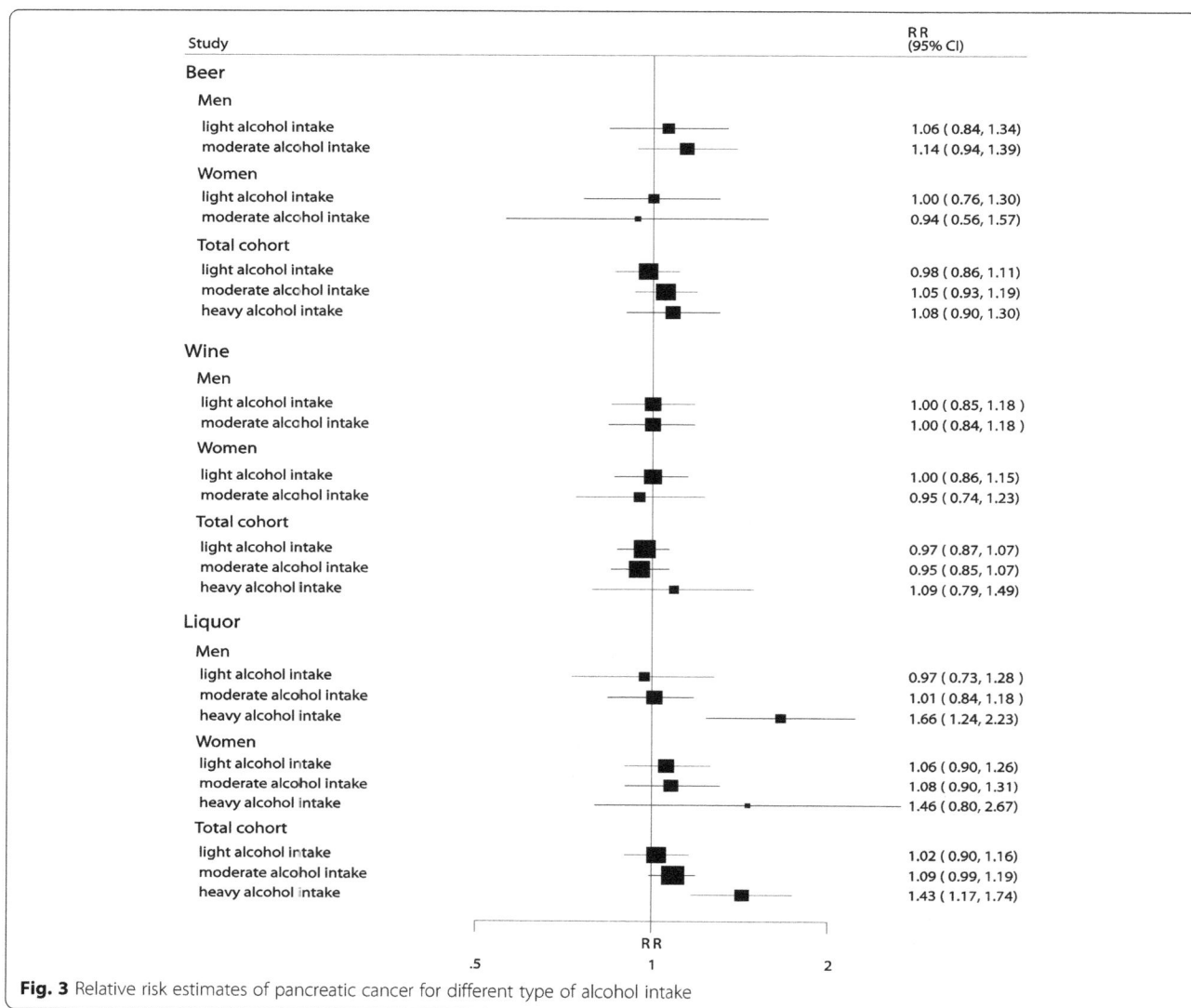

Fig. 3 Relative risk estimates of pancreatic cancer for different type of alcohol intake

confirmed by stratified analyses adjusted for these factors in future studies.

A previous pooled analysis [7] suggested that liquor intake greater than 45 g/day was associated with an increased risk of pancreatic cancer in men, but had no significant effect on the risk of pancreatic cancer in women, while no associations were noted for wine or beer intake. However, that study pooled only nested case–control studies, and prospective cohort studies were not included. Another important pooled analysis [8] suggested that alcohol intake greater than 30 g/day was associated with a modest increase in risk of pancreatic cancer. However, several important cohort studies were not included in this analysis. Finally, Tramacere et al. [6] suggested that moderate alcohol intake was not associated with the risk of pancreatic cancer, but high alcohol intake was associated with an increased risk of pancreatic cancer. It is notable that most of the epidemiological evidence is derived from retrospective case–control studies. In traditional case–control studies, information that reflects past exposure is collected after cancer is diagnosed, thus generating an inevitable recall bias that cannot be ignored. This bias may partly explain differences in the findings between prospective cohort studies and retrospective case–control studies. Furthermore, several adjustment factors are themselves considered to be leading risk factors for pancreatic cancer, but the primary aggregated results provide no information regarding their influence on pancreatic cancer causation. Considering the limitations of previous studies, we performed a meta-analysis of prospective cohort studies to determine the association between alcohol intake and the incidence of pancreatic cancer. Our study raised the probability that there are differences in this association based on pre-defined factors influencing pancreatic cancer.

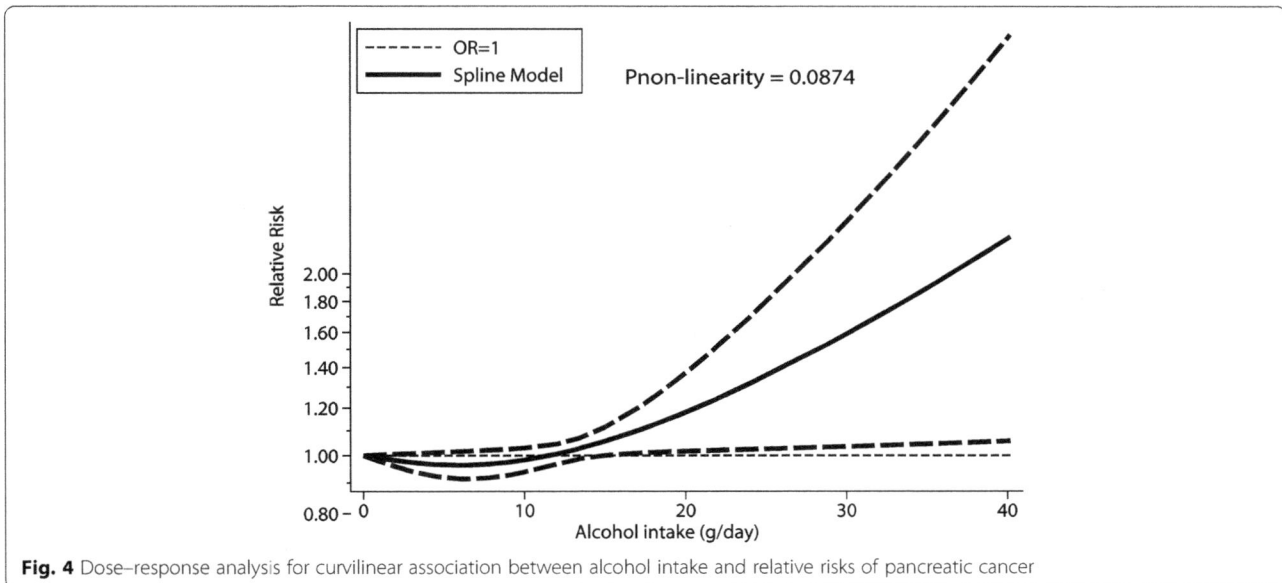

Fig. 4 Dose–response analysis for curvilinear association between alcohol intake and relative risks of pancreatic cancer

Most of our findings are in agreement with the results from several large cohort studies, showing the potential association between alcohol use and pancreatic cancer risk to be J-shaped. A study by Heinen et al. [34] suggested an increased risk of pancreatic cancer for persons with a high alcohol intake, but only observed that association during the first 7 years of follow-up. Jiao et al. [35] suggested that moderately increased pancreatic cancer risk correlated with high alcohol intake, especially liquor, but residual confounding by smoking status could not be ruled out. Gapstur et al. [16] suggested that alcohol intake, especially liquor intake greater than three drinks per day, was associated with the risk of pancreatic cancer development independent of smoking status. Our study found that low-to-moderate alcohol intake had no significant effect on pancreatic cancer risk, but that high alcohol intake especially high liquor intake, was associated with an increased risk of pancreatic cancer. There are some possible explanations for this. First, long-term high alcohol intake causes chronic alcoholic pancreatitis [44], which could affect the association between high alcohol intake and the risk of pancreatic cancer. Second, acetaldehyde, the main metabolite of alcohol, has been identified as a carcinogen in several in vitro, human, and animal studies [45, 46]. Finally, carcinogenic effects could differ according to the type of alcoholic beverages, where the association of liquor intake with pancreatic cancer risk may be due to a dosage effect because a drink of liquor contains a substantially higher concentration of alcohol than a drink of beer or wine [34, 47, 48].

Subgroup analyses suggested that high alcohol intake was associated with an increased risk of pancreatic cancer in several subpopulations. However, no significant association between alcohol intake and the risk of pancreatic cancer was found in each of the corresponding subpopulations. First, our study indicated that high liquor intake was associated with an increased risk of pancreatic cancer. The reason for this could be that the higher percentage of liquor intake in North America compared to populations from other countries. Second, we noted heavy alcohol intake was associated with increased risk of pancreatic cancer in men, while no significant effect was observed in women. This may have to do with the fact that far fewer women are heavy drinkers compared to men. Third, we noted alcohol intake was associated with an increased risk of pancreatic cancer if the duration of the follow-up was greater than 10 years for the total cohort or women, but that increase was only seen in men with a follow up of less than 10 years. A possible reason for this may be that more men are heavy drinkers, and the cumulative contribution of alcohol as a carcinogen accrues more quickly. Furthermore, follow up periods greater than 10 years in men included smaller cohorts with increased variability. Fourth, diabetes mellitus, BMI, and EI influenced the association between alcohol intake and the risk of pancreatic cancer. However, we could not determine the effects of these potential confounding factors on the risk of pancreatic cancer because they were analyzed in only a few studies. Finally, stratified analyses for several subpopulations may be unreliable due to the inclusion of smaller cohorts in these subsets. Therefore, we only performed subgroup analyses when studies adjusted for these factors, providing a relative result and a comprehensive overview.

Three strengths of our study should be highlighted. First, to lower the probability of selection and recall bias, which could be of concern in retrospective case–control

Table 2 Subgroup analysis of pancreatic cancer foralcohol intake versus the lowest intake

Subgroup		Light alcohol intake	Moderate alcohol intake	Heavy alcohol intake	Total alcohol intake
Country					
Men	US	0.92 (0.69–1.21)	0.92 (0.77–1.11)	1.22 (0.95–1.56)	1.02 (0.83–1.25)
	Europe	1.09 (0.88–1.36)	0.95 (0.62–1.46)	1.21 (0.84–1.76)	1.08 (0.90–1.30)
	Other	0.64 (0.25–1.64)	1.06 (0.64–1.76)	0.89 (0.61–1.30)	0.91 (0.68–1.22)
Women	US	1.00 (0.87–1.14)	1.04 (0.79–1.35)	1.27 (0.98–1.65)	1.05 (0.94–1.16)
	Europe	0.91 (0.50–1.64)	0.93 (0.75–1.15)	1.17 (0.70–1.97)	1.00 (0.82–1.23)
	Other	0.83 (0.60–1.13)	0.88 (0.56–1.38)	1.23 (0.66–2.29)	0.89 (0.70–1.13)
Total cohort	US	0.97 (0.88–1.08)	1.00 (0.93–1.08)	1.22 (1.14–1.30)*	1.06 (0.98–1.14)
	Europe	0.99 (0.85–1.15)	0.89 (0.80–1.00)	1.08 (0.91–1.27)	0.99 (0.90–1.10)
	Other	0.81 (0.60–1.09)	0.95 (0.67–1.34)	0.97 (0.70–1.34)	0.90 (0.75–1.08)
Duration of follow-up (years)					
Men	10 or more	1.01 (0.87–1.17)	0.89 (0.67–1.19)	1.07 (0.80–1.42)	1.00 (0.83–1.20)
	<10	0.92 (0.56–1.51)	0.96 (0.79–1.17)	1.30 (1.11–1.52)*	1.06 (0.89–1.27)
Women	10 or more	0.96 (0.83–1.11)	0.93 (0.67–1.29)	1.40 (1.01–1.94)*	1.01 (0.89–1.14)
	<10	0.98 (0.82–1.18)	1.01 (0.81–1.27)	1.04 (0.93–1.16)	0.99 (0.92–1.06)
Total cohort	10 or more	0.99 (0.89–1.09)	0.99 (0.91–1.08)	1.20 (1.07–1.34)*	1.02 (0.92–1.12)
	<10	0.93 (0.81–1.06)	0.93 (0.85–1.03)	1.12 (0.99–1.26)	1.01 (0.93–1.10)
Adjusted smoking status					
Men	Yes	0.98 (0.81–1.18)	0.94 (0.80–1.11)	1.19 (1.00–1.42)	1.04 (0.90–1.19)
	No	1.02 (0.73–1.43)	0.82 (0.49–1.37)	0.99 (0.59–1.67)	0.96 (0.75–1.23)
Women	Yes	0.97 (0.87–1.09)	0.93 (0.83–1.04)	1.07 (0.96–1.19)	0.99 (0.93–1.06)
	No	-	-	-	-
Total cohort	Yes	0.96 (0.89–1.05)	0.98 (0.92–1.04)	1.16 (1.06–1.26)*	1.02 (0.95–1.08)
	No	1.02 (0.73–1.43)	0.82 (0.49–1.37)	0.99 (0.59–1.67)	0.96 (0.75–1.23)
Adjusted BMI					
Men	Yes	0.98 (0.81–1.18)	0.93 (0.79–1.10)	1.19 (0.98–1.46)	1.03 (0.88–1.20)
	No	1.02 (0.73–1.43)	0.96 (0.66–1.40)	1.01 (0.70–1.47)	1.00 (0.81–1.23)
Women	Yes	0.94 (0.83–1.06)	0.90 (0.80–1.01)	1.07 (0.96–1.19)	0.97 (0.91–1.04)
	No	1.18 (0.88–1.59)	1.42 (0.74–2.73)	1.20 (0.54–2.68)	1.25 (0.99–1.58)
Total cohort	Yes	0.96 (0.87–1.05)	0.98 (0.93–1.04)	1.17 (1.06–1.30)*	1.02 (0.95–1.09)
	No	1.00 (0.83–1.21)	1.02 (0.80–1.31)	1.00 (0.77–1.28)	1.01 (0.87–1.17)
Adjusted DM					
Men	Yes	0.93 (0.74–1.16)	0.92 (0.77–1.10)	1.15 (0.91–1.45)	0.99 (0.83–1.18)
	No	1.08 (0.85–1.37)	1.00 (0.68–1.49)	1.11 (0.83–1.53)	1.06 (0.90–1.26)
Women	Yes	0.91 (0.80–1.04)	0.93 (0.74–1.17)	1.27 (0.99–1.64)	0.97 (0.87–1.07)
	No	1.18 (0.94–1.49)	1.13 (0.78–1.65)	1.03 (0.92–1.16)	1.11 (0.91–1.34)
Total cohort	Yes	0.91 (0.83–1.01)	1.00 (0.94–1.06)	1.20 (1.12–1.28)*	0.99 (0.91–1.07)
	No	1.11 (0.95–1.30)	1.02 (0.83–1.25)	1.05 (0.94–1.17)	1.06 (0.95–1.18)
Adjusted EI					
Men	Yes	0.89 (0.72–1.10)	0.87 (0.73–1.04)	1.21 (0.96–1.52)	0.98 (0.81–1.18)
	No	1.12 (0.92–1.36)	1.10 (0.82–1.48)	1.08 (0.84–1.40)	1.10 (0.94–1.29)
Women	Yes	0.97 (0.84–1.11)	0.94 (0.75–1.18)	1.36 (1.05–1.75)*	1.02 (0.92–1.13)
	No	0.97 (0.74–1.27)	1.11 (0.77–1.60)	1.02 (0.91–1.14)	1.00 (0.87–1.15)
Total cohort	Yes	0.94 (0.84–1.04)	0.89 (0.78–1.03)	1.30 (1.14–1.47)*	1.00 (0.92–1.10)

Table 2 Subgroup analysis of pancreatic cancer foralcohol intake versus the lowest intake *(Continued)*

	No	1.00 (0.89–1.14)	0.99 (0.87–1.13)	1.09 (0.99–1.21)	1.03 (0.94–1.13)
Study quality					
Men	8 or 9	0.97 (0.82–1.14)	0.90 (0.72–1.13)	1.09 (0.87–1.37)	0.98 (0.83–1.16)
	<8	1.20 (0.72–1.99)	0.96 (0.78–1.18)	1.22 (0.94–1.58)	1.17 (1.04–1.32)*
Women	8 or 9	0.96 (0.82–1.13)	0.99 (0.71–1.39)	1.48 (1.02–2.13)	1.01 (0.89–1.15)
	<8	0.98 (0.82–1.18)	0.98 (0.80–1.20)	1.04 (0.93–1.16)	0.99 (0.92–1.06)
Total cohort	8 or 9	0.95 (0.87–1.05)	1.00 (0.94–1.06)	1.18 (1.06–1.31)*	0.99 (0.90–1.09)
	<8	1.01 (0.85–1.19)	0.95 (0.84–1.08)	1.14 (0.99–1.30)	1.04 (0.96–1.13)

*BMI body mass index, *DM* diabetes mellitus, *EI* energy intake

studies, only prospective cohort studies were included. Second, the large sample size provided a more robust quantitatively assessment of the association of alcohol intake with the risk of pancreatic cancer, than that of any individual study. Third, the dose–response analysis included a wide range of alcohol intake rates, which allowed for an accurate assessment of the relationship between alcohol intake dosage and pancreatic cancer risk.

The limitations of our study are as follows. First, the adjusted models are different between included studies, and the factors included in these models might play an important role in pancreatic cancer development. Second, in a meta-analysis of published studies, publication bias is inevitable. Third, heterogeneity among studies can be another limitation of our meta-analysis. We applied a random-effect model that considers possible heterogeneity and preformed subgroup analyses based on different alcohol categories to further explore sources of heterogeneity.

Finally, the analysis used pooled data (individual data were not available), which restricted us from performing a more detailed relevant analysis and obtaining more comprehensive results.

Conclusion

Our study suggests that high alcohol intake, especially liquor intake, might play an important role in the risk of pancreatic cancer. According to dose–response meta-analysis, alcohol intake greater than 15 g/day seems to be associated with an increased pancreatic cancer incidence. Furthermore, this is a much lower level of intake than suggested in several of cohort studies, and this comparatively lower recommendation should be investigated further. Future studies should focus on specific populations and conduct stratified analyses of potential confounding factors to obtain a more detailed analysis of the association between alcohol intake and the risk of pancreatic cancer.

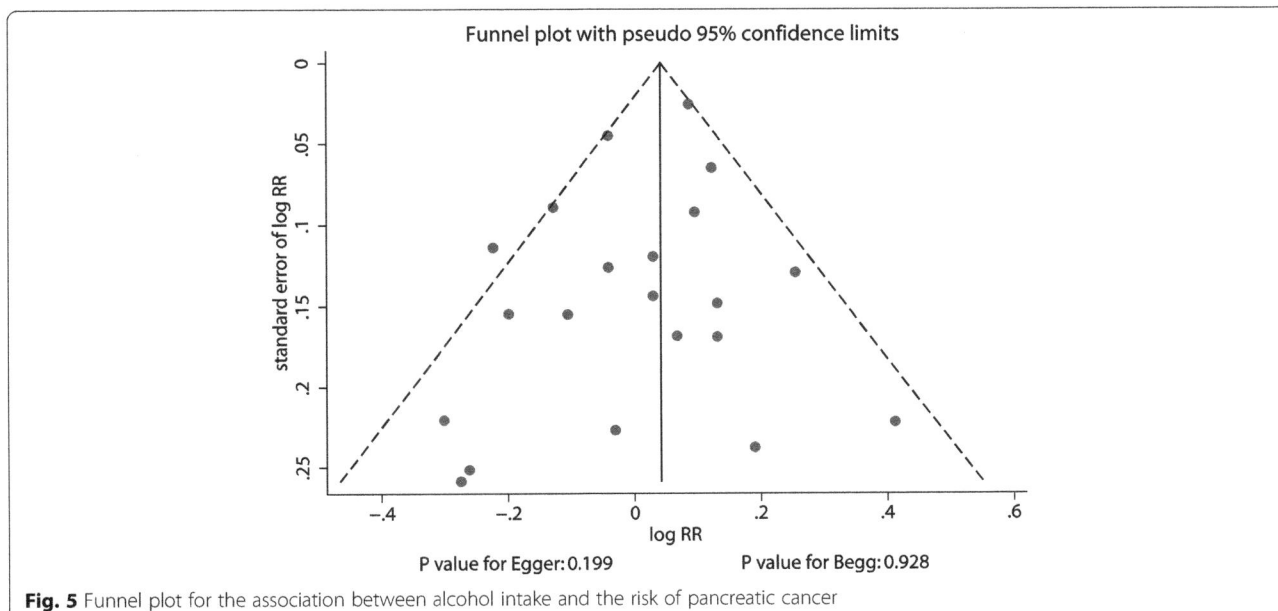

Fig. 5 Funnel plot for the association between alcohol intake and the risk of pancreatic cancer

Additional files

Additional file 1: MOOSE Checklist for Meta-analyses of Observational Studies.

Additional file 2: Figure S1. Relative risk estimates of light alcohol intake and the risk of pancreatic cancer in men, women, and total cohort.

Additional file 3: Figure S2. Relative risk estimates of moderate alcohol intake and the risk of pancreatic cancer in men, women, and total cohort.

Additional file 4: Figure S3. Relative risk estimates of alcohol intake versus the lowest alcohol intake and the risk of pancreatic cancer in men, women, and total cohort.

Additional file 5: Figure S4. Relative risk estimates of heavy alcohol intake and the risk of pancreatic cancer in men, women, and total cohort.

Additional file 6: Figure S5. Dose–response analysis for curvilinear association between alcohol intake and relative risks of pancreatic cancer in men and women.

Abbreviations
BMI: body mass index; CI: confidence interval; DM: diabetes mellitus; EI: energy intake; FHPC: family history of pancreatic cancer; HR: hazard ratio; NOS: Newcastle-Ottawa scale; PA: physical activity; RR: risk ratio.

Competing interests
The authors declare that they have no competing interests.

Authors' contributions
Designed research: W-YT, and F-HY. Conducted research: W-YT, G-YW, J-WW, X-M, and F-HY. Provided essential reagents or provided essential materials: F-HY. Analyzed data or performed statistical analysis: W-YT. Wrote paper: W-YT and F-HY. Had primary responsibility for final content: F-HY. Other: revised the paper: F-HY. All authors contributed to the planning, execution, and interpretation of the submitted manuscript and read and approved the final manuscript.

Acknowledgements
No funding was received for this work.

References

1. Ferlay J, Soerjomataram I, Ervik M, et al. GLOBOCAN 2012 v1.1, Cancer Incidence and Mortality Worldwide: IARC CancerBase No. 11 [Internet]. Lyon, France: International Agency for Research on Cancer; 2014. Available from: http://globocan.iarc.fr, accessed on 16/01/2015.
2. Everhart J, Wright D. Diabetes mellitus as a risk factor for pancreatic cancer. JAMA. 1995;273:1605–9.
3. Villeneuve PJ, Johnson KC, Hanley AJG, et al. Canadian cancer registries epidemiology research group. Alcohol, tobacco, and coffee consumption and the risk of pancreatic cancer: results from the Canadian Enhanced Surveillance System case–control project. Eur J Cancer Prev. 2000;9:49.
4. Patel AV, Rodriguez C, Bernstein L, et al. Obesity, recreational physical activity, and risk of pancreatic cancer in a large US cohort. Cancer Epidemiol Biomarkers Prev. 2005;14:459–66.
5. Pöschl G, Seitz HK. Alcohol and cancer. Alcohol Alcohol. 2004;39(3):155–65.
6. Tramacere I, Scotti L, Jenab M, et al. Alcohol drinking and pancreatic cancer risk: a meta-analysis of the dose-risk relation. Int J Cancer. 2010;126:1474–86.
7. Michaud DS, Vrieling A, Jiao L, et al. Alcohol intake and pancreatic cancer: a pooled analysis from the pancreatic cancer cohort consortium (PanScan). Cancer Causes Control. 2010;21(8):1213–25.
8. Genkinger JM, Spiegelman D, Anderson KE, et al. Alcohol intake and pancreatic cancer risk: a pooled analysis of fourteen cohort studies. Cancer Epidemiol Biomarkers Prev. 2009;18:765–76.

9. Rohrmann S, Linseisen J, Vrieling A, et al. Ethanol intake and the risk of pancreatic cancer in the European Prospective Investigation into Cancer and Nutrition (EPIC). Cancer Causes Control. 2009;20(5):785–94.
10. Lin Y, Tamakoshi A, Kawamura T, et al. Risk of pancreatic cancer in relation to alcohol drinking, coffee consumption and medical history: finding from the Japan collaborative cohort study for evaluation of cancer risk. In J Cancer. 2002;99:742–6.
11. Michaud DS, Giovannucci E, Willett WC, et al. Coffee and alcohol consumption and the risk of pancreatic cancer in two prospective United States Cohorts. Cancer Epidemiol Biomarkers Prev. 2001;10:429–37.
12. American Cancer Society. Cancer Facts and Figures. Atlanta, GA: American Cancer Society; 2009.
13. Kuzmickiene I, Everatt R, Virviciute D, et al. Smoking and other risk factors for pancreatic cancer: A cohort study in men in Lithuania. Cancer Epidemiol. 2013;37:133–9.
14. Baglietto L, Giles GG, English DR, et al. Alcohol consumption and risk of glioblastoma; evidence from the Melbourne Collaborative Cohort Study. Int J Cancer. 2011;128:1929–34.
15. Nakamura K, Nagata C, Wada K, et al. Cigarette smoking and other lifestyle factors in relation to the risk of pancreatic cancer death: a prospective cohort study in Japan. Jpn J Clin Oncol. 2011;41(2):225–31.
16. Gapstur SM, Jacobs EJ, Deka A, et al. Association of alcohol intake with pancreatic cancer mortality in never smokers. Arch Intern Med. 2011;171(5):444–51.
17. Stroup DF, Berlin JA, Morton SC, et al. Meta-analysis of observational studies in epidemiology: a proposal for reporting. Meta-analysis of observational studies in epidemiology (MOOSE) group. JAMA. 2000;283:2008–12.
18. Wells G, Shea B, O'Connell D. The Newcastle-Ottawa Scale (NOS) for assessing the quality of nonrandomised studies in meta-analyses. Ottawa (ON): Ottawa Hospital Research Institute; 2009. Available:http://www.ohri.ca/programs/clinical epidemiology/oxford.htm.
19. Higgins JP, Green S. Cochrane Handbook for Systematic Reviews of Interventions, Version 5.1.0. 2011; Available:www.cochrane-handbook.org.
20. Cooper H, Hedges LV, Valentine JC. Handbook of research synthesis and meta-analysis. Russell Sage Foundation; 2009.
21. Greenland S, Robins JM. Estimation of a common effect parameter from sparse follow-up data. Biometrics. 1985;41:55–68.
22. DerSimonian R, Laird N. Meta-analysis in clinical trials. Control Clin Trials. 1986;7:177–88.
23. Ades AE, Lu G, Higgins JP. The interpretation of random-effects metaanalysis in decision models. Med Decis Making. 2005;25:646–54.
24. Orsini N, Bellocco R, Greenland S. Generalized least squares for trend estimation of summarized dose–response data. Stata J. 2006;6:40–57.
25. Greenland S, Longnecker MP. Methods for trend estimation from summarized dose–response data, with applications to meta-analysis. Am J Epidemiol. 1992;135:1301–9.
26. Deeks JJ, Higgins JPT, Altman DG. Analyzing data and undertaking meta-analyses. In: Higgins J, Green S, editors. Cochrane Handbook for Systematic Reviews of Interventions 5.0.1. Oxford, UK: The Cochrane Collaboration; 2008. chap 9.
27. Higgins JPT, Thompson SG, Deeks JJ, Altman DG. Measuring inconsistency in meta-analyses. BMJ. 2003;327:557–60.
28. Higgins JP, Thompson SG. Quantifying heterogeneity in a meta-analysis. Stat Med. 2002;21:1539–58.
29. Tobias A. Assessing the influence of a single study in meta-analysis. Stata Tech Bull. 1999;47:15–7.
30. Egger M, Davey Smith G, Schneider M, Minder C. Bias in meta-analysis detected by a simple, graphical test. BMJ. 1997;315:629–34.
31. Begg CB, Mazumdar M. Operating characteristics of a rank correlation test for publication bias. Biometrics. 1994;50:1088–101.
32. Shibata A, Mack TM, Paganini-Hill A, et al. A prospective study of pancreatic cancer in the elderly. Int J Cancer. 1994;58:46–9.
33. Stolzenberg-Solomon RZ, Pietinen P, Barrett MJ, et al. Dietary and other methyl-group availability factors and pancreatic cancer risk in a cohort of male smokers. Am J Epidemiol. 2001;153:680–7.
34. Heinen MM, Verhage BAJ, Ambergen TAJ, et al. Alcohol consumption and risk of pancreatic cancer in the Netherlands Cohort Study. Am J Epidemiol. 2009;169:1233–42.
35. Jiao L, Silverman DT, Schairer C, et al. Alcohol use and risk of pancreatic cancer: the NIH-AARP Diet and Health Study. Am J Epidemiol. 2009;169:1043–51.

36. Harnack LJ, Anderson KE, Zheng W, et al. Smoking, alcohol, coffee, and tea intake and incidence of cancer of the exocrine pancreas: the Iowa Women's Health Study. Cancer Epidemiol Biomarkers Prev. 1997;6:1081–6.

37. Stevens RJ, Roddam AW, Spencer EA, et al. Factors associated with incident and fatal pancreatic cancer in a cohort of middle-aged women. Int J Cancer. 2009;124:2400–5.

38. Bandera EV, Freudenheim JL, Marshall JR, et al. Diet and alcohol consumption and lung cancer risk in the New York State Cohort (United States). Cancer Causes Control. 1997;8:828–40.

39. Calton BA, Stolzenberg-Solomon RZ, Moore SC, et al. A prospective study of physical activity and the risk of pancreatic cancer among women (United States). BMC Cancer. 2008;8:63.

40. Chang ET, Canchola AJ, Lee VS, et al. Wine and other alcohol consumption and risk of ovarian cancer in the California Teachers Study cohort. Cancer Causes Control. 2007;18:91–103.

41. Silvera SAN, Rohan TE, Jain M, et al. Glycemic index, glycemic load, and pancreatic cancer risk (Canada). Cancer Causes Control. 2005;16:431–6.

42. Prorok PC, Andriole GL, Bresalier RS, et al. Design of the Prostate, Lung, Colorectal and Ovarian (PLCO) cancer screening trial. Control Clin Trials. 2000;21:273S–309.

43. Larsson SC, Håkansson N, Giovannucci E, et al. Folate intake and pancreatic cancer incidence: a prospective study of Swedish women and men. J Natl Cancer Inst. 2006;98:407–13.

44. Dufour MC, Adamson MD. The epidemiology of alcohol-induced pancreatitis. Pancreas. 2003;27(4):286–90.

45. Gukovskaya AS, Mouria M, Gukovsky I, et al. Ethanol metabolism and transcription factor activation in pancreatic acinar cells in rats. Gastroenterology. 2002;122(1):106–18.

46. Pandol SJ, Periskic S, Gukovsky I, et al. Ethanol diet increases the sensitivity of rats to pancreatitis induced by cholecystokinin octapeptide. Gastroenterology. 1999;117(3):706–16.

47. Zheng W, McLaughlin JK, Gridley G, et al. A cohort study of smoking, alcohol consumption, and dietary factors for pancreatic cancer (United States). Cancer Causes Control. 1993;4(5):477–82.

48. Devos-Comby L, Lange JE. "My drink is larger than yours"? A literature review of self- defined drink sizes and standard drinks. Curr Drug Abuse Rev. 2008;1(2):162–76.

12

PET/CT incidental detection of second tumor in patients investigated for pancreatic neoplasms

Lucia Moletta[1], Sergio Bissol[2], Alberto Fantin[3], Nicola Passuello[1], Michele Valmasoni[1] and Cosimo Sperti[1*] (iD)

Abstract

Background: Positron Emission Tomography/computed tomography (PET/CT) is an imaging technique which has a role in the detection and staging malignancies (both in first diagnosis and follow-up). The finding of an unexpected region of FDG (Fluorodeoxyglucose) uptake can occur when performing whole-body FDG-PET, raising the possibility of a second primary tumor. The aim of this study was to evaluate our experience of second primary cancer incidentally discovered during PET/CT examination performed for pancreatic diseases, during the initial work-up or follow-up after surgical resection.

Methods: In this study, a retrospective evaluation of a prospectively collected data base was performed. Three hundred ninety- nine patients with pancreatic pathology were evaluated by whole body PET/CT imaging from January 2004 to December 2014. Among them, 348 patients were scanned before surgical resection and 51 during the course of their follow-up (pancreatic cancer). Median follow-up time was 29 months (range 14-124).

Results: Fifty-six patients (14%) had incidental uptake of FDG in their organs: 31 patients had focal uptake and 25 showed diffuse with or without focal uptake. All patients with focal uptake were investigated, and invasive malignancy was diagnosed in 22 patients: 14 colon, 4 lung, 1 larynx, 1 urothelial, 1 breast cancer, and 1 colon metastasis from pancreatic cancer. Twenty patients underwent resection, and 6 endoscopic removal of colonic polyps. Three patients were not operated for advanced disease, and two patients did not show any pathology (PET/CT false positive). Of the 10 patients investigated for diffuse uptake, no malignancy was found; none of these patients developed a second cancer during the follow-up.

Conclusions: As in other malignancies, unexpected FDG uptake can occur in patients having PET/CT investigation for pancreatic diseases. Focal uptake is likely to be a malignancy and deserves further investigations, although the stage and the poor prognosis of primary pancreatic cancer should be kept in mind. Some selected patients may benefit from the aggressive treatment of incidental lesions and show survival benefit.

Keywords: Incidentaloma, Pancreas, Pancreatic neoplasms, Positron emission tomography, Surveillance

Background

Positron Emission Tomography/computed tomography (PET/CT) is an imaging technique which has a role in the detection of malignancies and in cancer staging (both in first diagnosis and follow-up) [1, 2], including pancreatic neoplasms [3]. The finding of an unexpected region of FDG uptake can occur when performing whole-body FDG-PET; this raises the possibility of a second primary tumor [4]. In the past decade, incidental cancer has been detected by PET/CT in asymptomatic patients [5], patients with head neck cancer [6], oesophagogastric malignancies [7], lymphoma [8], and lung cancer [9]. Informations regarding PET/CT incidental cancer in patients with pancreatic neoplasms are still lacking. Aim of this study was to assess the frequency and significance of incidental findings reported by PET/CT scans in patients investigated for pancreatic lesions, both benign and malignant.

---
* Correspondence: csperti@libero.it
[1]Department of Surgery, Oncology and Gastroenterology, 3rd Surgical Clinic, University of Padua, Padua, Italy
Full list of author information is available at the end of the article

Methods

Patients who underwent PET/CT examination for staging or follow-up after resection of pancreatic tumors observed in our Department from January 2004 to December 2014, were identified from a prospectively collected database. The scans were reviewed and any incidental findings recorded. One person (SB) assessed all PET/CT reports. An incidental finding was defined as a significant area of FDG uptake in a site unlikely to be related to the pancreatic neoplasm. FDG uptake was described according to focal or diffuse pattern assessed by the nuclear medicine physician. Clinical, radiographic, endoscopic, surgical and pathological records, and follow-up imaging were used as evaluation of incidental PET findings. A validation of the diagnosis was based on the pathologic findings of a resected specimen, biopsy examination, or follow-up. When an extrapancreatic or focal uptake of 18-FDG was detected, an additional diagnostic work-up was performed. All suspected lesions underwent histological confirmation. 18F-FDG PET scans were performed using standard clinical protocols by a hybrid system (Biograph Sensation 16, Siemens, provided with a multislice CT and LSO crystals). A minimum fasting time of 6 h was prescribed and blood glucose levels less than 120 mg/dl before intravenous injection of a weight-based amount of 18-FDG (37 MBq/10 kg) were obtained. The CT scans were performed without oral and/or intravenous contrast medium. Cross-sections for attenuation correction of the emission images (when the PET tomograph without CT was used) were obtained with two transmission scans of the abdomen by 68 Ge/68 Ga rod sources before the administration of 18-FDG. When using the hybrid system, CT scan was done with a kCp of 120 and weight-based amperage of 120 mAs. PET scan (for both tomographs) began 90 min after the tracer's injection acquiring 2 beds (16 cm each) to cover upper abdomen area. Coronal, sagittal and transaxial sections were obtained for visual analysis. In the suspected neoplastic areas, a quantitative analysis was performed through the calculation of the maximum standardized uptake value (SUVmax, SUV = tissue tracer concentration/injected dose/body weight) which was analyzed by placing a circular region of interest (on transaxial sections) over the area of maximal focal 18-FDG uptake. We established a SUVmax cut-off of 2.5 or greater according to our previous experience. The PET scan was interpreted by a single observer (S.B.) without knowledge of the CT scan results.

Results

A total of 399 patients underwent PET/CT imaging during the study period: 348 in the initial work-up for pancreatic neoplasm, and 51 in the course of follow-up after resection for pancreatic cancer. Incidental FDG uptake was identified in 56 patients (14%): in these patients, pancreatic neoplasms included ductal adenocarcinoma (n = 32), intraductal papillary mucinous neoplasms (IPMNs, n = 21), cystic neoplasms (two mucinous tumors and 1 solid-pseudopapillary tumor). Forty-five patients underwent PET/CT at initial stage and 11 during the course of their follow-up after resection of pancreatic cancer. Thirty-one patients (55%) had focal uptake, while 25 (45%) showed diffuse with or without focal uptake. Focal uptake was observed in the colon (n = 21), lung (n = 4), rectum (n = 2), larynx (n = 1), urether (n = 1), breast (n = 1), duodenum (n = 1) (Table 1). Diffuse with or without focal uptake was observed in the colon (n = 20), rectum (n = 2), thyroid (n = 2), oesophagus

Table 1 Site of incidental findings, results of investigation, treatment and outcome of patients with PET/CT extra-pancreatic focal uptake of the radiotracer

Site	Total Number of Patients	Pathology	Number of patients	Treatment	Outcome N°	A / D (mo)
Colon	19	Adenocarcinoma	14	Colectomy	13	D
					1	A (61)
		Pancreatic cancer metastasis	1	CT	1	D (8)
		HGD	4	ER	4	D
Rectum	2	HGD	2	ER	1	D
					1	A (74)
Lung	4	Adenocarcinoma	3	Lobectomy	3	D
			1	CT	1	D (13)
Breast	1	Ductal Carcinoma	1	CT	1	D (7)
Ureter	1	Urothelial Cancer	1	Nephrectomy	1	D (21)
Duodenum	1	HGD	1	PD	1	A (72)
Larynx	1	Laryngeal Cancer	1	Laryngectomy	1	D (27)

D dead, *A* alive, *CT* chemotherapy, *ER* endoscopic resection, *PD* pancreaticoduodenectomy, *HGD* high grade dysplasia

Table 2 Site of incidental findings, results of investigation, reasons of non investigation of patients with pancreatic tumors who underwent PET/CT with diffuse uptake of the radiotracer

Site	Total Number of Patients	Investigated		Reason of Non Investigation	
		N°	Pathology	N°	Reason
Oesophagus	1	1	Oesophagitis	–	–
Stomach	1	1	Gastritis	–	–
Colon	20	5	1 Hyperplastic Polyps	8	Physiological uptake
				7	Advanced Disease
Rectum	2	1	Proctitis	–	–
Thyroid	2	2	Benign Goiter	–	–

($n = 1$), stomach ($n = 1$) (Table 2). The colon was the most common site of FDG uptake in all groups (Figs. 1, 2). All patients with focal uptake were investigated with colonoscopy ($n = 23$), contrast-enhanced CT ($n = 5$), gastroscopy ($n = 1$), mammography ($n = 1$), laryngoscopy ($n = 1$). Investigations were performed in 10 patients with diffuse uptake

(5 colonoscopy, 2 gastroscopy, 2 ultrasonography and fine-needle aspiration, 1 sigmoidoscopy).

Of the 31 patients investigated for focal FDG uptake (19 patients with primary malignant tumors and 12 benign pancreatic neoplasms), invasive malignancy was diagnosed in 22 patients: 14 colon adenocarcinoma, 4

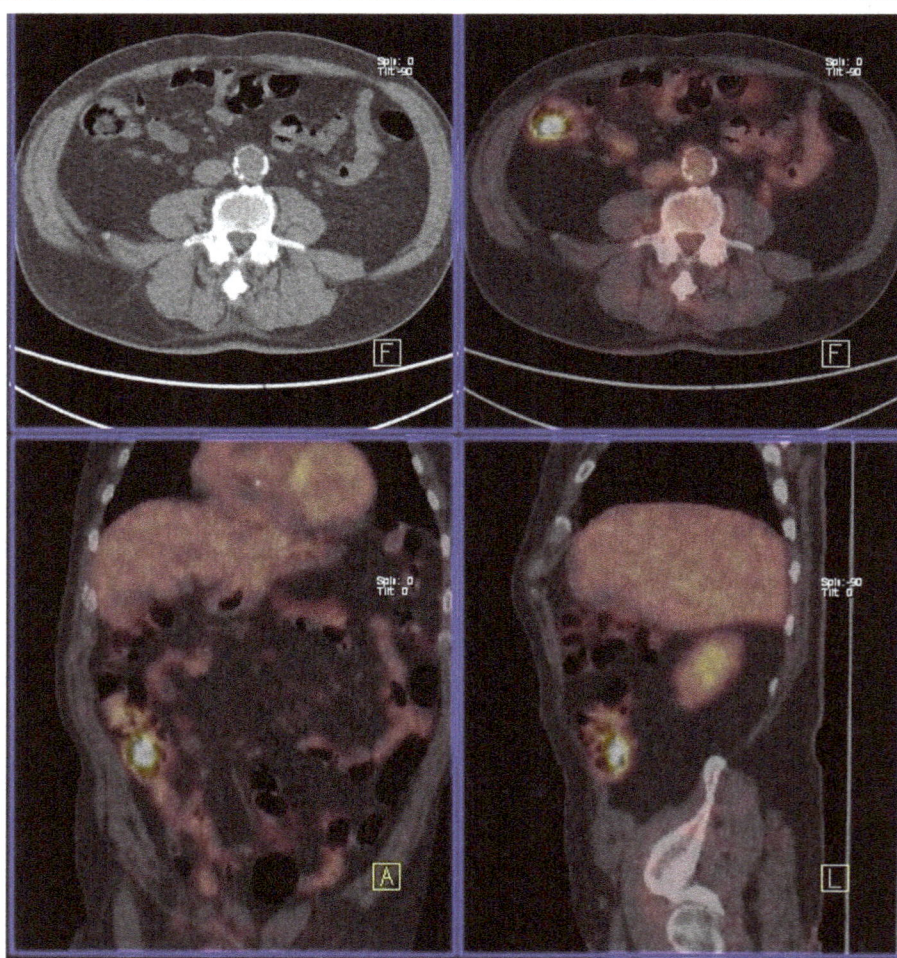

Fig. 1 PET/CT incidental detection of cancer of the ascending colon associated with branch-type IPMN of the pancreatic head (PET negative)

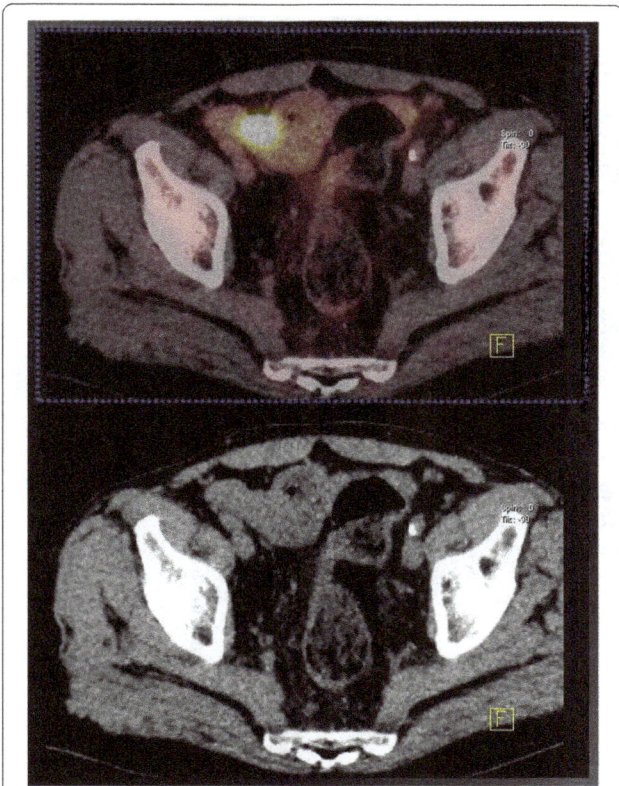

Fig. 2 PET/CT incidental detection of cancer of the sigmoid colon 39 months after pancreatico-duodenectomy for pancreatic cancer

lung adenocarcinoma (Fig. 3), 1 cancer of the larynx, 1 urothelial cancer (Fig. 4), 1 breast cancer, and 1 colon metastasis from pancreatic cancer. Among the remaining 9 patients, 7 showed colonic ($n = 6$) or duodenal ($n = 1$) polyps with high-grade dysplasia, and two patients did not show any pathology. Fourteen patients underwent colectomy, 6 endoscopic removal of colonic polyps, 3 lung lobectomy, 1 laryngectomy, 1 pancreaticoduodenectomy, and 1 nephrectomy. Five patients did not undergo surgery: three for advanced disease (1 lung cancer, 1 breast cancer, and 1 pancreatic cancer metastasis), and two for not evidence of disease (false positive). Among patients with pathological uptake of FDG during initial work-up for pancreatic cancer ($n = 7$ patients), in 5 patients detection of second tumor changed the operative management and a colectomy was associated with the pancreatic resection. The other two patients did not undergo pancreatic resection for advanced cancer. After a median follow-up of 29 months (range 14-96 months), 2 patients investigated for pancreatic cancer are alive and free of disease, 4 and 5 years after resection of lung cancer and colon cancer, respectively. The remaining patients died of progression of disease, with a median overall survival of 20 months (range 5-96 months), with 5 long survivors (survival > 60 months) .

Among the 12 patients investigated for benign pancreatic disease (9 IPMNs and 3 cystadenomas), 8 patients are alive and disease-free (median survival time 48 months) while 2 patients died for colon cancer ($n = 1$) and urothelial cancer ($n = 1$) 37 and 16 months after surgery, respectively. The remaining 2 patients died for causes unrelated to cancer.

Of the 10 patients investigated for diffuse uptake, hyperplastic colonic polyps were detected in 1 patient, proctitis in 1, gastritis in 1, oesophagitis in 1, thyroid goiter in 2, no abnormality in the remaining 4 patients (Table 2). None of these patients developed a second cancer during the entire follow-up. Quantitative analysis did not show significant difference between lesions with focal uptake (mean SUV = 6.4, range 3.0-12.5) and diffuse uptake (mean SUV 5.1, range 2.5-10.0).

A total of 51 patients underwent PET/CT during the follow-up after resection of pancreatic cancer. Eleven patients showed extrapancreatic focal uptake of FDG and 9 had resection of confirmed second cancer; one patient is alive 61 months after operation, while 8 patients died for recurrent pancreatic or colon cancer with a median survival time of 41 months (range 13-118 months). The remaining two patients did not have evidence of disease (colon) and are still alive and well after 1 and 3 years, respectively (Table 3).

Discussion

FDG-PET offers the unique opportunity to provide not only whole-body images, but also metabolic or functional informations regarding the tumor tissue. Moreover, the widespread availability of this imaging technique led to increasing number of incidental findings: this necessarily suggest further investigations in order to exclude malignancies. As previously reported by other studies dealing with PET/CT in different malignancies, we have observed an increasing number of extrapancreatic FDG uptake in patients with pancreatic neoplasms. So, we evaluated our experience of incidental findings of PET/CT performed for patients with neoplasms of the pancreas: to our knowledge this is the first study dedicated to this specific topic. An incidental finding was detected in 14% of the patients in our study, and it was further investigated in 72% of cases (all with focal and 10 out of 25 patients with diffuse uptake). Second malignant or premalignant lesions were confirmed in all but one patient who showed PET/CT with focal uptake: the remaining patient with a focal FDG uptake had a colonic metastasis from pancreatic cancer confirmed by pathologic examination. The number of incidental findings in our study appears higher than that reported by other authors [10, 11] but much greater incidence (more than 20%) has been reported for other types of primary neoplasms [9, 12].

Most of our PET/CT incidental findings were localized in the large bowel, in according with previous studies

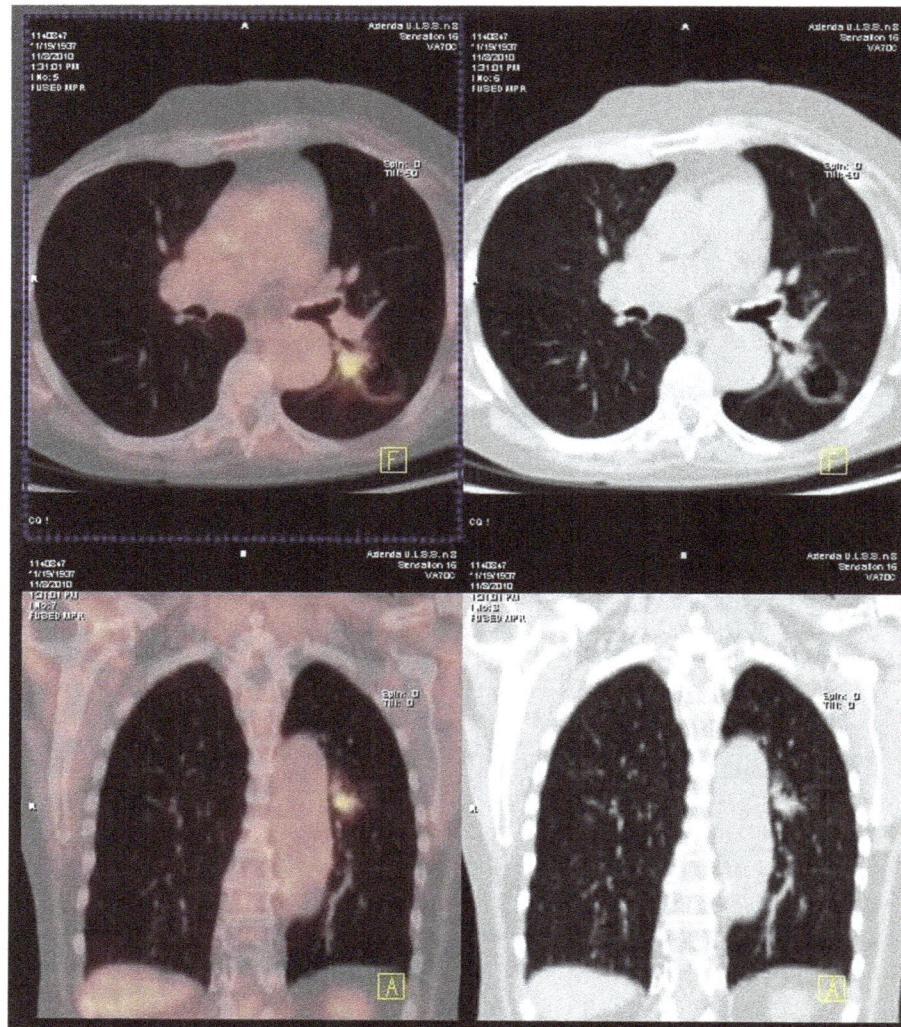

Fig. 3 PET/CT incidental detection of left pulmonary adenocarcinoma 31 months after distal pancreatectomy for pancreatic cancer

including patients with different primary tumors [13–15]. In our study a malignant or premalignant lesion was detected in 74% of patients who underwent endoscopy. A confirmed pathologic lesion was obtained in all but two patients with focal FDG uptake, while none of the patients investigated for diffuse FDG uptake showed unexpected tumors. This finding outlines the concept that when a focal uptake of FDG is detected, a high suspicion of malignancy is suggested, and further investigations are necessary [16–18]. One could argue that detection of a second tumor in patients with such an aggressive disease as pancreatic cancer does not modify the poor prognosis, and it is without a clinical significance. However, in our experience, some patients who underwent resection of a second neoplasm incidentally detected by PET/CT, showed prolonged survival: this is particularly true for

lesions incidentally detected in the follow-up of patients without recurrence after resection of pancreatic cancer. So, as we previously reported [19], PET/CT is useful not only for the staging of pancreatic malignancy, but also for the postoperative surveillance of resected pancreatic cancer. Moreover, it has been reported that IPMNs are at risk of association with extra-pancreatic malignancies [20, 21], but contrasting results are also suggested [22, 23]. In our study, 21 patients with benign IPMNs showed extra-pancreatic PET/CT incidental findings: in 11 patients a focal uptake of the radiotracer was evident, and a second malignancy was resected in 9.

In our Center, after an initial period when PET/CT was performed (whenever possible) in almost all patients with pancreatic cancer, we now perform it to stage resectable cancer and, when indicated, during the follow-

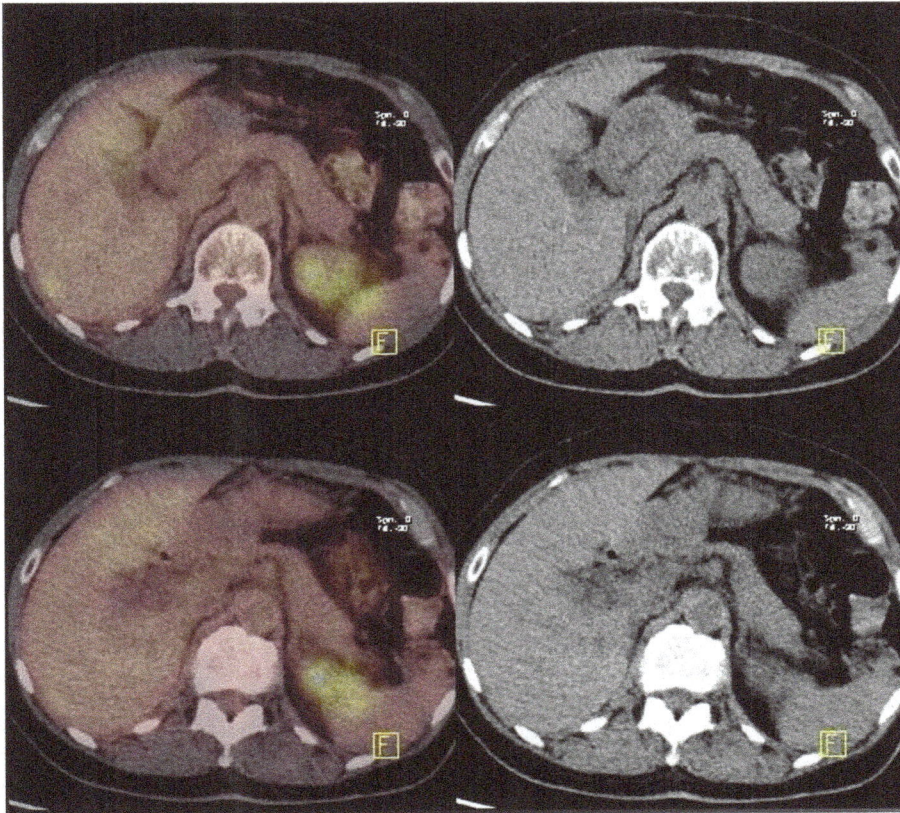

Fig. 4 PET/CT incidental detection of left ureteral cancer associated with IPMN (adenoma) of the pancreatic tail (PET negative)

up of resected patients. Moreover, we think that PET/CT can be an useful tool also during follow-up of selected patients with IPMNs. On the contrary, we have observed that PET/CT is unlikely to modify the management of patients with metastatic pancreatic cancer.

Conclusions

As in other tumors, our study reveals that unexpected FDG uptake is frequent in patients having PET/CT investigation for pancreatic neoplasms. Focal uptake is likely to be a malignancy and deserves accurate examination, although the stage and the poor prognosis of primary cancer should be kept in mind. Some selected patients (with benign IPMN, or in follow-up after resection of pancreatic cancer) may benefit from the aggressive treatment of incidental lesions and show survival benefit.

Abbreviations

18F-FDG: 18F-Fluorodeoxyglucose; A: Alive; CT: Chemotherapy; D: Dead; ER: Endoscopic resection; FP: False positive; HGD: High grade dysplasia; IPMN: Intraductal papillary mucinous neoplasms; PD: Pancreaticoduodenectomy; PET/CT: Positron emission tomography/computed tomography; SUV: Standardized uptake value

Authors' contributions

LM and CS conceived the study and drafted the manuscript; LM, AF, MV and NP collected and analyzed the data; SB made PET/CT interpretation. All authors read and approved the final manuscript.
University of Padua, Italy). All study participants provided informed written consent prior to study enrollment.

Table 3 Site of incidental findings, results of investigation of patients who underwent PET/CT with focal uptake of the radiotracer during the follow-up after resection of pancreatic tumors

Site	Total Number of Patients	Investigated	
		N°	Pathology
Lung	2	2	Cancer
Larynx	1	1	Cancer
Colon	7	7	5 Cancer + 2 FP[a]
Rectum	1	1	HGD polyp

FP false positive, HGD high grade dysplasia
[a] two patients with colonic focal uptake were investigated with colonoscopy and CT scan, which resulted negative for pathology in both cases

Competing interests

The Authors declare that they have no competing interests.

Author details

[1]Department of Surgery, Oncology and Gastroenterology, 3rd Surgical Clinic, University of Padua, Padua, Italy. [2]Department of Nuclear Medicine, Castelfranco Veneto General Hospital, Castelfranco Veneto, Treviso, Italy. [3]Gastroenterology Unit, University of Padua, Padua, Italy.

References

1. Hustinx R, Benard F, Alavi A. Whole-body FDG-PET imaging in the management of patients with cancer. Semin Nucl Med. 2002;32:35–46.
2. Pham KH, Ramawamy MR, Hawkins RA. Advances in positron emission tomography imaging in the GI tract. Gastrointest Endosc. 2002;55(Suppl 7): 553–63.
3. Van Hertum RI, Fawvaz RA. The role of nuclear medicine in the evaluation of pancreatic disease. Surg Clin North Am. 2001;8:345–58.
4. Sone Y, Sobajima A, Kawachi T, Kohara S, Kato K, Naganawa S. Ability of 18-fluorodeoxyglucose positron emission tomography/CT to detect incidental cancer. Bt. J Radiol. 2014;87:20140030.
5. Minamimoto R, Senda M, Jinnouchi S, Terauchi T, Yoshida T, Murano T, Fukuda H, Iinuma T, Uno K, Nishizawa S, Tsukamoto E, Iwata H, Inoue T, Oguchi K, Nakashima R, Inoue T. The current status of an FDG-PET cancer screening program in Japan, based on a 4-year (2006-2009), nationwide survey. Ann Nucl Med. 2013;27:46–57.
6. Haerle SK, Strobel K, Hany TF, Sidler D, Stoeckli SJ. 18-FDG-PET/CT versus panendoscopy for the detection of synchronous second primary tumors in patients with head and neck squarrous cell carcinoma. Head Neck. 2010;32: 319–25.
7. Adams HL, Janunoo SS. Clinical significance of incidental findings on staging positron emission tomography for oesophago-gastric malignancies. Ann R Coll Surg Engl. 2014;96:207–10.
8. Sato K, Ozaki K, Fujiwara S, Oh I, Matsuyama T, Ohmine K, Suzuki T, Mori M, Nagai T, Muroi K, Ozawa K. Incidental carcinomas detected by PET/CT scans in patients with malignant lymphoma. Int J Hematol. 2010;92:647–50.
9. Chopra A, Ford A, de Noronha R, Matthews S. Incidental findings on positron emission tomography/CT scans performed in the investigation of lung cancer. Br J Radiol. 2012;85:e229–37.
10. Ishimori T, Patel PV, Wahl RL. Detection of unexpected additional primary malignancies with PET/CT. J Nucl Med. 2005;46:752.757.
11. Israel O, Yefremov N, Bar-Shalom R, Kagana O, Frenkel A, Zet K, Fischer D. PET/CT detection of unexpected gastrointestinal foci of 18-FDG uptake: incidence, localization patterns and clinical significance. J Nucl Med. 2005; 46:758–62.
12. Vella-Bocaud J, Papathanassiou D, Bouche O, Prevost A, Lestra T, Dury S, Vallerand H, Perotin JM, Launois C, Eoissiere L, Brasseur M, Lebargy F, Deslee G. Incidental gastrointestinal 18F-Fluorodeoxyglucose uptake associated with lung cancer. BMC Pulm Med. 2015;15:152.
13. Andia GS, Soriano AP, Ortega Candil A, Cabrera Martin MN, Gonzalez Roiz JJ, Ortiz Zapata JJ, Cardona Arbonies J, Lapena Gutierrez L, Carreras Delgado JL. Clinical relevance of incidental finding of focal uptakes in the colon during 18-FDG PET/CT studies in oncologic patients without known colorectal carcinoma and evaluation of the impact on management. Rev Esp Med Nucl. 2012;31:15–21.
14. Goldin E, Mahamid M, Koslowsky B, Shteingart S, Dubner Y, Lalazar G, Wengrover D. Unexpected FDG-PET uptake in the gastrointestinal tract:

endoscopic and histopathological correlations. World J Gastroenterol. 2014; 20:4377–81.
15. Peng J, He Y, Xu J, Sheng J, Cai S, Zhang Z. Detection of incidental colorectal tumours with 18F-labelled 2-fluoro-2-deoxyglucose positron emission tomography/computed tomography scans: results of a prospective study. Color Dis. 2011;13:e374–8.
16. Tatidi R, Jadvar H, Bading JR, Conti PS. Incidental colonic fluorodeoxyglucose uptake : correlation with colonoscopic and histopathologic findings. Radiology. 2002;224:783–7.
17. Treglia G, Calcagni ML, Rufini V, Leccisotti L, Meduri GM, Spitilli MG, Dambra DP, De Gaetano AM, Giordano A. Clinical significance of incidental focal colorectal 18F-fluorodeoxyglucose uptake: our experience and a review of the literature. Color Dis. 2011;14:174–80.
18. Kunawudhi A, Wong AK, Alkasab TK, Mahmood U. Accuracy of FDG-PET/CT for detection of incidental premalignant and malignant colonic lesions-correlations with colonoscopic and histopathologic findings. Asian Pac J Cancer Prev. 2016;17:4143–7.
19. Sperti C, Pasquali C, Bissoli S, Chierichetti F, Liessi G, Pedrazzoli S. Tumor relapse after pancreatic cancer resection is detected earlier by 18-FDG PET than by CT. J Gastrointest Surg. 2010;14:131–40.
20. Reid-Lombardo KM, Mathis KL, Wood CM, Harmsen WS, Sarr MG. Frequency of extrapancreatic neoplasms in intraductal papillary mucinous neoplasms of the pancreas: implications for management. Ann Surg. 2010;251:64–9.
21. Larghi A, Panic N, Capurso G, Leoncini E, Arzani D, Salvia R, Del Chiaro M, Frulloni L, Arcidiacono PG, Zerbi A, Manta R, Fabbri C, Ventrucci M, Tarantino I, Piciucchi M, Carnuccio A, Boggi U, Costamagna G, Delle Fave G, Pezzili R, Bassi C, Bulajic M, Ricciardi W, Boccia S. Prevalence and risk factors of extrapancreatic malignancies in a large cohort of patients with intraductal papillary mucinous neoplasm (IPMN) of the pancreas. Ann Oncol. 2013;24:1907–11.
22. Kawakubo K, Tada M, Isayama H, Sasahira N, Nakai Y, Yamamoto K, Kogure H, Sasaki T, Hirano K, Ijichi H, Tateishi K, Yoshida H, Koike K. Incidence of extrapancreatic malignancies in patients with intraductal papillary mucinous neoplasms of the pancreas. Gut. 2011;60:1249–53.
23. Malleo G, Marchegiani G, Borin A, Capelli P, Accordini F, Butturini G, Pederzoli P, Bassi C, Salvia R. Observational study of the incidence of pancreatic and extraèpancreatic malignancies during surveillance of patients with branch-duct intraductal papillary mucinous neoplasm. Ann Surg. 2015;281:984–90.

13

Single-cell mRNA profiling reveals transcriptional heterogeneity among pancreatic circulating tumour cells

Morten Lapin[1,2,3]* [iD], Kjersti Tjensvoll[1,2], Satu Oltedal[1,2], Milind Javle[4], Rune Smaaland[1,2], Bjørnar Gilje[1,2] and Oddmund Nordgård[1,2]

Abstract

Background: Single-cell mRNA profiling of circulating tumour cells may contribute to a better understanding of the biology of these cells and their role in the metastatic process. In addition, such analyses may reveal new knowledge about the mechanisms underlying chemotherapy resistance and tumour progression in patients with cancer.

Methods: Single circulating tumour cells were isolated from patients with locally advanced or metastatic pancreatic cancer with immuno-magnetic depletion and immuno-fluorescence microscopy. mRNA expression was analysed with single-cell multiplex RT-qPCR. Hierarchical clustering and principal component analysis were performed to identify expression patterns.

Results: Circulating tumour cells were detected in 33 of 56 (59%) examined blood samples. Single-cell mRNA profiling of intact isolated circulating tumour cells revealed both epithelial-like and mesenchymal-like subpopulations, which were distinct from leucocytes. The profiled circulating tumour cells also expressed elevated levels of stem cell markers, and the extracellular matrix protein, SPARC. The expression of SPARC might correspond to an epithelial-mesenchymal transition in pancreatic circulating tumour cells.

Conclusion: The analysis of single pancreatic circulating tumour cells identified distinct subpopulations and revealed elevated expression of transcripts relevant to the dissemination of circulating tumour cells to distant organ sites.

Keywords: Circulating tumour cell, CTC, Single-cell isolation, mRNA, RT-qPCR, Pancreatic cancer

Background

Pancreatic cancer is one of few cancer types for which survival has not substantially changed over the last few decades. In Norway, the 5-year survival remains a meagre 7% [1], despite improvements in median survival demonstrated recently with novel multidrug treatments [2–4]. The poor survival associated with pancreatic cancer can be explained by the late clinical presentation, the aggressive disease trajectory, and the generally poor response to chemotherapy [5]. In addition, tumour biopsies are often inadequate for molecular testing, and there are few validated blood-based diagnostic or predictive biomarkers. Thus, there is a need for new biological markers that can improve diagnostics by identifying localized disease and that can predict tumour progression and resistance to systemic therapy. Circulating tumour cells (CTCs) have potential as a biomarker, because they represent a "snapshot" of the total tumour burden, and they provide information about the tumour of origin. Additionally, because they are associated with the migration of cancer to distant sites, they may also indicate the underlying biology of the metastatic process.

To date, the small number of studies on the clinical relevance of CTCs in pancreatic cancer have produced ambiguous results (reviewed in [6, 7]). In addition, they have been limited to analysing CTCs with only one or a few markers, which is insufficient to elucidate the complexity

* Correspondence: morten.lapin@sus.no
[1]Department of Haematology and Oncology, Stavanger University Hospital, N–4068 Stavanger, Norway
[2]Laboratory for Molecular Biology, Stavanger University Hospital, N–4068 Stavanger, Norway
Full list of author information is available at the end of the article

of CTC involvement in the metastatic process. Investigations into the mutational landscape of primary pancreatic carcinomas and metastases have shown that specific mutations are only present in a small subset of tumour cells, and that the mutational profile of metastases may be different from that of the primary tumour. Thus, heterogeneity exists among tumour cells and among tumour sites [8, 9]. Some of these cell subsets may also be clinically relevant, because they may harbour specific mutations associated with therapy resistance and disease progression. The heterogeneity among tumour cells is further expected to be apparent at both the transcriptional and translational levels. Thus, because the CTC population is a "snapshot" of the total tumour burden, its characterization in analyses at the single-cell level could provide valuable information. The CTC population is also affected by the epithelial-mesenchymal transition (EMT); a process which changes the phenotype and migratory properties of CTCs. Moreover, it has been suggested that the EMT is involved in the dissemination process [10]. Thus, single-cell analyses might reveal CTCs with different transcriptional and mutational profiles, and a characterization of these subtypes could identify CTC phenotypes that are involved in dissemination to distant organ sites. In a previous study, heterogeneous expression of RNA transcripts was demonstrated in CTCs with single-cell mRNA profiling in samples from a small cohort of patients with pancreatic cancer [11]. To our knowledge, no other study has described transcriptional heterogeneity among single pancreatic CTCs and its potential clinical relevance.

To characterize pancreatic CTCs molecularly at a single-cell level, we applied a multi-marker negative depletion strategy, known as MINDEC [12], to peripheral blood samples from patients with locally advanced or metastatic pancreatic cancer. With single-cell multiplex mRNA profiling, we demonstrated that CTCs from patients with pancreatic cancer comprised distinct, epithelial-like and mesenchymal-like subpopulations. In addition, the CTC population showed enriched expression of cancer stem cell (CSC) markers and the extracellular matrix (ECM) protein, *SPARC*.

Methods

Patient samples

Between March 2015 and January 2017, we included 21 patients with locally advanced (n = 2) or metastatic (n = 19) pancreatic cancer treated with chemotherapy (nab-paclitaxel plus gemcitabine or FOLFIRINOX) at Stavanger University Hospital. Peripheral venous blood samples were drawn at multiple time points, before (n = 8) and after (n = 48) the start of chemotherapy in 9-mL EDTA tubes, and processed within 2 h. The treatment response was defined with standard disease evaluations of images, based on the RECIST 1.1 criteria [13].

All patients and healthy controls provided written informed consent to participate in the study. The project was approved by the Regional Committee for Medical and Health Research Ethics (REK-Vest 2011/475).

Cell line cultivation and spiking

Human pancreatic cancer cell lines, ASPC-1 and PANC1, and the human mesothelioma cell line, SDM103T2, (all from ECACC) were cultured according to manufacturer recommendations, except that the culture media was supplemented with 100 units/mL penicillin and 0.5 mg/mL streptomycin (Penicillin-streptomycin, Sigma-Aldrich). Cells were harvested by adding 0.25% trypsin/EDTA (Sigma-Aldrich) for 3–5 min at 37 °C. For spiking experiments, 1000 cells were spiked into 9 mL of blood from a healthy volunteer.

CTC enrichment

All blood samples were processed with density gradient centrifugation using Lymphoprep™ density gradient medium (Axis Shield, Norway), according to manufacturer instructions. After centrifugation, mononuclear cells were resuspended in 1 mL isolation buffer (PBS supplemented with 2 mM EDTA and 0.1% BSA) and layered on top of 3 mL foetal bovine serum to remove residual platelets. Subsequently, the samples were centrifuged at 200×g for 15 min at room temperature, and platelets were removed with the supernatant. The samples were then resuspended in 100 µL isolation buffer and processed with the MINDEC strategy [12]. Briefly, each sample was labelled with biotinylated antibodies directed at CD45, CD16, CD19, CD163, and CD235a/GYPA. Then, streptavidin-coated super-paramagnetic beads (Depletion MyOne™ SA Dynabeads®, Life Technologies AS, Norway) were added, and magnetic force was applied to remove bead-bound leucocytes and any remaining erythrocytes. Unbound cells in the supernatant were collected for subsequent analyses.

Immuno-fluorescence labelling

Enriched cells were resuspended in 100 µL cold staining buffer (PBS supplemented with 2 mM EDTA and 0.5% BSA), with 25 µL FcR blocking reagent (Miltenyi Biotech), 2 µL Hoechst 33,342 (Molecular Probes), and 2 µL of each of the labelled antibodies EpCAM-FITC (clone HEA-125, Miltenyi Biotech), MCAM-FITC (clone OJ79c, AbD Serotec®), and CD45-DyLight550 (clone T29/33, Leinco Technologies, Inc.). Then, cells were incubated in darkness for 20 min at room temperature. Stained samples were washed with staining buffer, and subsequently resuspended in 150 µL cold staining buffer.

Single cell isolation

The stained cell suspensions were transferred to a microscope slide coated with Silanization Solution I (Sigma) and imaged with an Olympus XI 81 inverted microscope (20× magnification, Olympus LUCPLFLN 20×). Exposure times were fixed at 86 ms for Hoechst 33,342, 1400 ms for EpCAM-MCAM, and 1600 ms for CD45. Each sample was manually inspected to identify tumour cell-line cells or possible CTCs. Cells with a visible nucleus, no beads attached, expression of EpCAM-MCAM, no expression of CD45, and with a round or ovoid shape were classified as cell-line cells or CTCs (Fig. 1) and subjected to single cell isolation. A threshold for EpCAM-MCAM positivity had been established previously by processing blood samples from healthy volunteers [12]. The selected cells were transferred into 8.9 µL lysis buffer (9 parts Lysis Enhancer and 1 part Lysis Solution, Invitrogen) on a hydrophobic microscope slide with a MMI CellEctor cell manipulator (Molecular Machines & Industries). Then, cells were transferred into PCR tubes by manual pipetting, and subsequently they were frozen at −80 °C until further analysis. Possible CTC clusters (≥2 CTCs) were also isolated and analysed as a single entity.

Single-cell RT-qPCR

Reverse transcription and pre-amplification were performed with the CellsDirect™ One–Step qRT–PCR Kit (Invitrogen, Carlsbad, CA). Briefly, isolated single cells stored in lysis buffer were thawed on ice and lysed by incubation at 75 °C for 15 min. Subsequently, to each lysed cell, we added 5 µL DNAse I, Amplification Grade (1 U/µL) and 1.6 µL 10× DNase I buffer (both Invitrogen). The reactions were incubated at room temperature for 5 min. Next, 4 µL of 25 mM EDTA (Invitrogen) was added to each reaction, and the mixture was incubated at 70 °C for 10 min. Next, we added 1 µL SuperScript® III RT/Platinum® Taq Mix, 25 µL 2× Reaction mix (both Invitrogen), and 4.5 µL of 13 pooled 20× TaqMan assays (Applied Biosystems) at a 1:40 dilution. Single-cell mRNA was then reverse-transcribed to cDNA (50 °C for 15 min, 95 °C for 2 min), pre-amplified for 14 cycles (each cycle: 95 °C for 15 s, 60 °C for 4 min), and subsequently, diluted 1:5 in TE buffer.

Quantitative PCR was performed by mixing 2 µL of diluted pre-amplified cDNA with 9.25 µL nuclease-free H_2O, 12.5 µL TaqMan Gene Expression Master Mix, and 1.25 µL 20× TaqMan assay. The thermocycling protocol started at 95 °C for 10 min, and then ran 40 cycles of: 95 °C for 30 s and 60 °C for 1 min. All samples were run in duplicate.

The mRNA panel consisted of 13 markers (Table 1), including sequences for: epithelial (KRT8, KRT19, EPCAM, E-Cadherin) and mesenchymal/EMT (vimentin, N-Cadherin, ZEB1) markers to differentiate epithelial CTCs from CTCs that had undergone EMT; CSC markers (CD24, CD44, ALDH1A1), which were previously shown to be expressed on pancreatic tumour cells with increased metastatic potential (Ishizawa et al., 2010; Li et al., 2007; Rasheed et al., 2010); the ECM marker, SPARC, which was demonstrated to be highly expressed in pancreatic cancer CTCs, and when knocked down in mice, it suppressed cell migration and invasiveness Ting et al. [11]; a reference marker (HPRT1); and a leucocyte marker (CD45). Cells without detectable levels of either vimentin or SPARC mRNA, which were expected to be expressed in all cells, were considered to have poor quality RNA, inadequate for complete mRNA profiling.

Statistical analysis

The statistical analyses were performed with R version 3.3.0. All reported Cq-values were expressed as the mean ± standard deviation. The reported p-values were calculated with the unpaired t-test, unless otherwise stated. p-values less than 0.05 were considered statistically significant.

Missing data points were replaced with the highest Cq-value observed for a particular gene expression assay,

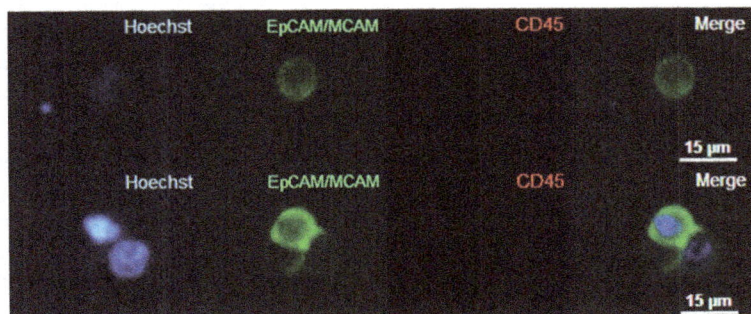

Fig. 1 Thumbnail gallery of analysed CTCs. Representative fluorescence images of a CTC (*top row*) and a CTC cluster (*bottom row*) isolated from the peripheral blood of a patient with pancreatic cancer. (*Left column*) Hoechst stain (blue) identifies nuclei; (*second column*) EpCAM-MCAM (*green*) identifies membranes of CTCs; (*third column*) CD45 (*red*) identifies leucocytes; (*right column*) superimposed images confirms intact cells. Images were acquired with 20× magnification. To enhance visibility, we adjusted the brightness and contrast equally for all microscopic images, and these adjustments were applied to the entire image

Table 1 mRNA panel used to analyse cell mRNA transcripts

Gene Symbol	Gene Name	ENSEMBL Gene ID	Amplicon length	Assay number
Epithelial transcripts				
KRT8	Keratin 8	ENSG00000170421	164	Hs01595539_g1
KRT19	Keratin 19	ENSG00000171345	96	AI70M8O (Custom assay)
EPCAM	Epithelial cell adhesion molecule	ENSG00000119888	64	Hs00158980_m1
CDH1	Cadherin 1; type 1, E-cadherin	ENSG00000039068	65	Hs01013953_m1
EMT-associated transcripts				
VIM	Vimentin	ENSG00000026025	73	Hs00185584_m1
CDH2	Cadherin 2; type 1, N-cadherin	ENSG00000170558	66	Hs00983056_m1
ZEB1	Zinc finger E-box binding homeobox 1	ENSG00000148516	63	Hs00232783_m1
Cancer stem cell transcripts				
CD24	CD24 molecule	ENSG00000272398	140	Hs02379687_s1
CD44	CD44 molecule	ENSG00000026508	70	Hs01075861_m1
ALDH1A1	Aldehyde dehydrogenase 1; family member A1	ENSG00000165092	61	Hs00946916_m1
Pancreas cancer-associated transcript				
SPARC	Secreted protein, acidic, cysteine-rich (osteonectin)	ENSG00000113140	76	Hs00234160_m1
Reference transcript				
HPRT1	Hypoxanthine phosphoribosyltransferase 1	ENSG00000165704	82	Hs02800695_m1
Leucocyte transcript				
PTPRC	Protein tyrosine phosphatase, receptor type C (CD45)	ENSG00000081237	57	Hs04189704_m1

plus a value of 1. This approach was designed to provide balanced weighting to negative observations, and it also took into account differences in PCR efficiency among the gene expression assays. All gene expression data were also mean-centred and z-score transformed by dividing the mean-centred expression by the standard deviation; this approach provided all measured mRNAs with equal weighting in the statistical analyses. Normalization by reference marker was not performed, due to the stochastic expression of mRNAs in single cells [14, 15].

To explore associations between cell groups, we performed unsupervised hierarchical clustering and principal component analysis (PCA). Unsupervised hierarchical clustering (*Hclust* function in heatmap.2) and heatmap visualization were performed with the *heatmap.2* function supplied with the Gplots package in R. The unsupervised hierarchical clustering was performed with agglomerative hierarchical clustering with average (UPGMA) linkage and a distance metric equal to 1 minus the Pearson correlation. The PCA was performed with the *princomp* function in R. Figures from the PCA were constructed with the first three components, because components 1 and 2 only explained 63% of the variance.

Correlation matrix plots of correlations between the different mRNAs measured were constructed with the *corrplot* function supplied with the Corrplot package in R; it used the *cor* function to compute correlations. The correlation matrix was computed separately for CTCs, epithelial pancreatic cancer cell lines, ASPC-1 and PANC1, and the mesenchymal cell line SDM103T2, with Spearman rank correlations. Associated *p*-values were computed with the *cor.mtest* function in R. The Bonferroni correction of *p*-values was performed to adjust for multiple testing in the rank correlation matrix.

Results

Isolation and characterization of pancreatic CTCs

CTCs were detected in 33/56 (59%) peripheral blood samples from 21 patients treated for locally advanced or metastatic pancreatic cancer. Based on immunofluorescence staining, we selected 48 morphologically intact CTCs and 3 morphologically intact CTC clusters (containing ≤3 CTCs) by micromanipulation. Of these, 30/51 (59%) had sufficient RNA quality for mRNA analysis; the remaining 21/51 (41%) cells and CTC clusters had degraded RNA, despite appearing morphologically intact. In total, 18/30 (60%) cells were identified as CTCs, based on expression of epithelial and/or mesenchymal markers. For comparison, we also isolated 12 leucocytes from a healthy volunteer, and 16 single cells from each of the cell lines, PANC1, ASPC-1, and SDM103T2—all of which had been spiked into healthy blood and subjected to CTC enrichment prior to isolation.

The isolated single cells were subjected to mRNA profiling with a multi-marker mRNA panel (Table 1) designed to capture inherent heterogeneity in pancreatic CTCs. The panel consisted of sequences that identified specific epithelial markers (*KRT8*, *KRT19*, *EPCAM*, E-Cadherin); mesenchymal/EMT markers (Vimentin, N-Cadherin, *ZEB1*); CSC markers (*CD24*, *CD44*, and *ALDH1A1*); an ECM marker (*SPARC*), a reference marker (*HPRT1*), and a leucocyte marker (*CD45*).

Cluster analysis defines pancreatic CTCs in epithelial-like and mesenchymal-like subgroups The mRNA data (Additional file 1) from all single cells were z-score adjusted and analysed with unsupervised hierarchical clustering to visualize similarities and dissimilarities (Fig. 2a). Unlike the cell-line cells, which expressed most markers in the mRNA panel at high levels, each of the CTCs expressed few markers, and generally, at lower levels than observed with cell-line cells. Based on mRNA expression patterns, the CTCs could be divided into two groups: one epithelial-like CTC cluster (CTC-E) and one mesenchymal-like CTC cluster (CTC-M). These clusters were distinct from leucocytes and cancer cell-line cells, though more closely related to the former than to the latter. From two of the patient samples, we isolated more than one CTC with sufficient mRNA quality. Two CTCs were isolated from sample PC22B3, one in each CTC group. Five CTCs were isolated from sample PC35B1, all in the CTC-E group.

The leucocytes analysed formed a separate cluster, and most of the isolated cell-line cells analysed formed separate clusters. A few cells from each cancer cell line were

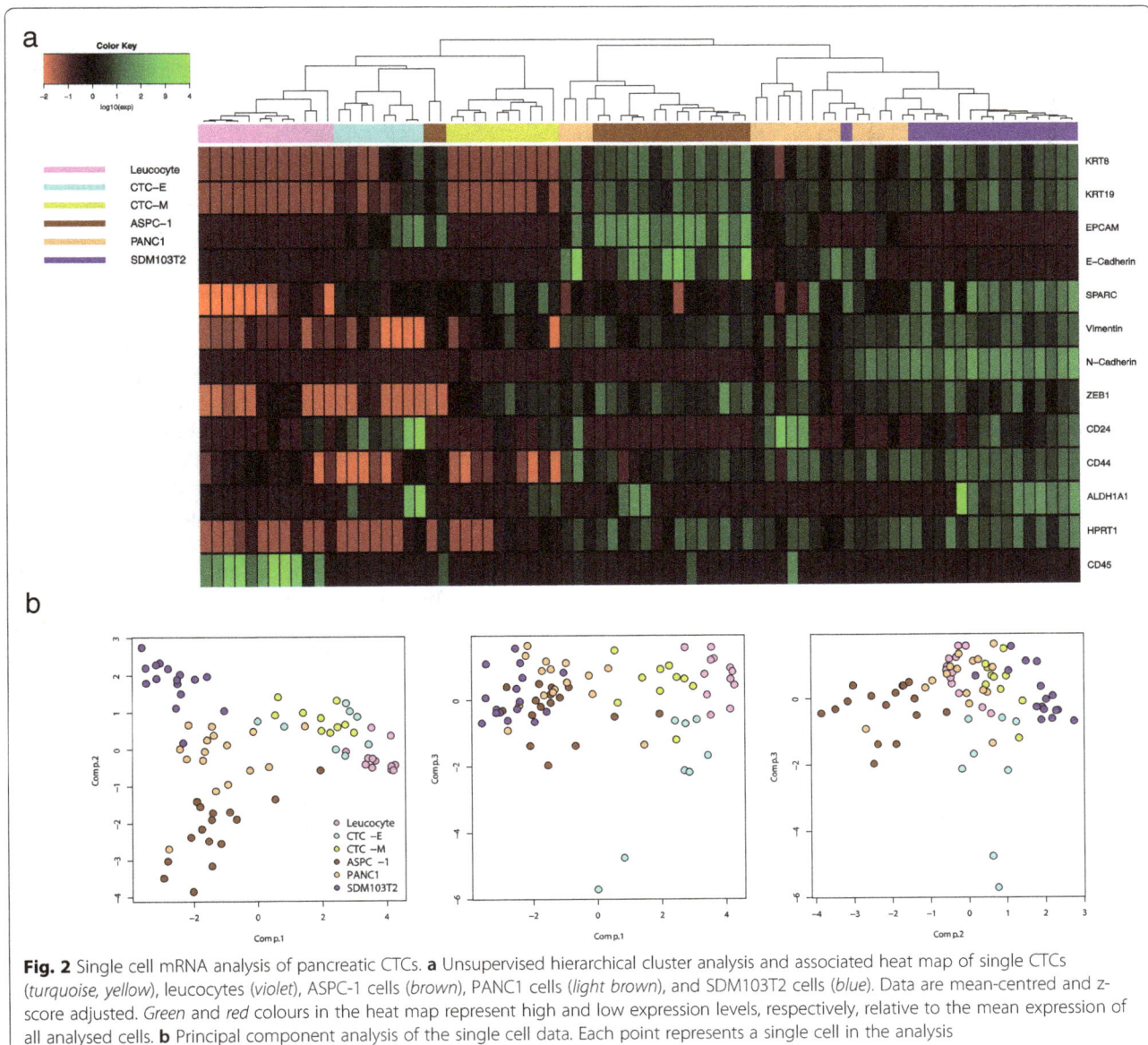

Fig. 2 Single cell mRNA analysis of pancreatic CTCs. **a** Unsupervised hierarchical cluster analysis and associated heat map of single CTCs (*turquoise, yellow*), leucocytes (*violet*), ASPC-1 cells (*brown*), PANC1 cells (*light brown*), and SDM103T2 cells (*blue*). Data are mean-centred and z-score adjusted. *Green* and *red* colours in the heat map represent high and low expression levels, respectively, relative to the mean expression of all analysed cells. **b** Principal component analysis of the single cell data. Each point represents a single cell in the analysis

markedly different from all the other cell-line cells (Fig. 2a); thus, heterogeneity among single cells was observed even among apparently homogenous cancer cell-line cells. A PCA of the expression data confirmed the findings from the hierarchical clustering analysis (Fig. 2b); leucocytes, cancer cell-line cells, and the CTC subgroups formed separate clusters.

Expression of epithelial, mesenchymal, and CSC markers in pancreatic CTCs Further characterization of the CTC subgroups revealed that cells in the CTC-E subgroup expressed the epithelial markers, KRT8, KRT19, and EPCAM, and they showed elevated expression of the CSC marker, CD24. These cells also lacked, or showed lower expression, of the mesenchymal markers, vimentin, ZEB1, and N-Cadherin. In contrast, cells in the CTC-M subgroup expressed the mesenchymal marker, ZEB1, showed elevated expression of vimentin compared to the cells in the CTC-E subgroup, and lacked expression of epithelial markers. Several CTCs co-expressed epithelial and mesenchymal markers; most co-expressed epithelial markers and vimentin, but a few CTCs co-expressed epithelial markers and the mesenchymal marker, ZEB1. These cells with an intermediate phenotype did not form a separate cluster in the hierarchical clustering analysis, but were identified in either the CTC-E or CTC-M cluster, according to their levels of mesenchymal marker expression. The CSC markers, CD24, CD44, and ALDH1A1 were expressed in cells found in both the CTC-E and the CTC-M subgroups, and each subgroup contained cells that co-expressed two or more CSC markers. Both CD24 and ALDH1A1 expression levels were elevated in CTCs compared to leucocytes and pancreatic cancer cell-line cells. In contrast, CD44 expression was similar in CTCs and leucocytes, but lower in CTCs than in cell-line cells. CD24 expression was detected in all profiled cells in the CTC-E subgroup, and expression was elevated compared to CD24 expression in the CTC-M subgroup ($p < 0.001$; Mann-Whitney U). Expression of the characteristic "cadherin switch" [16] proteins, E-Cadherin and N-Cadherin, was undetectable in most CTCs isolated: each of these markers was detected in only one CTC. All CTCs lacked expression of the leucocyte marker, CD45, but it was detected in all but one leucocyte.

A correlation analysis of the CTC mRNA levels (Fig. 3) showed high internal correlations between individual epithelial markers and between individual mesenchymal markers. Negative correlations were demonstrated between these groups, which indicated that increased expression of mesenchymal markers was associated with downregulation of epithelial markers. This finding supported the hypothesis that those CTCs were undergoing EMT. Interestingly, CSC markers were only correlated with the epithelial markers.

High SPARC expression was found in pancreatic CTCs and correlated with EMT markers

The ECM marker, SPARC, was analysed because previous studies showed that it was elevated in pancreatic CTCs. The expression of SPARC was high in all isolated CTCs and cancer cell-line cells analysed, and it was nearly absent in leucocytes. On average, the expression of SPARC in CTCs was higher than in the pancreatic cancer cell lines, PANC1 ($p = 0.053$) and ASPC-1 ($p = 0.004$), even though the general distributions of most measured mRNAs were much lower in the CTCs than in the cell-line cells. Furthermore, we noted a trend towards higher SPARC expression in the CTC-M subgroup than in the CTC-E subgroup ($p = 0.101$; Mann-Whitney U). Correlation analysis of CTC mRNA levels (Fig. 3) revealed that SPARC expression was moderately correlated with the EMT markers, vimentin (Spearman correlation = 0.62, $p = 0.0003$) and ZEB1 (Spearman correlation = 0.55, $p = 0.01$), and moderately negatively correlated with the epithelial markers, KRT8 (Spearman correlation = −0.63, $p = 0.014$) and EPCAM (Spearman correlation = −0.65, $p = 0.004$). These correlations were not observed in the pancreatic cancer cell-line cells (Additional file 2) or in the mesenchymal cancer cell-line cells (Additional file 3).

Clinical relevance of CTC-E and CTC-M detection

CTCs with sufficient mRNA quality were isolated from 13 samples obtained from 8 patients. The CTC-E phenotype was present in four samples obtained from four patients. For three of these patients follow-up data was available. These three patients had a median survival, from the time of inclusion, of 10.6 months (95% CI: 0–22.2). In contrast, the CTC-M phenotype was encountered more frequently; it was present in 10 samples obtained from seven patients. In four of these patients, the CTC-E phenotype was not present at any time point during follow-up. The median survival of these four patients, from the time of inclusion, was 18.5 months (95% CI: 14.8–22.2). The difference in survival between patients where the CTC-E phenotype was present during follow-up and patients where only the CTC-M phenotype was present was borderline significant (log-rank test: $p = 0.093$). Interestingly, both patients that provided more than one isolated CTC in a single sample died within 3 months after CTC detection. In total, 3 of 4 patients with CTC-E positive samples progressed at the same time or shortly after the positive sample were identified, and they died within 3 months. In contrast, although some patients progressed after a CTC-M positive sample was identified, only 1 of 5 patients died shortly after providing a sample positive only for CTC-M. This patient was hospitalized with sepsis and died from toxicity due to the chemotherapy.

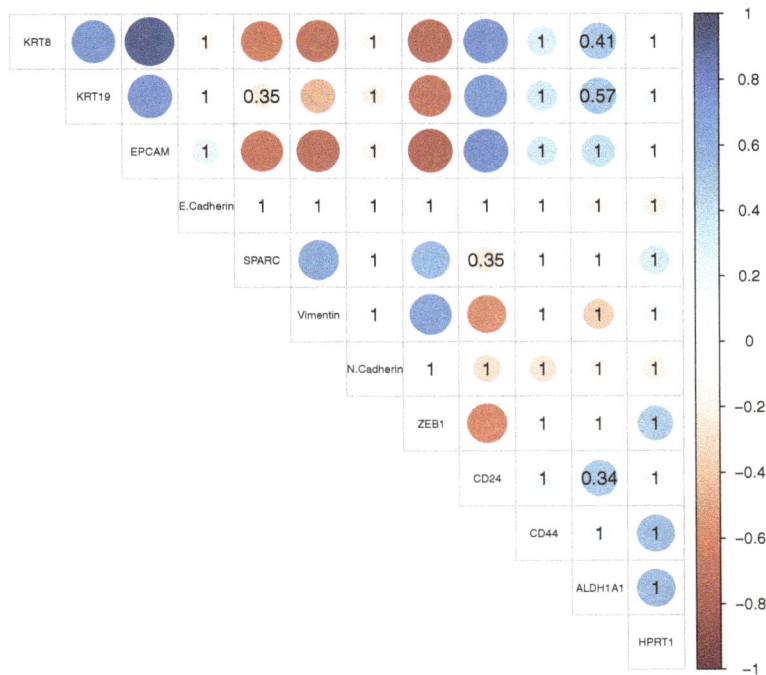

Fig. 3 Correlation plots of mRNA expression levels in single pancreatic CTCs. Matrix shows pairwise Spearman rank correlations between expression levels of the indicated mRNAs in pancreatic CTCs. Blue and red colours represent positive and negative correlations, respectively, according to scale bar (*right*). The circle size represents the magnitude of the correlation. The values in the matrix represent *p*-values that did not reach significance. All *p*-values were corrected for multiple testing with the Bonferroni correction

Discussion

With our previously established CTC enrichment strategy, MINDEC [12], and single-cell mRNA profiling, we isolated and garnered gene expression data from single human pancreatic CTCs. In total, we isolated and profiled 18 CTCs from 13 patient samples. Although the mRNA panel was small, with only 13 markers, the CTC clustering analysis revealed two distinct subpopulations, CTC-E and CTC-M. These subpopulations were distinct from both leucocytes and cell-line cells. Ting et al. previously stratified mouse pancreatic CTCs into classic (epithelial), proliferative, and platelet-associated subgroups, based on mRNA expression [11]. However, to our knowledge, this study was the first to describe a subgroup of human pancreatic CTCs enriched for mesenchymal markers, based on mRNA expression. However, previous studies have described CTCs with mesenchymal and intermediate epithelial-mesenchymal phenotypes, based on protein expression [17, 18].

A large number of the CTCs isolated (41%) had low quality RNA, inadequate for mRNA profiling. We suspected that these cells might have lost viability during the enrichment process. However, mRNA profiles were obtained for all isolated cell-line cells after the spiking experiments. Thus, we suspected that it was more likely that CTCs with degraded RNA lost viability in the bloodstream, prior to sampling and enrichment. Similar numbers of CTCs with insufficient mRNA quality were also reported by other groups that employed other enrichment methods [11, 19].

Both *CD24* and *CD44* were frequently expressed in CTCs, but CTCs did not express higher *CD44* levels than leucocytes. *ALDH1A1* was expressed in several CTCs, and several cells also co-expressed two or three CSC markers. Sorted pancreatic tumour cells ALDH-positive, dual CD24- and CD44-positive, and triple CD24-, CD44-, and ALDH-positive were previously demonstrated to be highly tumourigenic compared to unsorted tumour cells. As few as 100 of the sorted cells were necessary to produce tumours after xenotransplantation in immuno-compromised mice [20–22]. Although we measured mRNA levels, which do not necessarily translate to protein levels, the prevalence of CSC markers in CTCs suggested that these cells may have high metastatic potential. Accordingly, the high prevalence of CSC markers in pancreatic CTCs might explain the high metastatic frequency of pancreatic tumours, despite the low number of CTCs reported [17, 23, 24].

SPARC was highly expressed in all isolated CTCs compared to cell-line cells and leucocytes, particularly in the CTC-M group. This finding suggested that *SPARC* upregulation might be related to the ability of CTCs to spread and invade distant sites. *SPARC* mRNA levels were previously demonstrated to be highly elevated in both chronic pancreatitis (16-fold increase) and pancreatic cancers (31-fold increase), compared to normal pancreatic tissue [25]. Elevated SPARC protein levels were also demonstrated to promote invasiveness of pancreatic tumour cells. In contrast to our findings, Ting et al., in a mouse model, found that SPARC expression was highest in epithelial–like CTCs [11]. They also demonstrated that SPARC was highly expressed in human pancreatic CTCs, and they provided evidence of the invasiveness and metastatic potential of SPARC-expressing tumour cells. In contrast, our results suggested that SPARC expression was associated with mesenchymal markers and CTCs undergoing EMT, because SPARC expression was positively correlated with vimentin and ZEB1 and negatively correlated with KRT8 and EPCAM. Consistent with our results, evidence from melanoma and breast carcinoma studies pointed to SPARC as an inducer of EMT [26, 27].

It should be taken into consideration that our single-cell mRNA analyses might have been affected by burst transcription in single cells. This process causes the levels of specific mRNAs to fluctuate over time [14, 15], and it is the primary cause of differences in mRNA expression levels between apparently identical cells. The nature of burst transcription precludes the normalization of quantitative RT-PCR data from single cells against a reference transcript [28]. Nevertheless, it was demonstrated that the magnitude of the noise caused by burst transcription was smaller than the variation caused by gene regulation [29].

The number of CTCs we isolated from each patient sample in this study was consistent with previous reports on pancreatic CTCs [17, 23, 24]. The low number of detectable CTCs in pancreatic cancer is most likely due to their uptake by the liver, which occurs when the venous drainage from the gastrointestinal tract passes through the liver, which is prone to metastatic spread in pancreatic cancer. Catenacci et al. reported that the number of CTCs in patients with pancreaticobiliary cancers was more than 100-fold higher in portal vein blood compared to peripheral blood. That finding suggested that enumerating CTCs in peripheral blood from patients with pancreatic tumours might be difficult compared to other solid cancers [24]. Ideally, portal vein blood would be the best source of blood for CTC analysis in patients with pancreatic cancer. However, acquisition of portal vein blood is an invasive procedure that would be hard to recommend for a patient group with high morbidity.

Several previous investigations of pancreatic CTCs have failed to support the clinical utility of CTC analysis in pancreatic cancer. However, the consensus opinion was that CTC analysis in pancreatic cancer is clinically relevant (reviewed in [6, 7]). Although some previous studies were limited by small patient cohorts, it is apparent that, in most studies, CTCs were detected with only a single or few markers, which either targeted epithelial- or cancer-specific transcripts or proteins. Thus, those results did not elucidate the complexity of the identified CTCs. In this study, we showed that CSC and mesenchymal transcripts were detected in the majority of isolated CTCs. Similar to our findings, a previous study described a subgroup of CTCs with a mesenchymal profile and CTCs that expressed CSC transcripts in patients with breast cancer [30]. In a recent study by Poruk et al., the expression of CSC markers on the surface of pancreatic epithelial CTCs was associated with shorter disease-free and overall survival [31]. Evidence from research on colorectal and breast cancer has also suggested that the identification of mesenchymal CTCs and transient CTCs undergoing EMT may provide additional prognostic information, compared to the information provided by epithelial CTCs alone [32–34]. The prognostic value of mesenchymal CTCs in pancreatic cancer is not clear; however, in a study by Poruk et al., the detection of vimentin on CK-positive CTCs was associated with disease recurrence [18]. Our data demonstrated that the CTC-E group expressed higher levels of stem cell markers than the CTC-M group. We also found indications that CTC-Es may predict survival better than CTC-Ms. However, due to the small patient numbers in that analysis, we urge careful interpretation; these results should be validated in a larger patient cohort.

Recent evidence has also suggested that CTC clusters might be a better prognostic marker than CTCs. Chang et al. detected CTC clusters in patients with pancreatic cancer and found them to be independent predictors of progression-free and overall survival [35]. We isolated three CTC clusters from three different patient samples, but only one cluster had sufficient mRNA quality for analysis. These low numbers prevented us from drawing any conclusions about whether CTC clusters might yield additional clinical information.

The major limitation of our study was the small mRNA panel used. This panel was designed to differentiate between epithelial and mesenchymal CTCs, and to assess the presence of potential tumourigenic CTCs, based on CSC marker expression. In hindsight, the mRNA panel could well have included more markers to provide a better characterization of CTCs. In a recent study on mRNA heterogeneity in single CTCs, Gorges et al. included markers associated with resistance to cancer therapy and tumour progression in their mRNA panel. Those markers were readily detected in breast and prostate cancer CTCs [30]. Inclusion of such markers in our mRNA panel might have provided a means to identify the CTC groups responsible for metastasis. In addition, such markers might have provided information on tumour progression and the effect of therapy. However, future single-cell analyses of pancreatic CTCs might be best served by performing RNA sequencing, which could avoid dependence on small, selective mRNA panels [11]. Other limitations to our study included the low numbers of analysed CTCs and the lack of patients with localized disease in our patient cohort. Moreover, it would have been interesting to analyse CTCs in early-stage cancer samples, for instance after surgery, to determine whether specific CTC subpopulations also have prognostic value for these patients.

Conclusions

In conclusion, our analysis of single pancreatic CTCs identified distinct epithelial-like and mesenchymal-like subpopulations and revealed elevated expression of CSC markers and the EMT-associated marker, *SPARC*. These transcripts might be relevant in the dissemination of CTCs to distant organ sites. In addition, our preliminary results suggested that epithelial-like CTCs may be a better predictor of survival than mesenchymal-like CTCs. That finding warrants future investigations in larger studies.

Abbreviations
CSC: Cancer stem cells; CTC: Circulating tumour cell; CTC-E: Epithelial-like CTC; CTC-M: Mesenchymal-like CTC; ECM: Extracellular matrix; EMT: Epithelial-mesenchymal transition

Acknowledgments
Not applicable.

Funding
This project was supported by the Folke Hermansen Fund, the Norwegian Cancer Society, and the Western Norway Health Authorities. The project was part of a strategic programme called "Personalized medicine-biomarkers and clinical studies", which was supported by the Western Norway Regional Health Authority. The funding bodies had no role in the design of the study, in the collection, analysis, and interpretation of data, or in writing of the manuscript.

Authors' contributions
ML and O.N. designed the study; ML performed CTC enrichment, performed single-cell isolation, performed single-cell RT-pre-Amp and qPCR, analysed data, performed statistical analysis, and drafted the manuscript; KT contributed to result interpretation and statistical analysis; SO performed density gradient centrifugation on patient samples; MJ contributed to result interpretation; BG, and RS recruited patients and provided patient samples and data; ON supervised the study and contributed to result interpretation and statistical analysis; All authors reviewed, commented on, and approved the manuscript.

Competing interests
The authors declare no competing interests.

Author details
[1]Department of Haematology and Oncology, Stavanger University Hospital, N–4068 Stavanger, Norway. [2]Laboratory for Molecular Biology, Stavanger University Hospital, N–4068 Stavanger, Norway. [3]Department of Mathematics and Natural Sciences, University of Stavanger, N–4036 Stavanger, Norway. [4]Department of Gastrointestinal (GI) Medical Oncology, Division of Cancer Medicine, MD Anderson Cancer Center, The University of Texas, Houston, TX, USA.

References
1. Cancer Registry of Norway. Cancer in Norway 2015 - Cancer incidence, mortality, survival and prevalence in Norway. Oslo: Cancer Registry of Norway; 2016.
2. Conroy T, Desseigne F, Ychou M, Bouché O, Guimbaud R, Bécouarn Y, et al. FOLFIRINOX versus Gemcitabine for Metastatic Pancreatic Cancer. N Engl J Med. 2011;364:1817–25.
3. Goldstein D, El-Maraghi RH, Hammel P, Heinemann V, Kunzmann V, Sastre J, et al. nab-Paclitaxel Plus Gemcitabine for Metastatic Pancreatic Cancer: Long-Term Survival From a Phase III Trial. J Natl Cancer Inst. 2015;(2)107.
4. Von Hoff DD, Ervin T, Arena FP, Chiorean EG, Infante J, Moore M, et al. Increased Survival in Pancreatic Cancer with nab-Paclitaxel plus Gemcitabine. N Engl J Med. 2013;369:1691–703.
5. Vincent A, Herman J, Schulick R, Hruban RH, Goggins M. Pancreatic cancer. Lancet. 2011;378:607–20.
6. Tjensvoll K, Nordgard O, Smaaland R. Circulating tumor cells in pancreatic cancer patients: methods of detection and clinical implications. Int J Cancer. 2014;134:1–8.
7. Nagrath S, Jack RM, Sahai V, Simeone DM. Opportunities and Challenges for Pancreatic Circulating Tumor Cells. Gastroenterology. 2016;151:412–26.
8. Jones S, Zhang X, Parsons DW, Lin JC, Leary RJ, Angenendt P, et al. Core signaling pathways in human pancreatic cancers revealed by global genomic analyses. Science. 2008;321:1801–6.
9. Yachida S, Jones S, Bozic I, Antal T, Leary R, Fu B, et al. Distant metastasis occurs late during the genetic evolution of pancreatic cancer. Nature. 2010; 467:1114–7.
10. Tsai JH, Yang J. Epithelial-mesenchymal plasticity in carcinoma metastasis. Genes Dev. 2013;27:2192–206.
11. Ting DT, Wittner BS, Ligorio M, Vincent Jordan N, Shah AM, Miyamoto DT, et al. Single-cell RNA sequencing identifies extracellular matrix gene expression by pancreatic circulating tumor cells. Cell Rep. 2014;8:1905–18.
12. Lapin M, Tjensvoll K, Oltedal S, Buhl T, Gilje B, Smaaland R, et al. MINDEC-An Enhanced Negative Depletion Strategy for Circulating Tumour Cell Enrichment. Sci Rep. 2016;6:28929.
13. Eisenhauer EA, Therasse P, Bogaerts J, Schwartz LH, Sargent D, Ford R, et al. New response evaluation criteria in solid tumours: revised RECIST guideline (version 1.1). Eur J Cancer. 2009;45:228–47.
14. Elowitz MB, Levine AJ, Siggia ED, Swain PS. Stochastic gene expression in a single cell. Science. 2002;297:1183–6.
15. Raj A, Peskin CS, Tranchina D, Vargas DY, Tyagi S. Stochastic mRNA Synthesis in Mammalian Cells. PLoS Biol. 2006;4:e309.
16. Cavallaro U, Schaffhauser B, Christofori G. Cadherins and the tumour progression: is it all in a switch? Cancer Lett. 2002;176:123–8.
17. Khoja L, Backen A, Sloane R, Menasce L, Ryder D, Krebs M, et al. A pilot study to explore circulating tumour cells in pancreatic cancer as a novel biomarker. Br J Cancer. 2012;106:508–16.
18. Poruk KE, Valero V, 3rd, Saunders T, Blackford AL, Griffin JF, Poling J, et al. Circulating Tumor Cell Phenotype Predicts Recurrence and Survival in Pancreatic Adenocarcinoma. Ann Surg. 2016;264:1073–81.
19. Miyamoto DT, Zheng Y, Wittner BS, Lee RJ, Zhu H, Broderick KT, et al. RNA-Seq of Single Prostate CTCs Implicates Noncanonical Wnt Signaling in Antiandrogen Resistance. Science (New York, NY). 2015:349, 1351–1356.
20. Ishizawa K, Rasheed ZA, Karisch R, Wang Q, Kowalski J, Susky E, et al. Tumor-initiating cells are rare in many human tumors. Cell Stem Cell. 2010;7:279–82.
21. Rasheed ZA, Yang J, Wang Q, Kowalski J, Freed I, Murter C, et al. Prognostic significance of tumorigenic cells with mesenchymal features in pancreatic adenocarcinoma. J Natl Cancer Inst. 2010;102:340–51.
22. Li C, Heidt DG, Dalerba P, Burant CF, Zhang L, Adsay V, et al. Identification of pancreatic cancer stem cells. Cancer Res. 2007;67:1030–7.
23. Allard WJ, Matera J, Miller MC, Repollet M, Connelly MC, Rao C, et al. Tumor cells circulate in the peripheral blood of all major carcinomas but not in healthy subjects or patients with nonmalignant diseases. Clin Cancer Res. 2004;10:6897–904.
24. Catenacci DV, Chapman CG, Xu P, Koons A, Konda VJ, Siddiqui UD, et al.

Acquisition of Portal Venous Circulating Tumor Cells From Patients With Pancreaticobiliary Cancers by Endoscopic Ultrasound. Gastroenterology. 2015;149:1794–803. e1794

25. Guweidhi A, Kleeff J, Adwan H, Giese NA, Wente MN, Giese T, et al. Osteonectin influences growth and invasion of pancreatic cancer cells. Ann Surg. 2005;242:224–34.

26. Robert G, Gaggioli C, Bailet O, Chavey C, Abbe P, Aberdam E, et al. SPARC represses E-cadherin and induces mesenchymal transition during melanoma development. Cancer Res. 2006;66:7516–23.

27. Sangaletti S, Tripodo C, Santangelo A, Castioni N, Portararo P, Gulino A, et al. Mesenchymal Transition of High-Grade Breast Carcinomas Depends on Extracellular Matrix Control of Myeloid Suppressor Cell Activity. Cell Rep. 2016;17:233–48.

28. Stahlberg A, Rusnakova V, Forootan A, Anderova M, Kubista M. RT-qPCR work-flow for single-cell data analys s. Methods. 2013;59:80–8.

29. Colman-Lerner A, Gordon A, Serra E, Chin T, Resnekov O, Endy D, et al. Regulated cell-to-cell variation in a cell-fate decision system. Nature. 2005; 437:699–706.

30. Gorges TM, Kuske A, Rock K, Mauermann O, Muller V, Peine S, et al. Accession of Tumor Heterogeneity by Multiplex Transcriptome Profiling of Single Circulating Tumor Cells. Clin Chem. 2016;62:1504–15.

31. Poruk KE, Blackford AL, Weiss MJ, Cameron JL, He J, Goggins MG, et al. Circulating Tumor Cells Expressing Markers of Tumor Initiating Cells Predict Poor Survival and Cancer Recurrence in Patients with Pancreatic Ductal Adenocarcinoma. Clin Cancer Res. 2016. [Epub ahead of print].

32. Yokobori T, Iinuma H, Shimamura T, Imoto S, Sugimachi K, Ishii H, et al. Plastin3 is a novel marker for circulating tumor cells undergoing the epithelial-mesenchymal transition and is associated with colorectal cancer prognosis. Cancer Res. 2013;73:2059–69.

33. Satelli A, Brownlee Z, Mitra A, Meng QH, Li S. Circulating tumor cell enumeration with a combination of epithelial cell adhesion molecule- and cell-surface vimentin-based methods for monitoring breast cancer therapeutic response. Clin Chem. 2015;61:259–66.

34. Ueo H, Sugimachi K, Gorges TM, Bartkowiak K, Yokobori T, Muller V, et al. Circulating tumour cell-derived plastin3 is a novel marker for predicting long-term prognosis in patients with breast cancer. Br J Cancer. 2015;112:1519–26.

35. Chang MC, Chang YT, Chen JY, Jeng YM, Yang CY, Tien YW, et al. Clinical Significance of Circulating Tumor Microemboli as a Prognostic Marker in Patients with Pancreatic Ductal Adenocarcinoma. Clin Chem. 2016;62:505–13.

14

Anti-LRP/LR-specific antibody IgG1-iS18 impedes adhesion and invasion of pancreatic cancer and neuroblastoma cells

Thalia M. Rebelo, Carryn J. Chetty, Eloise Ferreira and Stefan F. T. Weiss[*]

Abstract

Background: Cancer has become a global burden due to its high incidence and mortality rates, with an estimated 14.1 million cancer cases reported worldwide in 2012 particularly as a result of metastasis. Metastasis involves two crucial steps: adhesion and invasion, and the non-integrin receptor; the 37-kDa/67-kDa laminin receptor precursor/ high affinity laminin receptor (LRP/LR) has been shown to be overexpressed on the surface of tumorigenic cells, thus being implicated in the enhancement of these two crucial steps. The current study investigated the role of LRP/LR on the aggressiveness of pancreatic cancer (AsPC-1) and neuroblastoma (IMR-32) cells with respect to their adhesive and invasive potential.

Methods: AsPC-1 and IMR-32 cells were utilized as the experimental cell lines for the study. Cell surface LRP/LR levels were visualised and quantified on the experimental and control (MCF-7) cell lines via confocal microscopy and flow cytometry, respectively. Total LRP/LR levels in the cell lines were assessed by Western blotting and the adhesive and invasive potential of the above-mentioned cell lines was determined before and after supplementation with the anti-LRP/LR specific antibody IgG1-iS18. Statistical significance of the data was confirmed via the use of the two-tailed student's *t*-test and Pearson's correlation coefficient.

Results: Flow cytometry revealed that AsPC-1 and IMR-32 cells displayed significantly higher cell surface LRP/LR levels in comparison to the MCF-7 control cell line. However, Western blotting and subsequent densitometric analysis revealed that all three tumorigenic cell lines displayed no significant difference in total LRP/LR levels. The treatment of AsPC-1 and IMR-32 cells with IgG1-iS18 caused a significant reduction in the adhesive and invasive potential of the cells to laminin-1 and through the ECM-like Matrigel™, respectively. Pearson's correlation coefficients indicated a high correlation, thus suggesting a directly proportional relationship between cell surface LRP/LR levels and the adhesive and invasive potential of AsPC-1 and IMR-32 cells.

Conclusion: These findings suggest that through the interference of the LRP/LR-laminin-1 interaction, the anti-LRP/LR specific antibody IgG1-iS18 may act as an alternative therapeutic tool for the treatment of metastatic pancreatic cancer and neuroblastoma.

Keywords: Metastasis, 37 kDa/67-kDa laminin receptor (LRP/LR), Adhesion, Invasion, Laminin-1, Metastasis, Pancreatic cancer, Neuroblastoma

Background

Cancer is defined as the uncontrolled proliferation of body cells due to the diminished levels of apoptosis or programmed cell death, thus resulting in abnormal cellular growth [1, 2]. Cancer is implicated as the primary cause of death in economically developed countries and the second leading cause of death in developing countries [3]. According to the World Cancer Research Fund (WCRF), 14.1 million cancer cases were reported worldwide in 2012 and this number is expected to increase to 24 million by the year 2035 [4]. Referring to the present study, two cancer types are of importance namely pancreatic cancer which is an aggressive cancer type as it is asymptomatic in the early stages and upon diagnoses the tumour is of an advanced stage, after metastasis has

---
* Correspondence: stefan.weiss@wits.ac.za
School of Molecular and Cell Biology, University of the Witwatersrand, Johannesburg, Republic of South Africa (RSA)

occurred. Pancreatic cancer was ranked as the 12th most diagnosed cancer in 2012 with approximately 338 000 cases being diagnosed. Neuroblastoma is an aggressive and malignant cancer type with 50% of all cases being classified as high risk upon diagnosis as the disease has metastasised. Neuroblastoma most commonly affects infants and young children and it was ranked as the 17th most diagnosed cancer types in 2012 with approximately 256 000 cases being diagnosed [4]. Due to these alarming statistics, it is therefore crucial to develop novel therapeutic strategies for the treatment of cancer and in particular metastatic pancreatic cancer and neuroblastoma.

The 37-kDa/67-kDa laminin receptor (LRP/LR) is a 295 amino acid, transmembrane receptor consisting of three domains; the N-terminal intracellular cytosolic domain, the transmembrane domain and the C-terminal extracellular domain which contains binding sites for laminin-1, carbohydrates, elastin, prion proteins and IgG antibodies [5–7]. The 37-kDa LRP is thought to be the precursor of the 67-kDa high-affinity laminin receptor LR, however the exact mechanism by which the precursor forms the receptor is unknown [8]. The receptor is seen to be overexpressed on the surface of tumorigenic cells such as cervical, lung, prostate and colon [9, 10], breast and oesophageal [11] and liver cancer cells [12], thus serving many physiological functions such as signal transduction, cell cycle progression, cell migration, cell-matrix adhesion, cell viability and proliferation [13–15]. LRP/LR is also associated with the process of Aβ- generation in Alzheimer's disease [16, 17] as well as enhancing telomerase activity which is seen to play a role in disease progression and chemotherapy resistance in some cancers [18]. LRP/LR overexpression directly promotes the adhesion and invasion of tumorigenic cell lines via the process of metastasis. Metastasis is responsible for secondary tumor formation thus accounting for 90% of cancer- associated deaths [11]. LRP/LR has a high binding affinity for the extracellular matrix (ECM) protein; laminin-1 [14]. Laminins make up the majority of the non-collagenous glycoprotein component when localized in the basement membrane [19]. Laminins support the promotion of the invasive phenotype of several tumorigenic cells as they are involved in significant biological activities such as cell attachment, growth and migration [19]. The main event responsible for tumor invasion is the interaction of cancer cells; in particular LRP/LR with laminin-1, therefore inducing proteolytic activity which involves type IV collagenase which hydrolyses type-IV collagen in the basal lamina, resulting in the metastatic spread of the cancer cells to distant tissues in the body [19].

Hindering the LRP/LR-laminin-1 interaction may be considered an essential tool in treating metastatic cancer. This may be achieved by blocking LRP/LR with IgG1-iS18. IgG1-iS18 is the full length version

immunoglobulin G1 (IgG1)-iS18 of the single-chain anti-LRP/LR antibody scFv iS18. It is a monoclonal anti-LRP/LR specific antibody which was designed to specifically target the LRP/LR-laminin-1 interaction and it is characteristic of having a high stability and long half-life of up to 21 days in blood. This approach has therefore been shown to significantly reduce the adhesive and invasive potential of several tumorigenic cells [10–12].

In this study, we investigated whether the anti-LRP/LR specific antibody IgG1-iS18 is capable of impeding the adhesive and invasive potential of pancreatic cancer (AsPC-1) and neuroblastoma (IMR-32) cells.

Methods
Cell culture
Poorly invasive, human breast adenocarcinoma (MCF-7) cells, human pancreatic adenocarcinoma (AsPC-1) cells and human neuroblastoma (IMR-32) cells were cultivated in Dulbecco's Modified Eagle Medium (DMEM), RPMI 1640 and Minimum Essential Media (MEM), respectively. Each cell culture medium was supplemented with 10% FCS and 1% penicillin/ streptomycin, with additional amino acids, vitamins and salts being added as required for complete growth media. All cell lines were cultivated at 37 °C and 5% CO_2.

Cells were seeded and sub-cultured at appropriate dilutions. The cultured cells were washed and detached using phosphate buffered saline (PBS) and 1X Trypsin/ Versene, respectively.

Reagents and antibodies
Laminin-1 (10 μg/ml) obtained from BD Biosciences was used for cell adhesion assays.

Matrigel™ matrix used in cell invasion assays was extracted from the Engelbreth-Holm-Swarm (EHS) mouse sarcoma a tumor rich in extracellular matrix proteins. Once isolated, the Matrigel™ constitutes of approximately 60% laminin, 30% collagen IV, 8% entactin and several growth factors. It was obtained from Corning Inc.

Chloramphenicol acetyltransferase (CAT) antibody was used as the negative control and it was obtained from Sigma-Aldrich.

IgG1-iS18 was used as the treatment antibody (positive control) and it was recombinantly produced in a mammalian expression system as described by Zuber et al., (2008).

Confocal microscopy
In order to qualitatively visualize the localization of LRP/LR on the cell surface, confocal microscopy was employed. The cells were first seeded onto coverslips and allowed to reach an approximate confluency of 75% before being fixed for 15 min in 4% paraformaldehyde (PFA). This was followed by five PBS washes and the addition of the primary antibody IgG1-iS18 (1:100)

diluted in 0.5% BSA. Post an overnight incubation at 4 °C, the coverslips were rinsed thrice in PBS/BSA. After the addition of the goat anti-human IgG FITC-coupled secondary antibody (abcam) that had been diluted in 0.5% BSA, a further 1 h incubation at 4 °C was allowed. Followed by three washes as before, Hoechst stain diluted in PBS was added and incubated for 10 min to allow for the staining of the nucleus. The cells were washed once with PBS and mounted onto a clean slide using GelMount (Sigma-Aldrich). A period of 2 h was allocated for setting to take place and the slides were then stored at 4 °C until visualisation. Importantly, controls included cells treated with the anti-CAT antibody (primary antibody) together with the FITC-coupled secondary antibody and cells treated with the secondary antibody only.

Flow cytometry- FACS™ analysis

In order to quantitatively determine cell surface LRP/LR levels, flow cytometry was employed. Trypsin/Versene (1X) was used to detach adherent cells, which were then centrifuged at 150 x g for 10 min. Cells were re-suspended and fixed in 4% PFA at 4 °C for 10 min. PFA was discarded and cells were re-suspended in PBS which allowed for the preparation of three cell suspensions, one to which the primary anti-LRP/LR specific IgG1-iS18 antibody was added, one to which anti-CAT antibody was added and one to which no antibody was added (serving as the unstained control). All suspensions were incubated in the dark for 1 h at room temperature. Following three PBS washes by centrifugation at 2700 x g for 5 min, the goat anti-human phycoerythrin (PE)-coupled secondary antibody (abcam) was added to each cell suspension and further incubated for 1 h at room temperature. After the 1 h incubation, suspensions were centrifuged at 2700 x g for 1 min and pellets washed three times in PBS as previously described. The cell suspensions were then analysed using the BD Accuri flow cytometer and software. The experiment was performed in triplicate.

SDS PAGE and Western blotting

Total LRP/LR levels were determined using sodium dodecyl sulphate polyacrylamide gel electrophoresis (SDS-PAGE) as well as Western blotting. To perform SDS-PAGE, 11 µg of total protein was used. Proteins that were separated according to size by SDS-PAGE were identified via Western blotting. The proteins resolved on the polyacrylamide gel were transferred onto the polyvinylidene fluoride (PVDF) membrane using 1X transfer buffer (20% Methanol in 192 mM glycine and 25 mM Tris) for 45 min at 350 mV and a semi-dry transferring apparatus. Blocking buffer (3% BSA in 1X PBS Tween) was then used to block the blotted membrane for 1 h in order to prevent non-specific binding of primary and secondary antibodies. Once blocked, the membrane was probed with anti- LRP/LR specific primary antibody IgG1-iS18 for 1 h. Prior to the incubation of the membrane in the goat anti-human IgG- Horse radish peroxidase (HRP) conjugated secondary antibody, three 1X PBS Tween (0.1% Tween in 1X PBS) washes were performed. A further three PBS Tween washes were performed after incubation in the secondary antibody, followed by the detection of HRP using an enhanced chemiluminescent Clarity™ Western ECL Blotting Substrate (BIORAD). The resulting fluorescence was detected and visualised using the Chemidoc apparatus (BIORAD). The experiment was executed in triplicate and quantification was performed via densitometric analysis using ImageJ™ software.

Adhesion assay

In order to analyse the adhesive potential of the tumorigenic cell lines to the basement membrane in vitro, laminin-1 (10 µg/ml) was used to coat 96- microwell plates, leaving uncoated wells to be used as negative controls. After coating of the wells for 1 h and washing with 1% BSA in the respective media, other protein binding sites on the well were blocked using 100 µl of 0.5% BSA for 1 h. Cells were trypsinised and diluted in serum-free culture media to a density of 4×10^5 cells/ml and added to the wells in order to assess the adhesive potential. Furthermore, the cells pre-incubated with IgG1-iS18 (0.2 mg/ml) and the anti-CAT antibody (0.2 mg/ml) as the negative control were added to the relevant wells in order to examine the effect the antibody might have on the adhesive potential of the cells. The plates were incubated at 37 °C for 1 h and thereafter the non-adherent cells were washed off with PBS and the adherent cells fixed with 4% PFA for 10 min. The adherent cells were stained with 0.1% crystal violet for 10 min. The stain was extracted using 2% SDS and the absorbance of the extracted dye at 550 nm was assayed as a measure of the adhesive potential using an ELISA reader. The experiments were performed in triplicate.

Invasion assay

In vitro analysis of the ability of the tumorigenic cell lines to invade the basement membrane in the absence of the anti-LRP/LR specific antibody IgG1-iS18 and when treated with the antibody was assessed using the ECM- like Matrigel™ invasion assay.

Serum-free cold culture medium was used to dilute the Matrigel™ and the diluted gel was dispensed into the upper chamber of a 24 transwell plate (Corning, 8 µm pores). The gel was allowed to solidify for 4 h at 37 °C. After being trypsinised and harvested, the cells were diluted in serum-free culture media at a density of 1×10^6 cells/ml. The cells were then incubated with IgG1-

iS18 (0.2 mg/ml) or anti- CAT antibody (0.2 mg/ml) as the negative control and loaded onto the upper-Matrigel™ covered chamber. The lower chamber was then filled with 500 μl of media containing 10% FCS for the test and FCS-free media for the control and incubated for 24 h at 37 °C. After removal of the lower and upper chamber media, the cells were fixed with 100 μl of 4% PFA for 15 min. Cells were then washed with 100 μl cold PBS and further stained using 0.5% toluidine blue dye for 2 min. Non-invasive cells were removed using a cotton swab. The dye was then extracted using 1% SDS and the absorbance measured at 620 nm using an ELISA reader. The experiments were performed in triplicate.

Statistical evaluation

The two-tailed student's t-test with a confidence interval of 95% was used in order to prove the statistical significance of the results obtained, with p-values of less than 0.05 being considered significant. The degree of association between LRP/LR levels and the adhesive/ invasive potential of the cell lines was measured using Pearson's

correlation coefficient. A positive coefficient was an indication of direct proportionality between the two variables; however a negative coefficient implied indirect/ inverse proportionality.

Results

Pancreatic cancer and neuroblastoma cells reveal LRP/LR on the cell surface

Cell surface LRP/LR was visualised in order to confirm that the tumorigenic cells did indeed display LRP/LR on their surface and therefore play a pivotal role in the occurrence of metastasis due to the LRP/LR- laminin-1 interaction. LRP/LR was revealed on the cell surface of the poorly invasive breast cancer control cell line as well as the two experimental cell lines as indicated by the green fluorescence in Fig. 1a. Cells were non- permeablized allowing for cell surface staining of LRP/LR and the secondary antibody was shown to be specific for anti-LRP/LR specific antibody IgG1-iS18 only, as depicted by the control images B) and C) in Fig. 1. The anti-CAT antibody was used as an effective negative control due to its ability to bind specifically to the

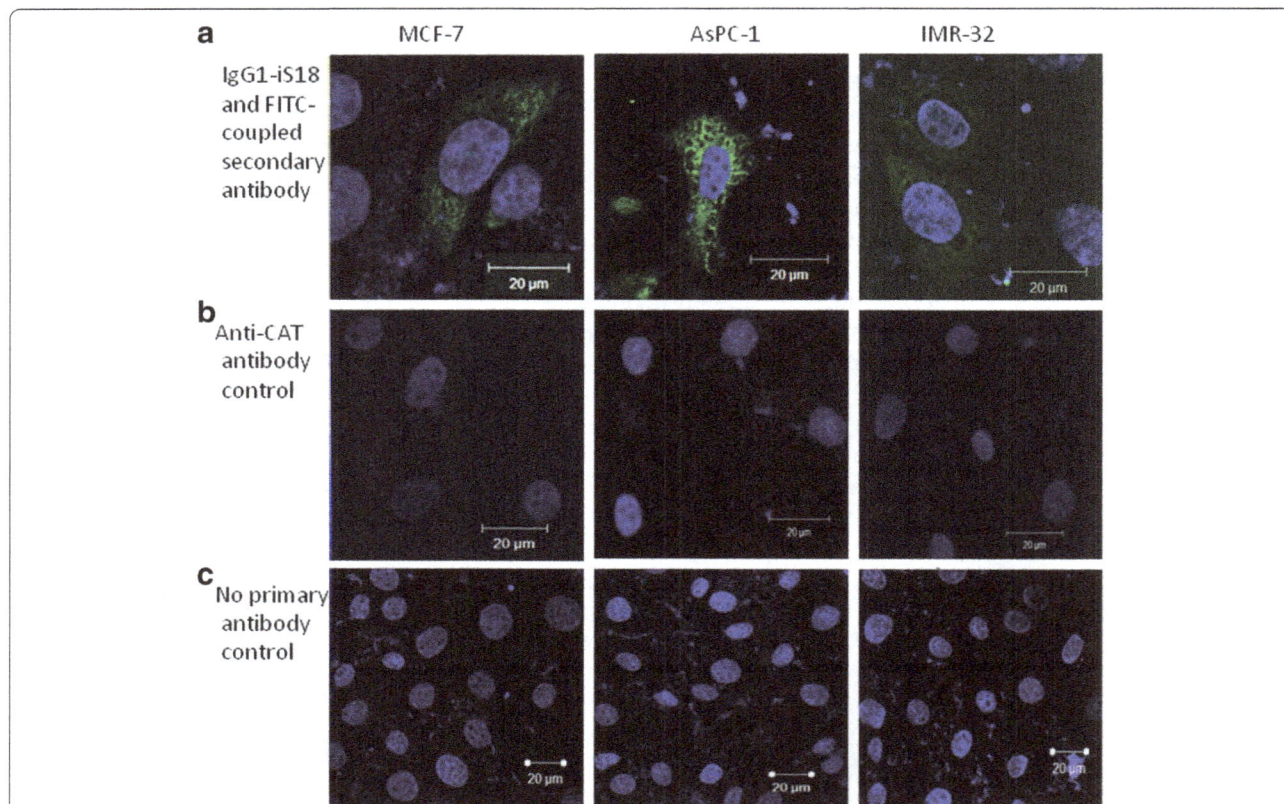

Fig. 1 Visualisation of cell surface LRP/LR levels of pancreatic cancer (AsPC-1) and neuroblastoma (IMR-32) cells. The cells were non-permeabilized in order to visualize the surface of the cancerous cells. **a** The cells were labelled with the primary antibody IgG1-iS18 which binds to LRP/LR and the FITC-coupled secondary antibody which is specific for the primary antibody thus exhibiting green fluorescence. **b** The cells were labelled with the anti-chloramphenicol acetyltransferase (CAT) antibody as the negative control. **c** The cells were labelled with the FITC coupled secondary antibody only, to indicate that no non-specific binding of the secondary antibody occurred

chloramphenicol acetyltransferase (CAT) bacterial protein which is absent in mammalian cells.

High percentages of tumorigenic cells reveal LRP/LR on the cell surface

As confirmed by confocal microscopy, the cells do indeed display LRP/LR on their cell surface, however further quantification of the endogenous expression of cell surface LRP/LR levels was required. Flow cytometry was therefore employed for this quantification. A high percentage of cells within the specific cell population that express LRP/LR on their cell surface were revealed for all three cell lines. This is indicated by the shift between the black (unlabelled) and red (IgG1-iS18 and PE) peaks, as seen in Fig. 2a. Due to the surface staining of the cells with anti-LRP/LR specific antibody IgG1-iS18 and a relevant fluorochrome-conjugated secondary antibody, a change in the

fluorescence intensity was observed. Approximately 98.33% of the poorly invasive MCF-7 cells displayed cell surface LRP/LR whilst 97.18% of the AsPC-1 cells and 81.82% of the IMR-32 cells displayed LRP/LR on the cell surface. A shift in fluorescence intensity was not observed in Fig. 2b, thus indicating that the CAT protein was indeed absent on the surface of the three cell lines under study.

Pancreatic cancer and neuroblastoma cells display significantly higher cell surface LRP/LR levels in comparison to the poorly-invasive breast cancer cells

The shift in fluorescence intensity was further analysed using median statistics as a means of determining the amount of cell surface LRP/LR present within the cell population. Identical concentrations of primary (IgG1-iS18) and secondary (PE) antibody were used to label 20 000 cells within a specific cell population over the same

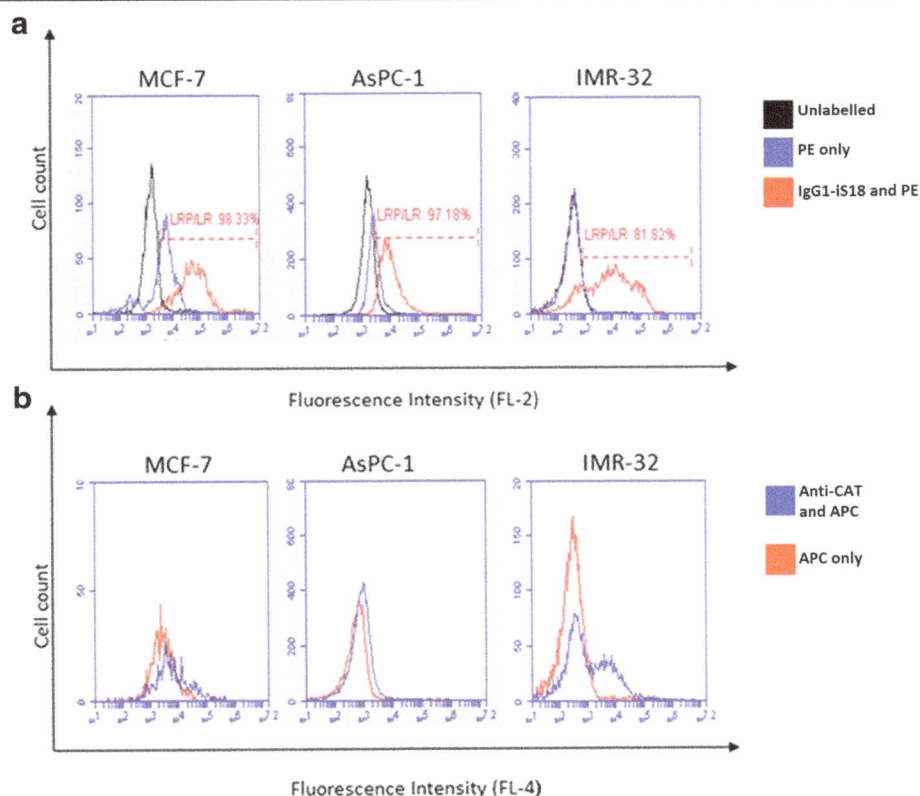

Fig. 2 Detection of LRP/LR levels on the surface of pancreatic cancer and neuroblastoma cells. a Quantification of LRP/LR on the surface of pancreatic cancer (AsPC-1) and neuroblastoma (IMR-32) cells. The black peak represents the unlabelled cells, whilst the blue peak represents the cells labelled with goat anti-human phycoerythin (PE)-coupled secondary antibody. The red peak represents the cells labelled with both anti-LRP/LR specific antibody IgG1-iS18 and the afore-mentioned secondary antibody. The inclusion of the unlabelled cells as a control, confirms that the secondary antibody does not bind non-specifically. The shift observed between the black and red peak indicates a change in fluorescence intensity thus the presence of LRP/LR on the cell surface of the cell lines under study. b Determination of chloramphenicol acetyltransferase protein levels on the surface of the three tumorigenic cell lines as a control. The blue peak represents cells that have been labelled with both anti-CAT primary antibody and goat anti-rabbit allophycocyanin (APC)-coupled secondary antibody, whilst the red peak represents the cells labelled with the afore-mentioned secondary antibody only. No distinct shift is seen between the blue and red peak, thereby indicating the absence of the CAT protein on the surface of the cell lines under study

time period. The median fluorescence intensity (MFI) is indicative of the differential expression of LRP/LR on the cell surface. A significant difference in surface LRP/LR levels were observed between the poorly invasive MCF-7 cells and the AsPC-1 cells as well as between the IMR-32 cells, as depicted in Fig. 3. When comparing the two experimental cell lines, there was a significant difference in surface LRP/LR levels observed with the IMR-32 cells exhibiting the highest percentage of cell surface LRP/LR.

Pancreatic cancer and neuroblastoma cells exhibit no significant difference in total LRP/LR levels in comparison to the poorly-invasive breast cancer control cell line

LRP/LR is not only located on the cell surface but it is also found in the nucleus, including the perinuclear region and in the cytosol. Total LRP/LR levels across the two tumorigenic cell lines as well in the poorly invasive MCF-7 cells were determined via Western blot analysis. Further insight on the relationship between the LRP/LR levels, both surface and total and the adhesive and invasive potential of the tumorigenic cells was obtained by performing densitometric analysis.

As seen in Fig. 4a, LRP/LR was expressed by the three cell lines, but a non- significant difference in total LRP/

LR levels were observed (Fig. 4b). The anti-LRP/LR specific antibody IgG1-iS18 only detected the 37-kDa laminin receptor precursor (LRP) form successfully and β-actin served as the loading control.

IgG1-iS18 significantly reduces the adhesive potential of pancreatic cancer and neuroblastoma cells

The initiation of invasion and ultimately metastasis occurs via the adhesion of a tumorigenic cell to the basement membrane through the LRP/LR- laminin-1 interaction. The LRP/LR-laminin-1 interaction results in the occurrence of additional interactions that enable basement membrane degradation. The tumorigenic cells were treated with IgG1-iS18 and anti-CAT (control) antibodies (0.2 mg/ml) and the absorbance readings taken were a representation of the extent of cell adhesion to laminin-1. The pancreatic cancer cells and the neuroblastoma cells revealed a higher adhesive potential than the poorly- invasive breast cancer (MCF-7) control cell line, with the IMR-32 cells displaying the highest adhesion to laminin-1 as shown in Fig. 5. However, when the cells were treated with the IgG1-iS18 antibody, there was a significant reduction in the adhesive potential of both AsPC-1 and IMR-32 cell lines.

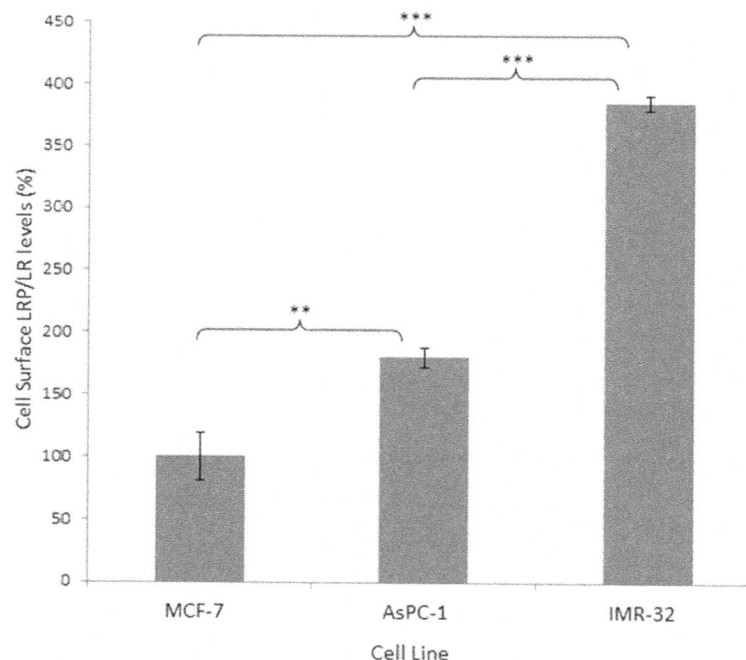

Fig. 3 Quantification of cell surface LRP/LR levels on pancreatic cancer (AsPC-1) and neuroblastoma (IMR-32) cells. The cells were labelled with the primary IgG1-iS18 antibody and the anti-human phycoerythrin (PE) secondary antibody. 20 000 cells were analysed across all three cell lines, with the median fluorescence intensity analysed as an indicator of the cell surface LRP/LR levels. In comparison to the MCF-7 control cell line, AsPC-1 cells exhibit an approximate 2-fold increase in cell surface LRP/LR whilst the IMR-32 cells exhibit an approximate 4-fold increase in cell surface LRP/LR. This data is representative of three experimental triplicates. The MCF-7 values were set to 100%. The error bars represent standard deviation and p-values *$p \leq 0.05$, **$p \leq 0.01$, ***$p \leq 0.001$

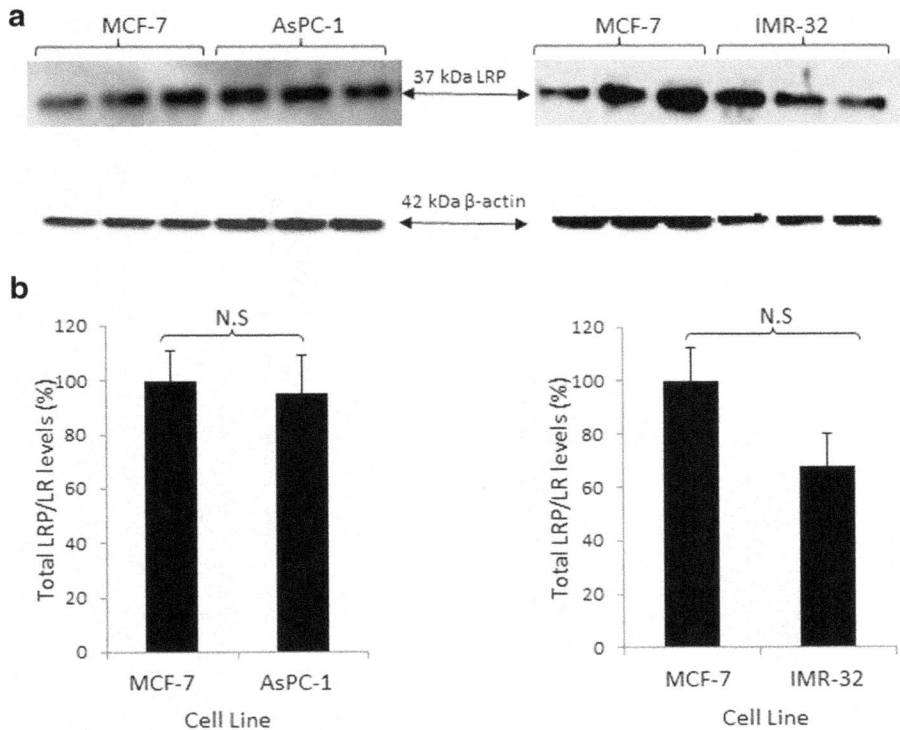

Fig. 4 Detection of total LRP levels in pancreatic cancer (AsPC-1) and neuroblastoma (IMR-32) cells. **a** Western blot analysis was performed to detect total 37-kDa LRP levels in all three cancer cell lines. β-actin was used as a loading control. **b** Densitometric quantification performed on these blots revealed that there was no significant difference in total LRP/LR levels between the poorly invasive MCF-7 cells and the two experimental cell lines: AsPC-1 and IMR-32. This data is representative of an average of three experiments. The values obtained from quantification of LRP were divided by the values obtained from β-actin quantification and the resultant values were used to construct the above graph. The MCF-7 values were set to 100%. The error bars represent standard deviation and Non-significant (N.S) p-value: $p > 0.05$

The adhesive potential of the tumorigenic cell lines were not significantly affected by the anti-CAT control antibody, as expected.

Invasion of pancreatic cancer and neuroblastoma cells is significantly reduced by IgG1-iS18

Invasion of the basement membrane by the tumorigenic cells is a pre-requisite for the translocation of the cell to secondary sites within the body via the process of metastasis. Matrigel™ invasion assays mimic the components of the basement membrane, allowing for the determination of the invasive potential of the respective cell lines. The three cell lines under study were treated with anti-LRP/LR specific antibody IgG1-iS18 and anti-CAT control antibody (0.2 mg/ml). AsPC-1 and IMR-32 cells proved to be significantly more invasive in comparison to the poorly-invasive MCF-7 control cell line (Fig. 6). Upon treatment with IgG1- iS18, the invasive potential of the pancreatic cancer and neuroblastoma cells were successfully reduced. The invasive potential of the tumorigenic cell lines were not significantly affected by the anti-CAT control antibody, as expected.

Discussion

Laminin is a key glycoprotein of the basement membrane and it is involved in the attachment, spreading, migration and differentiation of normal and neoplastic cells via the interaction with 37-kDa/67-kDa LRP/LR [20]. The overexpression of the 37-kDa/ 67-kDa LRP/LR in numerous tumorigenic cell lines has been implicated in the enhancement of the LRP/LR-laminin-1 interaction, as indicated by several studies [21, 22]. This enhanced interaction is therefore responsible for invasion of the basement membrane and consequent metastasis [21, 22]. Therefore, inhibiting the LRP/LR-laminin-1 interaction may be effective in impeding metastasis. This has recently been shown, where the anti-LRP/LR specific antibody IgG1-iS18 has significantly reduced the adhesive and invasive potential of cervical, lung, prostate, colon, oesophageal, breast and liver cancer cells [10–12]. In addition, Zuber et al. [23] showed that downregulation of LRP/LR with recombinant lentiviral plasmids expressing anti-LRP siRNAs, caused a reduction in invasive potential of tumorigenic HT1080 fibrosarcoma cells. The present study investigated the role of LRP/LR on the metastatic potential of pancreatic cancer (AsPC-1) and

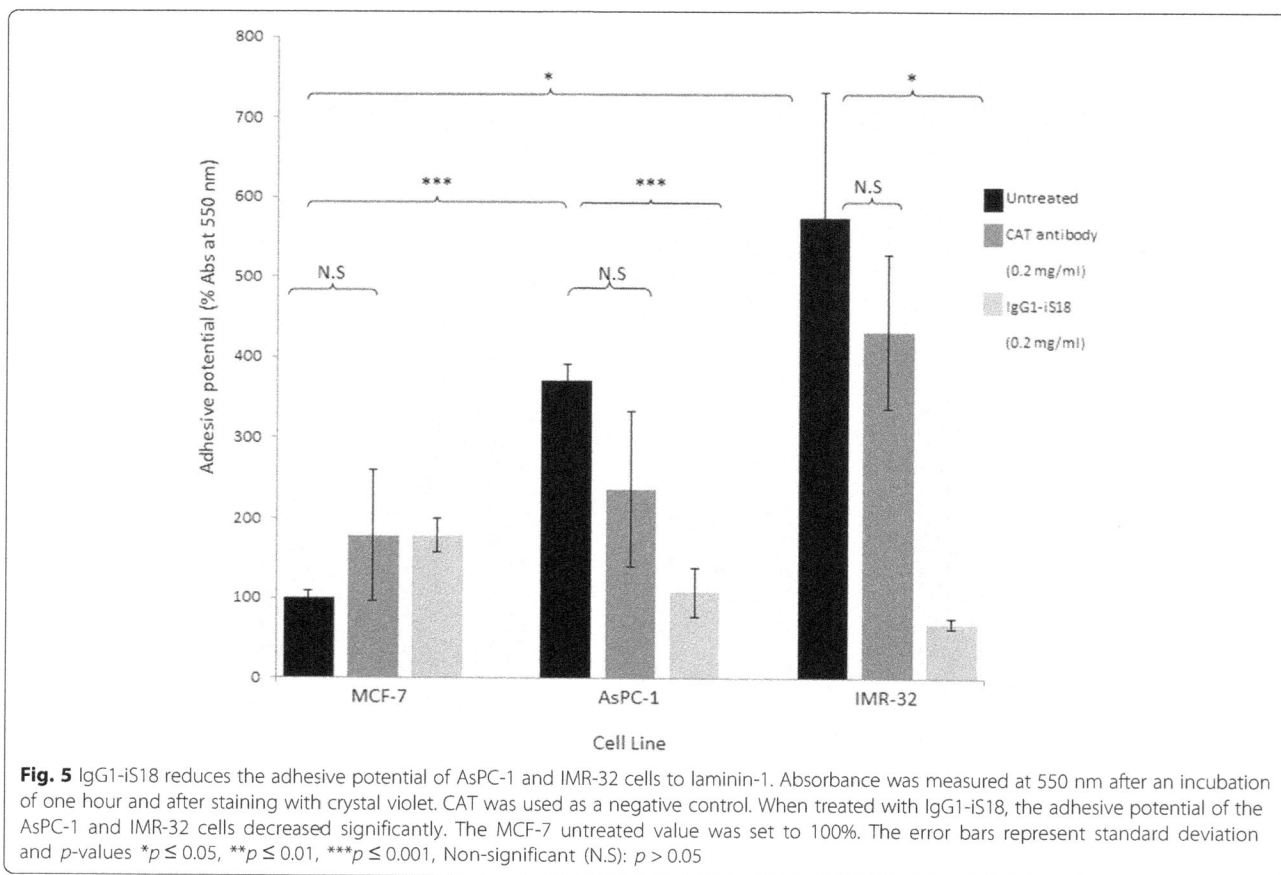

Fig. 5 IgG1-iS18 reduces the adhesive potential of AsPC-1 and IMR-32 cells to laminin-1. Absorbance was measured at 550 nm after an incubation of one hour and after staining with crystal violet. CAT was used as a negative control. When treated with IgG1-iS18, the adhesive potential of the AsPC-1 and IMR-32 cells decreased significantly. The MCF-7 untreated value was set to 100%. The error bars represent standard deviation and p-values *$p \leq 0.05$, **$p \leq 0.01$, ***$p \leq 0.001$, Non-significant (N.S): $p > 0.05$

neuroblastoma (IMR-32) cells with respect to adhesion and invasion and whether targeting the LRP/LR-laminin-1 interaction using the anti-LRP/LR specific antibody IgG1-iS18 may impede the metastatic potential of the two cancer cell lines.

All three cell lines displayed LRP/LR on the cell surface as revealed by confocal microscopy. This technique is limited by the fact that it is not quantitative, therefore further analysis using flow cytometry as well as fluorescence intensity was required in order to establish the level at which LRP/LR is displayed on the cell surface of the tumorigenic cell lines. A high percentage of cells with LRP/LR on their cell surface were displayed in the three cell lines under study. In comparison to the control cell line, it was observed that AsPC-1 cancer cells revealed significantly higher and IMR-32 cells revealed the highest cell surface LRP/LR levels. AsPC-1 and IMR-32 cancer cells are classified as metastatic, thus the high percentage of these cells displaying cell surface LRP/LR may be owing to their aggressiveness, with respect to their invasive potential.

All three cancer cell lines did display relatively similar percentages of cells that contain cell surface LRP/LR; however upon additional quantification of cell surface LRP/LR levels by analysis of fluorescence intensity, it

was observed that the level of LRP/LR displayed on the cell surface of the invasive cells in comparison to the poorly invasive cells was significantly higher.

Further analysis by Western blotting revealed the expression of the 37-kDa LRP in all three cancer cell lines, but upon densitometric analysis, the poorly invasive and invasive cell lines revealed similar total LRP/LR levels and no significant differences were therefore observed.

Total LRP/LR levels refer to cytosolic and nuclear LRP/LR in the tumorigenic cells, which serves to facilitate translational processes and maintain nuclear structures, respectively. Therefore, although there was no significant difference in total LRP/LR levels between the invasive and poorly invasive cell lines, cell surface LRP/LR levels are of importance for adhesion and consequent invasion of the cancer cell lines under study.

The correlation between cell surface LRP/LR levels to the adhesive and invasive potential of pancreatic cancer (AsPC-1) and neuroblastoma (IMR-32) cells was analysed and a high correlation was detected (Table 1). The respective correlation coefficients indicate a directly proportional and positive relationship between the two factors. This therefore confirms that the enhanced adhesive and invasive potential of the metastatic cancer cell lines under study is as a result of the high cell surface LRP/

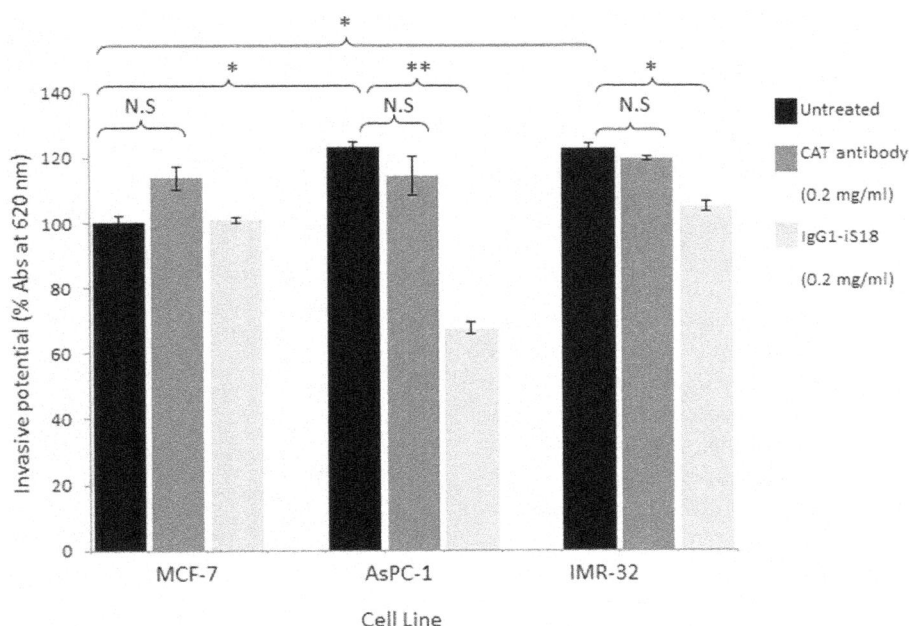

Fig. 6 IgG1-iS18 reduces the invasive potential of AsPC-1 and IMR-32 cells through the ECM-like Matrigel™. Absorbance was measured at 620 nm after an incubation of 24 h and after staining with toluidine blue. CAT was used as a negative control. When treated with IgG1-iS18, the invasive potential of the AsPC-1 and IMR-32 cells was significantly decreased, respectively. The MCF-7 untreated value was set to 100%. The error bars represent standard deviation and p-values *$p \leq 0.05$, **$p \leq 0.01$, ***$p \leq 0.001$, Non-significant (N.S): $p > 0.05$

LR levels [9]. The high correlation coefficients obtained for the adhesive to invasive potential serves as confirmation that the occurrence of adhesion is a pre-requisite for invasion. A non- significant difference in total LRP/LR levels between the cancer cell lines under study was observed and therefore only cell surface LRP/LR levels were taken into consideration in the calculations of Pearson's correlation coefficients.

The variation in the adhesive and invasive potential of both AsPC-1 and IMR-32 cell lines in comparison to the MCF-7 control cell line and how this variation may be due to differences in cell surface LRP/LR levels are demonstrated in the present study. Affirmation that the LRP/LR-laminin-1 interaction facilitates adhesion but also stimulates the secretion of enzymatic substances that degrade the basement membrane such as type IV collagenase (including matrix metalloproteinases, MMPs) is in agreement with reported results, thus suggesting the promotion of invasion and migration through the body [20]. Hence, the higher cell surface

Table 1 Pearson's correlation coefficients between cell surface LRP/LR levels and the adhesive and invasive potential of pancreatic cancer (AsPC-1) and neuroblastoma (IMR-32) cells

	LRP/LR levels to adhesive potential	LRP/LR levels to invasive potential	Adhesive to invasive potential
AsPC-1	0.996	0.981	0.994
IMR-32	0.761	0.993	0.833

LRP/LR levels detected for IMR-32 cells could be responsible for the higher adhesion of the metastatic cell to laminin-1 on the basement membrane. However, the neuroblastoma cells did not exhibit an increased invasive potential as anticipated from the high cell surface LRP/LR levels and adhesive potential. This could possibly be as a result of the expression of tissue inhibitors of metalloproteinases (TIMPs). TIMPs could therefore inhibit the activity of type IV collagenase [24], hence degradation of type IV collagen in the Matrigel is prevented, and thus preventing the invasion of IMR-32 cells in vitro [12]. The AsPC-1 cancer cells displayed high cell surface LRP/LR levels in comparison to the MCF-7 control cell line but lower expression levels than the IMR-32 cells. However, these elevated cell surface LRP/LR levels resulted in the enhanced adhesive and invasive potential of AsPC-1 cells.

It was further observed that the IgG1-iS18 antibody significantly decreased the adhesive potential of both AsPC-1 and IMR-32 cells. The invasive potential of both AsPC-1 and IMR-32 cells were also significantly reduced upon IgG1-iS18 application. The inhibition of adhesion; a mandatory step for invasion of the ECM as indicated by the high Pearson's correlation coefficients, may be the reason for the significant decrease in invasive potential.

These results suggest that the cleavage of the basal lamina is significantly enhanced by the LRP/LR-laminin-1 interaction, thus facilitating the process of invasion and migration. Furthermore, the exact mechanism by which the anti-LRP/LR specific antibody IgG1-iS18 impedes adhesion and invasion is not fully understood. However, it is possible that the two laminin binding domains (amino acid 160–180 and 205–229) on the 37-kDa/67-kDa laminin receptor LRP/LR may be directly blocked by the antibody or indirectly leading to conformational changes of the laminin binding domains, thereby changing the affinity of the binding domains for laminin.

Different cancer types exhibit different behavioural characteristics; therefore one cannot speculate that the IgG1-iS18 antibody will significantly impede the metastatic potential of all cancer types in the same manner. However, the results of the current study will indicate the use of the antibody as a possible therapeutic tool for the treatment of metastatic pancreatic cancer and neuroblastoma cells. Since LRP/LR is crucial for numerous physiological processes, targeting this receptor may prove difficult as its inhibition may further compromise the health of the patient. Therefore, studies concerning appropriate delivery systems for the IgG1-iS18 antibody should be conducted. Successful animal trials may further illustrate that this antibody is a possible therapeutic tool in the fight against metastatic cancer.

Conclusion

Anti-LRP/LR specific antibody IgG1-iS18 significantly affected the behaviour of AsPC-1 and IMR-32 cancer cells by impeding their adhesive and invasive potential in vitro, therefore suggesting that this antibody may act as a possible therapeutic tool for the treatment of metastatic pancreatic cancer and neuroblastoma. Future work will involve investigating the efficacy of the IgG1-iS18 antibody as a therapeutic tool for the prevention of several metastatic cancer types, using in vivo mouse xenograft models.

Abbreviations

APC: Allophycocyanin; AsPC-1: Human pancreatic adenocarcinoma; BCA: Bicinchroninic Acid; BSA: Bovine Serum Albumin; CAT: Chloramphenicol acetyltransferase; DMSO: Dimethyl sulfoxide; ECM: Extracellular Matrix; EDTA: Ethylenediaminetetraacetic acid; FCS: Fetal calf serum; FITC: Fluorescein isothiocyanate; HRP: Horse radish peroxidase; IgG: Immunoglobulin class G; IMR-32: Human neuroblastoma; LR: Laminin Receptor; LRP: Laminin Receptor Precursor; MCF-7: Human breast adenocarcinoma; PAGE: Polyacrylamide gel electrophoresis; PBS: Phosphate Buffered Saline; PE: Phycoerythrin; PFA: Paraformaldehyde; PVDF: Polyvinylidine fluoride; SDS: Sodium Dodecyl Sulfate

Acknowledgements

This work was supported by the National Research Foundation, the Republic of South Africa. Any opinions, findings and conclusions or recommendations expressed in this material are those of the authors, and therefore, the National Research Foundation does not accept any liability in this regard thereto. The funders had no role in study design, data collection and analysis, decision to publish or preparation of the manuscript. The research from which this publication emanated was co-funded by the South African Medical Research Council (SAMRC). We thank Affimed GmbH Heidelberg, Germany, for providing the IgG1-iS18 antibody.

Funding

The National Research Foundation (NRF), the Republic of South Africa, South African Medical Research Council (SAMRC).

Authors' contributions

SFTW conceptualized the study. TMR performed the experiments. TMR and CJC analysed the data. TMR wrote the paper. EF interpreted data and edited the manuscript. All authors participated in preparation and critical review of the final manuscript. All authors read and approved the final manuscript.

Competing interests

The authors declare that they have no competing interests in the manuscript.

References

1. Chao DL, Sanchez CA, Galipeau PC, Blount PL, Paulson TG, Cowan DS, et al. Cell proliferation, cell cycle abnormalities, and caner outcome in patients with Barrett's oesophagus: a long-term prospective study. Clin Cancer Res. 2008;14:6988–95.
2. Wong RS. Apoptosis in cancer: from pathogenesis to treatment. J Exp Clin Cancer Res. 2011;30:87.
3. Jemal A, Bray F, Melissa M, Ferlay J, Ward E, Forman D. Global Cancer Statistics. CA Cancer J Clin. 2011;61:69–90.
4. Worldwide data. http://www.wcrf.org/int/cancer-facts-figures/worldwide-data. Accessed 7 Apr 2015.
5. Gauczynski S, Peyrin J-M, Haïk S, Leucht C, Hundt C, Rieger R, Krasemann S, Deslys J-P, Dormont D, Lasmézas CI, Weiss S. The 237 kDa/67 kDa laminin receptor acts as the cell surface receptor for the cellular prionprotein. EMBO J. 2001;20:5863–75.
6. Hundt C, Peyrin J-M, Haïk S, Gauczynski S, Leucht C, Rieger R, Riley M-L, Deslys J-P, Dormont D, Lasmézas CI, Weiss S. Identification of interaction domains of the prion protein with its 37 kDa/67 kDalaminin receptor. EMBO J. 2001;20:5876–86.
7. Jovanovic K, Chetty CJ, Khumalo T, Da Costa DB, Ferreira E, Malindisa ST, et al. Novel patented therapeutic approaches targeting the 37 kDa/67 kDa laminin receptor for treatment of Cancer and Alzheimer's Disease. Expt Opin Ther Patents. 2015;25(5):567–82.
8. Buto S, Tagliabue E, Ardini E, Magnifico A, Ghirelli C, et al. Formation of the 67-kDa laminin receptor by acylation of the precursor. J Cell Biochem. 1998;69:244–51.
9. Omar A, Reusch U, Knackmuss S, Little M, Weiss SFT. Anti-LRP.LR specific antibody IgG1-iS18 significantly reduces adhesion and invasion of metastatic lung, cervix, colon and prostate cancer cells. J Mol Biol. 2012;419:102–9.
10. Vania L, Chetty CJ, Ferreira E , Weiss SFT. Anti-LRP/LR specific antibody IgG1-iS18 significantly impedes adhesion and invasion in early and late stage colorectal carcinoma cells. Mol Med. 2016; 22: 664–73.
11. Khumalo T, Reusch U, Knackmuss S, Little M, Veale RB, Weiss SFT. Adhesion and invasion of breast and oesophageal cancer cells are impeded by anti-LRP/LR-specific antibody IgG1-iS18. PLoS One. 2013;8(6):e66297.
12. Chetty C, Khumalo T, Da Costa DB, Reusch U, Knackmuss S, Little M, Weiss SFT. Anti-LRP/LR specific antibody IgG1-iS18 impedes adhesion and invasion of liver cancer cells. PLoS One. 2014. doi:10.1371/journal.pone.0096268.
13. Mbazima V, Da Costa DB, Omar A, Jovanovic K, Weiss SFT. Interactions between PrPᶜ and other ligands with the 37-kDa/67-kDa laminin receptor. Front Biosci. 2010;15:1150–63.
14. Omar A, Jovanovic K, Da Costa DB, Gonsalves D, Moodley K, Caveney R. Patented biological approaches for the therapeutic modulation of the 37-kDA/67-kDa laminin receptor. Expert Opin Ther Pat. 2011;21:35–53.
15. Vana K, Zuber C, Planz H, Kolodziejczak D, Zemora G, Bergmann AK, Weiss SFT. LRP/LR as an alternative promising target in therapy of prion diseases, Alzheimer's disease and cancer. Inf Disorder Drug Targets. 2009;9:69–80.
16. Da Costa DB, Jovanovic K, Gonsalves D, Moodley K, Reusch U, Knackmuss S, et al. Anti- LRP/LR specific antibody IgG1-iS18 and knock-down of LRP/LR by shRNAs rescue cells from Abeta42 induced cytotoxicity. Sci Rep. 2013;3:2702.
17. Jovanovic K, Loos B, Da Costa DB, Penny C, Weiss SFT. High resolution imaging study of interactions between the 37 kDa/67kDa Laminin Receptor and APP, beta-secretase and gamma-secretase in Alzheimer's disease. PLoS One. 2014;9(6):e100373.

18. Naidoo K, Malindisa ST, Otgaar TC, Bernert M, Da Costa Dias B, Ferreira E, et al. Knock-down of the 37 kDa/67kDa laminin receptor LRP/LR impedes telomerase activity. PLoS ONE. 2015; in press.

19. Givant-Horwitz V, Davidson B, Reich R. Laminin-Induced Signaling in Tumor cells: The Role of the M, 67, 000 Laminin Receptor. Cancer Res. 2004;64: 3572–9.

20. Liotta LA, Stetler SW. Tumor invasion and metastasis: an imbalance of positive and negative regulation. Cancer Res. 1991;51:50545–95.

21. Ardini E, Sporchia B, Pollegioni L, Modugno M, Ghirelli C, Castiglioni F. Identification of a novel function for 67-kDaq laminin receptor: increase in laminin degradation rate and release of motility fragments. Cancer Res. 2002;62:1321–5.

22. Ziober BL, Lin CS, Kramer RH. Laminin-binding integrins in tumor progression and metastasis. Semin Cancer Biol. 1996;7:119–28.

23. Zuber C, Mitteregger G, Schuhmann N, Rey C, Knackmuss S, Rupprecht W, Reusch U, Pace C, Little M, Kretzschmar HA, Hallek M, Büning H, Weiss S. Delivery of single-chain antibodies (scFvs) directed against the 37/67 kDa laminin receptor into mice via recombinant adeno-associated viral vectors for prion disease gene therapy. J Gen Virol. 2008;89(Pt 8):2055–61.

24. Stetler-Stevenson M, Mansoor A, Lim M, Fukushima P, Kehrl J, et al. Expression of matrix metalloproteinases and tissue inhibitors of metalloproteinases in reactive and neoplastic lymphoid cells. Blood. 1997;89: 1708–15.

15

Efficacy and safety of weekly *nab*-paclitaxel plus gemcitabine in Chinese patients with metastatic adenocarcinoma of the pancreas

Ruihua Xu[1], Xianjun Yu[2], Jihui Hao[3], Liwei Wang[4], Hongming Pan[5], Guohong Han[6], Jianming Xu[7], Yanqiao Zhang[8], Shujun Yang[9], Jia Chen[10], Jieer Ying[11], Guanghai Dai[12], Mingyu Li[13], Damir Begic[13], Brian Lu[13] and Lin Shen[14,15]*

Abstract

Background: This phase II bridging study assessed the safety and efficacy of *nab*-paclitaxel/gemcitabine (Metastatic Pancreatic Adenocarcinoma Clinical Trial [MPACT] regimen) in Chinese patients with metastatic pancreatic cancer (MPC).

Methods: This 3-part sequential study evaluated *nab*-paclitaxel 125 mg/m^2 plus gemcitabine 1000 mg/m^2 on days 1, 8, and 15 every 4 weeks. Part 1 evaluated safety. Part 2 evaluated efficacy using Simon's optimal 2-stage design: if >2 responses were observed in Stage 1 ($n = 28$), 54 additional patients would be enrolled in Stage 2. If >9 responses were observed, the study was complete. Otherwise, *nab*-paclitaxel/gemcitabine would be compared with gemcitabine alone in Part 3. The primary endpoint was overall response rate (ORR). Secondary endpoints included duration of response (DOR), overall survival (OS), and safety.

Results: Eighty-three patients were treated. The prespecified primary endpoint was met: the independently assessed ORR in Stages 1 + 2 was 35% (95% CI, 24.8–46.2); therefore, Part 3 was not initiated. The median DOR was 8.9 months (95% CI, 6.01–8.94). The median OS and progression-free survival were 9.2 (95% CI, 7.6–11.1) and 5.5 (95% CI, 5.29–7.16) months, respectively. The 12-month OS rate was 30%. In an updated analysis, the median OS was 9.3 months and the 12-month OS rate was 32%. Longer OS was observed in patients with baseline neutrophil-to-lymphocyte ratio ≤ 5 vs > 5. The most common grade ≥ 3 adverse events were leukopenia (35%), neutropenia (34%), anemia (15%), thrombocytopenia (10%), and fatigue (13%). Grade 3 peripheral neuropathy occurred in 7% of patients (no grade 4 reported).

Conclusions: The MPACT regimen of *nab*-paclitaxel/gemcitabine is efficacious in Chinese patients with MPC. No new safety signals were observed.

Keywords: *nab*-paclitaxel, Gemcitabine, MPACT, Pancreatic cancer, Metastatic, Chinese

Background

Pancreatic cancer is a growing health problem in China, where, similar to global trends, mortality nearly equals incidence [1, 2]. Epidemiological data from China's National Cancer Center Registry estimate that 79,400 people died from this disease in 2015 [3]. However, because these data are collected from multiple population-based cancer registries, they represent a small portion of the Chinese national population and may underestimate the true burden of pancreatic cancer. Similarly, a paucity of survival data exists for Chinese patients. A recent study from the Shanghai Cancer Registry reported a 5-year overall survival (OS) rate of 4.1% for all stages and tumor grades analyzed [4]. In China, approved treatment options for metastatic pancreatic cancer (MPC) are limited.

* Correspondence: linshenpku@163.com
[14]Peking University Cancer Hospital and Institute, No. 52 Fucheng Road, Haidian District, Beijing 100142, China
[15]Department of Gastrointestinal Oncology, Peking University Cancer Hospital and Institute, No. 52 Fucheng Road, Haidian District, Beijing 100142, China
Full list of author information is available at the end of the article

In the European Union and the United States, *nab*-paclitaxel in combination with gemcitabine has received approval for the first-line treatment of MPC [5, 6]. This approval was based on the global phase III Metastatic Pancreatic Adenocarcinoma Clinical Trial (MPACT), in which first-line *nab*-paclitaxel/gemcitabine treatment demonstrated a significantly better OS and overall response rate (ORR) than did gemcitabine alone in 861 patients from North America, Europe, and Australia [7, 8]. The combination of *nab*-paclitaxel/gemcitabine is also recommended for first-line treatment of patients with MPC by the National Comprehensive Cancer Network guidelines, which are often followed by Chinese physicians [9]. *nab*-Paclitaxel/gemcitabine may also be a suitable first-line treatment regimen for Chinese patients with MPC, despite known differences in cancer drug tolerability between Asian and white populations [10]. These differences may result from genetic or environmental factors, among other things, and one of the most commonly reported examples is increased chemotherapy-induced myelosuppression in Asian vs white patients [11–13]. Based on clinical trials in metastatic breast cancer, the safety profile of *nab*-paclitaxel monotherapy appears largely similar between Western and Chinese populations [14, 15]. However, limited data exist on the safety and tolerability of *nab*-paclitaxel/gemcitabine in Chinese patients. A phase I/II study evaluated this combination in Chinese patients with advanced pancreatic cancer, albeit at a dose and schedule different from that administered in MPACT [7, 8, 16]. Although the study did not meet its primary endpoint of identifying the maximum tolerated dose in Chinese patients, *nab*-paclitaxel 120 mg/m^2 (the highest dose tested) plus gemcitabine 1000 mg/m^2 on days 1 and 8 every 3 weeks was the recommended dosage/schedule for these patients. With respect to dose intensity, this regimen was comparable with the MPACT regimen and resulted in a tolerable safety profile [7, 16].

In this phase II study, the efficacy and safety of the *nab*-paclitaxel/gemcitabine regimen used in the MPACT study were evaluated in Chinese patients with MPC.

Methods

Study Population

Patients with histologically or cytologically confirmed metastatic pancreatic adenocarcinoma measurable by Response Evaluation Criteria in Solid Tumors (RECIST) version 1.0 were enrolled in this study. Key eligibility requirements included ≥18 years of age, no prior treatment for metastatic disease, Karnofsky performance status (KPS) ≥ 70, and adequate hematologic, renal, and liver function. Patients with known brain metastases or baseline peripheral neuropathy grade ≥ 2 were excluded.

This study was conducted in accordance with the Declaration of Helsinki and Good Clinical Practice Guidelines of the International Conference on Harmonisation. Informed consent was obtained from all patients prior to study entry. The trial is registered at ClinicalTrials.gov (NCT02135822).

Study Design

This phase II, multicenter, 3-part sequential study was conducted at 13 sites in China. Part 1 evaluated the dose of *nab*-paclitaxel/gemcitabine based on safety. In Part 1, 10 patients were to be enrolled and treated with *nab*-paclitaxel 125 mg/m^2 intravenously (IV) plus gemcitabine 1000 mg/m^2 IV once weekly for 3 weeks followed by a week of rest (qw 3/4). Safety data were evaluated after the last enrolled patient completed 2 treatment cycles or earlier if treatment was not tolerable or when ≥66% of patients tolerated ≥2 treatment cycles without dose delay or modification. If it was determined in Part 1 that *nab*-paclitaxel 125 mg/m^2 was the recommended dose for Part 2, the 10 patients from Part 1 were counted as a portion of the Part 2 enrollment. If the initial dose level in Part 1 was not tolerated, the Part 2 starting doses were to be reduced to *nab*-paclitaxel 100 mg/m^2 plus gemcitabine 800 mg/m^2.

Part 2 evaluated the efficacy of *nab*-paclitaxel/gemcitabine based on a single-arm, Simon's optimal 2-stage design [17]. Patients in Part 2 were treated with the *nab*-paclitaxel and gemcitabine dose levels selected from Part 1. In Stage 1, the planned enrollment was 28 patients. If >2 responses were observed, an additional 54 patients would be enrolled in Stage 2 for treatment at the same dose level. In Stage 2, if >9 of 82 responses were observed, the study would be complete. If an insufficient number of responses was observed after Stage 1 or Stage 2, the study would progress to Part 3.

Part 3 was designed to evaluate the efficacy and safety of *nab*-paclitaxel/gemcitabine vs gemcitabine alone based on a randomized 2-arm design. Planned total enrollment for Part 3 was 154 patients. Patients were to be randomized 1:1 to receive the Part 1 recommended dose of *nab*-paclitaxel followed by gemcitabine on days 1, 8, 15, 29, 36, and 43 or gemcitabine 1000 mg/m^2 IV alone weekly for 7 of 8 weeks (cycle 1). Subsequent treatments in both arms would occur on days 1, 8, and 15 of a 28-day cycle. Randomization would be stratified by liver metastasis and KPS score.

Study Assessment

The primary endpoint of the study was independently assessed ORR according to RECIST 1.0. Secondary endpoints included duration of response (DOR) according to RECIST 1.0, OS, safety, and tolerability. Exploratory endpoints were disease control rate (the percentage of patients achieving objective tumor response or stable disease for ≥16 weeks), serum carbohydrate antigen 19–9 levels and potential association with clinical outcomes, patient-reported quality of life using the European Organisation of Research and Treatment of Cancer Quality of

Life Questionnaire-Core 30, and tumor biomarker analysis. Ad hoc analyses included progression-free survival (PFS) and potential association of baseline neutrophil-to-lymphocyte ratio (NLR) and OS. Efficacy was evaluated in the intent-to-treat population, which included all enrolled patients. Response and progression were independently assessed by a central imaging reviewer, blinded to treatment, according to radiological review by computed tomography scan or magnetic resonance imaging every 8 weeks per RECIST 1.0. Treatment continued until unacceptable toxicity or disease progression. Safety was assessed on days 1, 8, 15, and 22 of each cycle by the investigator in all patients who received ≥1 dose of study drug. Adverse events (AEs) were classified by the Medical Dictionary for Regulatory Activities version 17.0 system, and severity was evaluated according to the National Cancer Institute's Common Terminology Criteria for Adverse Events version 3.0. Dose reductions, delays, premature discontinuations, and clinical laboratory data were also evaluated.

Sample Size and Statistical Analysis

In Part 2, Simon's optimal 2-stage design was used. The 1-sided hypothesis test on the ORR was H_0: ORR ≤ 7% vs H_1: ORR ≥ 19%. The hypotheses were based on the ORR results from MPACT; the observed ORR was 23% (2-sided 95% CI, 19%–27%) for the *nab*-paclitaxel/gemcitabine arm and 7% (2-sided 95% CI, 5%–10%) for gemcitabine alone. The planned sample size of 82 patients was estimated to provide 90% power at a 1-sided significance level of 0.05 [7]. The primary endpoint was analyzed based on the exact binomial distribution, and a 2-sided 95% CI was estimated using the Clopper-Pearson method. DOR, OS, OS by baseline NLR (cutoffs = 5 and median value), and PFS were analyzed by the Kaplan-Meier method. The data cutoff date was 1 June 2015. Data obtained using a cutoff date of 9 June 2016 were analyzed to determine updated OS rates. For the OS by baseline NLR subgroup analysis, the hazard ratio (HR) and 2-sided 95% CI were estimated using the nonstratified Cox proportional hazard model, and the survival distributions for the 2 baseline NLR groups were compared using the nonstratified log-rank test.

Results

Patients

In total, 83 patients were enrolled in Part 2. The baseline characteristics are described in Table 1. The median age was 57.0 years, and 19% of patients were aged ≥65 years. Most patients (70%) had a baseline KPS of 90 to 100. The median baseline carbohydrate antigen 19–9 level for all patients was 602.8 U/mL.

Efficacy Results

The initial dose administered to 15 patients in Part 1 was well tolerated; therefore, all patients in Part 2 were

Table 1 Baseline characteristics

Patient characteristics	$N = 83$
Age, median (range), years	57.0 (30–78)
≥ 65 years, %	19
Male, %	70
KPS, %	
90–100	70
70–80	30
Current site(s) of metastasis, %	
Hepatic/liver	83
Abdomen/peritoneal	53
Lung/thoracic	18
No. of metastatic sites, %	
1	35
2	43
3	19
4	2
CA 19–9, median (range), U/mL[a]	602.8 (0.93–1000)
Biliary stent, %	1

[a] CA 19–9 value above laboratory-defined upper limit of quantitation (1000 U/mL) is listed as 1000 U/mL

CA 19–9 carbohydrate antigen 19–9, *KPS* Karnofsky performance status

treated with *nab*-paclitaxel 125 mg/m^2 plus gemcitabine 1000 mg/m^2 qw 3/4. These 15 patients from Part 1 were included in Part 2. On the basis of combined results for Stages 1 and 2, the prespecified independently assessed ORR endpoint for Part 2 was met (35%; 95% CI, 24.8%–46.2%; Table 2). Although no complete responses were observed, there were 29 (35%) partial responses (PRs), and stable disease was achieved in 18 (22%) patients. Thirteen (16%) patients had progressive disease. The median DOR was 8.9 months (95% CI, 6.01–8.94), and the disease control rate was 55% (95% CI, 44.1%–66.3%; Table 2). Part 3 was not initiated per the study design (> 9 responses were observed in Part 2).

The median OS was 9.2 months (95% CI, 7.6–11.1; Fig. 1), and the 1-year OS rate was 30% (95% CI, 14%–47.6%); 15% of patients survived for ≥15 months. The median follow-up for OS was 8.9 months (range, 0.7–15.1 months). In an updated analysis approximately 1 year later, the median OS was 9.3 months, with a median follow-up of 14.6 months (range, 0.7–21.7 months). The 12-month OS rate was 32% in the follow-up analysis.

Baseline NLR ≤ 5 was associated with a longer OS vs NLR > 5, although this difference was not significant (median, 10.0 vs 8.3 months; HR, 0.617; 95% CI, 0.318–1.197; $P = 0.148$; Fig. 2). Because the n value in the >5 NLR arm was small ($n = 23$), a separate analysis using the median NLR baseline value (3.7) was performed; baseline NLR ≤ 3.7 ($n = 42$) vs > 3.7 ($n = 41$) was also associated with a longer OS, but the difference was not

Table 2 Efficacy

Outcome[a]	nab-P + Gem N = 83
ORR, n (%)	29 (35)
CR	0
PR	29 (35)
SD, n (%)	18 (22)
PD, n (%)	13 (16)
Not evaluable, n (%)	15 (18)
No postbaseline assessment, n (%)	8 (10)
DCR, n (%)[b]	46 (55)
DOR, median (95% CI), months	8.9 (6.01–8.94)
OS, median (95% CI), months	9.2 (7.6–11.1)
OS rate, %	
3 months	89
6 months	70
9 months	53
12 months	30
15 months	15
Progression-free survival, median (95% CI), months	5.5 (5.29–7.16)

CR complete response, DCR disease control rate, DOR duration of response, Gem gemcitabine, nab-P nab-paclitaxel, ORR overall response rate, OS overall survival, PD progressive disease, PR partial response, SD stable disease
[a]Percents may not add up to 100 due to rounding
[b]Defined as the percentage of patients achieving objective tumor response or SD for ≥16 weeks

significant (median, 10.0 vs 8.1 months; HR, 0.724; 95% CI, 0.398–1.319; P = 0.288). The median PFS was 5.5 months (95% CI, 5.29–7.16; Fig. 3).

Treatment Exposure

For all patients, the median duration of treatment was 4.8 months, and the median number of treatment cycles was 5 (range, 1–12). Forty-nine percent of patients had ≥1

nab-paclitaxel dose reduction, and 51% of patients had ≥1 gemcitabine dose reduction, most due to AEs. The most common AEs leading to dose reduction of nab-paclitaxel and gemcitabine were thrombocytopenia (14% and 20%), neutropenia (14% and 16%), and leukopenia (11% and 13%), respectively. At least 1 nab-paclitaxel or gemcitabine dose delay occurred in 37% of patients. The median cumulative doses of nab-paclitaxel and gemcitabine were 1500 and 12,000 mg/m^2, respectively. The median dose intensities of nab-paclitaxel and gemcitabine were 79 and 627 mg/m^2/week, respectively. The median percentages of per-protocol dose of nab-paclitaxel and gemcitabine were 85% and 84%, respectively.

Safety

Seventy-five percent of patients experienced ≥1 grade ≥ 3 AE (Table 3). The most common grade ≥ 3 AEs were leukopenia (35%), neutropenia (34%), anemia (15%), thrombocytopenia (10%), and fatigue (13%). Grade 3 peripheral neuropathy occurred in only 7% of patients (no grade 4 reported). Twenty-four percent of patients reported ≥1 serious treatment-emergent AE. Discontinuations due to AEs were relatively low (11%).

Discussion

In this phase II study, the MPACT regimen (nab-paclitaxel 125 mg/m^2 plus gemcitabine 1000 mg/m^2) was efficacious and safe as first-line treatment of Chinese patients with MPC. Per protocol, the study did not progress to Part 3 because >9 responses were observed during Part 2 and the study was considered complete. Although no complete responses were observed in this study, 35% of patients had a partial response, and the median DOR was 8.9 months, indicating a durable response. The median OS was 9.2 months, and the OS rate at 1 year was 30% (9.3 months and 32%, respectively, in an updated analysis). The regimen appeared to

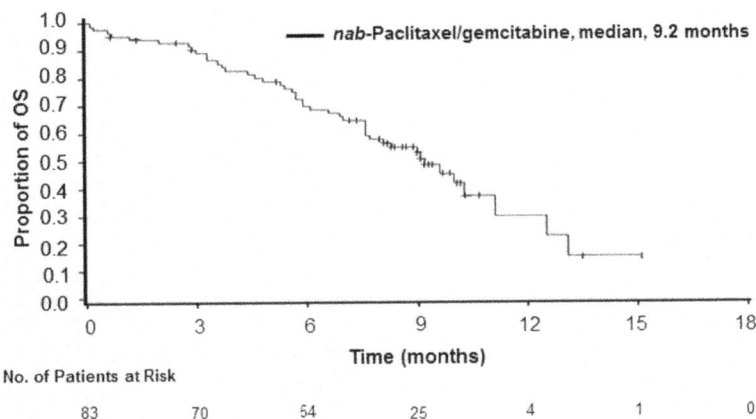

Fig. 1 Kaplan-Meier curve of overall survival (OS) in Chinese patients with metastatic pancreatic cancer (MPC)

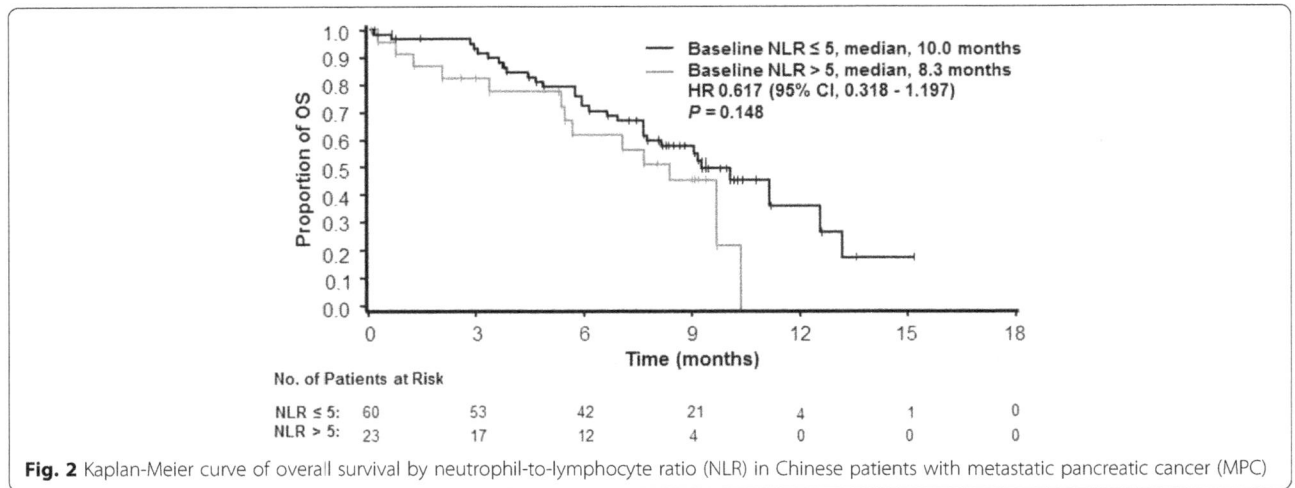

Fig. 2 Kaplan-Meier curve of overall survival by neutrophil-to-lymphocyte ratio (NLR) in Chinese patients with metastatic pancreatic cancer (MPC)

be well tolerated in Chinese patients with MPC, and no new safety signals were identified compared with those observed in the MPACT population [7].

Efficacy results in this study of Chinese patients were comparable with those reported in MPC trials using the same *nab*-paclitaxel/gemcitabine regimen in Western countries and Japan [7, 8, 18]. In the MPACT population, treatment with this *nab*-paclitaxel/gemcitabine regimen resulted in a median OS of 8.7 months compared with 9.2 months in the Chinese population (Table 4) [8]. Similar to the findings of MPACT, Chinese patients with a baseline NLR ≤ 5 had a longer OS compared with those with a baseline NLR > 5. The ORR was 23% in MPACT and 35% in the Chinese population, although treatment resulted in a slightly longer DOR in the global study (11.1 months in the MPACT population and 8.9 months in the Chinese population) [19]. In both populations, the median PFS was 5.5 months.

Although data from other studies of Chinese patients treated with *nab*-paclitaxel/gemcitabine are limited, a phase I/II study evaluated 3 different doses of *nab*-paclitaxel (80 mg/m^2, 100 mg/m^2, and 120 mg/m^2) in combination with gemcitabine 1000 mg/m^2, both given weekly for 2 weeks in a 21-day cycle in Chinese patients with advanced pancreatic cancer [16]. In that study, the maximum tolerated dose was not met; however, in the 12 patients treated with *nab*-paclitaxel 120 mg/m^2, the median OS and PFS were 12.2 and 5.2 months, respectively, and the ORR was 42%. Similar to the findings in our study, common grade 3/4 toxicities that were associated with the 120 mg/m^2 dose included neutropenia (17%) and thrombocytopenia (8%), and grade 3/4 sensory neuropathy occurred in only 1 patient. In a trial of Japanese patients with MPC, outcomes of treatment with the *nab*-paclitaxel/gemcitabine MPACT regimen were also higher/longer compared with the outcomes in the MPACT population [18]. These findings further support the use of the MPACT regimen for the treatment of Asian patients with MPC.

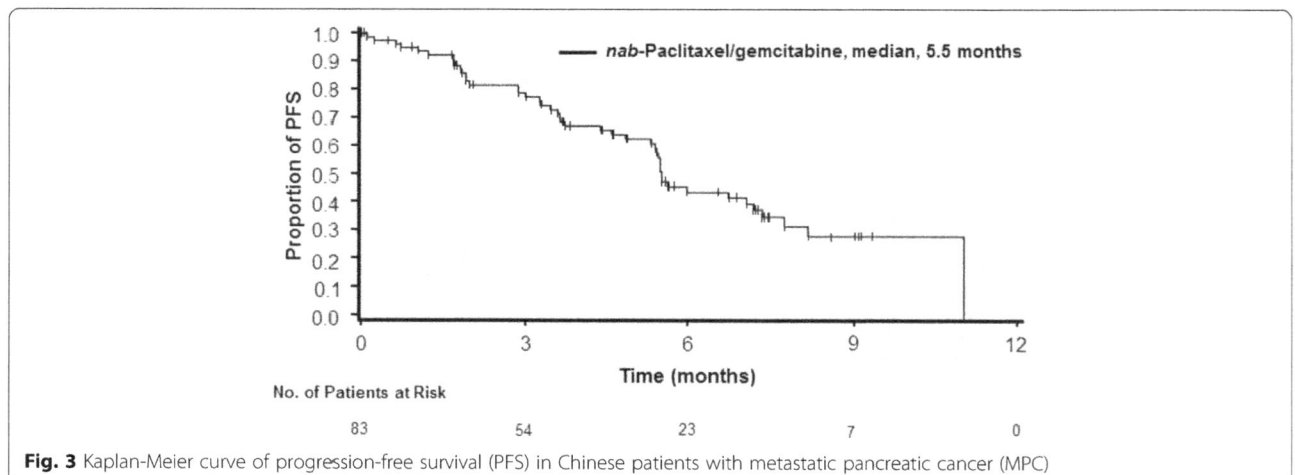

Fig. 3 Kaplan-Meier curve of progression-free survival (PFS) in Chinese patients with metastatic pancreatic cancer (MPC)

Table 3 Grade ≥ 3 treatment-emergent adverse events in ≥10% of patients

Grade ≥ 3 adverse events, n (%)	nab-P + Gem N = 83
Pts with at least 1 grade ≥ 3 AE	62 (75)
Hematologic AEs[a]	
Leukopenia	28 (35)
Neutropenia	27 (34)
Anemia	12 (15)
Thrombocytopenia	8 (10)
Nonhematologic AEs	
Fatigue	11 (13)

AE adverse event, Gem gemcitabine, nab-P nab-paclitaxel
[a]Based on laboratory values; n = 80 patients assessed

In the current study, the most common treatment-emergent grade ≥ 3 AEs were leukopenia, neutropenia, anemia, thrombocytopenia, and fatigue. Similarly, the most common grade ≥ 3 AEs in MPACT were neutropenia, leukopenia, thrombocytopenia, anemia, fatigue, and peripheral neuropathy [7]. The incidence of peripheral neuropathy was one noteworthy difference between these two trials. In the MPACT population, 17% of patients experienced grade ≥ 3 peripheral neuropathy compared with only 7% of Chinese patients in this study. The definitive reasons for this are unclear, and many factors, such as ethnic differences or regional variations in treatments for neuropathy, could be involved [20, 21]; this would be an interesting topic to investigate in the future. In addition, nab-paclitaxel treatment modifications due to AEs were less frequent in the MPACT population compared with the Chinese population [7]. nab-Paclitaxel dose reductions occurred in 41% and 49% of patients in MPACT and the Chinese study, respectively.

Table 4 Efficacy Outcomes of nab-paclitaxel plus gemcitabine in MPACT and the Chinese study

Parameter	MPACT [7, 8, 19]	Chinese Study
n	431	83
OS, median, months	8.7	9.2
NLR ≤ 5	9.1	10.0
NLR > 5	5.0	8.3
PFS, median, months[a]	5.5	5.5
ORR, %[a]	23	35
DCR, %	48	55
DOR, median, months	11.1	8.9

DCR disease control rate, DOR duration of response, NLR neutrophil-to-lymphocyte ratio, MPACT Metastatic Pancreatic Adenocarcinoma Clinical Trial, ORR overall response rate, OS overall survival, PFS progression-free survival
[a]Independently assessed

Results from this phase II study in Chinese patients are positive; however, several factors must be considered to put the data in perspective. Although this was a bridging study to assess the safety and efficacy of nab-paclitaxel/gemcitabine in Chinese patients, one limitation was the homogeneous population. However, the impact of this limitation may have been addressed by the study's multicenter sampling. In addition, efficacy was evaluated based on a single treatment arm rather than on a comparison of outcomes between 2 randomized groups. The results described here in Chinese patients are similar to those of the global MPACT study, though cross-trial comparisons should be interpreted with caution because of differences in factors such as patient population and usual supportive care. For example, in our study, a higher percentage of Chinese patients had a better baseline performance status (KPS of 90–100) than patients in the global MPACT population (70% vs 58%) [7]. Therefore, when comparing these 2 studies, it is possible that this difference could, in part, account for the improved efficacy outcomes observed in this study compared with the MPACT study. Further, although only the first 2 parts of the 3-part study design were executed, the null hypothesis was rejected as more than 9 of the 82 patients (planned sample size) responded. Although Part 3 would have provided more rigor to the overall statistical testing of nab-paclitaxel/gemcitabine vs gemcitabine in this disease setting, it would only have been triggered if sufficient activity was not observed vs known historical data in Part 2. Such adaptive trial designs are generally more efficient, requiring fewer patients to answer research questions. This unique study design was particularly beneficial and relevant in this disease setting and helped to avoid enrolling Chinese patients into an inferior treatment arm, as a large global study has established the significant clinical benefit of nab-paclitaxel/gemcitabine vs gemcitabine.

Conclusion

The nab-paclitaxel/gemcitabine regimen used in MPACT was efficacious and well tolerated in Chinese patients with MPC, supporting the use of this combination regimen in this patient population.

Abbreviations
AE: adverse event; DOR: duration of response; HR: hazard ratio; IV: intravenously; KPS: Karnofsky performance status; MPACT: Metastatic Pancreatic Adenocarcinoma Clinical Trial; MPC: metastatic pancreatic cancer; NLR: neutrophil-to-lymphocyte ratio; ORR: overall response rate; OS: overall survival; PFS: progression-free survival; PR: partial response; qw 3/4: the first 3 of 4 weeks; RECIST: Response Evaluation Criteria in Solid Tumors

Acknowledgements
The authors thank Richard Xue, Lotus Yung, and Xinyu Wei of Celgene Corporation for their support. Medical writing assistance was provided by Dena Jacob, PhD, of MediTech Media, funded by Celgene Corporation. The authors are fully responsible for all content and editorial decisions for this manuscript.

Funding

Funding received from Celgene Corporation. Celgene was involved in the development of the protocol and analysis of the data. All authors, including those authors listed as employees of Celgene were involved in the writing, review, and provided final approval of the manuscript.

Authors' contributions

ML, DB, BL analyzed and interpreted the patient data regarding all study endpoints and safety. RX, XY, JH, LW, HP, GH, JX, YZ, SY, JC, JY, GD, ML, DB, BL, and LS collected data, were contributors to the writing of the manuscript, reviewed, and provided final approval of the manuscript.

Authors' information

Not applicable

Competing interests

LS, RX, XY, JH, LW, HP, GH, JX, YZ, SY, JC, JY, and GD have nothing to disclose. ML, DB, and BL are employees of and have stock ownership in Celgene Corporation.

Author details

[1]Sun Yat-sen University Cancer Center, 651 Dongfeng East Road, Guangzhou 510060, China. [2]Fudan University Shanghai Cancer Center, No 270, Dongan Road, Shanghai 200032, China. [3]Tianjin Cancer Hospital, Huan-Hu-Xi Road, Tianjin 300060, China. [4]Renji Hospital, Shanghai Jiaotong University, 160 Pujian Lu, Shanghai 200127, China. [5]Sir Run Run Shaw Hospital, Zhejiang University, 3 East Qingchun Road, Hangzhou City 310016, China. [6]Xijing Hospital, W Rd, Xi'an, Changle 127, China. [7]307 Hospital of the People's Liberation Army, Beijing 100021, China. [8]Harbin Medical University Cancer Hospital, Haping Road No.150, Harbin, China. [9]Henan Cancer Hospital, Zhengzhou 450003, China. [10]Jiangsu Provincial Tumor Hospital, 300 Guangzhou Road, Nanjing 210029, China. [11]Zhejiang Cancer Hospital, 38 Guangji Road, Banshan Bridge, Hangzhou City 310022, China. [12]Chinese People's Liberation Army General Hospital No.28, Fuxing Road, Beijing, China. [13]Celgene Corporation, Summit, NJ, USA. [14]Peking University Cancer Hospital and Institute, No. 52 Fucheng Road, Haidian District, Beijing 100142, China. [15]Department of Gastrointestinal Oncology, Peking University Cancer Hospital and Institute, No. 52 Fucheng Road, Haidian District, Beijing 100142, China.

References

1. Lin QJ, Yang F, Jin C, Current FDL. Status and progress of pancreatic cancer in China. World J Gastroenterol. 2015;21(26):7988–8003.
2. World Health Organization. GLOBOCAN 2012: Estimated Cancer Incidence, Mortality and Prevalence Worldwide in 2012. http://globocan.iarc.fr/Pages/fact_sheets_cancer.aspx. Accessed 17 Sept 2015.
3. Chen W, Zheng R, Baade PD, Zhang S, Zeng H, Bray F, et al. Cancer statistics in China, 2015. CA Cancer J Clin. 2016;66(2):115–32.
4. Luo J, Xiao L, Wu C, Zheng Y, Zhao N. The incidence and survival rate of population-based pancreatic cancer patients: shanghai cancer registry 2004-2009. PLoS One. 2013;8(10):e76052.
5. Abraxane for injectable suspension (paclitaxel protein-bound particles for injectable suspension) (albumin-bound). Summit, NJ: Celgene Corporation. 2015.
6. European Medicines Agency. Summary of opinion: Abraxane. http://www.ema.europa.eu/docs/en_GB/document_library/Summary_of_opinion/human/000778/WC500155465.pdf. Accessed 21 Nov 2013.
7. Von Hoff DD, Ervin T, Arena FP, Chiorean EG, Infante J, Moore M, et al. Increased survival in pancreatic cancer with nab-paclitaxel plus gemcitabine. N Engl J Med. 2013;369(18):1691–703.
8. Goldstein D, El-Maraghi RH, Hammel P, Heinemann V, Kunzmann V, Sastre J, et al. Nab-paclitaxel plus gemcitabine for metastatic pancreatic cancer: long-term survival from a phase III trial. J Natl Cancer Inst. 2015;107(2) https://doi.org/10.1093/jnci/dju413.
9. NCCN Clinical Practice Guidelines in Oncology. Pancreatic Adenocarcinoma. V1.2016. Available at: http://www.nccn.org/professionals/physician_gls/f_guidelines.asp#site. Accessed 15 July 2012.
10. Ling WH, Lee SC. Inter-ethnic differences–how important is it in cancer treatment? Ann Acad Med Singap. 2011;40(8):356–61.
11. O'Donnell PH, Dolan ME. Cancer pharmacoethnicity: ethnic differences in susceptibility to the effects of chemotherapy. Clin Cancer Res. 2009;15(15):4806–14.
12. Ma B, Yeo W, Hui P, Ho WM, Johnson PJ. Acute toxicity of adjuvant doxorubicin and cyclophosphamide for early breast cancer – a retrospective review of Chinese patients and comparison with an historic western series. Radiother Oncol. 2002;62(2):185–9.
13. Dattani N, Altham D, Coady K. Neutropenia in Asian patients with solid tumors receiving chemotherapy: a retrospective case-control study. J Solid Tumors. 2016;6(2):25–9.
14. Gradishar WJ, Tjulandin S, Davidson N, Shaw H, Desai N, Bhar P, et al. Phase III trial of nanoparticle albumin-bound paclitaxel compared with polyethylated castor oil-based paclitaxel in women with breast cancer. J Clin Oncol. 2005;23(31):7794–803.
15. Guan Z-Z, Li QL, Feng F, Jiang Z, Shen Z, Yu S, et al. Superior efficacy of a Cremophor-free albumin-bound paclitaxel compared with solvent-based paclitaxel in Chinese patients with metastatic breast cancer. Asia Pac J Clin Oncol. 2009;5(3):165–74.
16. Zhang DS, Wang DS, Wang ZQ, Wang FH, Luo HY, Qiu MZ, et al. Phase I/II study of albumin-bound nab-paclitaxel plus gemcitabine administered to Chinese patients with advanced pancreatic cancer. Cancer Chemother Pharmacol. 2013;71(4):1065–72.
17. Simon R. Optimal two-stage designs for phase II clinical trials. Control Clin Trials. 1989;10(1):1–10.
18. Kasuga A, Ueno H, Ikeda M, Ueno M, Mizuno N, Ioka T, et al. Efficacy, safety and pharmacokinetics of weekly nab-paclitaxel plus gemcitabine in Japanese patients with metastatic pancreatic cancer (MPC): phase I/II trial. Presented at: APA/JPS 45th Anniversary Meeting; November 5–8, 2014; Big Island, HI, USA [abstr. 14200].
19. Shen L, Hao J, Wang L, Pan H, Han G, Xu J, et al. A phase II study of Chinese patients (pts) treated with nab-paclitaxel (nab-P) plus gemcitabine for metastatic pancreatic cancer (MPC). J Clin Oncol. 2016;34(4) [abstr. 327].
20. McQuade JL, Meng Z, Chen Z, Wei Q, Zhang Y, Bei W, et al. Utilization of and attitudes towards traditional Chinese medicine therapies in a Chinese cancer hospital: a survey of patients and physicians. Evid Based Complement Alternat Med. 2012;2012:504507.
21. Lee KH, Chang HJ, Han SW, DY O, Im SA, Bang YJ, et al. Pharmacogenetic analysis of adjuvant FOLFOX for Korean patients with colon cancer. Cancer Chemother Pharmacol. 2013;71(4):843–51.

16

Prognostic relevance of lactate dehydrogenase in advanced pancreatic ductal adenocarcinoma patients

Yuanyuan Xiao[1,2†], Wen Chen[3†], Zhihui Xie[3], Zhenyi Shao[3], Hua Xie[3], Guoyou Qin[1,4*] and Naiqing Zhao[1,4*]

Abstract

Background: The prognostic role of pretreatment serum lactate dehydronegase (LDH) has been well established in many malignant tumors, albeit it remains under-discussed in pancreatic cancer. In the present study, we aimed to assess the association between baseline LDH levels and overall survival (OS) in advanced pancreatic ductal adenocarcinoma (PDAC) patients who did and did not receive subsequent chemotherapy.

Methods: In total, 135 retrospectively determined patients with locally advanced or metastatic PDAC, who were diagnosed between 2012 and 2013, were analyzed. Baseline LDH levels were detected within 20 days after histopathological confirmation of the diagnosis. Multivariate Cox proportional hazards regression model was applied to estimate the adjusted hazards ratio (HR) for LDH levels and OS of PDAC. We used restricted cubic spline (RCS) to further investigate dose-effect relationship in the association.

Results: Having adjusted for possible confounders, we found that in advanced PDAC patients who went through subsequent chemotherapy, an elevated pretreatment LDH level ($\geq$250 U/L) had an adjusted HR of 2.47 (95% CI = 1.28–4.77) for death, but patients, who did not receive chemotherapy, had no significant HR (adjusted HR = 1.57; 95% CI = 0.83–2.96). RCS fitting results revealed a steep increase in HR for PDAC patients received chemotherapy with a baseline LDH > 500 U/L.

Conclusions: Pretreatment LDH levels had noticeable prognostic value in PDAC patients who received subsequent chemotherapy. Tackling elevated LDH levels before the initiation of chemotherapy might be a promising measure for improving OS of patients after treatment for their advanced PDAC. Studies with a large sample size and a prospective design are warranted to substantiate our findings.

Keywords: Lactate dehydrogenase, Advanced pancreatic ductal adenocarcinoma, Survival analysis, Restricted cubic spline

Background

In metabolic perspective, the most distinctive feature of cancer cells is the enhanced glycolytic activity even under sufficient oxygen supply, which is well known as the "Warburg effect" [1]. As a solid tumor which featured in hypoxia, some newly uncovered evidence has suggested that the "Warburg effect" may play a central role in the initiation, progression, and invasion of pancreatic cancer [2].

In the end of glycolysis process, lactate dehydrogenase (LDH) is involved as the catalyst in transforming pyruvate into lactate. It has been found that *LDHA* gene expression is up-regulated in many human malignant tumors, such as cancers of the esophagus [3], stomach [4], lung [5], colorectum [6], and more recently, pancreas [7].

The over-expression of *LDHA* inevitably promotes the production of LDH by cancer cells. Thus, the prognostic value of serum LDH levels in cancer has long been a topic of considerable research interest. Currently, the hazardous role of an elevated pretreatment LDH levels in survival of patients with small-cell lung cancer, naso-pharyngeal cancer, colon cancer, and aggressive lymphoid

* Correspondence: gyqin@fudan.edu.cn; nqzhao1954@163.com
†Equal contributors
[1]Department of Biostatistics, School of Public Health, Fudan University, 130 Dong'an Road, Shanghai, China
Full list of author information is available at the end of the article

cancers has been well established [8–13]. However, the association between serum LDH levels and pancreatic cancer survival has only been discussed at a very limited scale, although several published studies reached a consensus in supporting an inverse association [14–19]. Because published studies generally focused on advanced pancreatic cancer patients who received palliative chemotherapy, it is not clear whether the prognostic relevance of baseline LDH levels also exists in patients who are precluded from chemotherapy, which is another issue of potential clinical relevance, albeit it has never been discussed.

In the present study, we aimed to assess the association between baseline LDH levels and overall survival (OS) in advanced pancreatic ductal adenocarinoma (PDAC) patients who did and did not receive chemotherapy. Moreover, we further analyzed the dose-effect relationship in the association between LDH and OS of PDAC.

Methods

Study design

The study population consisted of 135 PDAC patients diagnosed between January 1, 2012 and December 31, 2013. All patients were retrospectively determined in a mega population-based electronic inpatients database originated from Shanghai metropolitan area, China. Other than histopathological confirmation, inclusion criteria for PDAC patients were: 1) locally advanced or metastasis occurred, already missed the opportunity for curative operation; 2) survival length, defined as time interval between the date of diagnosis and the date of death, surpassed 30 days; 3) vital information for analysis, such as age, sex, baseline (defined as within 20 days after PDAC confirmation) serum LDH and albumin test results, and chemotherapy regimens, was complete.

The outcome of interest was OS, and the date of death for PDAC patients was acquired through external matching with death registration system. The deadline of matching was set as January 31, 2015. The study protocol was reviewed and approved by Institutional Research Ethics Board of Fudan University, because of the retrospective nature, plus no individually identifiable or sensitive information was involved, informed consents from all patients had been waived.

General characteristics of 135 PDAC patients we studied are described in Table 1. The mean age of patients was 65.56 years, with a standard deviation of 10.91 years. The numbers of males and females were comparable. The longest survival length of PDAC patients was 965 days, and the shortest was 31 days. The median survival time was 214 days. Means of baseline LDH and albumin levels were 216.04 units/liter (U/L) and 38.61 g/L, respectively. Overall, 68 patients received subsequent

Table 1 General characteristics of PDAC patients analyzed ($N = 135$)

Characteristic	Mean (Std.)/ Median	Count (%)
Age (yrs)	65.56 (10.91)	-
Survival length (days)	214	-
Baseline LDH (U/L)	216.04 (90.96)	-
Baseline albumin (g/L)	38.61 (5.09)	-
Sex (Male)	-	65 (48.15)
Subsequent chemotherapy (Yes)	-	68 (50.37)
Gemcitabine only	-	12 (17.65)
Gemcitabine combined chemotherapy	-	50 (73.53)
Other chemotherapy regimen	-	6 (8.82)

chemotherapy, which accounted for 50.37%. Among the 68 patients who received chemotherapy, over 90% received gemcitabine alone or in combination with other agents and over 80% ($N = 116$) died before the pre-designated matching deadline.

Variables and definitions

A normal level of serum LDH is usually defined as less than 250 U/L. We used this cutoff-value to dichotomize PDAC patients into "normal LDH" and "elevated LDH" groups based on the baseline test results. Baseline serum albumin levels were defined as "normal" (≥ 35 g/L) and "decreased" (< 35 g/L) accordingly. Palliative chemotherapy was defined as the administration of one or more following medications that are commonly used for treatment of PDAC in China: gemcitabine, nab-Paclitaxel, 5-fluorouracil, Irinotecan, and Oxaliplatin.

Statistical analysis

Descriptive statistics were used to illustrate or compare characteristics within or between PDAC patients from different baseline LDH groups. Multivariate Cox proportional hazards regression model was applied to estimate the adjusted hazards ratio associated with LDH levels. Finally, considering the arbitrariness which might have been introduced by pre-designated cutoff for baseline LDH levels, a continuous variable, as well as the possibility of nonlinear relationship, we adopted restrictive cubic spline (RCS) to discuss the dose-effect relationship in the association between LDH and death hazards in PDAC patients who did and did not receive chemotherapy separately. We chose three knots to fit RCS: the 5th, 50th, and 95th percentiles of LDH levels.

All statistical analyses were executed by SAS (version 9.2, SAS Institute Inc., Cary, NC, USA), and the significance level for test or inference was set as two-tailed probability < 0.05.

Results

Overall survival of PDAC patients with different baseline LDH levels

By applying the aforementioned cutoffs for LDH and albumin levels, 30 (22.22%) patients recorded an elevated baseline LDH level, while 26 (19.26%) presented decreased baseline albumin level. There are significant distributional differences in age at diagnosis and albumin levels between PDAC patients with normal and elevated baseline LDH levels, and the OS was comparatively inferior for PDAC patients with elevated LDH levels (Table 2).

For subsequent chemotherapy, we sketched Kaplan-Meier survival curves with regard to baseline LDH levels: for both groups of patients, an elevated baseline LDH level was associated with significantly compromised OS (Fig. 1).

Independent association between baseline LDH levels and OS of PDAC

The serum LDH level is also an indicator of liver function, and because of anatomic vicinity, advanced pancreatic cancer usually metastases to the liver, leading to a decreased liver function in turn [20]. Therefore, when constructing multivariate Cox model, we further included the serum albumin level, a more sensitive indicator of liver function to adjust for possible confounding. Cox model fitting results are enumerated in Table 3. For advanced PDAC patients who underwent subsequent palliative chemotherapy, univariate Cox model found that pretreatment LDH level was significantly associated with deteriorated survival (crude HR = 2.34; 95% CI = 1.23–4.45), and this notable association was maintained in the multivariate model: compared with patients having a normally ranged LDH level, an elevated LDH level was associated with an HR of 2.47 (95% CI = 1.28–4.77). For PDAC patients who did not accept chemotherapy, initially a prominent association between baseline LDH levels and OS has been discerned (crude HR = 1.91; 95% CI = 1.04–3.47), but after adjustment for possible confounders, this association was insignificant (adjusted HR = 1.57; 95% CI = 0.83–2.96).

Dose-response association between baseline LDH and OS of PDAC

RCS fitting results disclosed that, in general, the dose-response trend between pretreatment LDH levels and HR was less apparent. In advanced PDAC patients who received chemotherapy, LDH levels higher than 500 U/L were associated with a significantly increased HR. On the contrary, in PDAC patients who did not receive chemotherapy, the change of baseline LDH levels showed an insignificant influence on OS (Fig. 2).

Discussion

In the present study, we discussed the influence of LDH levels measured right after cancer diagnosis on OS of patients with advanced PDAC. Based on multivariate Cox model and RCS, we observed that, for patients who received subsequent palliative chemotherapy, an elevated baseline LDH level was associated with nearly 2.5 folds hazards of death, whereas for patients who did not receive chemotherapy, this association was not statistically significant.

Serum LDH levels are widely accepted as indicators of tissue breakdown. In cancer patients, because of enhanced proliferation capacity, the cycle of cancer cells will be shortened, which in turn causes an increased risk of necrosis. Besides, vicinal normal tissues can be encroached upon and destructed by cancer cells [21]. All these mechanisms, along with enhanced glycolysis, may collectively contribute to increased serum LDH levels in cancer patients. In this sense, LDH levels can actually partly reflect tumor burden. It has been suggested that, high concentration of lactate can promote tumor progression and metastasis through up-regulation of tumor growth factors, such as vascular endothelial growth factor and hypoxia-inducible factor 1α, or through the direct enhancement of cellular motility [22]. More recently, Rong et al. found that LDH directly promotes the growth of pancreatic cancer cells [7]. Thus, it is reasonable to suspect that the significant inverse association between baseline LDH levels and survival we found in advanced PDAC patients who received chemotherapy can partly be attributed to tumor burden or pro-progression nature of LDH. As to the reason that why this association was not

Table 2 Distributional differences in general characteristics for PDAC patients of different baseline LDH levels

Characteristics	Normal baseline LDH (N = 105)	Elevated baseline LDH (N = 30)	p value
Age at diagnosis (Yrs, mean, std.)	65.04 (9.94)	67.37 (13.81)	0.02[a]
Sex (Male, %)	51 (48.57)	14 (46.67)	1.00[b]
Baseline albumin (Deceased, %)	16 (15.24)	10 (33.33)	0.04[b]
Subsequent chemotherapy (Yes, %)	55 (52.38)	13 (43.33)	0.41[b]
Survival length (Days, Median)	238	96	<0.01[c]

[a]By t test [b]By Fisher's exact test [c]By log-rank test

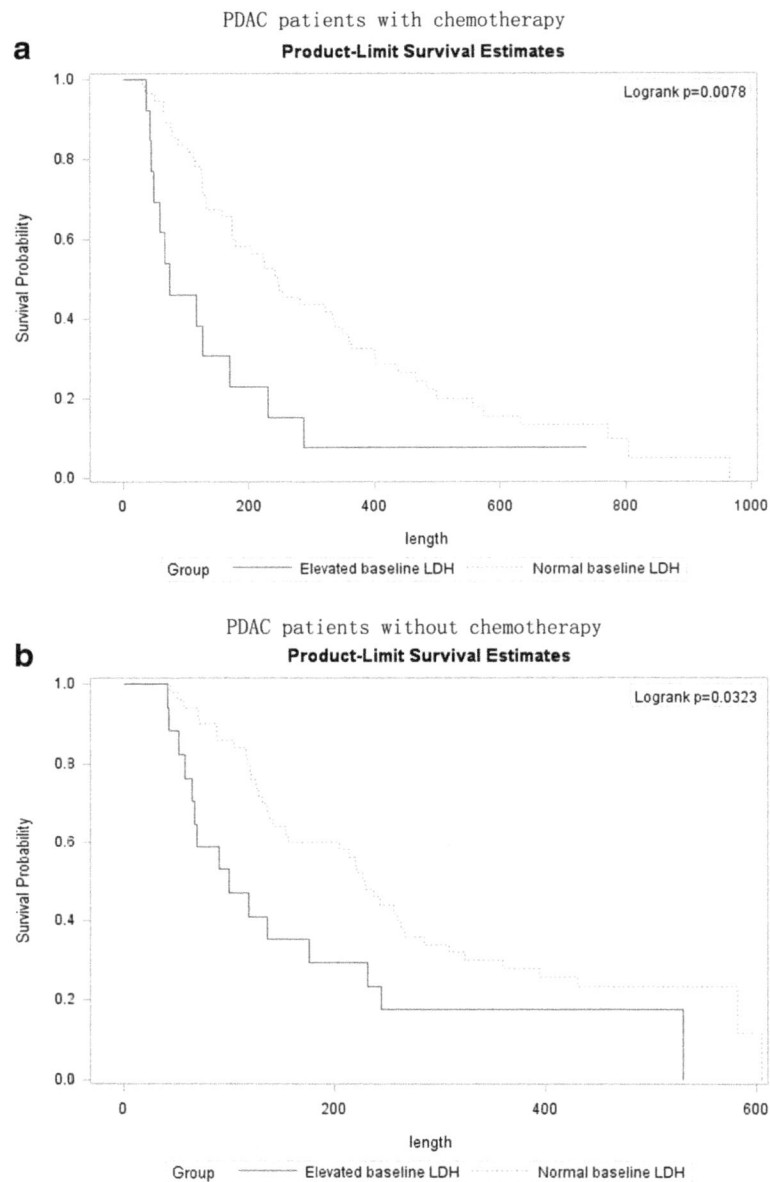

Fig. 1 Kaplan-Meier curves illustrating overall survival status by baseline LDH levels in two groups of advanced PDAC patients. **a** PDAC patients with chemotherapy; **b** PDAC patients withoutchemotherapy

Table 3 Multivariate Cox regression model fitting results by acceptance of chemotherapy in advanced PDAC patients

Independent variables	Chemotherapy group		Non-chemotherapy group	
	Crude HR (95% CI)	Adjusted HR (95% CI)	Crude HR (95% CI)	Adjusted HR (95% CI)
Age at diagnosis (+5 years)	1.09 (0.94–1.25)	1.06 (0.94–1.20)	1.17 (1.03–1.33)	1.14 (1.00–1.30)
Sex (Male)	0.64 (0.38–1.07)	0.67 (0.39–1.14)	0.90 (0.53–1.55)	0.89 (0.50–1.56)
Baseline albumin (Decreased)	3.14 (1.67–5.89)	3.27 (1.70–6.27)	1.24 (0.62–2.47)	1.06 (0.51–2.21)
Baseline LDH (Elevated)	2.34 (1.23–4.45)	2.47 (1.28–4.77)	1.91 (1.04–3.47)	1.57 (0.83–2.96)

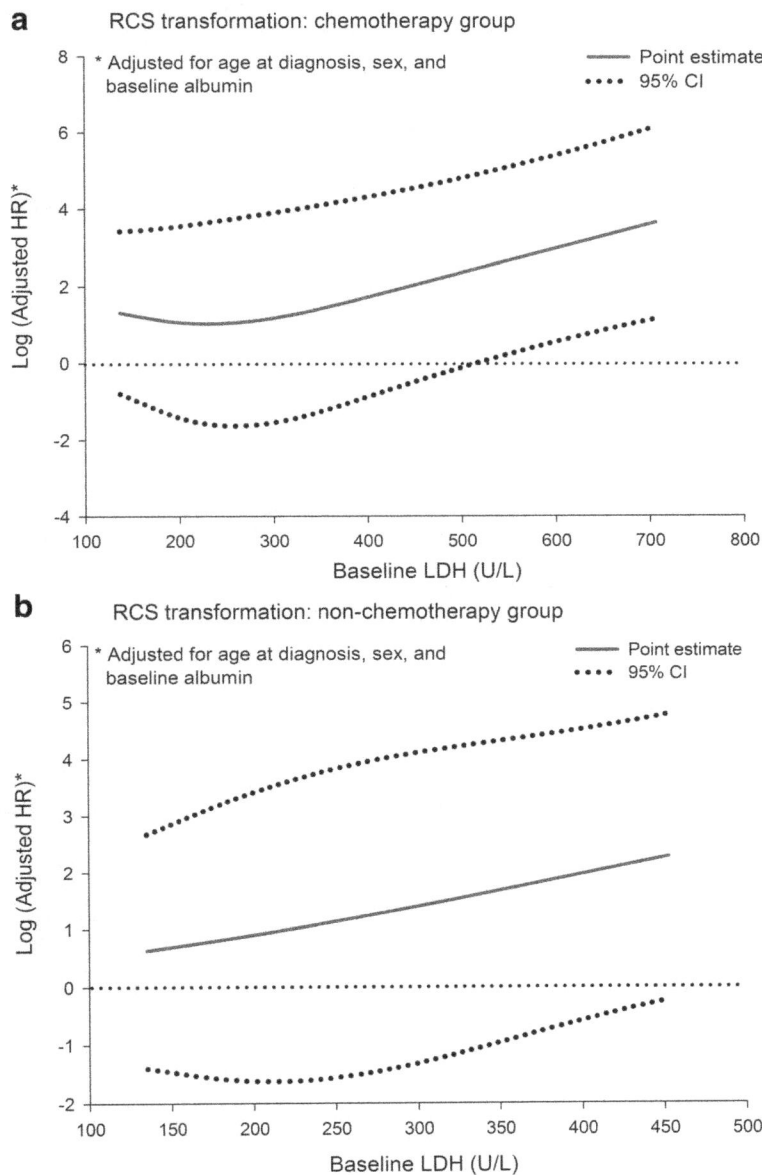

Fig. 2 RCS fitting results for baseline LDH and OS in two groups of advanced PDAC patients. **a** chemotherapy group; **b** non-chemotherapy group

recognizable in patients who did not receive chemotherapy, the most likely explanation is that, usually an end-stage disease and exhausted physical status are major hurdles that may prevent cancer patients from chemotherapy; therefore, in this group of patients, the plummeting health would inundate a comparatively weak influence of LDH in survival, if it indeed existed.

High serum LDH levels have been found to be associated with resistance to chemotherapy in many types of cancer, such as cancers of the colorectum [23, 24], breasts [25], and lung [26, 27], just to name a few. A popular theory for this phenomenon is that stromal cells inversely transform lactate into pyruvate, which fuels progression of cancer cells and strengthens their resistance to chemotherapeutic agents [1, 28]. One previously published in vitro study clearly demonstrated that, novel LDH inhibitors exhibited synergistic cytotoxic activity with gemcitabine [29]. Therefore, it might be true that the association between elevated pretreatment LDH levels and deteriorated survival in advanced PDAC patients who went through chemotherapy was actually the association between enhanced chemoresistance and increased hazards of death.

Nevertheless, either way suggests the promising role of baseline LDH levels in individualized treatment of

PDAC: for patients who are designated for chemotherapy, tackling elevated LDH levels before treatment may alleviate tumor stress and improve the efficacy of chemotherapeutic agents, thus gain survival benefit in the end. Currently, various effective LDH inhibitors are already available, and the inhibition of LDH has minimum impact on normal tissues and presents no major side effects [29–31]. More importantly, the reduction in LDH activity has been proved an effective anti-proliferation measure for several other types of cancer in vivo [32, 33]. For PDAC patients who are not suitable for chemotherapy, based on current evidence, the therapeutic value of LDH inhibition cannot be concluded yet.

Although the acceptance of chemotherapy can be an ideal surrogate for the disease stage and physical performance status, there lies a possibility that cost concern prevented some eligible PDAC patients from this available but expensive treatment, and this situation could introduce bias to the association between baseline LDH levels and OS in patients who did not receive chemotherapy. Nonetheless, this bias tended to derail the association away from the null, and even so, we still concluded an insignificant association in this group of patients.

Several limitations of the present study should be considered. At first, the risk of selection bias cannot be eliminated as we only chose advanced PDAC patients whose vital information was complete. Besides, although when estimating the association between baseline LDH levels and PDAC survival, we have successfully controlled for multiple possible confounders, residual confounding effect undoubtedly existed, and its extent is hard to estimate. Finally, all patients were originated from a localized region in China, thus the generalization of our study results should be made with caution. For future studies, from the genetic perspective, the association between LDH gene expression and OS of both advanced and resectable PDAC patients is a promising topic that deserves additional investigation. It is critically important to unveil the possible underlying mechanisms of our findings and to successfully implement effective intervention measures in improving the prognosis of PDAC patients.

Conclusions

In this retrospective study, we assessed the association between LDH levels measured right after cancer diagnosis and OS in a group of advanced PDAC patients. We found that an elevated pretreatment LDH level was associated with significantly deteriorated survival in PDAC patients who received subsequent chemotherapy, but this association was not statistically significant in PDAC patients who did not receive chemotherapy. Our findings suggest that, for PDAC patients, before the initiation of chemotherapy, tackling the enhanced LDH activity may ultimately improve survival. Prospective cohorts are warranted to validate our findings.

Abbreviations
HR: Hazard ratio; LDH: Lactate dehydrogenase; OS: Overall survival; PDAC: Pancreatic ductal adenocarcinoma; RCS: Restricted cubic spline

Acknowledgments
The authors would like to thank Professor Qingyi Wei of Duke Cancer Institute, who provided generous help in revising and proofreading this manuscript.

Funding
This study was supported by National Natural Science Foundation of China (No. 81273187), National Science and Technology Major Project of the People's Republic of China (2012ZX09303-013-014).

Authors' contributions
YX and NZ conceptualized the study. WC, ZX, ZS, and HX collected and sorted the data. YX, NZ, and GQ performed data analysis. YX drafted the manuscript, NZ, GQ, WC, ZX, ZS, and HX critically revised the paper. All authors had read and approved the final manuscript.

Competing interests
The authors declare that they have no competing interests.

Author details
[1]Department of Biostatistics, School of Public Health, Fudan University, 130 Dong'an Road, Shanghai, China. [2]School of Public Health, Kunming Medical University, Kunming, Yunnan, China. [3]Information Center, Shanghai Municipal Commission of Health and Family Planning, Shanghai, China. [4]Key Lab of Health Technology Assessment, Ministry of Health (Fudan University), Shanghai, China.

References
1. Gatenby RA, Gillies RJ. Why do cancers have high aerobic glycolysis? Nat Rev Cancer. 2004;4:891–9.
2. Zhao D, Zou SW, Liu Y, Zhou X, Mo Y, Wang P, et al. Lysine-5 acetylation negatively regulates lactate dehydrogenase A and is decreased in pancreatic cancer. Cancer Cell. 2013;23:464–76.
3. Yao F, Zhao T, Zhong C, Zhu J, Zhao H. LDHA is necessary for the tumorigenicity of esophageal squamous cell carcinoma. Tumour Biol. 2013; 34:25–31.
4. Sun X, Sun Z, Zhu Z, Guan H, Zhang J, Zhang Y, et al. Clinicopathological significance and prognostic value of lactate dehydrogenase A expression in gastric cancer patients. PLoS One. 2014;9:e91068.
5. Koukourakis MI, Giatromanolaki A, Sivridis E, Bougioukas G, Didilis V, Gatter KC, et al. Lactate dehydrogenase-5 (LDH-5) overexpression in non-small-cell lung cancer tissues is linked to tumour hypoxia, angiogenic factor production and poor prognosis. Br J Cancer. 2003;89:877–85.
6. Koukourakis MI, Giatromanolaki A, Sivridis E, Gatter KC, Harris AL. Lactate dehydrogenase 5 expression in operable colorectal cancer: strong association with survival and activated vascular endothelial growth factor pathway—a report of the Tumour Angiogenesis Research Group. J Clin Oncol. 2006;24:4301–8.
7. Rong Y, Wu W, Ni X, Kuang T, Jin D, Wang D, et al. Lactate dehydrogenase A is overexpressed in pancreatic cancer and promotes the growth of pancreatic cancer cells. Tumour Biol. 2013;34:1523–30.

8. Souhami RL, Bradbury I, Geddes DM, Spiro SG, Harper PG, Tobias JS. Prognostic significance of laboratory parameters measured at diagnosis in small cell carcinoma of the lung. Cancer Res. 1985;45:2878–82.

9. Cohen MH, Makuch R, Johnston-Early A, Ihde DC, Bunn Jr PA, Fossieck Jr BE, et al. Laboratory parameters as an alternative to performance status in prognostic stratification of patients with small cell lung cancer. Cancer Treat Rep. 1981;65:187–95.

10. Terpos E, Katodritou E, Roussou M, Pouli A, Michalis E, Delimpasi S, et al. High serum lactate dehydrogenase adds prognostic value to the international myeloma staging system even in the era of novel agents. Eur J Haematol. 2010;85:114–9.

11. Scartozzi M, Giampieri R, Maccaroni E, Del Prete M, Faloppi L, Bianconi M, et al. Pre-treatment lactate dehydrogenase levels as predictor of efficacy of first-line bevacizumab-based therapy in metastatic colorectal cancer patients. Br J Cancer. 2012;106:799–804.

12. Jin Y, Ye X, Shao L, Lin BC, He CX, Zhang BB, et al. Serum lactic dehydrogenase strongly predicts survival in metastatic nasopharyngeal carcinoma treated with palliative chemotherapy. Eur J Cancer. 2013;49:1619–26.

13. Ferraris AM, Giuntini P, Gaetani GF. Serum lactic dehydrogenase as a prognostic tool for non-Hodgkin lymphomas. Blood. 1979;54:928–32.

14. Haas M, Heinemann V, Kullmann F, Laubender RP, Klose C, Bruns CJ, et al. Prognostic value of CA 19-9, CEA, CRP, LDH and bilirubin levels in locally advanced and metastatic pancreatic cancer: results from a multicenter, pooled analysis of patients receiving palliative chemotherapy. J Cancer Res Clin Oncol. 2013;139:681–9.

15. Tas F, Karabulut S, Ciftci R, Sen F, Sakar B, Disci R, et al. Serum levels of LDH, CEA, and CA19-9 have prognostic roles on survival in patients with metastatic pancreatic cancer receiving gemcitabine-based chemotherapy. Cancer Chemother Pharmacol. 2014;73:1163–71.

16. Stocken DD, Hassan AB, Altman DG, Billingham LJ, Bramhall SR, Johnson PJ, et al. Modelling prognostic factors in advanced pancreatic cancer. Br J Cancer. 2008;99:883–93.

17. Faloppi L, Bianconi M, Giampieri R, Sobrero A, Labianca R, Ferrari D, et al. The value of lactate dehydrogenase serum levels as a prognostic and predictive factor for advanced pancreatic cancer patients receiving sorafenib. Oncotarget. 2015;6:35087–94.

18. Lo Re G, Santeufemia DA, Foltran L, Bidoli E, Basso SM, Lumachi F. Prognostic factors of survival in patients treated with nab-paclitaxel plus gemcitabine regimen for advanced or metastatic pancreatic cancer: A single institutional experience. Oncotarget. 2015;6:8255–60.

19. Haas M, Laubender RP, Stieber P, Holdenrieder S, Bruns CJ, Wilkowski R, et al. Prognostic relevance of CA 19-9, CEA, CRP, and LDH kinetics in patients treated with palliative second-line therapy for advanced pancreatic cancer. Tumour Biol. 2010;31:351–7.

20. Donahue TR, Kazanjian KK, Isacoff WH, Reber HA, Hines OJ. Impact of splenectomy on thrombocytopenia, chemotherapy, and survival in patients with unresectable pancreatic cancer. J Gastrointest Surg. 2010;14:1012–8.

21. Yamada Y, Nakamura K, Aoki S, Tobiume M, Zennami K, Kato Y, et al. Lactate dehydrogenase, Gleason score and HER-2 overexpression are significant prognostic factors for M1b prostate cancer. Oncol Rep. 2011;25:937–44.

22. Walenta S, Mueller-Klieser WF. Lactate: mirror and motor of tumor malignancy. Semin Radiat Oncol. 2004;14:267–74.

23. Lin JT, Wang WS, Yen CC, Liu JH, Yang MH, Chao TC, et al. Outcome of colorectal carcinoma in patients under 40 years of age. J Gastroenterol Hepatol. 2005;20:900–5.

24. Koukourakis MI, Giatromanolaki A, Sivridis E, Gatter KC, Trarbach T, Folprecht G, et al. Prognostic and predictive role of lactate dehydrogenase 5 expression in colorectal cancer patients treated with PTK787/ZK 222584 (vatalanib) antiangiogenic therapy. Clin Cancer Res. 2011;17:4892–900.

25. Zhou M, Zhao Y, Ding Y, Liu H, Liu Z, Fodstad O, et al. Warburg effect in chemosensitivity: targeting lactate dehydrogenase-A re-sensitizes taxol-resistant cancer cells to taxol. Mol Cancer. 2010;9:33.

26. Argiris A, Murren JR. Staging and clinical prognostic factors for small-cell lung cancer. Cancer J. 2001;7:437–47.

27. Tas F, Aydiner A, Demir C, Topuz E. Serum lactate dehydrogenase levels at presentation predict outcome of patients with limited-stage small-cell lung cancer. Am J Clin Oncol. 2001;24:376–8.

28. Koukourakis MI, Pitiakoudis M, Giatromanolaki A, Tsarouha A, Polychronidis A, Sivridis E, et al. Oxygen and glucose consumption in gastrointestinal adenocarcinomas: correlation with markers of hypoxia, acidity and anaerobic glycolysis. Cancer Sci. 2006;97:1056–60.

29. Maftouh M, Avan A, Sciarrillo R, Granchi C, Leon LG, Rani R, et al. Synergistic interaction of novel lactate dehydrogenase inhibitors with gemcitabine against pancreatic cancer cells in hypoxia. Br J Cancer. 2014;110:172–82.

30. Manerba M, Vettraino M, Fiume L, Di Stefano G, Sartini A, Giacomini E, et al. Galloflavin (CAS 568-80-9): a novel inhibitor of lactate dehydrogenase. ChemMedChem. 2012;7:311–7.

31. Granchi C, Roy S, De Simone A, Salvetti I, Tuccinardi T, Martinelli A, et al. N-Hydroxyindole-based inhibitors of lactate dehydrogenase against cancer cell proliferation. Eur J Med Chem. 2011;46:5398–407.

32. Xie H, Hanai J, Ren JG, Kats L, Burgess K, Bhargava P, et al. Targeting lactate dehydrogenase-A inhibits tumorigenesis and tumor progression in mouse models of lung cancer and impacts tumor-initiating cells. Cell Metab. 2014; 19:795–809.

33. Le A, Cooper CR, Gouw AM, Dinavahi R, Maitra A, Deck LM, et al. Inhibition of lactate dehydrogenase A induces oxidative stress and inhibits tumor progression. Proc Natl Acad Sci U S A. 2010;107:2037–42.

17

Long-term trends in pancreatic cancer mortality in Spain (1952–2012)

Daniel Seoane-Mato[1], Olivier Nuñez[2,3], Nerea Fernández-de-Larrea[2,3], Beatriz Pérez-Gómez[2,3], Marina Pollán[2,3], Gonzalo López-Abente[2,3] and Nuria Aragonés[2,3]*

Abstract

Background: Pancreatic cancer is acquiring increasing prominence as a cause of cancer death in the population. The purpose of this study was to analyze long-term pancreatic cancer mortality trends in Spain and evaluate the independent effects of age, death period and birth cohort on these trends.

Methods: Population and mortality data for the period 1952–2012 were obtained from the Spanish National Statistics Institute. Pancreatic cancer deaths were identified using the International Classification of Diseases ICD-6 to ICD-9 (157 code) and ICD-10 (C25 code). Age-specific and age-adjusted mortality rates were computed by sex, region and five-year period. Changes in pancreatic cancer mortality trends were evaluated using joinpoint regression analyses by sex and region. Age-period-cohort log-linear models were fitted separately for each sex, and segmented regression models were used to detect changes in period- and cohort-effect curvatures.

Results: In men, rates increased by 4.1% per annum from 1975 until the mid-1980s and by 1.1% thereafter. In women, there was an increase of 3.6% per annum until the late 1980s, and 1.4% per annum from 1987 to 2012. With reference to the cohort effects, there was an increase in mortality until the generations born in the 1950s in men and a subsequent decline detected by the change point in 1960. A similar trend was observed in women, but the change point occurred 10 years later than in men.

Conclusions: Pancreatic cancer mortality increased over the study period in both sexes and all regions. An important rise in rates -around 4% annually- was registered until the 1980s, and upward trends were more moderate subsequently. The differences among sexes in trends in younger generations may be linked to different past prevalence of exposure to some risk factors, particularly tobacco, which underwent an earlier decrease in men than in women.

Keywords: Pancreatic cancer, Tobacco smoking, Mortality, Age-period-cohort analysis, Change-points, Time trends, Spain

Background

Though, in terms of incidence, pancreatic cancer is not among the most frequent cancers, its high lethality places this malignant tumor among those that cause a higher number of deaths worldwide [1]. The overall prognosis of pancreatic cancer is extremely poor, with five-year relative survival rates around 6% in Europe [2].

In Spain, 6367 new pancreatic cancer cases were estimated to occur in 2012, with age adjusted incidence rates (European standard population) of 11.5 cases per 100,000 males and 7.6 cases per 100,000 females [1]. According to these data, this cancer has become the tenth most common cancer type registered among men and the sixth among women.

As regards to mortality, in 2012 pancreatic cancer ranked seventh as cause of cancer death among Spanish men, with age adjusted mortality rates of 10.7 per 100,000 inhabitants [3], being the third leading cause of oncologic deaths among men between 40 and 59 years [4]. In women, pancreatic cancer was the fourth most common cause of oncologic death, with rates around 6.8 per 100,000. In sum, pancreatic cancer is currently responsible for 5 and 7% of the total number of deaths due to cancer among Spanish males and females, respectively.

* Correspondence: nuria.aragones@salud.madrid.org
[2]Cancer and Environmental Epidemiology Unit, National Center for Epidemiology, Carlos III Institute of Health, Madrid, Spain
[3]Consortium for Biomedical Research in Epidemiology and Public Health (CIBER Epidemiología y Salud Pública, CIBERESP), Madrid, Spain
Full list of author information is available at the end of the article

The etiology of pancreatic cancer is unclear [5] and, as in other cancers, probably multifactorial. Several factors have been suggested as possible causes for this neoplasm, but their contribution, according to their relative risks, is small [6]. Between 3 and 7% of cases could be associated with genetic susceptibility. Regarding exogenous exposures, tobacco smoking (with strong evidence) and *Helicobacter pylori* infection (with moderate evidence) have been considered the major risk factors for pancreatic cancer, in terms of their population attributable fraction, in a recent review [6]. According to the American Institute for Cancer Research, there is also convincing evidence to consider body fatness as a risk factor for pancreatic cancer [7]. Other exposures or clinical entities that have been suggested to be associated with increased risk include high red meat consumption, type II Diabetes Mellitus, chronic pancreatitis, high alcohol consumption, hepatitis B virus infection and specific occupational exposures, such as certain pesticides, organic solvents, polycyclic aromatic hydrocarbons and nickel compounds [6–9]. On the other hand, several factors could have a preventive effect, as it is the case of allergic conditions, high fruit and vegetable consumption and physical activity [6–8].

This study aimed to monitor pancreatic cancer mortality trends since the middle of the twentieth century until recent years in Spain, using joinpoint regression models and age-period-cohort analyses to evaluate the independent effects of age, death period and birth cohort on these trends.

Methods

Mortality data for the calendar period 1952–2012 were obtained from the Spanish National Statistics Institute (*Instituto Nacional de Estadística*) at national level. During this period, different revisions of the International Classification of Diseases (ICD) have been used. Codes selected to identify deaths due to pancreatic cancer were adapted accordingly: code 157 in the ICD-6 to ICD-9 and code C25 in the ICD-10. Population data corresponding to censuses and municipal rolls for the mid-year of each quinquennium were also obtained from the Spanish National Statistics Institute.

From 1975 to 2012, mortality and population data are public and available at regional level, and were stratified by sex, five-year-age group (from 0 to 4 to 85+ years), calendar year and region (Autonomous Community). Age-adjusted mortality rates (AAMR) per 100,000 person-years were then calculated, by the direct method, for each sex, five-year calendar period and region, using the 1976 European Standard Population (ESP). Age-adjusted mortality rates were also calculated using the 2013 ESP to allow comparison with other works (Additional files 1 and 2) [10]. Additionally, annual age-adjusted mortality rates and their corresponding standard errors were calculated to study

time trends for each region and sex. We used the joinpoint regression analysis to evaluate the presence of change points in adjusted mortality rates over time by sex and region and to estimate the annual percent of change over the study period [11]. Ceuta and Melilla regions were excluded from this analysis, because of their small populations.

With respect to age-period-cohort models, first, age-specific mortality rates per 100,000 person-years were computed by sex and calendar period (using five-year periods) at the national level. Then, separate log-linear Poisson models were fitted to study the effect of age, period of death and birth cohort for each sex on mortality trends. To address the "non-identifiability" problem (i.e. the three factors -age, period and cohort- are linearly dependent), we used Osmond and Gardner's solution [12], as well as curvature effects and net drift as proposed by Holford [13]. The Osmond-Gardner solution splits net drift into cohort and period slopes, by minimizing any disagreement in parameter estimates between the full three-factor model and each of the two-factor models (age-period, age-cohort and period-cohort) according to their goodness of fit. Moreover, it allows to estimate two parameters not affected by the non-identifiability problem: (i) overall change over time (denominated net drift), which is the sum of the cohort and period slopes [13]; and (ii) deviation of any period or cohort estimates from the general trend (denominated curvature). Age groups < 30 years were excluded from this analysis due to the limited number of deaths. The open-ended category of persons aged 85 years and over was also excluded. We checked for extra-Poisson dispersion [14] and, where present, effects were calculated using a negative binomial distribution.

The presence of change points and 95% confidence intervals in the curvatures of the cohort and period effects was evaluated by fitting segmented models to the relationship between curvature effects and time. Details of the recursive algorithm used to estimate the segmented regression have been published elsewhere [15], and the procedure can be easily fitted using the R package "segmented" [16].

Results

As a geographic reference, Fig. 1 shows the location of the Spanish Autonomous Communities, with the regional distribution of pancreatic cancer mortality in both sexes in the last quinquennium (2008–2012). AAMRs (1976 ESP) by sex, Autonomous Community and calendar period are presented in Table 1. AAMRs have increased in both sexes in all regions, but not uniformly. The largest increases occurred before the 1990s in both sexes. Then, pancreatic cancer mortality rates have increased at a slower speed. No differences in this trend were observed between men and women. In both sexes, the highest increment took place between the 1978–1982 and the 1983–1987 quinquennia (18% in men and 23% in women), with more

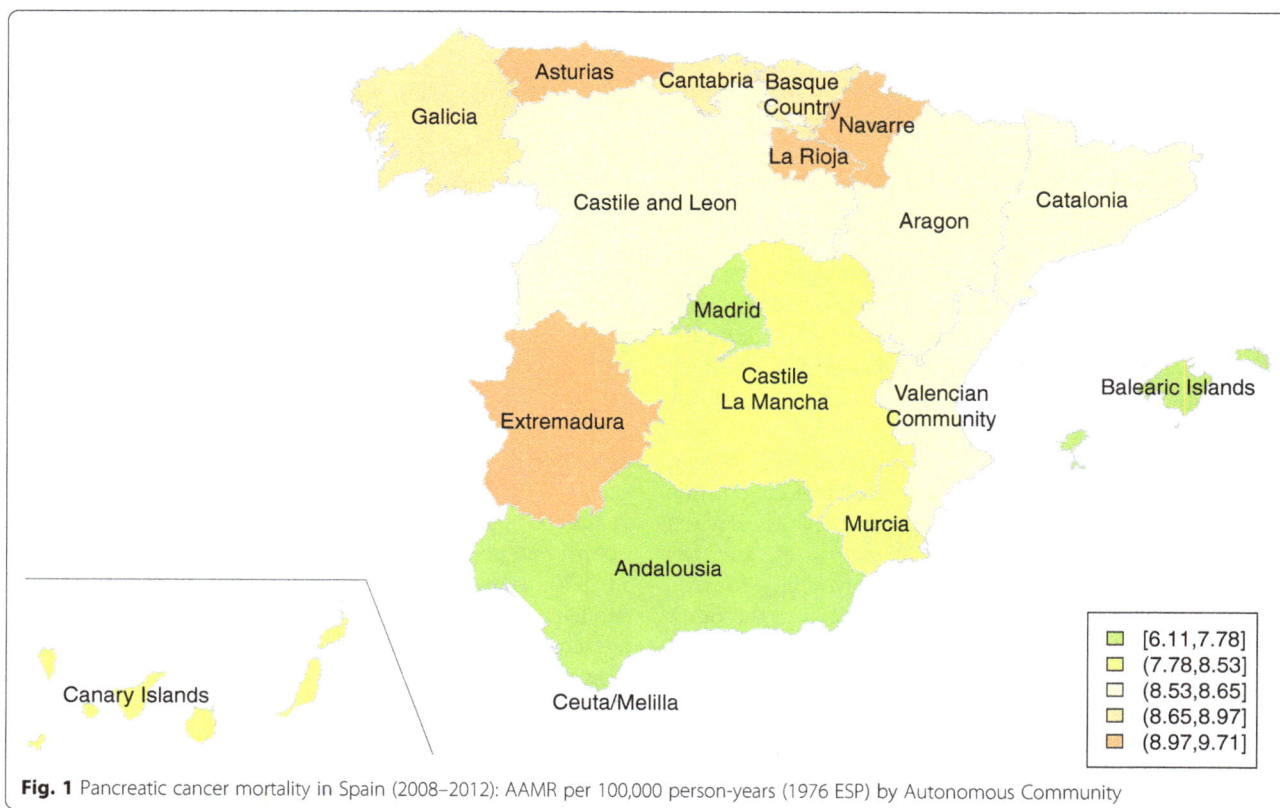

Fig. 1 Pancreatic cancer mortality in Spain (2008–2012): AAMR per 100,000 person-years (1976 ESP) by Autonomous Community

modest increments thereafter (between 5 and 11%). Differences among regions over the study period have been slightly reduced: while in the quinquennium 1978–1982 the ratio between the highest and lowest rates was around 1.8 in males and 1.7 in females, in 2008–2012 this ratio was around 1.3 in both sexes. In men, the highest rates in the quinquennium 2008–2012 were found in Asturias, La Rioja and Galicia, whereas in women the highest rates corresponded to Navarra, Asturias and Cantabria. Since a new European Standard Population has been published recently, AAMRs were recalculated using the 2013 ESP (Additional file 1: Figure S1 and Additional file 2: Table S1). Results are similar, though AAMRs tend to be higher when using the 2013 ESP, given the greater weight that this new standard population gives to older age groups.

The results from joinpoint regression analyses over the period 1975–2012 by Autonomous Community and sex, and in Spain as a whole are presented in Table 2. Both in men and women statistically significant upward trends were seen in nearly all Autonomous Communities. In men, there was an overall increase in the rates of 2% per annum. Joinpoint analysis detected a change point in the mid-1980s: during the first period, rates increased by 4.1% per annum and by 1.1% during the second period. In women, pancreatic cancer mortality rates experienced a marked increase of 3.6% per annum from 1975 until the

late 1980s, and then increased by 1.4% per annum from 1987 to the end of the study period. By region, some of them also showed a two-phase pattern, although with differences in the year when the change was estimated to have occurred. Meanwhile, in others no inflection points were detected and rates increased at the same speed through the study period. Asturias was the Autonomous Community with the smaller overall increase (the only one under 1%) in both sexes, though their mortality rates were among the highest of the country in all quinquennia. Figure 2 shows the evolution of smoothed pancreatic cancer death rates over time by sex and region. The presence of changes in trends is visible.

Figure 3 depicts age-specific rates by birth cohort, in men and women. In both sexes, clear increases over time are observed in all age groups over 45 years of age. However, in males younger than 45 years of age a trend to stabilization, or even a reduction, is observed, while among women this trend to stabilization is only observed for the 30–35 age group. Nevertheless, trends in the youngest age groups are based on a small number of deaths.

Table 3 presents the goodness of fit of the different age-period-cohort models. In men, period effect was the main contributor to the estimated trend in mortality, while in women the main contributor was the cohort effect. Figure 4 depicts cohort and period effects with the change

Table 1 Pancreatic cancer mortality in Spain (1978–2012) by sex, Autonomous Community and calendar period[a]

		1978–82	1983–87	1988–92	1993–97	1998–02	2003–07	2008–12
Men	Andalucía	5.34	6.18	6.71	7.37	7.57	8.29	9.34
	Aragón	5.91	7.57	9.39	8.95	9.83	10.38	11.17
	Asturias	8.81	11.67	10.26	9.79	11.10	11.64	12.37
	C.Valenciana	6.33	7.84	7.71	8.45	9.33	9.04	10.60
	Cantabria	7.88	9.49	10.78	10.74	10.33	11.79	10.81
	Castilla y León	6.43	7.36	8.39	9.38	9.06	10.46	10.59
	Castilla-la Mancha	4.86	5.96	6.78	7.18	7.74	8.68	9.26
	Cataluña	6.91	8.34	8.95	9.67	9.44	10.07	10.79
	Ceuta	5.14	10.31	11.69	14.56	13.21	13.66	9.54
	Extremadura	6.18	6.86	9.18	8.86	10.50	9.80	11.36
	Galicia	5.90	8.14	8.54	9.70	10.85	10.99	11.47
	Islas Baleares	6.57	7.89	9.17	7.99	9.38	9.81	9.57
	Islas Canarias	9.26	9.30	10.77	9.66	10.38	10.55	10.21
	La Rioja	7.77	8.01	10.43	9.67	9.08	10.46	12.17
	Madrid	5.93	5.76	7.99	7.92	9.31	9.52	9.19
	Melilla	1.68	2.09	0.87	3.77	8.49	8.34	8.39
	Murcia	6.16	6.33	6.48	7.73	9.06	9.66	10.21
	Navarra	6.49	8.25	9.89	10.98	11.37	10.87	11.30
	País Vasco	7.28	8.89	9.49	10.74	10.42	10.65	10.75
	Spain	6.33	7.49	8.31	8.81	9.32	9.77	10.32
Women	Andalucía	3.41	4.11	4.37	4.75	4.72	5.02	5.97
	Aragón	3.83	4.85	5.14	6.01	5.87	6.33	6.37
	Asturias	5.27	6.51	5.80	6.02	6.03	6.71	7.26
	C.Valenciana	3.17	4.37	4.75	5.34	5.45	6.03	6.69
	Cantabria	4.34	5.44	6.52	8.17	5.97	7.19	7.14
	Castilla y León	3.57	4.61	4.74	5.35	5.69	5.77	6.81
	Castilla-la Mancha	3.12	3.75	4.87	4.69	4.89	5.75	6.53
	Cataluña	3.97	4.80	5.21	5.28	5.88	6.12	6.69
	Ceuta	6.39	7.07	7.90	6.99	8.08	6.28	4.56
	Extremadura	4.18	4.12	4.92	5.55	5.39	6.15	6.88
	Galicia	3.35	4.36	4.50	5.47	5.89	6.16	6.58
	Islas Baleares	3.52	4.44	4.95	5.77	5.58	5.98	6.01
	Islas Canarias	3.74	5.06	6.24	6.42	6.58	6.91	6.69
	La Rioja	4.46	5.57	5.53	5.44	6.95	6.27	6.61
	Madrid	3.19	3.48	4.49	5.09	5.61	5.84	6.47
	Melilla	3.45	1.25	3.63	5.18	4.28	2.97	2.46
	Murcia	4.51	3.59	4.03	5.08	4.99	5.46	6.64
	Navarra	3.86	5.28	5.12	6.49	6.69	6.97	8.18
	País Vasco	3.86	5.25	5.74	5.81	6.47	6.44	6.80
	Spain	3.64	4.46	4.89	5.36	5.61	5.96	6.57

[a]Age-adjusted mortality rates per 100,000 person-years (1976 ESP)

Table 2 Pancreatic cancer mortality trend changes in Spain evaluated using joinpoint analysis by sex and Autonomous Community

		APC	N. of change points	Period 1 Years	APC 1	Period 2 Years	APC 2
Men	Andalucía	2.89[a]	1	1975-1978	17.66	1978-2012	1.68[a]
	Aragón	1.71[a]	0	-	-	-	-
	Asturias	0.84[a]	0	-	-	-	-
	C. Valenciana	2.14[a]	1	1975-1985	4.77[a]	1985-2012	1.19[a]
	Cantabria	0.84[a]	0	-	-	-	-
	Castilla y León	1.93[a]	1	1975-1990	3.39[a]	1990-2012	0.95[a]
	Castilla-la Mancha	2.00[a]	0	-	-	-	-
	Cataluña	1.79[a]	1	1975-1987	3.90[a]	1987-2012	0.80[a]
	Extremadura	1.80[a]	0	-	-	-	-
	Galicia	2.82[a]	1	1975-1985	6.93[a]	1985-2012	1.34[a]
	Islas Baleares	2.21[a]	1	1975-1986	6.51[a]	1986-2012	0.45
	Islas Canarias	2.37	1	1975-1978	29.02	1978-2012	0.30
	La Rioja	1.38[a]	0	-	-	-	-
	Madrid	1.62[a]	1	1975-2001	2.50[a]	2001-2012	-0.42
	Murcia	1.74[a]	0	-	-	-	-
	Navarra	1.39[a]	0	-	-	-	-
	País Vasco	1.03[a]	0	-	-	-	-
	Spain	1.99[a]	1	1975-1986	4.10[a]	1986-2012	1.11[a]
Women	Andalucía	1.57[a]	0	-	-	-	-
	Aragón	1.71[a]	0	-	-	-	-
	Asturias	0.94[a]	0	-	-	-	-
	C. Valenciana	2.78[a]	1	1975-1984	6.48[a]	1984-2012	1.61[a]
	Cantabria	2.23[a]	1	1975-1991	5.55[a]	1991-2012	-0.23
	Castilla y León	1.89[a]	0	-	-	-	-
	Castilla-la Mancha	2.34[a]	0	-	-	-	-
	Cataluña	1.52[a]	0	-	-	-	-
	Extremadura	1.65[a]	0	-	-	-	-
	Galicia	3.70[a]	1	1975-1977	38.72	1977-2012	1.99[a]
	Islas Baleares	1.54[a]	0	-	-	-	-
	Islas Canarias	1.76[a]	1	1975-1992	3.64[a]	1992-2012	0.18
	La Rioja	0.84	0	-	-	-	-
	Madrid	2.55[a]	1	1975-1994	3.61[a]	1994-2012	1.43[a]
	Murcia	1.65[a]	0	-	-	-	-
	Navarra	2.08[a]	0	-	-	-	-
	País Vasco	1.66[a]	1	1975-1989	3.03[a]	1989-2012	0.84[a]
	Spain	2.09[a]	1	1975-1987	3.56[a]	1987-2012	1.39[a]

APC Annual Percentage of Change

[a]Statistically significant trend as obtained from the segmented regression. Statistical tests were two sided. The significance level was considered as 0.05

points (listed in Table 4) detected on their curvatures. With respect to the cohort effect in men, there was an increase in mortality until the generations born in the 1950s and a subsequent decline with a detectable change point around 1960. In women, as can be seen from its flatter curvature (thin line), the cohort effect is less pronounced and the change point was placed a decade later, though this finding is difficult to assess as it is based on very few

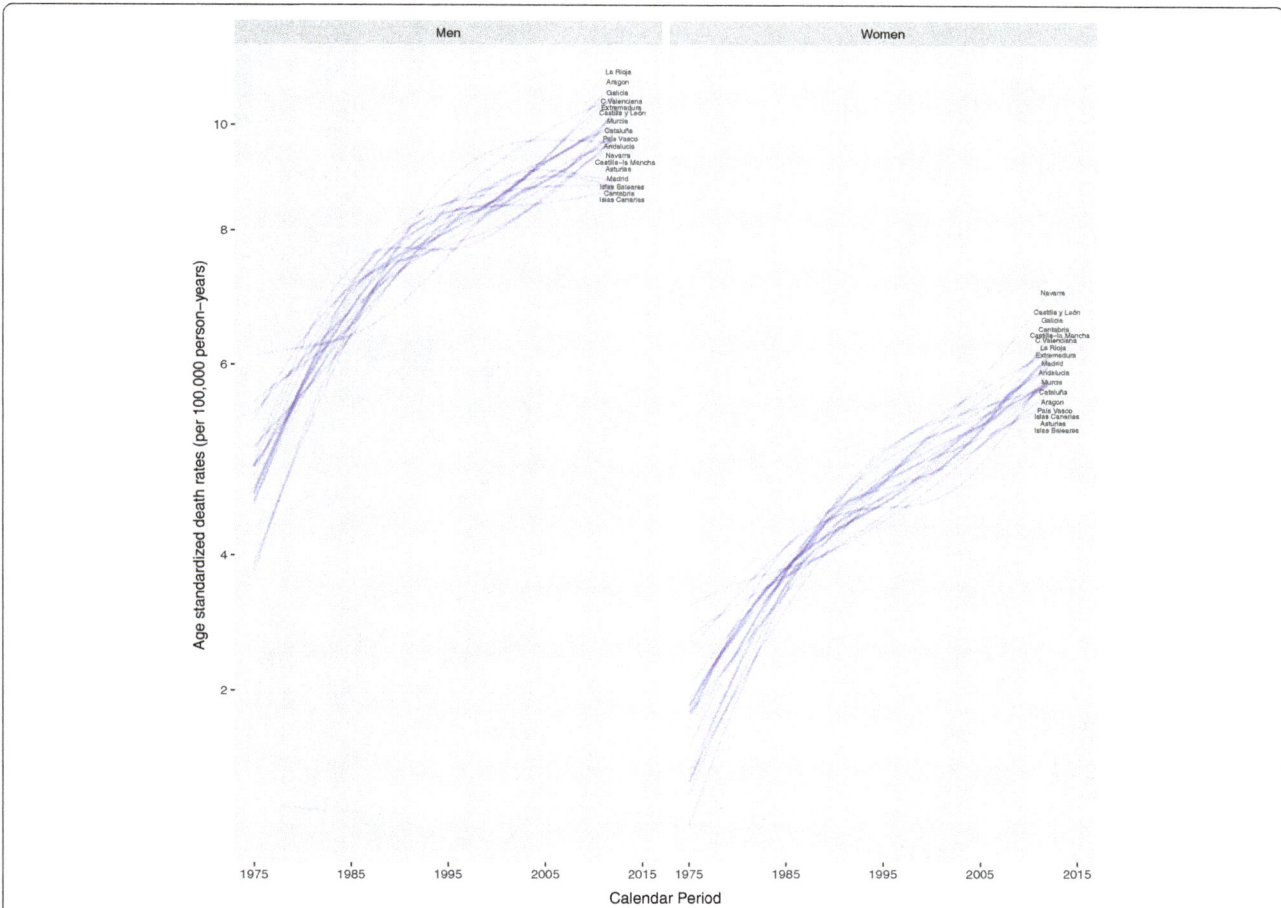

Fig. 2 Pancreatic cancer mortality trends in Spain (1975–2012), by sex and Autonomous Community. Age-adjusted smoothed mortality rates per 100,000 person-years (1976 ESP)

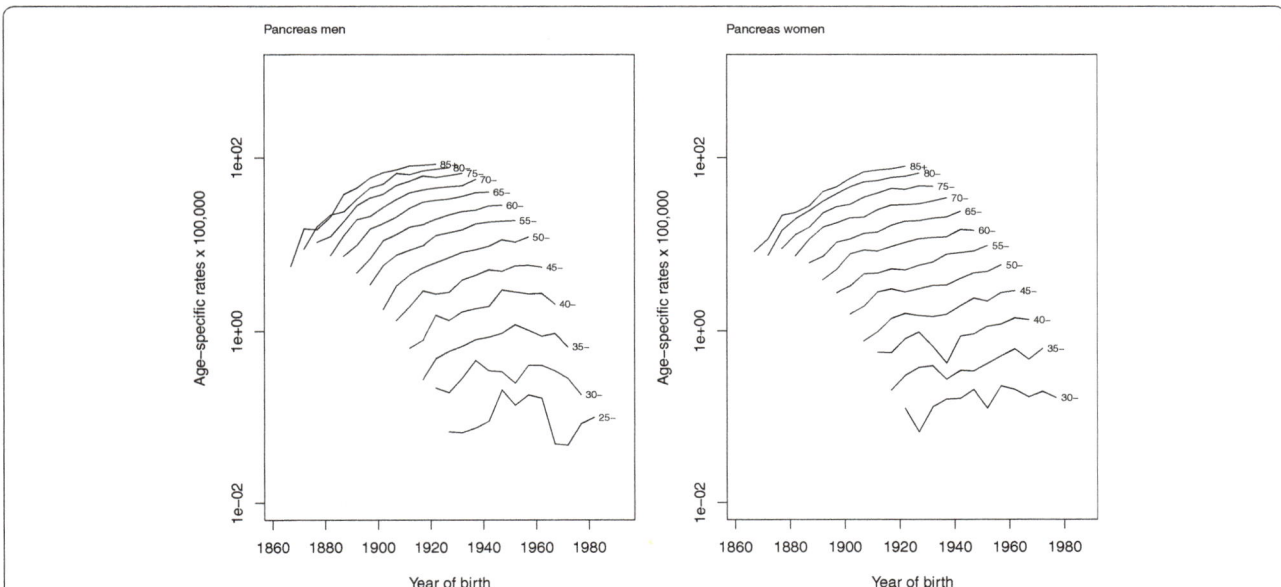

Fig. 3 AAMR per 100,000 person-years for pancreatic cancer by birth cohort and sex, Spain (1952–2012)

Table 3 Goodness of fit in age, period and cohort models for pancreatic cancer mortality by sex, Spain (1952–2012)

	Degrees of freedom	Deviance	% of change in deviance
Men			
Age	121	9980	–
Age + drift	120	1382	Reference
Age + period	110	354	74.4%
Age + cohort	100	509	63.2%
Age + period + cohort	90	109	92.1%
Women			
Age	121	6094	–
Age + drift	120	694	Reference
Age + period	110	327	52.9%
Age + cohort	100	153	78.0%
Age + period + cohort	90	82	88.2%

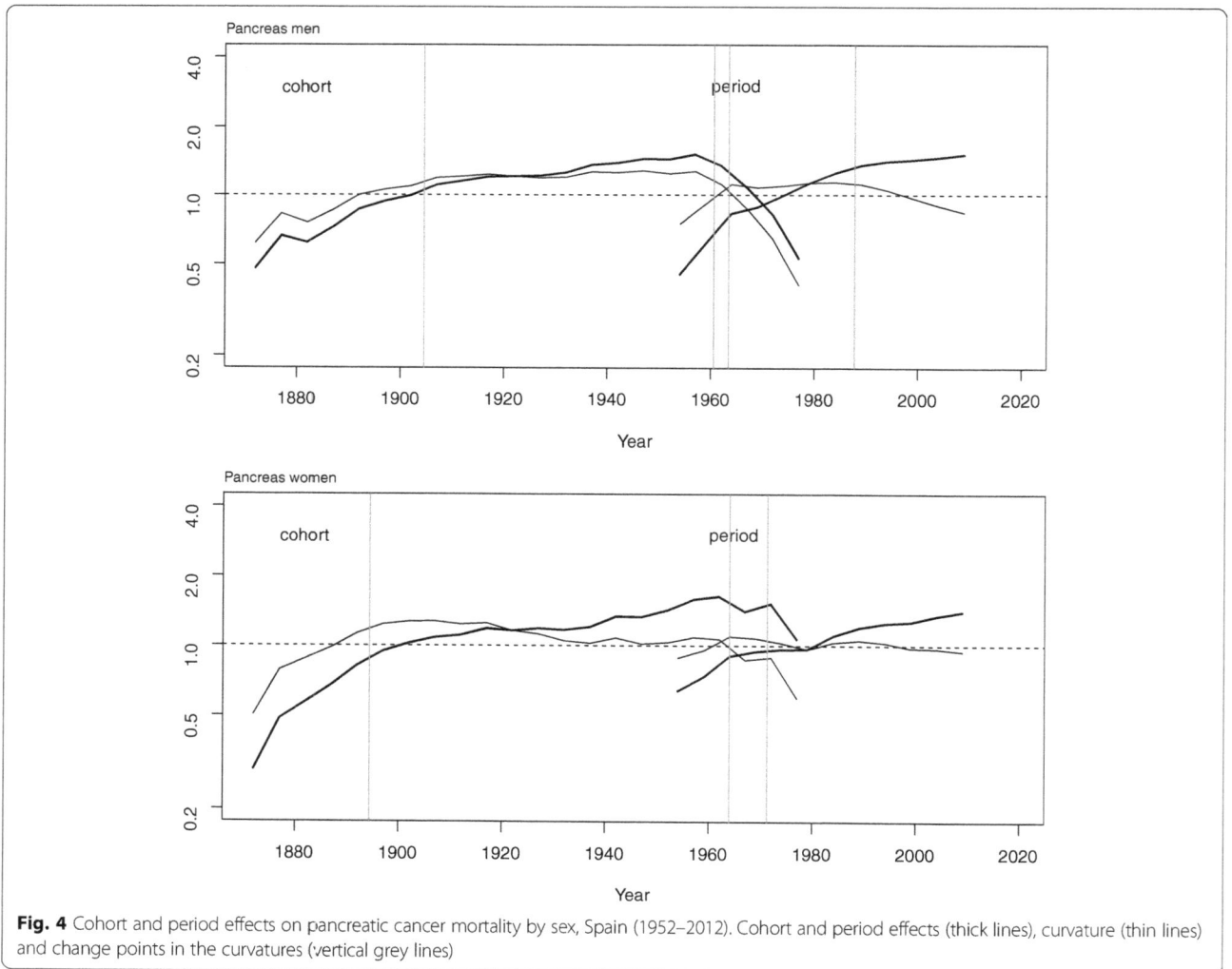

Fig. 4 Cohort and period effects on pancreatic cancer mortality by sex, Spain (1952–2012). Cohort and period effects (thick lines), curvature (thin lines) and change points in the curvatures (vertical grey lines)

Table 4 Cohort and period effect curvature change-points on pancreatic cancer mortality by sex, Spain (1952–2012)

	Changes in cohort effect[a]	
	Birth year (95% CI)	Birth year (95% CI)
Men	1904.6 (1898.7–1910.5)	1960.6 (1958.9–1962.3)
Women	1894.4 (1890.9–1897.8)	1971.2 (1968.9–1973.6)

	Changes in period effect[b]	
	Year of death (95% CI)	Year of death (95% CI)
Men	1963.5 (1961.7–1965.2)	1987.83 (1985.52–1990.14)
Women	1964.0 (1957.1–1970.9)	

[a]Year of birth with significant trend change as obtained from the segmented regression analysis of cohort curvatures from the three-factor model
[b]Year of death with significant trend change as obtained from the segmented regression analysis of period curvatures from the three-factor model

rates and deaths. For the period effect, there is a change in the general trend around 1962–1965 in both sexes, and a second change point in men around 1988, not visible in women.

Discussion

Our results show that pancreatic cancer mortality rates increased over the study period in Spain in both sexes and all regions. In general, this rise was similar in both sexes and in areas with higher and lower rates compared to Spain as a whole. In men, age-adjusted mortality rates annually grew on average by 4.1% in the period 1975–86, and by 1.1% between 1986 and 2012. In women there was a similar trend, with a bigger increase until the late 1980s (3.6% annually between 1975 and 1987) than in the years after (1.4% in the period 1987–2012).

The age-period-cohort analysis shows that, taking the mean rate for all cohorts as reference, the risk of dying from pancreatic cancer increased in generations born between 1870 and 1960 in men and women. This similarity in the trends could be related to changes in the exposure to risk factors linked to birth cohort and shared by both sexes. The rates observed in young men may indicate a levelling off in mortality in the most recent generations. Among women, this phenomenon is less clear, though the stabilization of the rates in the youngest age group could indicate that trend might soon parallel that of men.

For the period effect, there is a change in the general trend around 1962–1965 in males and females and a second change point in men around 1988. Though survival in pancreatic cancer is still very low, a slight improvement has been described in some countries in the last years [17–19], which could have contributed to the slower increase in the mortality rates since the 1990s observed in our study. The improvement in survival has been reported to be slightly higher in men [17]. This would be consistent with the different evolution in the period effect between men and women in the last years, with a lower annual increase of rates in men than in women since the 1990s.

In Europe, there are geographical differences in pancreatic cancer mortality trends. Mortality rates have increased in the last three decades in countries like France, Germany, Greece, Italy, Romania or Bulgaria, whereas in Sweden, the United Kingdom and Norway they have decreased (in the last two countries only in men). In Denmark, Ireland, Finland and Holland, mortality in men diminished until 1990s and then began to increase [20]. In the United States, white and black people show opposite trends: mortality rates in white men decreased from 1970 to 1995, and have increased since then; in white women, there was a slight increase between 1970 and 1984, a stabilization until the late 1990s, and an increase thereafter. On the other hand, in black men and women, rates increased until the late 1980s – early 1990s and have decreased since then [21]. In Canada, mortality rates between 1992 and 2009 declined in men and remained stable in women [22].

Understanding the reasons of the increase in pancreatic cancer mortality is challenging, given the complex and not well understood etiology of this neoplasm. In contrast with other cancer locations, like lung or cervical cancer, which are mainly associated with a unique risk factor, pancreatic cancer has been associated with multiple factors with modest effect sizes and, some of them, with high prevalence of exposure in the general population [6]. Probably, differences in latency periods among these factors may also have a different effect on pancreatic cancer trends, obscuring their specific contribution.

Among the risk factors for this cancer, the only universally accepted one is tobacco consumption [6]. Trends of pancreatic cancer mortality do not resemble those of other tumors strongly related to smoking, such as lung cancer, that is decreasing in males and increasing in females in Spain and in most developed countries. Nevertheless, the slower increase in pancreatic cancer mortality rates in the last decades could be influenced by the decreasing prevalence of tobacco consumption. In Spain, prevalence of smoking shows a decreasing trend in men since the late eighties (not previous data available), while in women, prevalence rose until the late nineties and then slightly decreased [23]. Accordingly, the continuous decrease of the rates in men cohorts born since the 1960s -not so evident in women-, could be related to the different evolution in the prevalence of smoking between sexes. Considering 2013 data, smoking prevalence in men over 34 years old had fell 9.8 percentage points in the last decade, while in women over 34 years old it had not decreased [24]. This would be consistent with a role of tobacco exposure in pancreatic cancer risk, but with the existence of other important contributing risk factors that would counterbalance the effect of the reduction in tobacco exposure.

Another suspected risk factor for pancreatic cancer is *Helicobacter pylori* infection [6]. Again, trends of pancreatic cancer mortality do not resemble those of gastric cancer, strongly associated with this infection and whose mortality rates are decreasing in both sexes. Nevertheless, according to Fig. 4, the higher increase in the risk in cohorts born until the late nineteenth century-early twentieth century and the decrease in those born since the 1960s or 1970s in men and women, respectively, is congruent with the epidemiology of *H. pylori* infection. Though this effect is not as clear as it is in gastric cancer [25], which could be explained by a weaker association between *H. pylori* infection and pancreatic cancer, there seems to be some coincidence in time between both tumors, especially in women.

Though with limited evidence, other factors have been suggested to play a role in the etiology of pancreatic cancer. Among proposed risk factors, extensive research has focused on the role of diet and anthropometric factors [26, 27]. As possible protective factors, a medical history of allergy, the consumption of fruits and vegetables, physical activity and parity have been suggested [6, 28–31]. The controversial evidence from epidemiologic studies, the diverging trends of this broad spectrum of factors and the different prevalence of exposure among regions make it not easy to disentangle the specific role of each factor in pancreatic cancer trends.

A different aspect that could have played a role in the observed upward trend in pancreatic cancer mortality is the introduction of Computerized Tomography in Spain during the late 1970s of the twentieth century, and the spreading of its use during the 1980s. In this sense, advances in diagnosis and better death certification would have yielded a rise in the period effect. However, trends become less pronounced from the 1980s onwards.

This study has some advantages and limitations that should be taken into account. Among its strengths, it involves the follow-up of the total Spanish population through 60 years. This is a dynamic cohort, with entries and exits across the study period, which encompasses generations born approximately from 1865 to 1975–1985 and thus constitutes a long time series. Also, survival of pancreatic cancer continues to be very low [2], and therefore, mortality statistics can be considered as a good proxy for incidence and are representative of the epidemiology of the disease. On the other hand, our results rely on the accuracy of death certificates and coding practices, and there could have been changes in their quality along the study period. However, cancer death certificates in Spain possess an accuracy comparable to that reported for other industrialized countries, and pancreatic cancer is among the cancer sites classified as well certified according to published quality indicators [32].

Conclusions

This study summarizes the trends in pancreatic cancer mortality in Spain, allowing for a detailed analysis of the influence of age, period and cohort effects in each sex. Like in other developed countries, pancreatic cancer mortality has been increasing over the last decades. However, differences have been identified between sexes. In men, mortality rates show a stabilization or even a decrease since the early 1990s, mainly among post-1960 birth cohorts, while in women, a stabilization in the trend is observable only among the youngest generations (born after the late 1970s). These differences may partially mirror the evolution of some established risk factors for pancreatic cancer, such as tobacco exposure, in men and women. Further research on the causes of pancreatic cancer is needed. In the meanwhile, recommendations to reduce exposure to preventable risk factors that have been associated with pancreatic cancer, such as tobacco smoking, obesity, diet and lack of physical activity may serve to reduce the impact of this and other chronic and malignant diseases.

Abbreviations
AAMR: Age-adjusted mortality rates; ESP: European Standard Population; ICD: International Classification of Diseases

Funding
The study was funded by a research grant from the Spanish Health Research Fund (FIS PI11/00871). The funding body had no role in the design of the study and collection, analysis, and interpretation of data and in writing the manuscript.

Authors' contributions
DSM analyzed and interpreted the data and drafted the manuscript. ON analyzed the data, formatted the figures and revised the manuscript. NFL, BPG and MP interpreted the results and revised the manuscript. GLA designed the study, analyzed and interpreted the results, formatted the figures and revised the manuscript. NA designed the study, interpreted the results and drafted the manuscript. All authors read and approved the final manuscript.

Competing interests
The authors declare that they have no competing interests.

Author details
[1]Research Unit, Spanish Society of Rheumatology, Madrid, Spain. [2]Cancer and Environmental Epidemiology Unit, National Center for Epidemiology, Carlos III Institute of Health, Madrid, Spain. [3]Consortium for Biomedical Research in Epidemiology and Public Health (CIBER Epidemiología y Salud Pública, CIBERESP), Madrid, Spain.

References

1. Ferlay, J. et al. GLOBOCAN 2012 v1.0, Cancer incidence and mortality worldwide: IARC CancerBase No. 11 [Internet]. (International Agency for Research on Cancer, 2013).
2. De Angelis R, et al. Cancer survival in Europe 1999-2007 by country and age: results of EUROCARE–5-a population-based study. Lancet Oncol. 2014; 15:23–34.
3. Instituto de Salud Carlos III. Mortalidad por Cáncer en España (2012). *http://www.isciii.es/ISCIII/es/contenidos/fd-servicios-cientifico-tecnicos/fd-vigilancias-alertas/fd-epidemiologia-ambiental-y-cancer/mortalidad-cancer-en-espana.shtml* (2014).
4. López-Abente, G., Núñez, O., Pérez-Gómez, B., Aragonés, N. & Pollán, M. La situación del cáncer en España: Informe 2015. (Centro Nacional de Epidemiología, 2015).
5. Hidalgo M. Pancreatic cancer. N Engl J Med. 2010;362:1605–17.
6. Maisonneuve P, Lowenfels AB. Risk factors for pancreatic cancer: a summary review of meta-analytical studies. Int J Epidemiol. 2015;44:186–98.
7. American Institute for Cancer Research. World Cancer Research Fund. Food, physical activity and the prevention of cancer: a global perspective. (AICR, 2007).
8. Ekbom A, Trichopoulos D. Pancreatic Cancer. In: Hans-Olov Adami, David Hunter, and Dimitrios Trichopoulos. In: Textbook of Cancer Epidemiology. Second ed. Oxford (United Kingdom): Oxford University Press; 2008.
9. Fritschi L, et al. Occupational exposure to N-nitrosamines and pesticides and risk of pancreatic cancer. Occup Environ Med. 2015;72:678–83.
10. Pace, M. et al. Revision of the European standard population. Report of the Eurostat's task force. (Publications Office of the European Union, 2013).
11. Kim HJ, Fay MP, Feuer EJ, Midthune DN. Permutation tests for joinpoint regression with applications to cancer rates. Stat Med. 2000;19:335–51.
12. Osmond C, Gardner MJ. Age, period and cohort models applied to cancer mortality rates. Stat Med. 1982;1:245–59.
13. Holford TR. Understanding the effects of age, period, and cohort on incidence and mortality rates. Annu Rev Public Health. 1991;12:425–57.
14. Breslow NE. Extra-Poisson variation in log-linear models. Appl Stat. 1984;33: 38–44.
15. Muggeo VM. Estimating regression models with unknown break-points. Stat Med. 2003;22:3055–71.
16. Muggeo VM. Segmented: segmented relationships in regression models. R package version. 2004;0:1–4.
17. Søreide K, Aagnes B, Møller B, Westgaard A, Bray F. Epidemiology of pancreatic cancer in Norway: trends in incidence, basis of diagnosis and survival 1965-2007. Scand J Gastroenterol. 2010;45:82–92.
18. Lefebvre A-C, et al. Pancreatic cancer: incidence, treatment and survival trends–1175 cases in calvados (France) from 1978 to 2002. Gastroentérologie Clin Biol. 2009;33:1045–51.
19. Riall TS, et al. Pancreatic cancer in the general population: improvements in survival over the last decade. J Gastrointest Surg. 2006;10:1212–1223; discussion 1223–1224.
20. Bosetti C, et al. Cancer mortality in Europe, 2005-2009, and an overview of trends since 1980. Ann Oncol. 2013;24:2657–71.
21. Ma J, Siegel R, Jemal A. Pancreatic cancer death rates by race among US men and women, 1970-2009. J Natl Cancer Inst. 2013;105:1694–700.
22. Fung S, Forte T, Rahal R, Niu J, Bryant H. Provincial rates and time trends in pancreatic cancer outcomes. Curr Oncol. 2013;20:279–81.
23. Instituto Nacional de Estadística. Encuesta Nacional de Salud (serie histórica). Portal estadístico [Internet]. Ministerio de Sanidad, Servicios Sociales e Igualdad [cited 30/06/2017]. Available from: http://pestadistico.inteligenciadegestion.msssi.es/publicoSNS/Comun/ArbolNodos.aspx?idNodo=42.
24. Observatorio Español de la Droga y las Toxicomanías. Estadísticas 2015. Alcohol, tabaco y drogas ilegales en España [Internet]. Ministerio de Sanidad, Servicios Sociales e Igualdad. 2016 [cited 30/06/2017]. Available from: http://www.pnsd.msssi.gob.es/profesionales/sistemasInformacion/informesEstadisticas/pdf/INFORME_2015.pdf.
25. Seoane-Mato D, et al. Trends in oral cavity, pharyngeal, oesophageal and gastric cancer mortality rates in Spain, 1952-2006: an age-period-cohort analysis. BMC Cancer. 2014;14:254.
26. Shen Q-W, Yao Q-Y. Total fat consumption and pancreatic cancer risk: a meta-analysis of epidemiologic studies. Eur J Cancer Prev. 2015;24:278–85.
27. Genkinger JM, et al. Dairy products and pancreatic cancer risk: a pooled analysis of 14 cohort studies. Ann Oncol. 2014;25:1106–15.
28. Behrens G, et al. Physical activity and risk of pancreatic cancer: a systematic review and meta-analysis. Eur J Epidemiol. 2015;30:279–98.
29. Farris MS, Mosli MH, McFadden AA, Friedenreich CM, Brenner DR. The association between leisure time physical activity and pancreatic Cancer risk in adults: a systematic review and meta-analysis. Cancer Epidemiol Biomark Prev. 2015;24:1462–73.
30. Guan H-B, Wu L, Wu Q-J, Zhu J, Gong T. Parity and pancreatic cancer risk: a dose-response meta-analysis of epidemiologic studies. PLoS One. 2014;9: e92738.
31. Zhu B, et al. Parity and pancreatic cancer risk: evidence from a meta-analysis of twenty epidemiologic studies. Sci Rep. 2014;4:5313.
32. Pérez-Gómez B, et al. Accuracy of cancer death certificates in Spain: a summary of available information. Gac Sanit. 2006;20(Suppl 3):42–51.

18

Deficiency in hormone-sensitive lipase accelerates the development of pancreatic cancer in conditional KrasG12D mice

Mu Xu[1†], Hui-Hua Chang[1,3†], Xiaoman Jung[1], Aune Moro[1], Caroline Ei Ne Chou[1], Jonathan King[1], O. Joe Hines[1], James Sinnett-Smith[2,3], Enrique Rozengurt[2,3] and Guido Eibl[1,3*]

Abstract

Background: Hormone sensitive lipase (HSL) is a neutral lipase that preferentially catalyzes the hydrolysis of diacylglycerol contributing to triacylglycerol breakdown in the adipose tissue. HSL has been implicated to play a role in tumor cachexia, a debilitating syndrome characterized by progressive loss of adipose tissue. Consequently, pharmacological inhibitors of HSL have been proposed for the treatment of cancer-associated cachexia. In the present study we used the conditional KrasG12D (KC) mouse model of pancreatic ductal adenocarcinoma (PDAC) with a deficiency in HSL to determine the impact of HSL suppression on the development of PDAC.

Methods: $KC;Hsl^{+/+}$ and $KC;Hsl^{-/-}$ mice were fed standard rodent chow for 20 weeks. At sacrifice, the incidence of PDAC was determined and inflammation in the mesenteric adipose tissue and pancreas was assessed histologically and by immunofluorescence. To determine statistical significance, ANOVA and two-tailed Student's t-tests were performed. To compare PDAC incidence, a two-sided Fisher's exact test was used.

Results: Compared to $KC;Hsl^{+/+}$ mice, $KC;Hsl^{-/-}$ mice gained similar weight and displayed adipose tissue and pancreatic inflammation. In addition, $KC;Hsl^{-/-}$ mice had reduced levels of plasma insulin and leptin. Importantly, the increased adipose tissue and pancreatic inflammation was associated with a significant increase in PDAC incidence in $KC;Hsl^{-/-}$ mice.

Conclusions: HSL deficiency is associated with adipose tissue and pancreatic inflammation and accelerates PDAC development in the KC mouse model.

Keywords: Pancreatic cancer, Hormone sensitive lipase, Adipose tissue inflammation, Pancreatic inflammation, Animal model

Background

Hormone sensitive lipase (HSL) is an intracellular, neutral lipase that catalyzes the hydrolysis of triacylglycerol, diacylglycerol, monoacylglycerol, cholesteryl esters, and retinyl esters [1]. Its activity against diacylglycerol is several-fold higher than against triacylglycerol and monoacylglycerol. Adipose triglyceride lipase (ATGL) and HSL are therefore the major enzymes contributing to triacylglycerol breakdown in the adipose tissue [2]. Interestingly, an increase in the level and activity of HSL has been implicated in the pathogenesis of cachexia [3, 4], a debilitating syndrome characterized by progressive loss of adipose tissue via increased lipolysis [2–5]. Consequently, pharmacological inhibitors of HSL have been proposed for the treatment of cancer-associated cachexia [4] and a number of compounds have been synthesized and characterized [6, 7]. However, the impact of HSL suppression on cancer development has not been examined.

Pancreatic ductal adenocarcinoma (PDAC) is an extremely aggressive disease with an overall 5-year survival rate of about 8% [8]. Currently, it is the fourth leading

* Correspondence: GEibl@mednet.ucla.edu
†Mu Xu and Hui-Hua Chang contributed equally to this work.
¹Departments of Surgery, David Geffen School of Medicine, University of California, Los Angeles, 10833 Le Conte Ave, CHS 72-236, Los Angeles, CA 90095, USA
³CURE: Digestive Diseases Research Center, University of California at Los Angeles, Los Angeles, USA
Full list of author information is available at the end of the article

cause of cancer deaths in both men and women [8]. PDAC mortality is projected to increase, and before the year 2030 it is expected to become the second leading cause of cancer-related deaths [9]. Cachexia is a prominent condition in PDAC that severely restricts therapeutic options. Therefore, the development of pharmacological agents that can attenuate or reverse cachexia in the context of PDAC is of clinical importance. Administration of inhibitors of HSL have been proposed in the management of cachexia [4] but the precise effect of chronic HSL suppression on the progression of PDAC has never been examined.

HSL null mice appear phenotypically normal (with the exception of infertility in males due to severe oligo- or azoospermia) and are resistant to diet-induced and genetic obesity [10]. In order to assess the role of HSL in PDAC development, we generated conditional Kras^{G12D} mice with HSL deficiency. We found that KC mice with HSL deficiency, compared to KC mice with functional HSL, had similar weight gain and enhanced adipose tissue (AT) and pancreatic inflammation. Surprisingly, KC mice with HSL deficiency exhibited an increased incidence of PDAC. Our results strongly indicate that HSL deficiency is sufficient to accelerate PDAC development in KC mice and therefore imply that chronic suppression of HSL has an unrecognized tumor promoting effect in the KC model.

Methods

Conditional KrasG12D mouse model with HSL deficiency

The conditional KrasG12D (KC) mouse model from Hingorani and colleagues was used for this study [11]. In the KC (*LSL-KrasG12D;p48-Cre*) strain, expression of oncogenic KrasG12D is activated by Cre-mediated excision of LoxP-Stop-LoxP (LSL) in pancreatic lineages during early embryonic development when the *Ptf1a/p48* promoter is active. HSL deficient mice were kindly provided by Fredric Kraemer at Stanford University [10]. *Hsl$^{+/-}$* mice were crossed into *p48-Cre$^{+/-}$* and *LSL-KrasG12D$^{+/-}$* mice to obtain *p48-Cre$^{+/-}$;Hsl$^{+/-}$* and *LSL-KrasG12D$^{+/-}$;Hsl$^{+/-}$* double mutants. The double mutant mice were crossed to generate the desired triple mutant genotypes: *LSL-KrasG12D$^{+/-}$;p48-Cre$^{+/-}$;Hsl$^{+/+}$ (KC;Hsl$^{+/+}$), LSL-KrasG12D$^{+/-}$;p48-Cre$^{+/-}$;Hsl$^{+/-}$ (KC;Hsl$^{+/-}$), and LSL-KrasG12D$^{+/-}$;p48-Cre$^{+/-}$;Hsl$^{-/-}$ (KC;Hsl$^{-/-}$)* (Figs. 1a, b). Mice were fed regular chow beginning at one month of age until 20 weeks of age. We

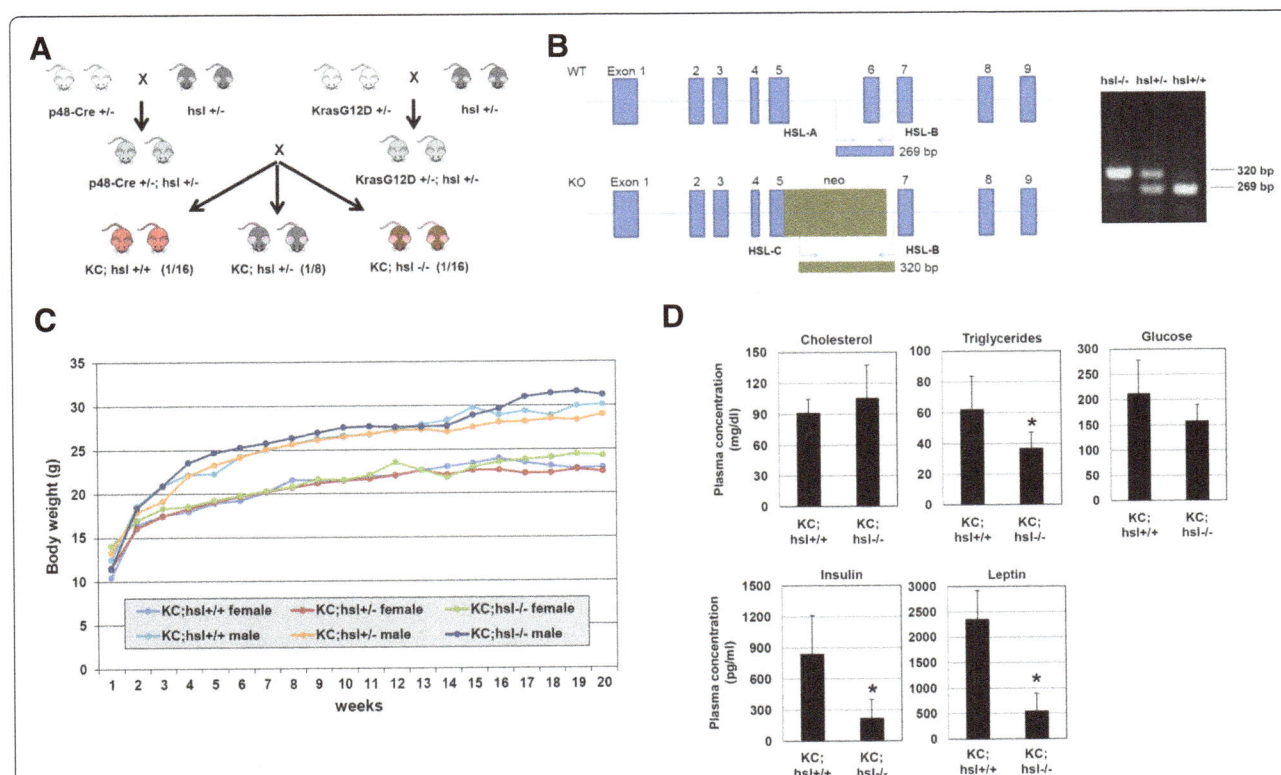

Fig. 1 a Breeding scheme to generate *KC;Hsl$^{+/+}$*, *KC;Hsl$^{+/-}$*, and *KC;Hsl$^{-/-}$* mice. **b** Exon structure of wildtype and HSL deficient mice. Replacing portions of exon 5 and the entire exon 6 with a neo cassette renders mice functionally HSL deficient [10]. Representative genotyping result showing a single 320 bp band in *Hsl$^{-/-}$* mice, a single 269 bp band in *Hsl$^{+/+}$* mice, and a double band (320 bp and 269 bp) in *Hsl$^{+/-}$* mice. **c** Weight curves of female and male *KC;Hsl$^{+/+}$* (n = 9 males+ 14 females), *KC;Hsl$^{+/-}$* (n = 20 males+ 23 females), and *KC;Hsl$^{-/-}$* (n = 10 males+ 10 females) mice fed standard rodent chow for 20 weeks. **d** Plasma levels of cholesterol, triglycerides, glucose, insulin, and leptin in *KC;Hsl$^{+/+}$* and *KC;Hsl$^{-/-}$* mice at 6 months (at sacrifice). N = 6

analyzed 23 $KC;Hsl^{+/+}$, 43 $KC;Hsl^{+/-}$, and 20 $KC;Hsl^{-/-}$ mice. Animal studies were approved by the Chancellor's Animal Research Committee of the University of California, Los Angeles (UCLA) in accordance with the National Institutes of Health Guide for the Care and Use of Laboratory Animals. All mice were sacrificed under general anesthesia with isoflurane. None of the animals died without euthanasia.

Genotyping analysis

The *LSL-KrasG12D*, *p48-Cre*, and *Hsl* alleles were genotyped by polymerase chain reaction (PCR) analysis as described elsewhere [10, 12].

Blood metabolic panel

Blood samples were collected from mice by intracardiac puncture at euthanasia. Blood chemistry (plasma cholesterol, glucose, and triglycerides levels) was obtained by the DLAM Pathology & Laboratory Medicine Services at UCLA. Levels of plasma insulin and leptin were determined using the MILLIPLEX MAP Mouse Adipokine Magnetic Bead Panel - Endocrine Multiplex Assay (EMD Millipore, Billerica, MA) based on the manufacturer's instructions.

Adipose tissue inflammation

Formalin-fixed AT was paraffin-embedded and sectioned. Hematoxylin and eosin (H.E.)-stained sections were analyzed on a Nikon Eclipse 90i microscope (Nikon, Melville, NY) equipped with NIS AR4.2 software (Nikon). Crown-like structures (CLS) representing inflammatory foci [13, 14] were quantified and described as number per high-power field (hpf). A CLS was defined as one adipocyte surrounded by inflammatory cells at least partially. For each tissue sample, ten images were taken, and the number of CLS per 10 randomly selected adipocytes were quantified.

Cytokine array

Mesenteric fat homogenates from $KC;Hsl^{+/+}$ and $KC;Hsl^{-/-}$ mice were profiled using the Mouse Cytokine Antibody Array, C1000 (RayBiotech, Norcross, GA) following the manufacturer's instructions. The membrane-based proteomic array detects relative levels of 96 different cytokines and chemokines. The complete list of cytokines and chemokines analyzed can be found here: https://www.raybiotech.com/c-series-mouse-cytokine-array-c1000-2/. Following exposure to horseradish peroxidase (HRP) the membranes were imaged using the ChemiDoc™ Touch Imaging System (Bio-Rad Laboratories, Hercules, CA), and the intensity of signals normalized to the internal positive controls was quantified with Multi Gauge V3.0 software (Fujifilm Life Sciences, Tokyo, Japan).

Pancreas histology

Formalin-fixed, paraffin-embedded pancreatic tissue sections were stained with hematoxylin and eosin and histologically analyzed in a blinded fashion. Murine pancreatic intraepithelial neoplasia (PanINs) and invasive PDAC were classified according to histopathologic criteria as previously described [15–17].

Quantification of lipid content

Tissue content of triglycerides (TG), phospholipids (PL), and free fatty acids (FFA) and the fatty acid (FA) profile in each lipid fraction was analyzed by the Vanderbilt Mouse Metabolic Phenotyping Center. Briefly, phospholipids, diglycerides, triglycerides, and cholesteryl esters in the extracted lipids were separated by thin layer chromatography, scraped from the plates and methylated. The methylated FA were then extracted and analyzed on an Agilent 7890A gas chromatograph. FA methyl esters were identified by comparing the retention times to those of known standards. Inclusion of lipid standards with odd chain FAs allowed quantitation of lipids in the sample. Dipentadecanoyl phosphatidylcholine (C15:0), diheptadecanoin (C17:0), trieicosenoin (C20:1), and cholesteryl eicosenoate (C20:1) were the standards used.

Immunohistochemistry

Paraffin was removed with xylene and graded alcohol. Heat-induced antigen retrieval was performed with citrate buffer, and endogenous peroxidase activity was blocked with 3% hydrogen peroxide. Slides were then incubated overnight with polyclonal rabbit primary antibodies against HSL (Novus Biologicals, Littleton, CO) or monoclonal rabbit primary antibodies against Ki67 (Cell Signaling Technologies, Danvers, MA). Control images were prepared using isotype matched rabbit IgG (Cell Signaling Technologies). Images were analyzed on a Nikon Eclipse 90i microscope equipped with NIS AR4.2 software (Nikon). Ki67 staining was quantified by counting Ki67 positive cells (stromal and epithelial) in 10 high-power fields per tissue section.

Immunofluorescence

Paraffin was removed with xylene and graded alcohol. Antigen retrieval was performed by using Antigen Unmasking Solution (Vector Laboratories, Burlingame, CA) plus ethylenediaminetetraacetic acid (EDTA). Endogenous peroxidase activity was blocked with 1% hydrogen peroxide. Slides were then incubated overnight with monoclonal rabbit anti-F4/80 antibody (clone SP115, Novus Biologicals) and monoclonal mouse anti-TNF-α (tumor necrosis factor alpha) antibody (clone SPM543, Novus Biologicals). Anti-rabbit IgG antibodies conjugated with Alexa Fluor 555 (Thermo Fisher Scientific, Canoga Park, CA) and anti-mouse IgG antibodies conjugated with Alexa Fluor 488 (Thermo Fisher Scientific) were added at room temperature for one hour. Images were analyzed on a Nikon Eclipse 90i microscope equipped with NIS AR4.2 software (Nikon). F4/80 and TNF-α positive cells were counted in 10 hpf per tissue section and analyzed as 0 (no staining), + (1–5 cells/hpf), ++ (5–10 cells/hpf), and +++ (> 10 cells/hpf).

Western blot analysis

Mouse tissue samples were homogenized in radio-immunoprecipitation assay (RIPA) buffer containing mixture of protease and phosphatase inhibitors (Roche Applied Science, Basel, Switzerland). Tissue homogenates were resolved by SDS-PAGE, electrophoretically transferred onto nitrocellulose membranes, and then immunoblotted for the proteins of interest using the following primary antibodies: Peroxisome proliferator-activated receptor gamma (PPAR-γ) and p44/42 MAPK from Cell Signaling Technologies, and HSL from Novus Biologicals. After incubation with secondary antibodies, the immune-reactive bands detected with enhanced chemiluminescence reagents were imaged and analyzed by the ChemiDoc™ Touch Imaging System (Bio-Rad Laboratories).

PCR analysis of *Hsl*

Total RNA from tissue or cell lysates were extracted using RNA purification kits (Biomiga, Inc., San Diego, CA). Reverse transcription was performed with the iScript reverse transcription supermix (Bio-Rad Laboratories). The synthesized cDNA was used as template for the PCR analysis of *Hsl* gene expression. The iTaq™ Supermix (Bio-Rad Laboratories) was used for amplifications. All reactions were performed on the Bio-Rad iQ™5 system. Primers for mouse *Hsl*: forward, 5′- GCAGTGGTGTGTAACTAGG ATTG-3′, and reverse, 5′- CGCTGAGGCTTTGA TCTTGC -3′ (spanning exons 1 and 2).

Statistical analysis

Data are presented as mean ± SD. Statistical significance was determined by one-way (or two-way) ANOVA and two-tailed Student's *t*-tests assuming unequal variances. For the comparison of PDAC incidence, a two-sided Fisher's exact test was performed. Significance (*p*-value less than 0.05) was indicated with an asterisk (*).

Results

Weight gain and metabolic parameters in KC mice with HSL deficiency

After weaning female and male *KC;Hsl*$^{+/+}$, *KC;Hsl*$^{+/−}$, and *KC;Hsl*$^{−/−}$ mice were fed regular rodent chow for 20 weeks. Although females gained less weight than male mice, *KC;Hsl*$^{+/+}$, *KC;Hsl*$^{+/−}$, and *KC;Hsl*$^{−/−}$ mice within each gender group gained weight similarly throughout the study period (Fig. 1c), which is in accordance with previous reports [10, 18]. Compared to

KC;Hsl$^{+/+}$ mice, *KC;Hsl*$^{−/−}$ mice showed reduced plasma TG levels, while cholesterol levels were unchanged (Fig. 1d). Our studies demonstrated reduced plasma insulin levels in *KC;Hsl*$^{−/−}$ mice with normal glucose concentrations (Fig. 1d), suggesting enhanced insulin sensitivity. Furthermore, *KC;Hsl*$^{−/−}$ mice had reduced plasma levels of leptin (Fig. 1d), a hormone secreted primarily by adipocytes of white adipose tissue (WAT).

KC mice with HSL deficiency display enhanced AT inflammation

We have previously reported an enhanced depot-specific AT inflammation during diet-induced obesity (DIO) in KC mice [14]. In the present study, histological examination revealed increased WAT (mesenteric depot) inflammation in *KC;Hsl*$^{−/−}$ mice as assessed by quantification of CLS (Fig. 2a). The increase in CLS was accompanied by an enhanced presence of TNF-α expressing F4/80-positive cells (macrophages) in the mesenteric WAT of *KC;Hsl*$^{−/−}$ mice as assessed by immunofluorescence (Fig. 2b). Detailed tissue lipid analysis revealed decreased TG content in mesenteric WAT of *KC;Hsl*$^{−/−}$ mice as well as reduced expression of pro-adipogenic PPAR-γ (Fig. 2c), confirming the impairment of adipogenesis in HSL null mice [18]. The anti-adipogenic phenotype associated with HSL deficiency is consistent with the role of HSL in providing intrinsic ligands for PPARγ through release of FAs [19]. The PL content in mesenteric WAT was unchanged in *KC;Hsl*$^{−/−}$ mice, reflecting the lack of phospholipase activity of HSL. Despite the physiological role of HSL in FA release, the levels of FFA in the mesenteric WAT of *KC;Hsl*$^{−/−}$ mice were unaltered (Fig. 2c). Due to limited amount of tissue available for each analysis, we did not measure the intracellular levels of diacylglycerols, which are known to accumulate in tissues of *Hsl*$^{−/−}$ mice due to the importance and preference of HSL to hydrolyze diacylglycerols [20]. Using a Mouse Cytokine Antibody Array, multiple changes in cytokines and chemokines were detected in the mesenteric WAT of *KC;Hsl*$^{−/−}$ mice (Fig. 2d). Significant elevations of adhesion molecules (e.g. ICAM-1, L-selectin) and chemokines (e.g. MIP-1 gamma, CCL5, CCL22) were found (Fig. 2d) that may reflect AT inflammation with recruitment and infiltration of immune cells into the mesenteric WAT.

KC mice with HSL deficiency have an increased incidence of PDAC

Consistent with previous reports [21], HSL was expressed in pancreatic islets of wild type (WT) mice (Fig. 3a). Interestingly, immunohistochemistry showed strong HSL expression in PanIN lesions of *KC;Hsl*$^{+/+}$ and *KC;Hsl*$^{−/−}$ mice (Fig. 3a), which has never been described before. Expression of HSL in PanIN cells was confirmed by PCR analysis of primary PanIN cells

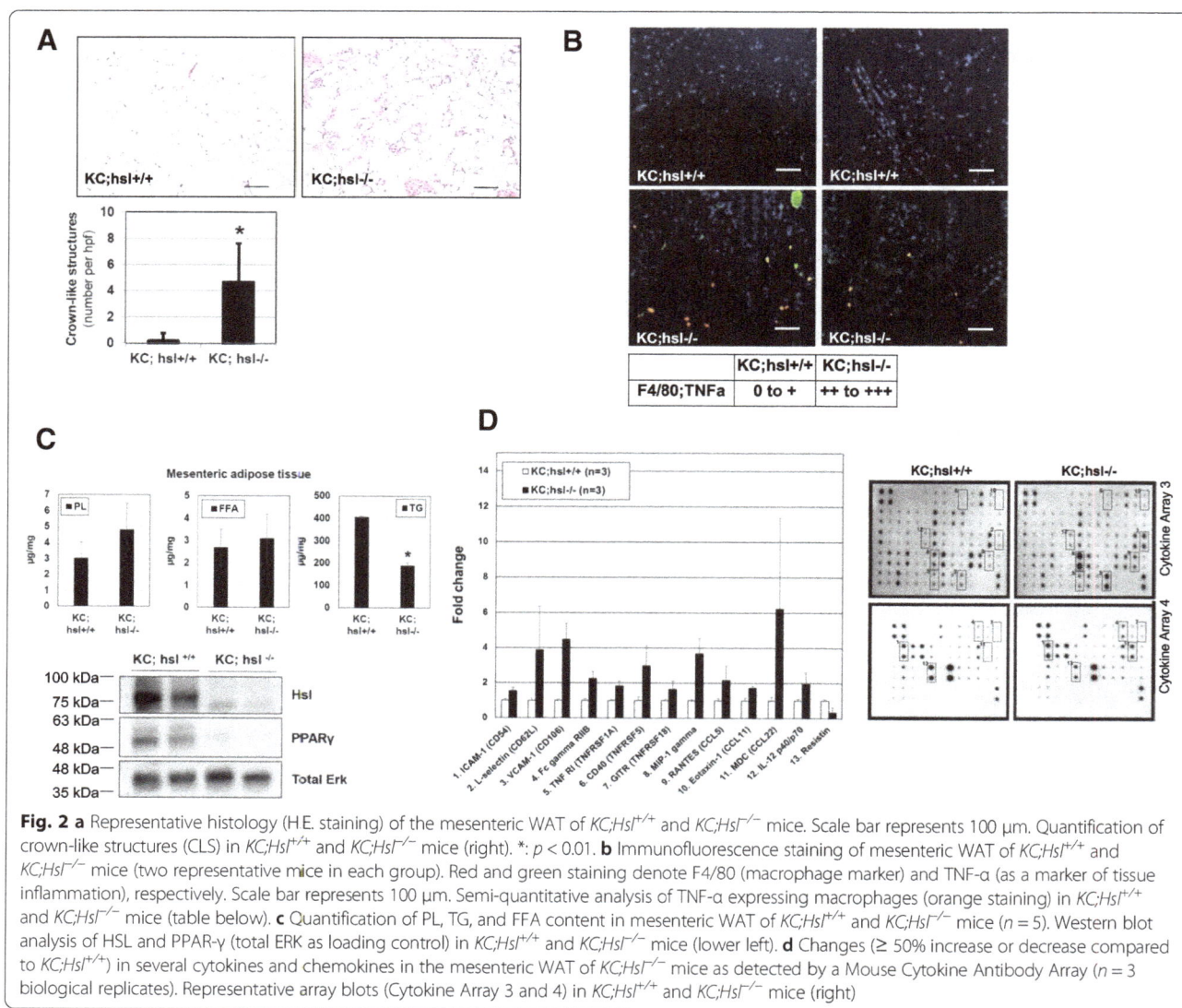

Fig. 2 a Representative histology (H.E. staining) of the mesenteric WAT of *KC;Hsl*$^{+/+}$ and *KC;Hsl*$^{-/-}$ mice. Scale bar represents 100 μm. Quantification of crown-like structures (CLS) in *KC;Hsl*$^{+/+}$ and *KC;Hsl*$^{-/-}$ mice (right). *: $p < 0.01$. **b** Immunofluorescence staining of mesenteric WAT of *KC;Hsl*$^{+/+}$ and *KC;Hsl*$^{-/-}$ mice (two representative mice in each group). Red and green staining denote F4/80 (macrophage marker) and TNF-α (as a marker of tissue inflammation), respectively. Scale bar represents 100 μm. Semi-quantitative analysis of TNF-α expressing macrophages (orange staining) in *KC;Hsl*$^{+/+}$ and *KC;Hsl*$^{-/-}$ mice (table below). **c** Quantification of PL, TG, and FFA content in mesenteric WAT of *KC;Hsl*$^{+/+}$ and *KC;Hsl*$^{-/-}$ mice ($n = 5$). Western blot analysis of HSL and PPAR-γ (total ERK as loading control) in *KC;Hsl*$^{+/+}$ and *KC;Hsl*$^{-/-}$ mice (lower left). **d** Changes ($\geq$ 50% increase or decrease compared to *KC;Hsl*$^{+/+}$) in several cytokines and chemokines in the mesenteric WAT of *KC;Hsl*$^{-/-}$ mice as detected by a Mouse Cytokine Antibody Array ($n = 3$ biological replicates). Representative array blots (Cytokine Array 3 and 4) in *KC;Hsl*$^{+/+}$ and *KC;Hsl*$^{-/-}$ mice (right)

isolated from KC mice (with functional HSL) and cultured in vitro (Fig. 3b). Despite the functional HSL deficiency in *KC;Hsl*$^{-/-}$ mice (by virtue of replacing portions of exon 5 and the entire exon 6 with a neo cassette), the antibodies used in the present study seem to be able to detect the non-functional HSL protein in *KC;hsl*$^{-/-}$ mice. It is unclear whether the apparent lower expression of HSL in *KC;Hsl*$^{-/-}$ WAT and pancreatic lysates (Fig. 2c and 3b) is caused by an actual decreased expression or by a lower affinity of the antibody to the non-functional HSL protein. Detailed pancreatic tissue lipid analysis demonstrated markedly reduced TG and FFA content in *KC;Hsl*$^{-/-}$ mice (Fig. 3c). Again, the PL content was unaltered in the pancreas of *KC;Hsl*$^{-/-}$ mice (Fig. 3c).

The most salient feature of this study is that *KC;Hsl*$^{-/-}$ mice displayed a significantly increased PDAC incidence at 20 weeks (Fig. 4a). While none of the *KC;Hsl*$^{+/+}$ mice developed invasive PDAC at six months of age, 25% (5/

20) of *KC;Hsl*$^{-/-}$ mice had cancer ($p = 0.016$). The increased PDAC incidence in *KC;Hsl*$^{-/-}$ mice was thereby associated with an elevated proliferation of PanIN and stromal cells (Fig. 4b) as assessed by Ki67 immunostaining. Furthermore, *KC;Hsl*$^{-/-}$ mice displayed enhanced pancreatic inflammation as evident histologically and by an increase in TNF-α expressing F4/80-positive macrophages assessed by immunofluorescence (Fig. 4c).

Patients with PDAC and low expression of *LIPE* have unfavorable prognosis

To assess the significance of HSL expression in human PDAC, we determined the importance of the expression of the gene encoding HSL as a prognostic marker of survival in patients with PDAC. We used a recently published interactive open-access database (www.proteinatlas.org/pathology) to perform correlation analyses based on mRNA expression levels of *LIPE* (the gene encoding HSL)

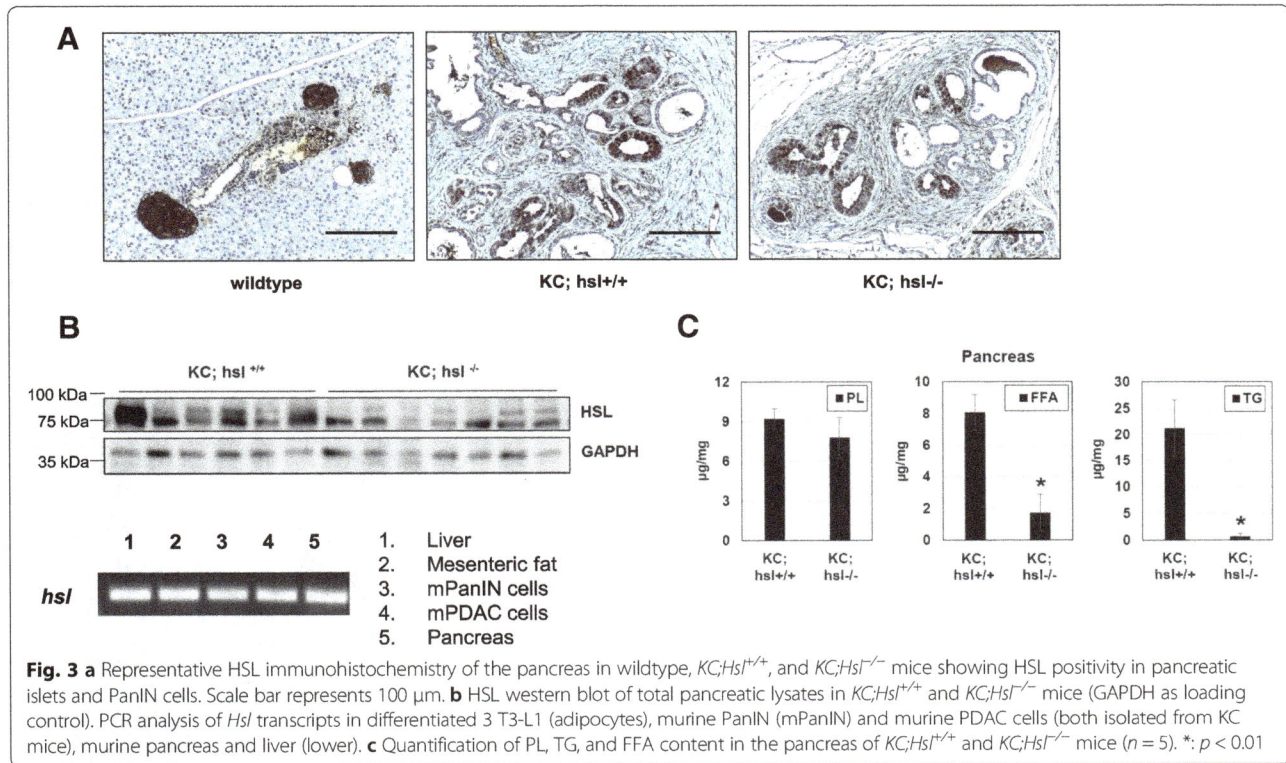

Fig. 3 a Representative HSL immunohistochemistry of the pancreas in wildtype, $KC;Hsl^{+/+}$, and $KC;Hsl^{-/-}$ mice showing HSL positivity in pancreatic islets and PanIN cells. Scale bar represents 100 µm. **b** HSL western blot of total pancreatic lysates in $KC;Hsl^{+/+}$ and $KC;Hsl^{-/-}$ mice (GAPDH as loading control). PCR analysis of *Hsl* transcripts in differentiated 3 T3-L1 (adipocytes), murine PanIN (mPanIN) and murine PDAC cells (both isolated from KC mice), murine pancreas and liver (lower). **c** Quantification of PL, TG, and FFA content in the pancreas of $KC;Hsl^{+/+}$ and $KC;Hsl^{-/-}$ mice (n = 5). *: p < 0.01

in PDAC tissue and the clinical outcome (survival) of the patients. The data in the Pathology Atlas is based on the analysis of transcriptomics and survival in 176 PDAC patients. As illustrated in the Kaplan-Meier plot in Fig. 5, none of the patients of the population with lower levels of *LIPE* mRNA expression (n = 69) survived for 5 years while 42% of the population (n = 107) with the higher levels of *LIPE* mRNA survived for 5 years or more.

Discussion

A striking feature of the results presented here is that KC mice lacking HSL ($KC;Hsl^{-/-}$) mice displayed a significant increase in PDAC incidence. To our knowledge, it is the first time that HSL deficiency has been linked to an increased cancer risk. In humans, carriers of a frameshift deletion of exon 9 in the *LIPE* gene, encoding for HSL, were characterized by metabolic dysfunction, including dyslipidemia, hepatic steatosis, systemic insulin resistance, and diabetes [22]. In the adipose tissue from carriers with the mutation, impaired lipolysis and inflammation were observed [22]. In our study, the exact mechanism(s) involved in promoting PDAC remains incompletely understood. HSL deficiency in KC mice was accompanied by enhanced inflammation in the AT and pancreas. While CLS is a well-characterized feature of adipose tissue inflammation (macrophages surrounding necrotic adipocytes), additional analysis is warranted to further identify inflammatory cell subpopulations. It has

been postulated that an increased heterogeneity of adipocytes with necrotic cell death of hypertrophic adipocytes and subsequent infiltration of macrophages may play an important role in inducing WAT inflammation in the context of HSL deficiency [10, 23]. Lipid analysis of the mesenteric WAT in $KC;Hsl^{-/-}$ mice has revealed a decreased TG content, in agreement with previous reports [24]. The mechanistic link between HSL deficiency and TG reduction in WAT was suggested to be a compensatory downregulation of FA esterification enzymes, leading to reduced cellular TG synthesis [25]. This observation is consistent with the reported impairment of white adipocyte differentiation and decreased WAT mass in HSL null mice [18]. The anti-adipogenic phenotype may also be mediated by a decrease in PPAR-γ expression and activity through the reduced intracellular release of FAs, acting as endogenous PPAR-γ ligands, in HSL null mice [19]. This is corroborated by our finding of reduced PPAR-γ expression in the mesenteric WAT of $KC;Hsl^{-/-}$ mice. FFA levels in the mesenteric WAT were not significantly altered in $KC;Hsl^{-/-}$ mice, which can be explained by the presence of additional lipases in the WAT, i.e. adipose triglyceride lipase, which preferentially catalyzes the conversion of triacylglycerol to diacylglycerol and thereby maintaining a FFA pool in WAT [24].

In addition to AT inflammation, $KC;Hsl^{-/-}$ mice also had enhanced pancreatic inflammation as demonstrated

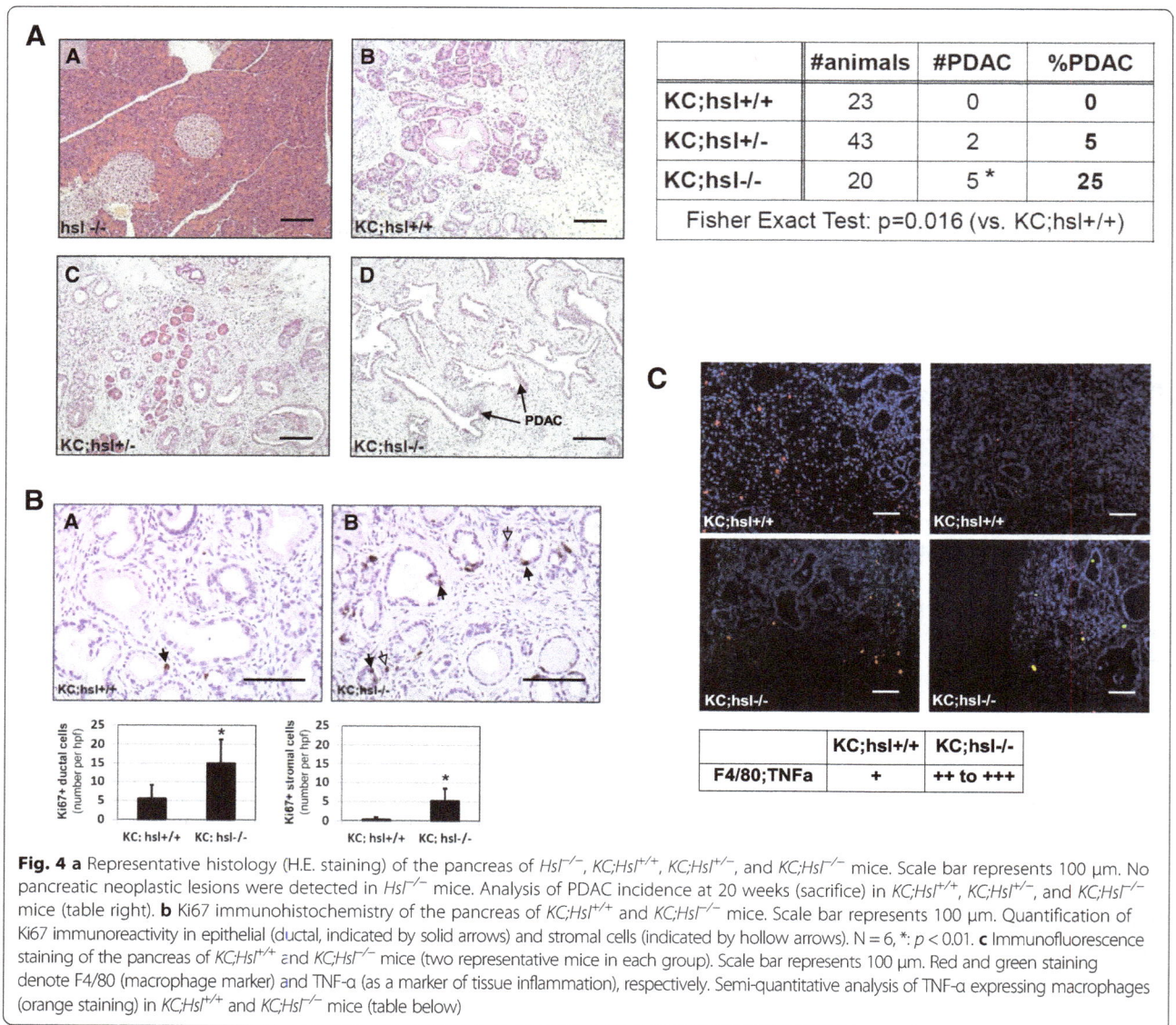

	#animals	#PDAC	%PDAC
KC;hsl+/+	23	0	0
KC;hsl+/-	43	2	5
KC;hsl-/-	20	5 *	25
Fisher Exact Test: p=0.016 (vs. KC;hsl+/+)			

	KC;hsl+/+	KC;hsl-/-
F4/80;TNFa	+	++ to +++

Fig. 4 a Representative histology (H.E. staining) of the pancreas of $Hsl^{-/-}$, $KC;Hsl^{+/+}$, $KC;Hsl^{+/-}$, and $KC;Hsl^{-/-}$ mice. Scale bar represents 100 μm. No pancreatic neoplastic lesions were detected in $Hsl^{-/-}$ mice. Analysis of PDAC incidence at 20 weeks (sacrifice) in $KC;Hsl^{+/+}$, $KC;Hsl^{+/-}$, and $KC;Hsl^{-/-}$ mice (table right). **b** Ki67 immunohistochemistry of the pancreas of $KC;Hsl^{+/+}$ and $KC;Hsl^{-/-}$ mice. Scale bar represents 100 μm. Quantification of Ki67 immunoreactivity in epithelial (ductal, indicated by solid arrows) and stromal cells (indicated by hollow arrows). N = 6, *: $p < 0.01$. **c** Immunofluorescence staining of the pancreas of $KC;Hsl^{+/+}$ and $KC;Hsl^{-/-}$ mice (two representative mice in each group). Scale bar represents 100 μm. Red and green staining denote F4/80 (macrophage marker) and TNF-α (as a marker of tissue inflammation), respectively. Semi-quantitative analysis of TNF-α expressing macrophages (orange staining) in $KC;Hsl^{+/+}$ and $KC;Hsl^{-/-}$ mice (table below)

histologically and by an increased number of TNF-α producing macrophages in the pancreas. It is currently unclear what mechanisms elicited the pancreatic inflammation seen in $KC;Hsl^{-/-}$ mice. It is possible that HSL deficiency causes enhanced inflammation primarily in the visceral WAT adjacent to the pancreas with an increased production and secretion of pro-inflammatory cytokines, which could elicit a subsequent inflammatory reaction in the pancreas of KC mice. This is supported by our finding that HSL deficiency failed to cause pancreatic inflammation in WT mice. It is conceivable that the robust visceral WAT inflammation in $KC;Hsl^{-/-}$ mice reinforces and amplifies the oncogenic and inflammatory signaling in KrasG12D harboring pancreatic cells, thereby leading to substantial pancreatic inflammation and accelerated PDAC development.

However, we cannot rule out an important role of pancreatic HSL in mediating pancreatic inflammation and tumorigenesis. Indeed, we detected strong HSL expression in pancreatic islets and PanIN lesions and reduced expression of *LIPE* (the gene encoding HSL) in pancreatic tissue of patients with PDAC is associated with decreased overall survival [26]. HSL deficiency in pancreatic islets may thereby explain the observed reduction in insulin of $KC;Hsl^{-/-}$ mice in our study, as HSL has been described to be important in glucose-stimulated insulin secretion in pancreatic beta cells [27]. HSL deficiency in the pancreas was accompanied by reduced TG and FFA levels, indicating a prominent role of HSL (and a possible absence of additional neutral lipases) in FFA release from intracellular TG depots in the pancreas. It is plausible that in the

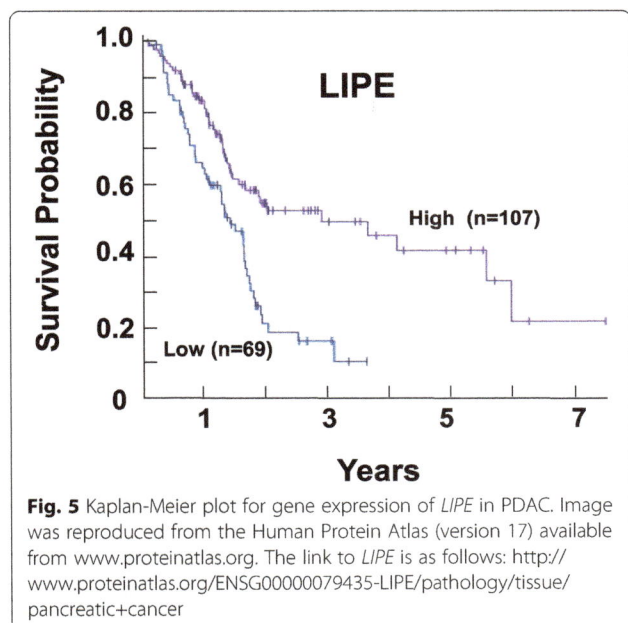

Fig. 5 Kaplan-Meier plot for gene expression of *LIPE* in PDAC. Image was reproduced from the Human Protein Atlas (version 17) available from www.proteinatlas.org. The link to *LIPE* is as follows: http://www.proteinatlas.org/ENSG00000079435-LIPE/pathology/tissue/pancreatic+cancer

presence of oncogenic KRAS these lipid changes locally in the pancreas in *KC;Hsl*$^{-/-}$ mice are driving promotional factors of pancreatic inflammation and PDAC development. These possibilities are not mutually exclusive and the lack of HSL in both visceral WAT and in the pancreas of KC could cooperate in accelerating PDAC development.

Conclusion

Our data demonstrated that HSL deficiency in KC mice leads to inflammation of mesenteric WAT and the pancreas and importantly accelerated PDAC formation. Collectively, our results revealed an unexpected tumor-suppressive role of HSL and emphasize the need of caution in targeting HSL for tumor cachexia or dyslipidemia, as chronic suppression of this enzyme may lead to increased incidence of PDAC.

Abbreviations

PPAR-γ: Peroxisome proliferator-activated receptor gamma; TNF-α: Tumor necrosis factor-alpha; AT: Adipose tissue; CLS: Crown like structures; DIO: Diet-induced obesity; FA: Fatty acid; FFA: Free fatty acid; HPF: High power field; HSL: Hormone sensitive lipase; PanIN: Pancreatic intraepithelial neoplasia; PCR: Polymerase chain reaction; PDAC: Pancreatic ductal adenocarcinoma; PL: Phospholipids; TG: Triglycerides; WAT: White adipose tissue

Acknowledgements
We thank Andrea Schmidt, Kathleen Hertzer, and Alex Stark for their excellent technical assistance with the animal studies.

Funding
GE is supported by P01CA163200 and the Hirshberg Foundation for Pancreatic Cancer Research. MX was supported by T32DK07180 and the SSAT Mentored Research Award. ER is supported by P01CA163200, R01DK100405 and P30DK41301, Department of Veterans Affair Grant 1I01BX001473 and funds from the endowed Ronald S. Hirschberg Chair of Pancreatic Cancer Research. The MMPC Lipid Core was supported by DK59637. The funders had no role in study design, data collection and analysis, decision to publish, or preparation of the manuscript.

Authors' contributions
MX performed the animal experiment, immunohistochemistry, and analyzed the data. HHC performed the animal experiments, western blots, and analyzed the data. XJ performed the animal experiments, tissue harvest, immunohistochemistry, and immunofluorescence. AM performed the animal experiments, monitored the animals daily, and helped with tissue harvest. CENC was involved with tissue harvest, processing, genotyping analyses, and western blots. JK contributed important intellectual content. OJH contributed important intellectual content. JSS performed the Kaplan-Meier plot for gene expression of *LIPE* in PDAC. ER made substantial contributions to analysis and interpretation of data, and has been critically involved in revising the manuscript. GE made substantial contributions to conception and design, analysis and interpretation of data, drafting the manuscript and revising it. All authors have read and approved the final manuscript.

Competing interests
The authors declare that they have no competing interests.

Author details
[1]Departments of Surgery, David Geffen School of Medicine, University of California, Los Angeles, 10833 Le Conte Ave, CHS 72-236, Los Angeles, CA 90095, USA. [2]Departments of Medicine, David Geffen School of Medicine, University of California, Los Angeles, Los Angeles, CA, USA. [3]CURE: Digestive Diseases Research Center, University of California at Los Angeles, Los Angeles, USA.

References

1. Kraemer FB, Shen WJ. Hormone-sensitive lipase: control of intracellular tri-(di-)acylglycerol and cholesteryl ester hydrolysis. J Lipid Res. 2002;43(10): 1585–94.
2. Das SK, Hoefler G. The role of triglyceride lipases in cancer associated cachexia. Trends Mol Med. 2013;19(5):292–301.
3. Tisdale MJ. Mechanisms of Cancer Cachexia. Physiol Rev. 2009;89(2):381–410.
4. Das SK, Eder S, Schauer S, Diwoky C, Temmel H, Guertl B, Gorkiewicz G, Tamilarasan KP, Kumari P, Trauner M, et al. Adipose triglyceride lipase contributes to Cancer-associated Cachexia. Science. 2011;333(6039):233–8.
5. Agustsson T, Rydén M, Hoffstedt J, van Harmelen V, Dicker A, Laurencikiene J, Isaksson B, Permert J, Arner P. Mechanism of increased lipolysis in Cancer Cachexia. Cancer Res. 2007;67(11):5531–7.
6. Ogiyama T, Yamaguchi M, Kurikawa N, Honzumi S, Terayama K, Nagaoka N, Yamamoto Y, Kimura T, Sugiyama D, Inoue S-I. Design, synthesis, and pharmacological evaluation of a novel series of hormone sensitive lipase inhibitor. Bioorg Med Chem. 2017;25(17):4817–28.
7. Vasilieva E, Dutta S, Malla RK, Martin BP, Spilling CD, Dupureur CM. Rat hormone sensitive lipase inhibition by Cyclipostins and their analogs. Bioorg Med Chem. 2015;23(5):944–52.
8. Siegel RL, Miller KD, Jemal A. Cancer statistics, 2017. CA Cancer J Clin. 2017; 67(1):7–30.
9. Rahib L, Smith BD, Aizenberg R, Rosenzweig AB, Fleshman JM, Matrisian LM. Projecting Cancer incidence and deaths to 2030: the unexpected burden of thyroid, liver, and pancreas cancers in the United States. Cancer Res. 2014; 74(11):2913–21.
10. Osuga J, Ishibashi S, Oka T, Yagyu H, Tozawa R, Fujimoto A, Shionoiri F, Yahagi N, Kraemer FB, Tsutsumi O, et al. Targeted disruption of hormone-sensitive lipase results in male sterility and adipocyte hypertrophy, but not in obesity. Proc Natl Acad Sci U S A. 2000;97(2):787–92.
11. Hingorani SR, Petricoin EF, Maitra A, Rajapakse V, King C, Jacobetz MA, Ross S, Conrads TP, Veenstra TD, Hitt BA, et al. Preinvasive and invasive ductal pancreatic cancer and its early detection in the mouse. Cancer Cell. 2003; 4(6):437–50.
12. Funahashi H, Satake M, Dawson D, Huynh NA, Reber HA, Hines OJ, Eibl G. Delayed progression of pancreatic intraepithelial neoplasia in a conditional Kras(G12D) mouse model by a selective cyclooxygenase-2 inhibitor. Cancer Res. 2007;67(15):7068–71.
13. Subbaramaiah K, Howe LR, Bhardwaj P, Du B, Gravaghi C, Yantiss RK, Zhou XK, Blaho VA, Hla T, Yang P, et al. Obesity is associated with inflammation and elevated aromatase expression in the mouse mammary gland. Cancer Prev Res (Phila). 2011;4(3):329–46.

14. Hertzer KM, Xu M, Moro A, Dawson DW, Du L, Li G, Chang HH, Stark AP, Jung X, Hines OJ, et al. Robust early inflammation of the Peripancreatic visceral adipose tissue during diet-induced obesity in the KrasG12D model of pancreatic Cancer. Pancreas. 2016;45(3):458–65.

15. Hruban RH, Adsay NV, Albores-Saavedra J, Compton C, Garrett ES, Goodman SN, Kern SE, Klimstra DS, Kloppel G, Longnecker DS, et al. Pancreatic intraepithelial neoplasia: a new nomenclature and classification system for pancreatic duct lesions. Am J Surg Pathol. 2001;25(5):579–86.

16. Chang HH, Moro A, Takakura K, Su HY, Mo A, Nakanishi M, Waldron RT, French SW, Dawson DW, Hines OJ, et al. Incidence of pancreatic cancer is dramatically increased by a high fat, high calorie diet in KrasG12D mice. PLoS One. 2017;12(9):e0184455.

17. Dawson DW, Hertzer K, Moro A, Donald G, Chang HH, Go VL, Pandol SJ, Lugea A, Gukovskaya AS, Li G, et al. High-fat, high-calorie diet promotes early pancreatic neoplasia in the conditional KrasG12D mouse model. Cancer Prev Res (Phila). 2013;6(10):1064–73.

18. Kraemer FB, Shen WJ. Hormone-sensitive lipase knockouts. Nutr Metab (Lond). 2006;3:12.

19. Shen WJ, Yu Z, Patel S, Jue D, Liu LF, Kraemer FB. Hormone-sensitive lipase modulates adipose metabolism through PPARgamma. Biochim Biophys Acta. 2011;1811(1):9–16.

20. Haemmerle G, Zimmermann R, Hayn M, Theussl C, Waeg G, Wagner E, Sattler W, Magin TM, Wagner EF, Zechner R. Hormone-sensitive lipase deficiency in mice causes diglycerice accumulation in adipose tissue, muscle, and testis. J Biol Chem. 2002;277(7):4806–15.

21. Mulder H, Holst LS, Svensson H, Degerman E, Sundler F, Ahren B, Rorsman P, Holm C. Hormone-sensitive lipase, the rate-limiting enzyme in triglyceride hydrolysis, is expressed and active in beta-cells. Diabetes. 1999;48(1):228–32.

22. Albert JS, Yerges-Armstrong LM, Horenstein RB, Pollin TI, Sreenivasan UT, Chai S, Blaner WS, Snitker S, O'Connell JR, Gong DW, et al. Null mutation in hormone-sensitive lipase gene and risk of type 2 diabetes. N Engl J Med. 2014;370(24):2307–15.

23. Wang SP, Laurin N, Himms-Hagen J, Rudnicki MA, Levy E, Robert MF, Pan L, Oligny L, Mitchell GA. The adipose tissue phenotype of hormone-sensitive lipase deficiency in mice. Obes Res. 2001;9(2):119–28.

24. Zimmermann R, Lass A, Haemmerle G, Zechner R. Fate of fat: the role of adipose triglyceride lipase in lipolysis. Biochim Biophys Acta. 2009;1791(6):494–500.

25. Zimmermann R, Haemmerle G, Wagner EM, Strauss JG, Kratky D, Zechner R. Decreased fatty acid esterification compensates for the reduced lipolytic activity in hormone-sensitive lipase-deficient white adipose tissue. J Lipid Res. 2003;44(11):2089–99.

26. Uhlen M, Zhang C, Lee S, Sjöstedt E, Fagerberg L, Bidkhori G, Benfeitas R, Arif M, Liu Z, Edfors F, et al. A pathology atlas of the human cancer transcriptome. Science. 2017;357(6352):eaan2507.

27. Shen WJ, Liang Y, Wang J, Harada K, Patel S, Michie SA, Osuga J, Ishibashi S, Kraemer FB. Regulation of hormone-sensitive lipase in islets. Diabetes Res Clin Pract. 2007;75(1):14–26.

19

Pancreatic cancer as a sentinel for hereditary cancer predisposition

Erin L. Young[1], Bryony A. Thompson[2,3], Deborah W. Neklason[2,4], Matthew A. Firpo[2,5], Theresa Werner[2,6], Russell Bell[1], Justin Berger[7], Alison Fraser[7], Amanda Gammon[2], Cathryn Koptiuch[2], Wendy K. Kohlmann[2], Leigh Neumayer[8], David E. Goldgar[2,9], Sean J. Mulvihill[2,5], Lisa A. Cannon-Albright[2,4,10] and Sean V. Tavtigian[1,2*] (iD)

Abstract

Background: Genes associated with hereditary breast and ovarian cancer (HBOC) and colorectal cancer (CRC) predisposition have been shown to play a role in pancreatic cancer susceptibility. Growing evidence suggests that pancreatic cancer may be useful as a sentinel cancer to identify families that could benefit from HBOC or CRC surveillance, but to date pancreatic cancer is only considered an indication for genetic testing in the context of additional family history.

Methods: Preliminary data generated at the Huntsman Cancer Hospital (HCH) included variants identified on a custom 34-gene panel or 59-gene panel including both known HBOC and CRC genes for respective sets of 66 and 147 pancreatic cancer cases, unselected for family history. Given the strength of preliminary data and corresponding literature, 61 sequential pancreatic cancer cases underwent a custom 14-gene clinical panel. Sequencing data from HCH pancreatic cancer cases, pancreatic cancer cases of the Cancer Genome Atlas (TCGA), and an unselected pancreatic cancer screen from the Mayo Clinic were combined in a meta-analysis to estimate the proportion of carriers with pathogenic and high probability of pathogenic variants of uncertain significance (HiP-VUS).

Results: Approximately 8.6% of unselected pancreatic cancer cases at the HCH carried a variant with potential HBOC or CRC screening recommendations. A meta-analysis of unselected pancreatic cancer cases revealed that approximately 11.5% carry a pathogenic variant or HiP-VUS.

Conclusion: With the inclusion of both HBOC and CRC susceptibility genes in a panel test, unselected pancreatic cancer cases act as a useful sentinel cancer to identify asymptomatic at-risk relatives who could benefit from relevant HBOC and CRC surveillance measures.

Keywords: HBOC, Lynch syndrome, Colorectal cancer, Pancreatic cancer, Genetic testing

Background

Over the last few years, massively parallel sequencing converged with targeted capture using array synthesized baits to enable panel testing of most known cancer susceptibility genes [1–4]. These panel tests have since replaced Sanger sequencing of limited sets of syndromic genes, thereby revolutionizing the genetic testing landscape for Hereditary Breast and Ovarian cancer (HBOC) and Colorectal cancer (CRC) predisposition. A great

benefit for these predictive genetic tests is to identify carriers of pathogenic medically-actionable variants in asymptomatic individuals, notably the at-risk relatives of the sentinel cancer patient.

Methods for prevention or early detection of pancreatic cancer have limited utility, [5, 6] so utilizing germline predisposition testing to identify individuals with modest to moderate increases in pancreatic cancer susceptibility is also limited in utility. Current guidelines recommend genetic testing only in pancreatic cancer patients with additional family history matching the patterns indicative of hereditary breast and ovarian cancer, colorectal cancer predisposition such as FAP or Lynch syndrome, or melanoma [7–11]. However, studies have

---
* Correspondence: sean.tavtigian@hci.utah.edu
[1]Department of Oncological Sciences, University of Utah School of Medicine, Salt Lake City, United States
[2]Huntsman Cancer Institute, University of Utah School of Medicine, Salt Lake City, United States
Full list of author information is available at the end of the article

found that these criteria will miss 50% of pancreatic cancer patients who harbor actionable pathogenic variants [12, 13]. Therefore, pancreatic cancer may be a useful sentinel cancer for identification of carriers of pathogenic variants in HBOC and CRC susceptibility genes, whose relatives can benefit from surveillance, medical, and surgical strategies for prevention, risk reduction, or early detection [7, 14–22].

To estimate the percentage of pancreatic cancer cases that carry variants with potential medical management impact for at-risk relatives, we applied panel testing to 274 pancreatic cancer patients ascertained at the Huntsman Cancer Hospital (HCH) in Salt Lake City, UT, unselected for family cancer history. To demonstrate generalizability of the results in pancreatic cancer cases, we performed a meta-analysis including published panel tests of unselected pancreatic cancer cases.

Methods

Subjects and ethics statement

This study was approved by the Institutional Review Board of the University of Utah. All participants gave written consent, which included DNA sampling for molecular studies and access to medical records.

An initial set of pancreatic cancer cases ($n = 66$) were selected on the minimal requirements of personal history of cancer and having at least two grandparents in the genealogy data represented in the Utah Population Database (UPDB). These patients were screened with a 34-gene custom research panel. Individual family members were then linked to statewide cancer, demographic, and medical information [23]. Ages at diagnosis and family cancer history were obtained from the UPDB after sequencing and variant evaluation. Additional subjects were selected on the basis of being newly diagnosed pancreatic cancer cases ascertained at the HCH from July 2014 to April 2017 ($n = 224$). The pancreatic cancer cases ascertained during the interval July 2014–November 2015 ($n = 151$) were screened with a 59-gene custom research panel, and the cases ascertained during the interval December 2015–April 2017 ($n = 73$) were screened with a 14-gene custom clinical panel.

Next-generation sequencing library preparation and custom targeted capture

For research panel testing, blood-derived genomic DNA (100 ng) was sheared using a Covaris S2 instrument (Covaris, Woburn, MA, United States). Genomic libraries were prepared using the Ovation Ultralow Library System (NUGEN # 0329) according to the manufacturer's instructions. Library enrichment for a 34 or 59-gene custom panel was done with the Roche SeqCap EZ Choice Library (cat# 06266339001) and the SeqCap EZ Reagent Kit Plus v2 (NimbleGen #06–953–247-001)

using the manufacturer's protocol. Individual libraries were combined into pools of 6–12 prior to hybridization, and then super-pooled for up to 96 samples per sequencing lane. Captured libraries were sequenced on an Illumina HiSeq2000 channel using the HiSeq 101 Cycle Paired-End sequencing protocol.

On the strength of preliminary data from this study, HCH began systematically offering clinical panel predisposition testing beginning December 2015, without regard to family history. From December 2015 to April 2017, clinical testing was offered to 73 sequential pancreatic cancer cases. Sixty-one pancreatic cancer patients accepted clinical testing with the 14-gene custom panel that was conducted by Invitae. The 12 individuals that declined were in poor health and/or did not see value in undergoing a genetic test. A complete list of genes captured is included in Additional file 1: Table S1.

Sequences from the Utah cohort with ≥100X mean coverage and 154 pancreatic cancer cases from the Cancer Genome Atlas (TCGA) [24] were analyzed using the USeq (useq.sourceforge.net) in-house pipeline, according to the Genome Analysis Toolkit (GATK v.3.3–0) best practices recommendations [25]. Variants with a mapping quality score less than 20 were excluded. ANNOVAR was used for variant functional annotation followed by conversion to Human Genome Variation Society (HGVS) nomenclature using Mutalyzer [26, 27].

Sequence variant evaluation

Truncating variants not present in the final exon of a gene were considered pathogenic. The following filters were used to exclude variants from further analysis: minor allele frequency ≥ 0.1% in one or more populations from the Exome Aggregation Consortium (ExAC) database; [28] synonymous/intronic variants with no predicted effect on splicing via MaxEntScan; [29] variants reported as probable-non-pathogenic/non-pathogenic by more than one source with no conflicting reports in ClinVar (www.ncbi.nlm.nih.gov/clinvar).

Variants of uncertain significance (VUS) were included if in silico predictions were suggestive of being relatively high probabilities of pathogenicity VUS (HiP-VUS). HiP-VUS had estimated prior probabilities of pathogenicity > 0.8 based on calibrated in silico predictions from publicly available databases for the mismatch repair (MMR) genes (hci-lovd.hci.utah.edu), or *BRCA1/2* (http://priors.hci.utah.edu/PRIORS/). HiP-VUS of this type were weighted according to their sequence analysis-based prior probability of pathogenicity (Prior_P) score. The VUS from the remaining genes were denoted HiP-VUS and included if at least three of the four missense analysis programs Align-GVGD, MAPP, Polyphen-2, and CADD predicted a severe score [30–34]. This filter corresponds with an OR = 3.27 when comparing early-onset breast cancer cases with matched controls [33]. Based on the likelihood ratios identified for *BRCA1/2*, [35] this grouping was assigned a weight of 0.81. Canonical splice acceptor/donor variants predicted to impact splicing were given the weight of 0.97 if the effect of the variant had not been demonstrated experimentally [36]. Pathogenic variants and HiP-VUS detected by the 34–/59-gene panels were confirmed via Sanger sequencing. VUS reported by the Mayo Clinic [37] plus the non-TCGA ExAC (excluding the Finnish and undescribed populations), were graded with the same weights and severity to generate a bioinformatically equivalent set of HiP-VUS. An overview of the datasets and methods used for evaluation is shown (Fig. 1).

Statistical analysis

STATA V.13.1 (StataCorp, College Station, Texas, USA) was used to conduct meta-analyses, and calculate carrier percentages and 95% confidence intervals. The meta-analyses to compare the carrier frequencies between different pancreatic cancer cohorts were conducted using Metaprop under a random effects model, and Freeman-Tukey transformation to stabilize the variances over the studies [38]. The weighted proportions of variant carriers in the unselected pancreatic cancer cases were compared to the corresponding proportions in the non-TCGA ExAC population to estimate Standardized Incidence Ratios (SIR) [39]. Tests of significance and confidence intervals were estimated based on a Poisson

distribution [40]. For the meta-analysis and SIR calculation, the genes were split into subgroups of high- and moderate-risk cancer susceptibility genes. High- and moderate-risk were defined as genes with a cumulative risk at age 80 > 32% or between 19 and 32%, respectively, for the cancer with which they are most closely associated [2]. The R package ggplot2 was used to plot the meta-analyses and SIRs [41].

Results

Identification of pathogenic variants and HiP-VUS in pancreatic cancer patients, unselected for family history

In an initial set of 66 pancreatic cancer cases unselected for family history of cancer, 4 pathogenic variants were identified in *BRCA2*, *MSH6*, *PALB2*, and *STK11*. After filtering VUS, 2 HiP-VUS in *ATM* remained (Table 1). After weighting, 8.5% of these pancreatic cancer cases carried a variant with potential medical management impact for relatives.

Two series of cases were used for internal replication. From a set of 147 pancreatic cancer cases undergoing an in-house custom 59-gene panel, 6 pathogenic variants were identified in *ATM*, *BRCA1*, *BRCA2*, *MRE11A*, and *PALB2*, and 6 HiP-VUS in *ATM*, *BRCA2*, *CHEK2*, *MSH6*, and *TP53*. In addition to in silico predictions, *CHEK2* p.(T476 M) was found to be damaging in a functional assay for *CHEK2* variants, and was thus weighted more strongly towards being pathogenic [42]. Subsequently, an additional set of pancreatic cancer

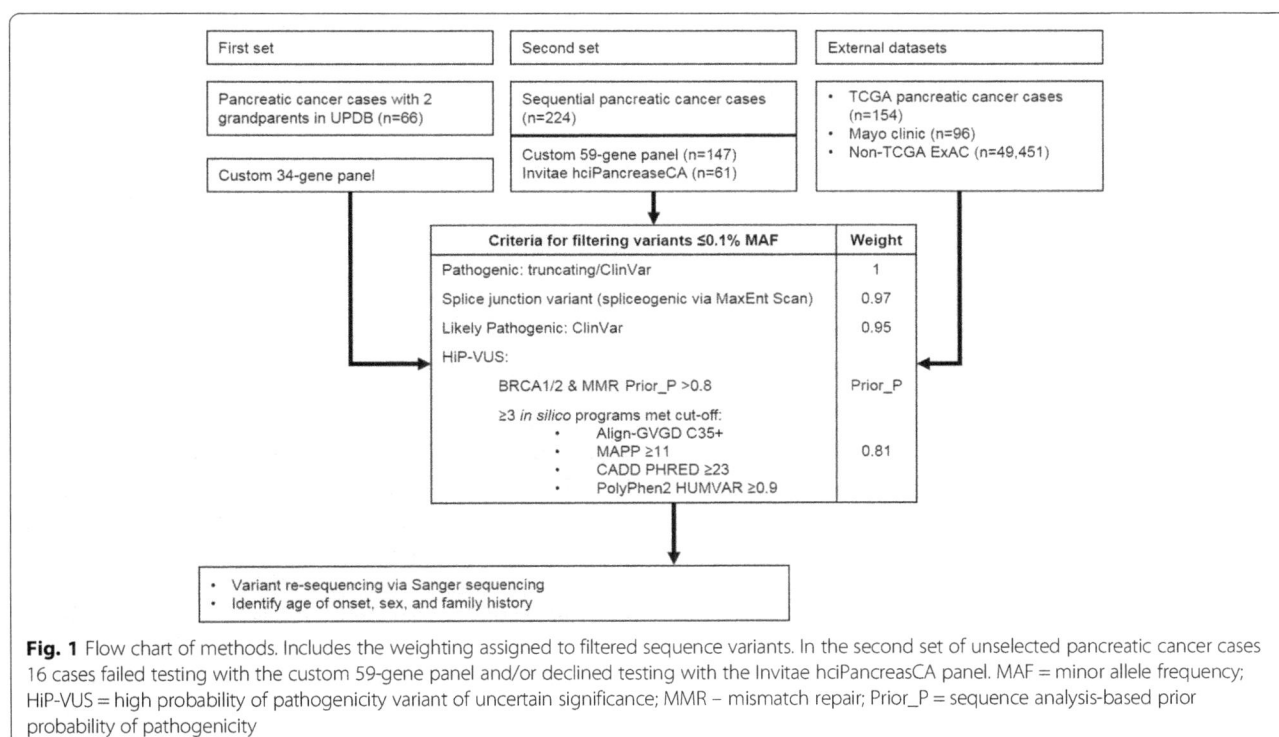

First set	Second set	External datasets
Pancreatic cancer cases with 2 grandparents in UPDB (n=66)	Sequential pancreatic cancer cases (n=224)	• TCGA pancreatic cancer cases (n=154) • Mayo clinic (n=96) • Non-TCGA ExAC (n=49,451)
Custom 34-gene panel	Custom 59-gene panel (n=147) Invitae hciPancreaseCA (n=61)	

Criteria for filtering variants ≤0.1% MAF	Weight
Pathogenic: truncating/ClinVar	1
Splice junction variant (spliceogenic via MaxEnt Scan)	0.97
Likely Pathogenic: ClinVar	0.95
HiP-VUS:	
BRCA1/2 & MMR Prior_P >0.8	Prior_P
≥3 *in silico* programs met cut-off: • Align-GVGD C35+ • MAPP ≥11 • CADD PHRED ≥23 • PolyPhen2 HUMVAR ≥0.9	0.81

• Variant re-sequencing via Sanger sequencing
• Identify age of onset, sex, and family history

Fig. 1 Flow chart of methods. Includes the weighting assigned to filtered sequence variants. In the second set of unselected pancreatic cancer cases 16 cases failed testing with the custom 59-gene panel and/or declined testing with the Invitae hciPancreasCA panel. MAF = minor allele frequency; HiP-VUS = high probability of pathogenicity variant of uncertain significance; MMR – mismatch repair; Prior_P = sequence analysis-based prior probability of pathogenicity

Table 1 Pathogenic variants and high probability of pathogenicity variants of uncertain significance (HiP-VUS) identified from a custom 34- or 59-gene panel and a clinical 14-gene panel in pancreatic cancer cases, unselected for family history

Gene	HGVS Notation	Sex: Age of Onset	Carrier Weight
Custom 34-gene panel (*n* = 66)			
ATM	c.7327C > G p.(R2443G)	M: 60s	0.81
ATM	c.8734A > G p.(R2912G)	F: 60s	0.81
BRCA2	c.3873del p.(Q1291Hfs*2)	M: 50s	1
MSH6	c.3261dup p.(F1088Lfs*5)	F: 50s	1
PALB2	c.1240C > T p.(R414*)	F: 60s	1
STK11	c.738C > A p.(Y246*)	M: 40s	1
	Carrier Frequency: 5.62/66 = 8.52% (3.87–17.7%)		
Custom 59-gene panel (*n* = 147)			
ATM	c.1564_1565del p.(E522lfs*43)	M: 50s	1
ATM	c.8734A > G p.(R2912G)	M: 70s	0.81
BRCA1	c.68_69del p.(E23Vfs*17)	M: 70s	1
BRCA2	c.3974_3975insTGCT p.(T1325Cfs*4)	M: 70s	1
BRCA2	c.8447G > A p.(G2816D)	F: 60s	0.81
CHEK2	c.1159A > G p.(T387A)	M: 80s	0.81
CHEK2	c.1427C > T p.(T476 M)	F: 50s	0.99[a]
MRE11A	c.923dupT p.(M309Hfs*8)	M: 50s	1
MRE11A	c.1516G > T p.(E506*)	F: 60s	1
MSH6	c.3851C > T p.(T1284 M)	F: 60s	0.94
PALB2	c.2167_2168del p.(M723Vfs*21)	M: 60s[c]	1
RAD50	c.3641G > A p.(R1214H)	F: 50s	-[a]
TP53	c.847C > T p.(R283C)	M: 60s	0.81
Clinical 14-gene panel (*n* = 61)			
ATM	c.1402_1406delAAGAG p.(K468Vfs*17)	F:40s	1
ATM	c.2426C > A p.(S809*)	F:80s[d]	1
ATM	c.3993 + 1G > A (splice donor)	M:70s[e]	-[b]
BRCA2	c.6275_6276delTT p.(L2092Pfs*7)	M:70s	1[b]
CDKN2A	c.301G > T p.(G101 W)	F:60s[f]	1
CHEK2	c.349A > G p.(R117G)	F:70s	0.95
MSH6	c.1444C > T p.(R482*)	F:70s[g]	1
TP53	c.1015G > A p.(E339K)	F:70s	0.81
	Carrier Frequency: 17.89/208 = 8.60% (5.50–13.20%)		

HGVS Human Genome Variation Society
[a,b]The same individual carried both variants, so carrier weight was combined and only counted once. Additional cancers: [c]CRC in 40s; [d]lung in 80s and CRC in 60s; [e]prostate (Gleason 7) in 70s; [f]melanoma in 40s and cervical in 30s; [g]breast in 50s, endometrial in 50s, and urethral in 70s

cases (*n* = 61) were tested with the 14-gene clinical panel, which identified 6 pathogenic variants and 2 HiP-VUS in 7 patients (Table 1). All pathogenic variants and HiP-VUS were identified in genes included in the original 34-gene panel. After weighting carriers, 8.6% of the pancreatic cancer cases from the latter two sets, unselected for family history, carried a variant with potential medical impact. A full list of rare variants with corresponding *in silico* information is available in Additional file 1: Table S2.

Post-variant evaluation of genetic testing eligibility

In order to estimate the proportion of pancreatic cancer cases with pathogenic variants or HiP-VUS that would have qualified for genetic testing, the family histories were compared to NCCN guidelines [43]. Pedigree data regarding familial cancer were available from UPDB for the carriers of pathogenic variants and HiP-VUS in 6 of the initial set of 66 pancreatic cancer patients (Additional file 2: Figure S1). Self-reported family history information was also available for the final set of 61 patients that underwent the Invitae clinical panel, including the 7 carriers of pathogenic variants or HiP-VUS. Among the 13 identified carriers, the STK11 carrier had a clinical diagnosis of Peutz-Jegher syndrome with multiple affected relatives, and 9 additional patients met criteria for HBOC or Lynch syndrome genetic testing. Thus, more than 23% of these carriers would not have qualified for testing under current guidelines.

Once a pathogenic variant is identified, cascade testing for that variant can occur on biological relatives to identify individuals who would benefit from HBOC or CRC preventive measures. For three of the five pancreatic cancer cases with positive results with the clinical panel, 17 biological relatives have undergone cascade genetic testing thus far, 10 of whom have tested positive for the family pathogenic variant. Of note, 21 (29%) pancreatic cancer cases who underwent the clinical panel passed away since the beginning of the study, 17 of whom had undergone testing. This suggests that having a family member(s) present during pre-test counseling and delegated to receive results may be beneficial in the context of utilization of pancreatic cancer as a sentinel for HBOC or Lynch syndrome.

Meta-analysis of carrier proportions across studies

The HCH sets of pancreatic cancer cases were combined with a published study of unselected pancreatic cancer cases from the Mayo Clinic ($n = 96$), [37] plus the pancreatic cancer cases from TCGA ($n = 154$), in a meta-analysis (Fig. 2; Additional file 1: Table S3; Additional file 3: Table S4). Among unselected

pancreatic cancer cases, 3.9% ($p = 2.1 \times 10^{-13}$) carried a clearly pathogenic variant in a high-risk cancer susceptibility gene which includes pancreatic cancer in its tumor spectrum [8]. Weighed inclusion of HiP-VUS increased the proportion to 5.1% ($p = 6.8 \times 10^{-18}$). For the moderate-risk homologous recombination repair (HRR) breast cancer genes ATM, BARD1, CHEK2, and NBN, [2, 44] 3.3% ($p = 7.2 \times 10^{-04}$) of unselected pancreatic cancer cases carried a clearly pathogenic variant, and weighted inclusion of HiP-VUS increased the proportion to 5.1% ($p = 2.3 \times 10^{-08}$). Including all the high-risk genes and the moderate-risk HRR breast cancer genes, 7.9% ($p = 1.4 \times 10^{-12}$) of unselected pancreatic cancer cases carry a clearly pathogenic variant, and 10.4% ($p = 9.1 \times 10^{-17}$) carry either a clearly pathogenic variant or weighted HiP-VUS with elevated probability of pathogenicity that could enable the at-risk relatives to qualify for preventive HBOC or CRC measures.

Further, the gene burdens observed in the Utah, Mayo, and TCGA were compared to the non-TCGA ExAC ($n = 49,451$, excluding the Finnish and other subpopulations) as a population sample to determine SIR for subgroups of genes (Fig. 3, Additional file 3: Table S5). As a group, the high-risk susceptibility genes had a SIR = 2.6 ($p = 1.6 \times 10^{-05}$). The moderate-risk HRR genes had a slightly lower SIR = 2.3 ($p = 2.0 \times 10^{-05}$).

Discussion

From the 16 pathogenic and 11 HiP-VUS carriers identified through systematic panel testing of pancreatic

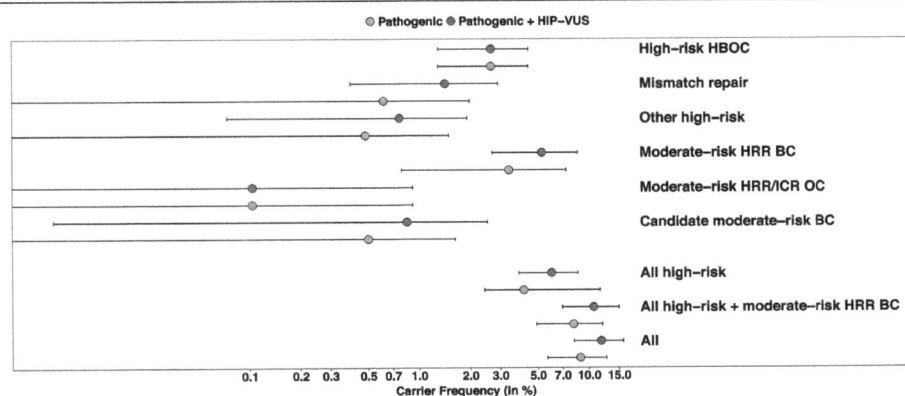

Fig. 2 Proportion of carriers of pathogenic variants and high probability of pathogenicity variants of uncertain significance (HiP-VUS) in unselected pancreatic cancer. Results based on a meta-analysis of the unselected pancreatic cancer cases from the Huntsman Cancer Hospital (HCH), the Mayo Clinic, and the pancreatic cancer cases from The Cancer Genome Atlas (TCGA). Carrier frequency point estimates and 95% confidence intervals for groups of genes are presented on a log-scale. A list of genes contained within each analysis group is provided in Additional file 1: Table S1. The breakdown of results by study is described in Additional file 1: Table S3. HBOC = Hereditary Breast and Ovarian Cancer; HRR = Homologous Recombination and Repair; ICR = Interstrand Crosslink Repair; OC = Ovarian Cancer; BC = Breast Cancer

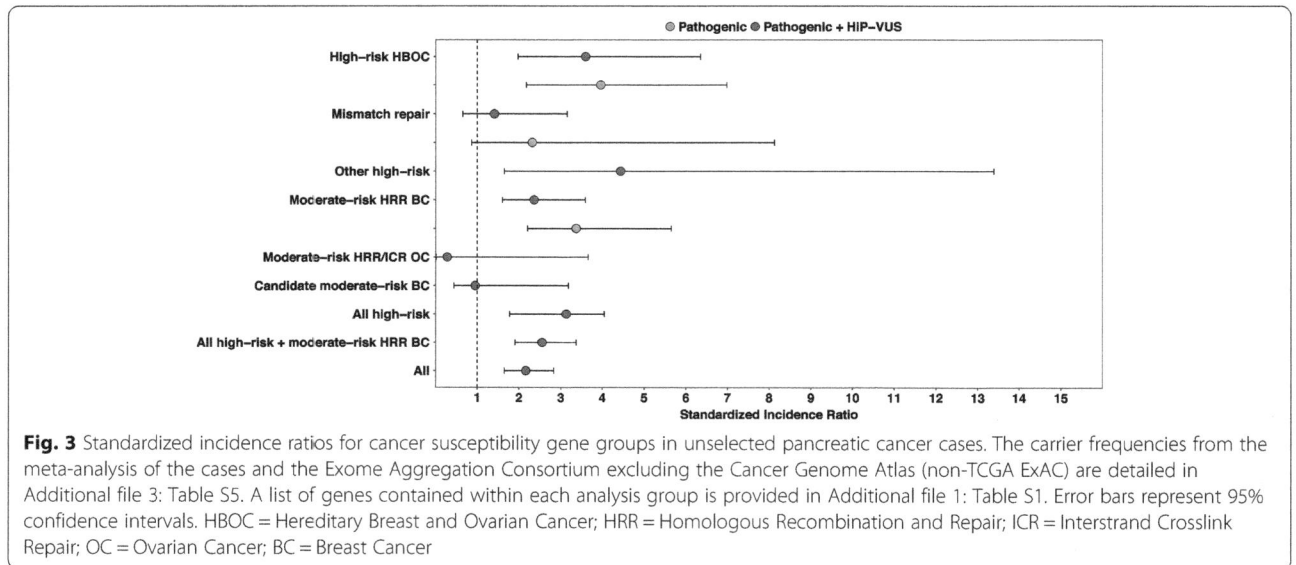

Fig. 3 Standardized incidence ratios for cancer susceptibility gene groups in unselected pancreatic cancer cases. The carrier frequencies from the meta-analysis of the cases and the Exome Aggregation Consortium excluding the Cancer Genome Atlas (non-TCGA ExAC) are detailed in Additional file 3: Table S5. A list of genes contained within each analysis group is provided in Additional file 1: Table S1. Error bars represent 95% confidence intervals. HBOC = Hereditary Breast and Ovarian Cancer; HRR = Homologous Recombination and Repair; ICR = Interstrand Crosslink Repair; OC = Ovarian Cancer; BC = Breast Cancer

cancer cases unselected for family history, we estimate that 2.7% (95% CI: 1.4–4.4) carry a pathogenic allele of a high-risk HBOC gene (*BRCA1, BRCA2*, or *PALB2*) and 1.3% (95% CI: 0.3–2.8) of probands carry a pathogenic allele of a Lynch Syndrome (LS)-associated MMR gene (*MLH1, MSH2, PMS2*, or *MSH6*). Adding other high-risk genes such as *TP53, CDKN2A*, and *STK11* results in 5.1% (95% CI: 3.3–7.2) of pancreatic cancer cases with a sequence variant that would alter medical management of healthy at-risk relatives: i.e. MRI in addition to mammography or early colonoscopy (Fig. 2) [7, 9, 45–47]. An additional 5.1% (95% CI: 2.4–8.5) are estimated to carry a pathogenic allele of a moderate-risk breast cancer susceptibility gene (i.e., *ATM, BARD1, CHEK2*, or *NBN*) bringing the total proportion of estimated carriers to 10.4% (95% CI: 6.5–14.9). Here we note that *ATM* and *CHEK2* have recently been added to NCCN's list of genes with associated medical action for breast cancer [7]. Focusing on individual genes, the top four genes with potential medical impact for at-risk relatives, based on weighted counts, were *ATM* (identified in 7 cases), *BRCA2* (4 cases), *CHEK2* (3 cases), and *MSH6* (3 cases).

The precedent for testing all pancreatic cancer patients comes from what has been accepted and learned from universal testing of all CRCs for LS. Universal LS testing, with immunohistochemical (IHC) or microsatellite instability (MSI)-based pre-screen of tumors followed by germline testing for indicated individuals, is recommended for newly diagnosed CRC cases [45, 48]. This strategy may soon be overtaken by germline DNA panel testing for LS due to 1) rapid decline of panel testing cost, 2) superiority of specificity and sensitivity, and 3)

evidence that pre-screening delays genetic testing, which results in a subsequent ∼ 50% loss in follow up by patients [49–56]. Indeed, a health economics analysis recently published by Erten et al. [56] concluded that universal testing of CRC patients for LS based on sequencing alone will become more cost effective than the two-step test when the cost of MMR gene sequencing drops to or below $609 USD, echoing a similar finding by Gould-Suarez et al. [56, 57]. Based on our results, universal testing of pancreatic cancer patients using a panel test would identify pathogenic variants or HiP-VUS in MMR genes at a frequency similar to what is detected with universal screening of CRC patients, 1.3 and 1.2% respectively [56].

In a recent study, 11.8% of unselected patients with metastatic prostate cancer were found to carry pathogenic variants in DNA-repair genes [58]. Pritchard et al. suggest that this proportion of metastatic prostate cancer cases is high enough to utilize metastatic prostate cancer as a sentinel for cancer predisposition testing. The 11.8% proportion observed in metastatic prostate cancer is similar to the 10.4% observed in this meta-analysis of pancreatic cancer cases. For these patients, universal panel testing offers critical time and convenience advantages over step-wise testing strategies, resulting in decreased loss to follow up or mortality and correspondingly increased benefit to at-risk relatives.

Lastly, there are an increasing number of options for targeted treatments based on germline mutations. PARP inhibitors show promise in pancreatic cancer, include olaparib and rucaparib (which are FDA approved in ovarian cancer), as well as veliparib (or ABT-888) which is in clinical trials [59]. Most patients with pathogenic germline *BRCA1*, *BRCA2*, or *PALB2* variants would be expected to respond. Solid tumors with MMR deficiency often respond to immunotherapy [60]. The US Food and Drug Administration (FDA) has granted accelerated approval to pembrolizumab (Keytruda) for pediatric and adult patients with microsatellite unstable cancers, a hallmark molecular feature of Lynch syndrome related cancers [59]. The availability of targeted treatments increases the utility of testing for pancreatic cancer patients themselves, in addition to the prevention and screening benefits for relatives.

Conclusions

Our study adds to the increasing body of evidence that pancreatic cancer is an indicator of hereditary cancer predisposition. Identifying cases who carry mutations in genes associated with clinical recommendations will allow relatives to benefit from screening and prevention strategies for the range of cancer risks conferred. Increasingly, the finding of a germline mutation in pancreatic cancer patients may also impact their treatment. The benefits of genetic testing of all pancreatic cancer cases mirrors other cancers for which routine evaluation has become standard of care. Significant morbidity and poor prognosis may make this a uniquely challenging population to offer genetic counseling and testing. Research on the inherited basis of pancreatic cancer should be paired with psychosocial and behavioral studies to determine how best to incorporate genetic testing into the care of these patients and to ensure that findings are optimally used to benefit families.

Abbreviations

CRC: colorectal cancer; ExAC: Exome Aggregation Consortium; FDA: US Food and Drug Administration; GATK: Genome Analysis Toolkit; HBOC: hereditary breast and ovarian cancer; HCH: Huntsman Cancer Hospital; HGVS: Human Genome Variation Society; HiP-VUS: high probabilities of pathogenicity variants of uncertain significance; IHC: immunohistochemical; LS: Lynch Syndrome; MMR: mismatch repair; MSI: microsatellite instability; SIR: Standardized Incidence Ratios; TCGA: the Cancer Genome Atlas; UPDB: Utah Population Database; VUS: Variants of uncertain significance

Acknowledgements

We acknowledge and appreciate the families for their continued support and participation in our studies. We would like to thank Angela K. Snow and Nykole R. Sutherland for contributions of sequencing. We would also like to thank Ken R. Smith and the Utah Population Database team for enabling this project. The results published here are in part based upon data generated by The Cancer Genome Atlas managed by the NCI and NHGRI. Information about TCGA can be found at http://cancergenome.nih.gov. The authors would also like to thank the Exome Aggregation Consortium and the groups that provided exome variant data for comparison. A full list of contributing groups can be found at http://exac.broadinstitute.org/about

Funding

This research was supported by United States National Institutes of Health (NIH) National Cancer Institute (NCI) grant R01CA164138; NCI grant P30CA042014 (support of Genetic Counseling Shared Resource), by the Utah Genome Project; by the Canadian Institutes of Health Research (CIHR) for the CIHR Team in Familial Risks of Breast Cancer program; by the Government of Canada through Genome Canada and the Canadian Institutes of Health Research, and the Ministère de l'enseignement supérieur, de la recherche, de la science, et de la technologie du Québec through Génome Québec; by NIH NCI Cancer Center Support Grant P30CA042014; and by the Huntsman Cancer Foundation.
BAT is a National Health and Medical Research Council CJ Martin Early Career Fellow. ELY was supported by the National Institutes of Health under Ruth L. Kirschstein National Research Service Award T32HG008962 from the National Human Genome Research Institute. The content is solely the responsibility of the authors and does not necessarily represent the official views of the National Institutes of Health.

Authors' contributions

ELY and SVT were involved in all aspects of manuscript. BAT was involved in DNA sequencing, analysis and interpretation of data, the meta-analysis and additional statistical analysis. DWN made substantial contributions to the study concept and design, and acquisition of data. MAF, TW, RB, LN, DEG, SJM, LACA were involved in analysis and interpretation of data as well as significant contributions of intellectual content. AG, CK, WKK are genetic counselors at the Familial Cancer Assessment Clinic at the Huntsman Cancer Hospital, and were involved in the acquisition of pancreatic cancer patients for both the research and clinical multigene panel. Additionally, they identified pancreatic cancer patients that met NCCN eligibility for genetic testing and drafted and edited substantial portions of manuscript creation pertaining to NCCN guidelines. JB and AF were crucial in identifying pancreatic cancer patients in UPDB with the correct requirements as well as generating pedigrees for those pancreatic cancer cases that carried a P/LP variant or HiP-VUS. All authors have read and approved the final manuscript.

Competing interests

The authors declare that they have no competing interests.

Author details

[1]Department of Oncological Sciences, University of Utah School of Medicine, Salt Lake City, United States. [2]Huntsman Cancer Institute, University of Utah School of Medicine, Salt Lake City, United States. [3]Centre for Epidemiology and Biostatistics, School of Population and Global Health, University of Melbourne, Melbourne, Australia. [4]Division of Genetic Epidemiology, Department of Internal Medicine, University of Utah, Salt Lake City, United States. [5]Department of Surgery, University of Utah School of Medicine, Salt Lake City, United States. [6]Division of Oncology, Department of Medicine, University of Utah, Salt Lake City, United States. [7]Population Sciences, Huntsman Cancer Institute, University of Utah, Salt Lake City, United States. [8]Department of Surgery and Arizona Cancer Center, University of Arizona, Tucson, United States. [9]Department of Dermatology, University of Utah School of Medicine, Salt Lake City, United States. [10]George E. Wahlen Department of Veterans Affairs Medical Center, Salt Lake City, United States.

References

1. Walsh T, Lee MK, Casadei S, Thornton AM, Stray SM, Pennil C, et al. Detection of inherited mutations for breast and ovarian cancer using genomic capture and massively parallel sequencing. Proc. Natl. Acad. Sci. U. S. A. 2010 ;107:12629–12633. Available from: http://www.pubmedcentral.nih.gov/articlerender.fcgi?artid=2906584&tool=pmcentrez&rendertype=abstract. [cited 2010 Dec 8]
2. Easton DF, Pharoah PDP, Antonious AC, Tischkowitz M, Tavtigian SV, Nathanson KL, et al. Gene-panel sequencing and the prediction of breast-Cancer risk. N Engl J Med. 2015;372:2243–57.
3. Hall MJ, Forman AD, Pilarski R, Wiesner G, Giri VN. Gene panel testing for inherited cancer risk. J Natl Compr Canc Netw. 2014;12:1339–46. Available from: http://www.ncbi.nlm.nih.gov/pubmed/25190699
4. Salo-Mullen EE, O'Reilly EM, Kelsen DP, Ashraf AM, Lowery MA, Yu KH, et al. Identification of germline genetic mutations in patients with pancreatic cancer. Cancer. 2015;121:4382–8. Available from: http://doi.wiley.com/10.1002/cncr.29664

5. Harinck F, Poley JW, Kluijt I, Fockens P, Bruno MJ, Dutch Research Group of Pancreatic Cancer Surveillance in High-Risk Individuals. Is early diagnosis of pancreatic cancer fiction? Surveillance of individuals at high risk for pancreatic cancer. Dig. Dis. 2010;28 670–8. Available from: http://www.ncbi.nlm.nih.gov/pubmed/21088419

6. Chari ST, Kelly K, Hollingsworth MA, Thayer SP, Ahlquist DA, Andersen DK, et al. Early detection of sporadic pancreatic cancer: summative review. Pancreas. 2015;44:693–712. Available from: http://www.pubmedcentral.nih.gov/articlerender.fcgi?artid=4467589&tool=pmcentrez&rendertype=abstract

7. Daly MB, Pilarski R, Axilbund JE, Berry M, Buys SS, Crawford B, et al. Genetic/familial high-risk assessment: breast and ovarian, version 2.2015. J Natl Compr Cancer Netw. 2016;14:153–62. Available from: http://www.ncbi.nlm.nih.gov/pubmed/26850485

8. Whitcomb DC, Shelton CA, Brand RE. Genetics and genetic testing in pancreatic cancer. Gastroenterology. 2015;149:1–13. Available from: http://linkinghub.elsevier.com/retrieve/pii/S0016508515010896

9. Leachman SA, Carucci J, Kohlmann W, Banks KC, Asgari MM, Bergman W, et al. Selection criteria for genetic assessment of patients with familial melanoma. J Am Acad Dermatol. 2009;61:1–14.

10. Kastrinos F, Mukherjee B, Tayob N, Wang F, Sparr J, Raymond VM, et al. Risk of pancreatic cancer in families with lynch syndrome. JAMA. 2009;302:1790–5. Available from: http://www.ncbi.nlm.nih.gov/pubmed/29151953

11. Bujanda L, Herreros-Villanueva M. Pancreatic Cancer in lynch syndrome patients. J Cancer. 2017;8:3667–74. Available from: http://www.ncbi.nlm.nih.gov/pubmed/29151953

12. Mandelker D, Zhang L, Kemel Y, Stadler ZK, Joseph V, Zehir A, et al. Mutation Detection in Patients With Advanced Cancer by Universal Sequencing of Cancer-Related Genes in Tumor and Normal DNA vs Guideline-Based Germline Testing. JAMA. 2017;318:825. Available from: http://jama.jamanetwork.com/article.aspx?doi=10.1001/jama.2017.11137

13. Shindo K, Yu J, Suenaga M, Fesharakizadeh S, Cho C, Macgregor-Das A, et al. Deleterious germline mutations in patients with apparently sporadic pancreatic adenocarcinoma. J Clin Oncol. 2017;JCO2017723502 Available from: http://www.ncbi.nlm.nih.gov/pubmed/28767289

14. Catts ZA-K, Baig MK, Milewski B, Keywan C, Guarino M, Petrelli N. Statewide Retrospective Review of Familial Pancreatic Cancer in Delaware, and Frequency of Genetic Mutations in Pancreatic Cancer Kindreds. Ann. Surg. Oncol. 2016;99. Available from: http://link.springer.com/10.1245/s10434-015-5026-x

15. Kim DH, Crawford B, Ziegler J, Beattie MS. Prevalence and characteristics of pancreatic cancer in families with BRCA1 and BRCA2 mutations. Fam. Cancer. 2009;8:153–8. Available from: http://www.ncbi.nlm.nih.gov/pubmed/18855126

16. Grant RC, Selander I, Connor AA, Selvarajah S, Borgida A, Briollais L, et al. Prevalence of germline mutations in Cancer predisposition genes in patients with pancreatic Cancer. Gastroenterology. 2015;148:556–64. [cited 2015 Jan 22]; Available from: http://www.ncbi.nlm.nih.gov/pubmed/25479140

17. Holter S, Borgida A, Dodd A, Grant R. Semotiuk K, Hedley D, et al. Germline BRCA mutations in a large clinic-based cohort of patients with pancreatic adenocarcinoma. J Clin Oncol. 2015;33:3124–9.

18. Hahn SA, Greenhalf B, Ellis I, Sina-Frey M, Rieder H, Korte B, et al. BRCA2 germline mutations in familial pancreatic carcinoma. J Natl Cancer Inst. 2003;95:214–21. Available from: http://www.ncbi.nlm.nih.gov/pubmed/12569143

19. Easton DF, Matthews FE, Ford D, Swerdlow AJ, Peto J. Cancer mortality in relatives of women with ovarian cancer: the OPCS study. Office of Population Censuses and Surveys. Int J Cancer. 1996;65:284–94. Available from: http://www.ncbi.nlm.nih.gov/pubmed/8575846

20. Lal G, Liu G, Schmocker B, Kaurah P, Ozcelik H, Narod SA, et al. Inherited predisposition to pancreatic adenocarcinoma: role of family history and germ-line p16, BRCA1, and BRCA2 mutations. Cancer Res. 2000;60:409–16. Available from: http://www.ncbi.nlm.nih.gov/pubmed/10667595

21. Humphris JL, Johns AL, Simpson SH, Cowley MJ, Pajic M, Chang DK, et al. Clinical and pathologic features of familial pancreatic cancer. Cancer. 2014;120:1–7. [cited 2014 Oct 25]; Available from: http://www.ncbi.nlm.nih.gov/pubmed/25313458

22. Lucas AL, Frado LE, Hwang C, Kumar S, Khanna LG, Levinson EJ, et al. BRCA1 and BRCA2 germline mutations are frequently demonstrated in both high-risk pancreatic cancer screening and pancreatic cancer cohorts. Cancer. 2014;120:1–8. [cited 2014 May 7]; Available from: http://www.ncbi.nlm.nih.gov/pubmed/24737347

23. Skolnick M. The Utah genealogical database: a resource for genetic epidemiology. Banbury Rep. 1980;4:285–97.

24. Tomczak K, Czerwińska P, Wiznerowicz M. The Cancer genome atlas (TCGA): an immeasurable source of knowledge. Wspolczesna Onkol. 2015;1A:A68–77.

25. DePristo MA, Banks E, Poplin R, Garimella KV, Maguire JR, Hartl C, et al. A framework for variation discovery and genotyping using next-generation DNA sequencing data. Nat. Genet. 2011;43:491–8. Available from: http://dx.doi.org/10.1038/ng.806

26. Wildeman M, van Ophuizen E, den Dunnen JT, Taschner PEM. Improving sequence variant descriptions in mutation databases and literature using the Mutalyzer sequence variation nomenclature checker. Hum Mutat. 2008;29:6–13. Available from: http://www.ncbi.nlm.nih.gov/pubmed/16835861

27. Wang K, Li M, Hakonarson H. ANNOVAR: functional annotation of genetic variants from high-throughput sequencing data. Nucleic Acids Res. 2010;38:e164. Available from: http://www.ncbi.nlm.nih.gov/pubmed/20601685

28. Lek M, Karczewski KJ, Minikel EV, Samocha KE, Banks E, Fennell T, et al. Analysis of protein-coding genetic variation in 60,706 humans. Nature. 2016;536:285–91. Available from: http://www.nature.com/doifinder/10.1038/nature19057

29. Yeo G, Burge CB. Maximum entropy modeling of short sequence motifs with applications to RNA splicing signals. J Comput Biol. 2004;11:377–94. [cited 2013 Feb 13]; Available from: http://www.ncbi.nlm.nih.gov/pubmed/15285897

30. Tavtigian SV, Deffenbaugh a M, Yin L, Judkins T, Scholl T, Samollow PB, et al. Comprehensive statistical study of 452 BRCA1 missense substitutions with classification of eight recurrent substitutions as neutral. J Med Genet. 2006;43:295–305. [cited 2013 Nov 7]; Available from: http://www.pubmedcentral.nih.gov/articlerender.fcgi?artid=2563222&tool=pmcentrez&rendertype=abstract

31. Adzhubei I, Jordan DM, Sunyaev SR. Predicting Functional Effect of Human Missense Mutations Using PolyPhen-2. Curr. Protoc. Hum. Genet. 2013; Chapter 7:–Unit7.20. [cited 2013 Feb 5]; Available from: http://www.ncbi.nlm.nih.gov/pubmed/23315928

32. Kircher M, Witten DM, Jain P, O'Roak BJ, Cooper GM, Shendure J. A general framework for estimating the relative pathogenicity of human genetic variants. Nat. Genet. 2014;46:310–5. [cited 2014 Mar 3]; Available from: http://www.nature.com/doifinder/10.1038/ng.2892

33. Young EL, Feng BJ, Stark AW, Damiola F, Durand G, Forey N, et al. Multigene testing of moderate-risk genes: be mindful of the missense. J Med Genet. 2016;53:366–76. Available from: http://jmg.bmj.com/lookup/doi/10.1136/jmedgenet-2015-103398%5Cn http://www.ncbi.nlm.nih.gov/pubmed/26787654

34. E a S, Sidow A. Physicochemical constraint violation by missense substitutions mediates impairment of protein function and disease severity. Genome Res. 2005;15:978–86. [cited 2013 Feb 5] Available from: http://www.pubmedcentral.nih.gov/articlerender.fcgi?artid=1172042&tool=pmcentrez&rendertype=abstract

35. Tavtigian SV, Byrnes GB, Goldgar DE, Thomas A. Classification of rare missense substitutions, using risk surfaces, with genetic- and molecular-epidemiology applications. Hum Mutat. 2008;29:1342–54. Available from: http://www.ncbi.nlm.nih.gov/pubmed/18951461

36. Vallée MP, Di STL, Nix DA, Paquette AM, Parsons MT, Bell R, et al. Adding In Silico Assessment of Potential Splice Aberration to the Integrated Evaluation of BRCA Gene Unclassified Variants. Hum. Mutat. 2016; Available from: http://www.ncbi.nlm.nih.gov/pubmed/26913838

37. Hu C, Hart SN, Bamlet WR, Moore RM, Nandakumar K, Eckloff BW, et al. Prevalence of Pathogenic Mutations in Cancer Predisposition Genes among Pancreatic Cancer Patients. Cancer Epidemiol Biomark Prev. 2016;25:207–11. Available from: http://cebp.aacrjournals.org/cgi/doi/10.1158/1055-9965.EPI-15-0455

38. Freeman MF, Tukey JW. Transformations related to the angular and the square root. Ann Math Stat. 1950;21:607–11.

39. Lek M, Karczewski K, Minikel E, Samocha K, Banks E, Fennell T, et al. Analysis of protein-coding genetic variation in 60,706 humans. bioRxiv. 2015:1–26. Available from: http://biorxiv.org/content/early/2015/10/30/030338.abstract

40. Rosner B. Fundamentals of biostatistics. 2nd ed. Boston: Duxbury Press; 1986.

41. Wickham H. ggplot2: elegant graphics for data analysis. Springer-Verlag New York; 2009.

42. Roeb W, Higgins J, King M. Response to DNA Damage of CHEK2 Missense Mutations in Familial Breast Cancer. Hum. Mol. Genet. 2012;21:2738–44. [cited 2012 Apr 9] Available from: http://www.ncbi.nlm.nih.gov/pubmed/22419737

43. Daly MB, Pilarski R, Berry M, Buys SS, Farmer M, Friedman S, et al. NCCN

guidelines insights: genetic/familial high-risk assessment: breast and ovarian, version 2.2017. J Natl Compr Cancer Netw. 2017;15:9–20. Available from: http://www.jnccn.org/content/15/1/9.long

44. Couch FJ, Shimelis H, Hu C, Hart SN, Polley EC, Na J, et al. Associations Between Cancer Predisposition Testing Panel Genes and Breast Cancer. JAMA Oncologia. 2017;3:1190–6. Available from: http://oncology. jamanetwork.com/article.aspx?doi=10.1001/jamaoncol.2017.0424

45. Provenzale D, Jasperson K, Ahnen DJ, Aslanian H, Bray T, Cannon JA, et al. Colorectal Cancer screening, version 1.2015. J Natl Compr Cancer Netw. 2015;13:959–68. quiz 968. Available from: http://www.jnccn.org/content/13/ 8/959.full.pdf

46. Villani A, Tabori U, Schiffman J, Shlien A, Beyene J, Druker H, et al. Biochemical and imaging surveillance in germline TP53 mutation carriers with Li-Fraumeni syndrome: a prospective observational study. Lancet. Oncol. 2011;12:559–67. Available from: http://www.ncbi.nlm.nih.gov/ pubmed/21601526

47. van der Post RS, Vogelaar IP, Carneiro F, Guilford P, Huntsman D, Hoogerbrugge N, et al. Hereditary diffuse gastric cancer: updated clinical guidelines with an emphasis on germline CDH1 mutation carriers. J Med Genet. 2015;52:361–74. Available from: http://www.pubmedcentral.nih.gov/ articlerender.fcgi?artid=4453626&tool=pmcentrez&rendertype=abstract

48. Evaluation of Genomic Applications in Practice and Prevention (EGAPP) Working Group. Recommendations from the EGAPP Working Group: genetic testing strategies in newly diagnosed individuals with colorectal cancer aimed at reducing morbidity and mortality from Lynch syndrome in relatives. Genet. Med. 2009;11:35–41. Available from: http://www. pubmedcentral.nih.gov/articlerender.fcgi?artid=2743612&tool= pmcentrez&rendertype=abstract

49. Hartman DJ, Brand RE, Hu H, Bahary N, Dudley B, Chiosea SI, et al. Lynch syndrome-associated colorectal carcinoma: Frequent involvement of the left colon and rectum and late-onset presentation supports a universal screening approach. Hum. Pathol. 2013;44:2518–28. Available from: http:// dx.doi.org/10.1016/j.humpath.2013.06.012

50. Heald B, Plesec T, Liu X, Pai R, Patil D, Moline J, et al. Implementation of universal microsatellite instability and immunohistochemistry screening for diagnosing lynch syndrome in a large academic medical center. J Clin Oncol. 2013;31:1336–40.

51. Kidambi TD, Blanco A, Myers M, Conrad P, Loranger K, Terdiman JP. Selective versus universal screening for lynch syndrome: a six-year clinical experience. Dig. Dis. Sci. 2014;60:2463–9. Available from: http://dx.doi.org/10. 1007/s10620-014-3234-z

52. Musulén E, Sanz C, Muñoz-Mármol AM, Ariza A. Mismatch repair protein immunohistochemistry: A useful population screening strategy for Lynch syndrome. Hum. Pathol. 2014;45:1388–96. Available from: http://dx.doi.org/ 10.1016/j.humpath.2014.02.012

53. Hampel H, Frankel WL, Martin E, Arnold M, Khanduja K, Kuebler P, et al. Feasibility of screening for lynch syndrome among patients with colorectal cancer. J Clin Oncol. 2008;26:5783–8. Available from: http://www.ncbi.nlm. nih.gov/pubmed/20045164

54. Chang SC, Lin PC, Yang SH, Wang HS, Liang WY, Lin JK. Taiwan hospital-based detection of lynch syndrome distinguishes 2 types of microsatellite instabilities in colorectal cancers. Surgery. 2010;147:720–8. Available from: http://dx.doi.org/10.1016/j.surg.2009.10.069

55. Hampel H, Frankel WL, Martin E, Arnold M, Khanduja K, Kuebler P, et al. Screening for the lynch syndrome (hereditary nonpolyposis colorectal cancer). N. Engl. J Med. 2005;352:1851–60. Available from: http://www.ncbi. nlm.nih.gov/pubmed/19038878

56. Erten MZ, Fernandez LP, Ng HK, McKinnon WC, Heald B, Koliba CJ, et al. Universal versus targeted screening for lynch syndrome: comparing ascertainment and costs based on clinical experience. Dig Dis Sci. 2016; Available from: http://www.ncbi.nlm.nih.gov/pubmed/27384051

57. Gould-Suarez M, El-Serag HB, Musher B, Franco LM, Chen GJ. Cost-effectiveness and diagnostic effectiveness analyses of multiple algorithms for the diagnosis of lynch syndrome. Dig Dis Sci. 2014;59:2913–26.

58. Pritchard CC, Mateo J, Walsh MF, De Sarkar N, Abida W, Beltran H, et al. Inherited DNA-Repair Gene Mutations in Men with Metastatic Prostate Cancer. N Engl J Med. 2016:NEJMoa1603144. Available from: http://www. nejm.org/doi/10.1056/NEJMoa1603144

59. https://clinicaltrials.gov/. Available from: https://clinicaltrials.gov/. Accessed 1 June 2018.

60. Czink E, Kloor M, Goeppert B, Fröhling S, Uhrig S, Weber TF, et al. Successful immune checkpoint blockade in a patient with advanced stage microsatellite-unstable biliary tract cancer. Mol. Case Stud. 2017;3:a001974. Available from: http://molecularcasestudies.cshlp.org/lookup/doi/10.1101/ mcs.a001974

20

A multicenter phase 4 geriatric assessment directed trial to evaluate gemcitabine +/− nab-paclitaxel in elderly pancreatic cancer patients (GrantPax)

Johannes Betge[1] (ID), Jing Chi-Kern[1], Nadine Schulte[1], Sebastian Belle[1], Tobias Gutting[1], Elke Burgermeister[1], Ralf Jesenofsky[1], Martin Maenz[2], Ulrich Wedding[3], Matthias P. Ebert[1*] and Nicolai Haertel[1*]

Abstract

Background: In the group of elderly patients (≥70 years) with metastatic pancreatic ductal adenocarcinoma (mPDAC), it is not known who benefits from intensive 1st line nab-paclitaxel/gemcitabine (nab-p/gem) combination chemotherapy or who would rather suffer from increased toxicity. We aim to determine whether treatment individualization by comprehensive geriatric assessments (CGAs) improves functional outcome of the patients.

Methods/Design: GrantPax is a multicenter, open label phase 4 interventional trial. We use a CGA to stratify elderly patients into three parallel treatment groups ($n = 45$ per arm): 1) GOGO (nab-p/gem), 2) SLOWGO (gem mono) or 3) FRAIL (best supportive care). After the 1st cycle of chemotherapy (or 4 weeks in FRAIL group) another CGA and safety assessment is performed. CGA-stratified patients may not decline in their CGA performance in response to the first cycle of chemotherapy (primary objective), measured as a loss of 5 points or less in Barthels activities of daily living. Based on the second CGA, patients are re-assigned to their definite treatment arm and undergo further CGAs to monitor the course of treatment. Secondary endpoints include CGA scores during the course of therapy (CGA1–4), response rates, safety and survival rates.

Discussion: GrantPax is the first trial implementing a CGA-driven treatment to personalize therapy for elderly patients with pancreatic cancer. This may lead to standardization of therapy decisions for elderly patients and may optimize standard of care for this increasing group of patients.

Keywords: Pancreatic cancer, Elderly, Comprehensive geriatric assessment, Nab-paclitaxel, Personalized medicine, Geriatric oncology

Background

In the developed countries, pancreatic cancer is the fifth leading cause of cancer-related death [1]. Pancreatic adenocarcinomas usually show rapid progression and limited response rates to chemotherapy, leading to a poor prognosis. Hence, median survival of patients with metastasized disease is only three to six months [2].

The incidence of pancreatic cancer increases with age, 70% presenting over the age of 65 years [3]. In Germany, mean age at diagnosis is 71 years in men and 75 years in women [4]. Elderly patients differ in psychosocial, functional and biological characteristics compared to younger patients [5]. Specifically, differences in stem cell biology, the functional decline of organs with age and significant co-morbidities may lead to enhanced toxicities [6, 7]. However, elderly patients are a very heterogeneous group of patients, since the physiologic and medical changes of aging are poorly reflected in chronologic age. There is rising evidence that comprehensive geriatric assessments (CGAs) as

* Correspondence: matthias.ebert@medma.uni-heidelberg.de;
nicolai.haertel@medma.uni-heidelberg.de
[1]Department of Medicine II, Medical Faculty Mannheim, University Hospital Mannheim, Heidelberg University, Theocor-Kutzer-Ufer 1-3, 68167 Mannheim, Germany
Full list of author information is available at the end of the article

well as condensed geriatric screening tools are able to predict treatment-related toxicity and outcome [6, 8–10]. In addition to performance status, these tools improve the assessment of co-morbidities, psychosocial and cognitive issues and functional aspects, all of which can impact the clinical course of elderly pancreatic cancer patients [6, 10].

Gemcitabine has been the standard chemotherapy for first-line treatment of pancreatic adenocarcinomas but only modestly increased median overall survival [11]. Recent studies convincingly demonstrated that nab-paclitaxel in combination with gemcitabine is an effective treatment regimen for metastatic pancreatic cancer [12, 13]. The pivotal phase III study (MPACT) demonstrated clinical superiority of a nab-p/gemcitabine combination over gemcitabine alone with respect to ORR (23% vs. 7%), PFS (5.5 months vs. 3.7 months) and OS (8.7 months vs. 6.6 months) [12, 13]. Data of the MPACT trial indicated that nab-p/gemcitabine may not be feasible in PDAC patients ≥75 years. However, the MPACT trial lacked a geriatric assessment to properly evaluate the health status and functional reserve of elderly pancreatic cancer patients. In contrast, retrospective data from routine clinical setting presented by Giordano et al. [14] suggest similar benefits of (selected) elderly and young patients from gemcitabine and nab-paclitaxel combination therapy. However, to date it is not clear which elderly patients will benefit from intensified combination treatment and how to select them.

This study is based on the hypothesis that personalized, geriatric assessment directed treatment algorithms can identify elderly patients, who benefit from nab-paclitaxel/gemcitabine combination therapy. A stratified treatment approach shall result in patient groups with a stable or improving CGA performance during the first cycle of treatment. As a result, more elderly patients may receive the combined treatment in the future, who have so far been excluded from such regimens due to an age cut-off. Conversely, a burdensome chemotherapy treatment may be spared in vulnerable patients even though they might fall into the appropriate age bracket.

Methods/design

Study design

This study is designed as a multicenter, open label, phase IV interventional study to describe the impact of comprehensive geriatric assessment (CGA) on the course of treatment of elderly pancreatic cancer patients. CGA includes various tests and scoring systems (compare below) to stratify patients as "GO-GO", "SLOW-GO" or "FRAIL" patients. Depending on the test results, patients receive either chemotherapy (GO-GO group: nab-paclitaxel/gemcitabine; SLOW-GO group: gemcitabine monotherapy) or best supportive care (FRAIL group). After the first cycle of chemotherapy (4 weeks) a subsequent CGA and a

safety assessment is performed to assess the primary objective and assign patients to their definite treatment arm (Fig. 1).

Study objectives

The primary objective is that CGA-stratified patients do not decline in their CGA performance in response to chemotherapy measured as a loss of five points or less in the Barthel's activities of daily living, (ADL1 vs. ADL2 during core CGA assessment). Thereby we aim to evaluate if treatment stratification by CGA leads to identification of those elderly patients, who benefit from combined nab-paclitaxel/gemcitabine therapy.

Secondary objectives

- Evaluation of the predictive value of the CGA (CGA 1 + 2) testing for the incidence of ≥ grade 3 hematological and/ or non-hematological toxicities;
- Predictive value of the assessed geriatric tests for treatment discontinuation;
- Response rates;
- Safety (nab-p/gemcitabine combination and gemcitabine alone);
- Survival rates including progression-free survival (PFS) and overall survival (OS);
- Percentage of patients receiving therapy in each treatment group;
- Percentage of patients improving in the CGA during therapy;
- Quality of life (QoL) and time to QoL deterioration.

Measurements

CGAs will be performed before (during screening, all treatment arms) and after the first chemotherapy cycle (CGA 1 + 2). Patients in the FRAIL arm will be assessed after 28 days for their 2nd CGA (CGA 2). Additional CGAs are performed after the 3rd and 6th cycle of chemotherapy and/or end of treatment. CGA 3 and 4 are performed in parallel with tumor restaging procedures. The ideal -albeit potentially unobtainable- time points for CGAs (CGA 3 + 4) in the FRAIL patients are Day 84 (± 14 days) and Day 168 (± 14 days) respectively.

A full CGA comprises the following assessments tools:

- Functional tests include the Instrumental Activities of Daily Living (IADL) according to Lawton/Browdy [15] and the Activities of Daily Living (ADL, Barthel's index) [16].
- Screening tests include the G8-Questionaire [17] and the non-hematological Chemotherapy Risk Assessment Scale for High-age patients (CRASH) to assess toxicity [18];

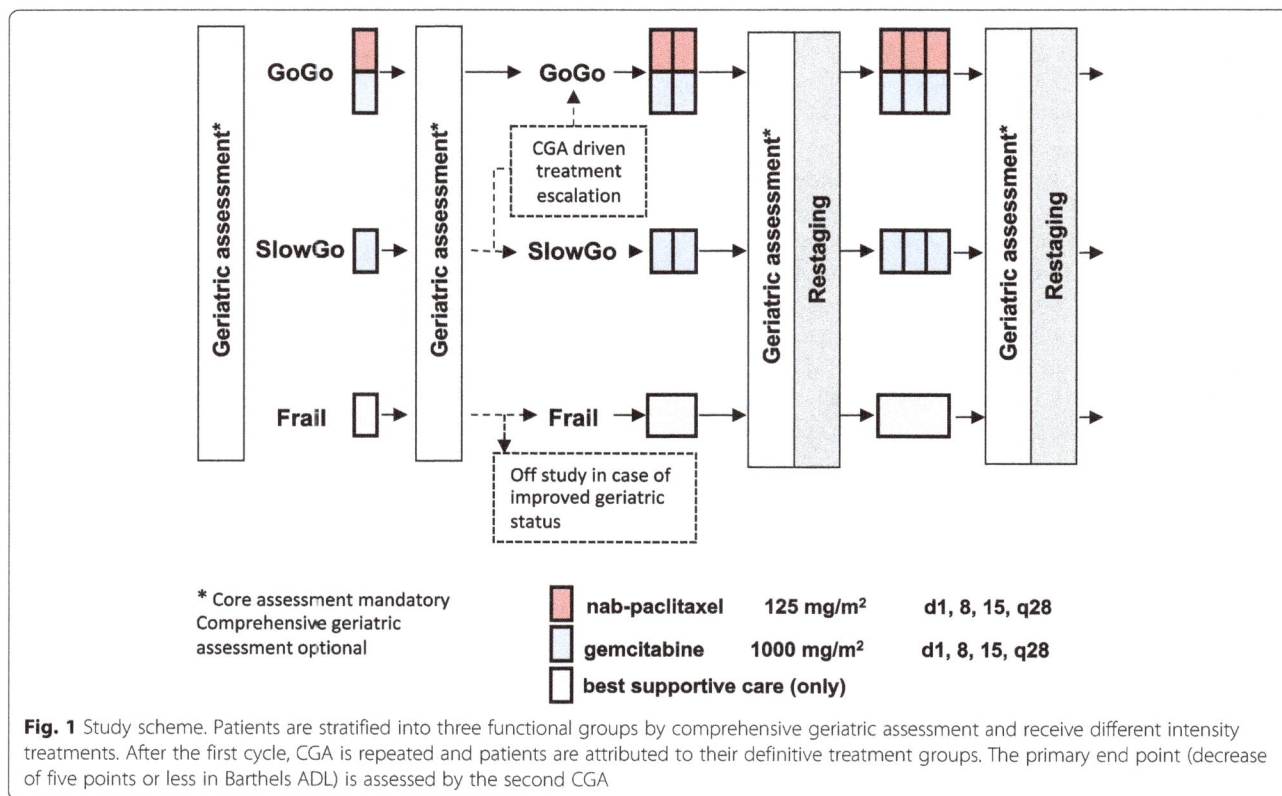

Fig. 1 Study scheme. Patients are stratified into three functional groups by comprehensive geriatric assessment and receive different intensity treatments. After the first cycle, CGA is repeated and patients are attributed to their definitive treatment groups. The primary end point (decrease of five points or less in Barthels ADL) is assessed by the second CGA

- Comorbidities are evaluated using the Charlson Comorbidity Index [19];
- Mini mental state examinations (MMSE) are performed to assess cognitive deficiencies [20];
- The Geriatric Depression Scale 15 (GDS15) is performed for analysis of affective co-morbidities [21];
- A nutritional assessment is done with the help of mini nutritional assessment (MNA) [22];
- As biological test, the timed get up test (chair stand test) is used [23];
- Finally, geriatric syndromes are evaluated by the treating physician and a trained geriatric nurse.

Full CGA will only be performed during the screening/baseline assessment (CGA1). Thereafter only the core CGA is mandated for all following assessments, while all additional assessment tools of the full CGA are optional. CGA core assessment for treatment decision and escalation during CGA1 and CGA2 consist of Eastern Cooperative Oncology Group (ECOG) performance status, ADL, IADL and G8-Questionnaire (Table 1).

Treatment assignment according to core CGA

Depending on the patients' performance during the baseline core CGA, patients are assigned to treatment as shown in Table 1. Definitive assignment is going to be confirmed by investigators decision.

After the first cycle of chemotherapy, the treatment regimen will be re-assessed based on the results of the 2nd core CGA assessment. CGA improvement and treatment related toxicity ≤ grade 1 according to CTC-criteria can lead to cross over to the GO-GO or SLOW-GO arm (escalation). The indication to escalate has to be confirmed by investigators decision. Of note, FRAIL subjects that become eligible for a mono-chemotherapy are withdrawn from the study and may commence any chemotherapy at the discretion of the treating physician. This is owed to the less strict inclusion criteria of this observational cohort. Therefore, technically no treatment escalation within this study from FRAIL to SLOW-GO is permitted. A central CGA review is conducted by telephone conference with the study investigator to relay changes in the CGA2 results, in particular CGA differences that result in treatment modifications. In case of toxicities to nab-paclitaxel or gemcitabine, schedules for dose delay and dose modification will apply.

Table 1 Treatment assignment based on core CGA testing

	GO-GO arm	SLOW-GO arm	FRAIL arm
ECOG	0–1	≤ 2	≥ 3
G8-Questionaire	> 14 points	≤ 14 points	< 14 points
ADL (Barthel)	= 100	≤ 100	< 100
IADL	= 8 (f) / = 5 (m)	≤ 8 (f) / ≤ 5 (m)	< 8 (f) / < 5 (m)

Primary and secondary end points

Primary endpoint

Evaluation of loss of five points or less in the Activity of Daily Living (Barthel's ADL) after first cycle of chemotherapy or after 4 weeks of best supportive care (BSC) compared to the initial ADL for each treatment group.

Secondary endpoints

- CGA scores before and after 1st treatment cycle or day 28 of BSC (CGA1 + 2; further CGA scores 3 + 4 – if available after 3rd and 6th cycle or D84 and D168 in FRAIL patients)
- Response rates
- Adverse events
- PFS, OS
- Percentage of patients receiving at least one chemotherapy in each treatment group and percentage of patients escalating treatment;
- Duration of treatment
- Cumulative dose of administered chemotherapy medication
- Quality of life (time to QoL deterioration, defined as loss of 10 points in Quality of Life Questionaire C30 (QLQ-C30))
- Discrepancy between CGA strata estimation by the investigator and true CGA assessment.

Data collection

Data for this study will be recorded via eCRF by the site from the source documents according to standard operational procedures. Data are reviewed and checked for omissions, apparent errors, and values requiring further clarifications using computerized (automatic) and/or manual procedures. Accurate and reliable data collection will be assured by verification and cross–check of the eCRF against the investigator's records by the study monitor. Data will be recorded and reported until the last subject will have completed the trial.

Statistical analysis and sample size

Despite of the descriptive nature of this study with its multiple CGA-driven decision processes, a formal statistical testing is planned after the 1st chemotherapy cycle. The primary endpoint will be analyzed separately in each CGA-defined treatment arm (GOGO, SLOWGO, FRAIL). Based on literature data it is assumed that without CGA approximately 20% of patients will experience a functional decline after the 1st chemotherapy cycle. With CGA this rate is expected to be considerably decreased to about 6% [8, 24]. Under this assumption it shall be shown with 80% power at one-sided significance level alpha of 0.05 that the proportion of patients with functional decline (Barthel's ADL) is less than 20%. Applying an exact one-sample test

for one binomial population, this requires the inclusion of 43 patients with a maximum number of 2 patients with ADL decline per group. Accounting for an additional 5% drop-out rate during the first treatment cycle, a total of $n = 45$ patients are to be recruited into each treatment arm. Hence, a total of 135 eligible patients will be enrolled in this study. It is expected that this number of patients can be recruited within 24 months by 6 sites in Germany. Inclusion and exclusion criteria of the GO-GO / SLOW-GO and FRAIL arms are shown in Table 2.

Study protocol

Our study protocol is in accordance with the SPIRIT guidelines for reporting clinical trials. We included a supplemental table containing a short study synopsis that includes all items from the World Health Organization Trial Registration Data Set (Additional file 1: Table S1).

Approval

The GrantPax trial is an Arbeitsgemeinschaft Internistische Onkologie (AIO) trial of the German Cancer Society, approved by the working group geriatric oncology (AIO-GER-0115). The study was approved by the Ethics Committee II at Medical Faculty Mannheim, Heidelberg University, Mannheim, Germany [2016-003F-MA], providing approval for all study sites in agreement with local ethics committees. Written informed consent is obtained from all participants. Amendments to the protocol have to undergo approval from the applicable competent authority and the ethics committees.

Trial status

GrantPax commenced recruitment in June 2016 and is at the moment recruiting patients. We estimate completion of the study by June 2019.

Discussion

It is not clear which elderly pancreatic cancer patient benefits from intensified combination treatment with gemcitabine and nab-paclitaxel and how to select those patients. GrantPax is the first trial worldwide evaluating a CGA-driven treatment allocation to personalize cancer therapy for elderly patients with mPDAC. The aim is to stratify patients into groups with different functional status to allow patients to receive different intensities of treatment (nab-paclitaxel/gemcitabine, gemcitabine monotherapy, BSC). This personalization of treatment shall result in a stable or improving functional performance, which is measured as a decrease in ADL of ≤5 points. Ultimately, this may allow for more elderly patients to receive intensive chemotherapy and thereby improve survival, but spare vulnerable patients a burdensome treatment. This approach has been successfully tested in elderly patients with lung cancer [2, 25].

Table 2 Inclusion and exclusion criteria

	GOGO and SLOWGO Arms	NOGO Arm
Inclusion criteria		
Patients ≥70 years of age	+	+
Histologically or cytologically confirmed metastatic adenocarcinoma of the pancreas.	+	+
No prior chemotherapy (except fluoruracil or gemcitabine in an adjuvant setting at least > 6 months prior enrollment).	+	+
Cooperation and willingness to complete all aspects of the study	+	+
Written informed consent to participate in the study	+	+
At least one measurable lesion of disease according to RECIST 1.1 criteria.	+	
Adequate end organ function (renal function: serum creatinine ≤1.5 × ULN or GFR≥30mL/min, hematopoietic function: white blood cell (WBC) count ≥3000/µL, absolute neutrophil count (ANC)≥1500/µL, platelets ≥105/µL, hemoglobin level>9.0g/dL, liver function: total bilirubin ≤1.5 × ULN, AST / ALT ≤3.0 × ULN)	+	
Exclusion criteria		
Patient has received any other investigational product within 28days prior study entry	+	+
Patient is < 5years free of another primary malignancy (except: not currently clinically significant nor requiring active intervention)	+	+
Patient with any significant history of non-compliance to medical regimens or with inability to grant reliable informed consent	+	+
Any psychiatric illness that would affect the patient's ability to understand the demands of the clinical trial	+	+
Parallel participation in another clinical trial or participation in another clinical trial within the last 30days or 7 half-lifes of a study medication, whichever is of longer duration, prior study start	+	+
Patient has a severe and/or uncontrolled medical disease (i.e. uncontrolled active infection, uncontrolled hypertension/diabetes or cardiac disease).	+	
Hypersensitivity against gemcitabine or nab-paclitaxel.	+	
Major surgery ≤28 days prior to study entry.	+	
Patient has a known diagnosis of human immunodeficiency virus (HIV) infection.	+	

In routine practice, estimation of the functional capacity of a patient depends on the experience and judgment of the oncologist. This judgment seems to be fair in the majority of cases, exemplified by the FOCUS2 trial, in which only

18% of colorectal cancer patients initially attributed to a reduced-dose regimen by the oncologist could tolerate an afterwards escalated dose regimen over longer time [26]. Nevertheless, the trial also exemplifies that there is a significant number of elderly patients over-treated by standard combination regimens, while there are certainly others that are under-treated and withheld from chemotherapy due to fear of enhanced side effects in elderly individuals. A standardized method for treatment allocation to elderly patients is lacking. GrantPax is the first trial to prospectively ascertain data on this matter in patients with pancreatic cancer.

Balducci and Extermann [6] defined three groups of elderly patients: functionally independent patients without co-morbidities that may receive standard cancer therapy, intermediate patients who may benefit from reduced chemotherapy and frail patients (dependent in activities of daily living, comorbidities, geriatric syndromes) that are candidates for best supportive care only [6]. Patients falling in each of these categories can be designated as GOGO, SLOWGO and FRAIL, respectively. A geriatric assessment for all elderly cancer patients has been recommended by different international societies but has not yet been implemented in routine practice [10, 27, 28]. There is evidence that geriatric assessments in oncology can support oncologist's treatment decisions and improve patients' quality of life, management of toxicities and also overall survival. However, previous studies were mainly small retrospective analyses [29]. Data on elderly patients with pancreatic cancer are especially limited [30, 31]. Also, there are only limited data available yet on how the functional status of elderly patients evolves under chemotherapy. Hoppe et al. [8] observed a functional decline in 16,7% of 364 elderly patients receiving first line chemotherapy for different solid tumors. Based on this data, the primary objective in our study is to reach a stable functional status by treatment stratification. A functional decline in less than 6% of patients was set as primary endpoint.

Currently, the safety and efficacy of dose-adjusted FOLFIRINOX in elderly patients with metastatic pancreatic cancer is assessed in the phase II PAMELA-70 trial (NCT02143219). Importantly, this trial evaluates the tolerance of the treatment by analysis of toxicity, but also by decrease of the patients' ADL. However, a CGA or a stratification of the patients by functional status is not included in this trial. Regarding Gem/NabP combination therapy, a retrospective analysis suggested that the combination was effective in elderly patients and exhibited a different, but tolerable toxicity profile [32, 33]. GrantPax prospectively evaluates this combination in elderly patients using CGA to stratify patients based on functional status.

To date, it is not clear which geriatric functional tests should be performed for treatment allocation in mPDAC patients receiving first line chemotherapy. The geriatric core assessment in the GrantPax trial consists of the ADL/

IADL, the G8 questionnaire and ECOG performance status. ADL and IADL are the most commonly used functional tests in geriatrics, ECOG is well known and established among oncologists. G8 is a screening tool that is recommended by consensus statements and has prognostic relevance [9, 10], however, no data are yet available on changes of the G8 score (and other geriatric tests) during chemotherapy in patients with mPDAC.

A potential problem regarding CGAs is the known inter-observer variability of ADL and IADL. We aim to minimize this problem by letting the same observer perform the CGA in each study center. Furthermore, there are no official cut-off values to discriminate between GOGO and SLOWGO or SLOWGO and FRAIL, potentially leading to overlaps and inconclusive classifications. Cut-off values exist for the G8, but not for ADL or IADL. Therefore, the final classification into one of the arms is the investigators decision.

A CGA is time consuming and therefore expensive, it is therefore questionable if it can be performed in routine practice. In the future, a condensed assessment with patient reports may be most practical. The GrantPax trial will evaluate which geriatric tests and screening tools are of the best predictive value with its secondary end points.

In conclusion, Grantpax is the first trial to evaluate the impact of a CGA based treatment stratification on functional decline of elderly pancreatic cancer patients under chemotherapy.

Abbreviations

ADL: Activities of daily living; CGA: Comprehensive geriatric assessments; CRASH: Chemotherapy risk assessment scale for high-age patients; ECOG: Eastern Cooperative Oncology Group; GDS15: Geriatric depression scale 15; IADL: Instrumental activities of daily living; MMSE: Mini mental state examinations; MNA: Mini nutritional assessment; Nab-P/Gem: Nab-paclitaxel/gemcitabine; ORR: Objective response rate; OS: Overall survival; PDAC: Pancreatic ductal adenocarcinoma; PFS: Progression-free survival; QLQ-C30: Quality of life questionaire C30

Funding

Grantpax is an investigator-initiated trial that is sponsored by the non-profit AIO-Studien gGmbH (Berlin, Germany) with funding from Celgene Corporation. Celgene had no role in the study design, and has no role in data collection, management, data analysis and interpretation, or decision to submit results for presentation or publication. Research in the Department of ME is supported by grants from the State of Baden-Württemberg for "Center of Geriatric Biology and Oncology (ZOBEL) - Perspektivförderung" and "Biology of Frailty - Sonderlinie Medizin". JB is supported by the Translational Physician Scientist (TraPS) Program of the Medical Faculty Mannheim and the State of Baden-Württemberg. We acknowledge financial support by Deutsche Forschungsgemeinschaft within the funding programme Open Access Publishing, by the Baden-Württemberg Ministry of Science, Research and Arts and by Ruprecht-Karls-Universität Heidelberg.

Authors' contributions

NH and MPE designed the study. ME is principal investigator of the GrantPax trial, NH is substitute principle investigator. JB, JCK, NS, SB, RJ, TG, EB and UW are members of the study team and made substantial contributions to conception and design. MM is representative of the AIO Studien gGmbH (Kuno-Fischer-Str. 8, 14,057 Berlin, Germany, info@aio-studien-ggmbh.de) and substantially contributed to conception and design. The AIO-Studien gGmbH is sponsor of the study and responsible for study management, logistics and monitoring and counseled in study design. JB and NH drafted the manuscript. All authors read and approved the final manuscript.

Competing interests

The GrantPax trial is sponsored by the non-profit AIO-Studien gGmbH and received funding from Celgene Corporation, Summit, NJ, USA, under study contract. Celgene had no role in the study design, and has no role in data collection, management, data analysis and interpretation, or decision to submit results for presentation or publication.
NH participated at advisory boards organized by the Celgene Corporation (presentation incl.)
JB has received a travel grant from Celgene to the ASCO 2017 meeting.
The authors declare that they have no competing interest.

Author details

[1]Department of Medicine II, Medical Faculty Mannheim, University Hospital Mannheim, Heidelberg University, Theodor-Kutzer-Ufer 1-3, 68167 Mannheim, Germany. [2]AIO-Studien gGmbH, Berlin, Germany. [3]Department of Medicine II, University Hospital Jena, Jena, Germany.

References

1. Torre LA, Bray F, Siegel RL, Ferlay J, Lortet-Tieulent J, Jemal A. Global cancer statistics, 2012. CA Cancer J Clin. 2015;65:87–108.
2. Sant M, Allemani C, Santaquilani M, Knijn A, Marchesi F, Capocaccia R. EUROCARE-4. Survival of cancer patients diagnosed in 1995–1999. Results and commentary. Eur J Cancer. 2009;45(6):931–91.
3. Ilic M, Ilic I. Epidemiology of pancreatic cancer. World J Gastroenterol. 2016; 22:9694–705.
4. Kaatsch P, Spix C, Hentschel S, Katalinic A, Luttmann S, Stegmaier C, et al. Krebs in Deutschland 2009/2010. Berlin: Robert Koch-Institut; 2013.
5. Higuera O, Ghanem I, Nasimi R, Prieto I, Koren L, Feliu J. Management of pancreatic cancer in the elderly. World J Gastroenterol. 2016;22(2):764–75.
6. Balducci L, Extermann M. Management of cancer in the older person: a practical approach. Oncologist. 2000;5(3):224–37.
7. Dale W, Mohile SG, Eldadah BA, Trimble EL, Schilsky RL, Cohen HJ, et al. Biological, clinical, and psychosocial correlates at the interface of cancer and aging research. J Natl Cancer Inst. 2012;104(8):581–9.
8. Hoppe S, Rainfray M, Fonck M, Hoppenreys L, Blanc J-F, Ceccaldi J, et al. Functional decline in older patients with cancer receiving first-line chemotherapy. J Clin Oncol. 2013;31(31):3877–82.
9. Kenis C, Decoster L, Van Puyvelde K, De Grève J, Conings G, Milisen K, et al. Performance of two geriatric screening tools in older patients with cancer. J Clin Oncol. 2014;32(1):19–26.
10. Pallis AG, Fortpied C, Wedding U, Van Nes MC, Penninckx B, Ring A, et al. EORTC elderly task force position paper: approach to the older cancer patient. Eur J Cancer. 2010;46(9):1502–13.
11. Burris HA, Moore MJ, Andersen J, Green MR, Rothenberg ML, Modiano MR, et al. Improvements in survival and clinical benefit with gemcitabine as first-line therapy for patients with advanced pancreas cancer: a randomized trial. JCO. 1997;15:2403–13.
12. Hoff Von DD, Ervin T, Arena FP, Chiorean EG, Infante J, Moore M, et al. Increased survival in pancreatic Cancer with nab-paclitaxel plus gemcitabine. N Engl J Med. 2013;369(18):1691–703.
13. Goldstein D, El-Maraghi RH, Hammel P, Heinemann V, Kunzmann V, Sastre J, Scheithauer W, Siena S, Tabernero J, Teixeira L, Tortora G, Van Laethem JL, Young R, Penenberg DN, Lu B, Romano A, Von Hoff DD. Nab-Paclitaxel Plus Gemcitabine for Metastatic Pancreatic Cancer: Long-Term Survival From a Phase III Trial. J Natl Cancer Inst. 2015;107(2). https://doi.org/10.1093/jnci/dju413
14. Giordano G, Vaccaro V, Lucchini E, Musettini G, Bertocchi P, Bergamo F, et al. Nab-paclitaxel (nab-P) and gemcitabine (G) as first-line chemotherapy (CT) in advanced pancreatic cancer (APDAC) elderly patients (pts): a "real-life" study. J Clin Oncol. 2015;33:424.

15. Lawton MP, Brody EM. Assessment of older people: self-maintaining and instrumental activities of daily living. Gerontologist. 1969;9(3):179–86.

16. Mahoney FI, Barthel DW. Functional evaluation: the Barthel index. Md State Med J. 1965;14:61–5.

17. Bellera CA, Rainfray M, Mathoulin-Pélissier S, Mertens C, Delva F, Fonck M, et al. Screening older cancer patients: first evaluation of the G-8 geriatric screening tool. Ann Oncol. 2012;23(8):2166–72.

18. Extermann M, Boler I, Reich RR, Lyman GH, Brown RH, DeFelice J, et al. Predicting the risk of chemotherapy toxicity in older patients: the chemotherapy risk assessment scale for high-age patients (CRASH) score. Cancer. 2011;118(13):3377–86.

19. Charlson ME, Pompei P, Ales KL. MacKenzie CR. A new method of classifying prognostic comorbidity in longitudinal studies: development and validation. J Chronic Dis. 1986;40(5):373–83.

20. Folstein MF, Folstein SE, McHugh PR. Mini-mental state. J Psy Res. 1975;12: 189–98.

21. Lesher EL, Berryhill JS. Validation of the geriatric depression scale--short form among inpatients. J Clin Psychol. 1994;50(2):256–60.

22. Vellas B, Villars H, Abellan G, Soto ME, Rolland Y, Guigoz Y, et al. Overview of the MNA--its history and challenges. J Nutr Health Aging. 2006;10(6):456–63.

23. Podsiadlo D, Richardson S. The timed "up & go": a test of basic functional mobility for frail elderly persons. J Am Geriat Soc. 2015;39:142–8.

24. Brain EGC, Mertens C, Girre V, Rousseau F, Blot E, Abadie S, et al. Impact of liposomal doxorubicin-based adjuvant chemotherapy on autonomy in women over 70 with hormone-receptor-negative breast carcinoma: a French geriatric oncology group (GERICO) phase II multicentre trial. Crit Rev Oncol Hematol. 2011;80:160–70.

25. Corre R, Greillier L, Le Caër H, Audigier-Valette C, Baize N, Bérard H, et al. Use of a comprehensive geriatric assessment for the Management of Elderly Patients with Advanced non-Small-Cell Lung Cancer: the phase III randomized ESOGIA-GFPC-GECP 08-02 study. J Clin Oncol. 2016; 34(13):1476–83.

26. Seymour MT, Thompson LC, Wasan HS, Middleton G, Brewster AE, Shepherd SF, et al. Chemotherapy options in elderly and frail patients with metastatic colorectal cancer (MRC FOCUS2): an open-label, randomised factorial trial. Lancet. 2011;377(9779):1749–59.

27. Papamichael D, Audisio RA, Glimelius B, de Gramont A, Glynne-Jones R, Haller D, et al. Treatment of colorectal cancer in older patients: International Society of Geriatric Oncology (SIOG) consensus recommendations 2013. Ann Oncol. 2014;26:463–76.

28. Hurria A, Wildes T, Blair SL, Browner IS, Cohen HJ, Deshazo M, et al. Senior adult oncology, version 2.2014: clinical practice guidelines in oncology. J Natl Compr Cancer Netw. 2014;12(1)82–126.

29. O'Donovan A, Mohile SG, Leech M. Expert consensus panel guidelines on geriatric assessment in oncology. Eur J Cancer Care. 2015;24(4):574–89.

30. Maréchal R, Demols A, Van Laethem J-L. Adjuvant pharmacotherapy in the Management of Elderly Patients with pancreatic Cancer. Drugs Aging. 2013; 30(3):155–65.

31. Berger AK, Abel U, Komander C, Harig S, Jäger D, Springfeld C. Chemotherapy for advanced pancreatic adenocarcinoma in elderly patients (≥70 years of age): a retrospective cohort study at the National Center for tumor diseases Heidelberg. Pancreatology. 2014;14(3):211–5.

32. Giordano G, De Vita F, Melisi D, Vaccaro V, Zaniboni A, Zagonel V, et al. Analysis of activity, efficacy and safety of first line nab paclitaxel (nab-P) and gemcitabine (G) in advanced pancreatic cancer (APDAC) frail and elderly patients (pts). Eur J Cancer. 2015;51:S445.

33. Giordano G, Pancione M, Olivieri N, Parcesepe P, Velocci M, Di Raimo T, et al. Nano albumin bound-paclitaxel in pancreatic cancer: current evidences and future directions. World J Gastroenterol. 2017;23(32):5875–86.

21

Pancreatic adenocarcinoma: insights into patterns of recurrence and disease behavior

Ibrahim H. Sahin[1], Harold Elias[2], Joanne F. Chou[3], Marinela Capanu[3] and Eileen M. O'Reilly[3,4,5]*

Abstract

Background: Pancreatic ductal adenocarcinoma (PDAC) is one of the most aggressive cancers with high metastatic potential. Clinical observations suggest that there is disease heterogeneity among patients with different sites of distant metastases, yielding distinct clinical outcomes. Herein, we investigate the impact of clinical and pathological parameters on recurrence patterns and compare survival outcomes for patients with a first site of recurrence in the liver versus lung from PDAC following original curative surgical resection.

Methods: Using the Memorial Sloan Kettering Cancer Center ICD billing codes and tumor registry database over a 10 years period (January 2004–December 2014), we identified PDAC patients who underwent resection and subsequently presented with either liver or lung recurrence. Time from relapse to death (TRD) was calculated from date of recurrence to date of death. Using the Kaplan-Meier method, TRD was estimated and compared by recurrence site using log-rank test.

Results: The median overall follow-up was 37.3 months among survivors in the entire cohort. Median TRD in this cohort was 10.7 months (95%CI: 8.9–14.6 months). Patients with first site of lung recurrence had a more favorable outcome compared to patients who recurred with liver metastasis as the first site of recurrence (median TRD of 15 versus 9 months respectively, $P = 0.02$). Moderate to poorly or poor differentiation was associated more often with liver than lung recurrence (40% vs 21% respectively, $P = 0.047$). A trend to increased lymph node metastasis in the lung recurrence cohort was observed.

Conclusion: PDAC patients who recur with a first site of lung metastasis have an improved clinical outcome compared to patients with first site of liver recurrence. Our data suggests there may be epidemiologic and pathologic determinants related to patterns of recurrence in PDAC.

Keywords: Pancreatic cancer, Lung, Liver, Metastasis, Pre-metastatic niche, Exosomes, Disease behavior, Recurrence pattern, Survival outcomes, Tumor differentiation, Alcohol use, Disease heterogeneity, Chemokine receptors

Background

Pancreatic ductal adenocarcinoma (PDAC) has remained a major obstacle for physicians and scientists, due to its distinct underlying molecular behavior and de novo resistance to conventional and targeted therapies. For advanced PDAC, the best survival results are achieved with combination cytotoxic agents such as fluorouracil, irinotecan and oxaliplatin (FOL-FIRINOX) [1] or gemcitabine based multi-agent chemotherapeutics [2]. However, the 5-year survival for metastatic disease is 2% which has improved by 1% over the last two decades [3] suggesting limited progress in management of metastatic PDAC. Although gemcitabine-based adjuvant therapy has reduced the recurrence rate of PDAC [4], the 5-year survival of patients who underwent curative resection is estimated to be 27% [3], indicating frequent recurrence in long term follow up ultimately leading to disease-related mortality.

* Correspondence: oreillye@mskcc.org
[3]Memorial Sloan Kettering Cancer Center, 300 East 66th Street, Office 1021, New York, NY 10065, USA
[4]David M. Rubenstein Center for Pancreatic Cancer Research, 300 East 66th Street, Office 1021, New York, NY 10065, USA
Full list of author information is available at the end of the article

The evidence to date indicates that metastasis is a very sophisticated molecular and cellular process involving distinct signaling pathways that includes crosstalk between cancer cells and the tumor microenvironment [5]. The pre-metastatic niche formation in the host organ may also influence the molecular and clinical behavior of cancer cells [6], indicating that there may be multiple elements that lead to the distinct course of the disease. For example, exosomes, membrane-bound protein and RNA carriers which act as a conduit for cell signals in the tissue microenvironment, may have important functions in the formation of pre-metastatic niche [7]. Tumor-derived exosomes may optimize the distant pre-metastatic microenvironment prior to the occurrence of tumor seeding. A study suggested that mesenchymal-like renal cancer stem cells expressing CD105 release exosomes that facilitate angiogenesis and foster the development of lung metastasis [8]. PDAC-derived exosomes that are received by Kupffer cells have been also shown to create a pre-metastatic niche formation in the liver by recruiting bone marrow-derived macrophages [9]. Collectively, these data indicate that there are inter-site signaling networks between tumor cells and the future host organ to condition the pre-metastatic niche, thereby suggesting that metastasis is an organ-specific, programmed process rather than a random event.

One notable clinical observation is that the heterogeneity of disease behavior of distant recurrent disease following potentially curative surgery, leads to further challenges in optimizing treatment and predicting clinical outcome. In the study reported herein, we focus on patterns of liver and lung recurrence of PDAC and examine the impact of first site of recurrence on disease behavior and post-relapse survival outcomes. We further investigate the potential contributions of epidemiologic and pathologic characteristics on the metastatic pattern of PDAC.

Methods
Study population
The institutional cancer registry for Memorial Sloan Kettering Cancer Center and ICD billing codes were queried for PDAC patients (AJCC Stage I/II) who underwent frontline surgical resection and developed either lung or hepatic metastasis as a first-site of recurrence during the 10-year period from January 1, 2004 through December 31, 2014. All patients identified in this query had pathologic confirmation of PDAC diagnosis. Adjudication of metastatic disease was determined by expert clinicians based on a biopsy from metastatic site (where available) and associated clinical and radiologic features. Patients who developed local recurrence, peritoneal carcinomatosis, concurrent multi-organ metastasis or other

distant organ dissemination prior to lung and liver metastasis were excluded from the cohort. Patients with the presence of concurrent liver and lung metastasis were also excluded from this analysis. Most of the patients included in the study ultimately developed multisite metastases as their disease progressed. This study was reviewed and approved by the Memorial Sloan Kettering Cancer Center Institutional Review and Privacy Board (IRB) on an annual basis.

Data collection
Demographic, clinical and pathologic information was obtained from the institutional electronic medical record using the chart review method. The data were collected by trained personnel. Recurrent metastatic disease was defined as the detection of a new distant lesion in the presence of unequivocal clinical and biomarker correlation with or without pathologic confirmation. Microscopic tumor involving the resection margin was considered a positive tumor margin. Tissue diagnosis from the metastatic site along with radiologic and clinical assessment of expert physicians were considered in the decision for adjudication of the site of recurrence of disease. The data, including date of diagnosis, medical and surgical history, pathologic information including tumor differentiation, vascular and perineural invasion, tumor margin status, lymph node status, tumor location and pathologic stage along with social history were obtained by detailed electronic medical record review.

Statistical analysis
Clinical and pathological characteristics were summarized using frequency and percentages for categorical covariates and mean and standard deviation (SD) for continuous variables and compared between site of recurrence using Fisher's exact test or Wilcoxon rank-sum test. The time from relapse to death (TRD) was calculated from the date of recurrence to the date of death. Patients alive at the end of the study period were censored at 01/01/2016. TRD was estimated using the Kaplan-Meier method and compared for recurrence sites of liver and lung metastasis using log-rank test. Statistical analyses were performed using SAS Version 9.4 (SAS Institute, INC., Cary, NC, USA). P-values were 2-sided and < 0.05 were considered statistically significant.

Results
A total of $N = 302$ PDAC patients with recurrent/metastatic disease in the liver or lung after initial curative surgery, were identified over the 10-year study period by using ICD and billing codes. After a detailed chart review, $N = 149$ patients were found to have either only liver or lung metastases as the first site of recurrence

(Fig. 1). In this cohort of $N = 149$ patients, the majority of the patients were Caucasian and had a normal Body-Mass Index (BMI) at the time of recurrence (Table 1). Most of the patients in the entire cohort had AJCC stage IIB disease at the time of surgical resection and had either a pancreatic head or body tumor. All patients had adenocarcinoma. Eighty percent ($N = 117$) of the patients had lymph node positive disease, 70% ($N = 103$) had vascular invasion, 90.6% ($N = 135$) had perineural invasion. Liver metastasis was the more common site of recurrence ($N = 102$) compared to patients with lung metastasis ($N = 47$). The most common adjuvant therapy administered after initial primary tumor resection was single agent gemcitabine (84%). Other adjuvant therapies utilized in the overall cohort were, fluoropyrimidine-based therapy and fluoropyrimidine-based chemoradiation. The majority of patients received multi-agent regimens at the time of recurrence in various combinations including, FOLFRINOX (5-fluorouracil, oxaliplatin, irinotecan, leucovorin) and gemcitabine-based regimens. In the entire cohort, approximately half of the patients were smokers and had a history of either social or regular alcohol use (Table 2).

We observed $N = 140$ deaths by January 2016 with a median follow up 37.3 months among survivors. The median TRD was 10.7 months in the overall cohort (95%CI: 8.9–14.6). The median TRD in PDAC patients with lung recurrence as the first site of metastasis compared to patients who recurred initially with liver metastasis was 15 [95%CI 11–18] versus 9 [95%CI: 7–11] months respectively ($P = 0.02$; Fig. 2). One-year and 2 year-survival rates from time of relapse were 38.2% [95% CI: 28–47%] and 17.5% [95% CI: 11–26%] in the liver metastasis cohort and 61.7% [95% CI: 46–74%] and 24.9% [95% CI: 13–38%] in the lung metastasis cohort. In a comparative analysis, underweight status (BMI < 18) was noted to be more common in the lung metastasis group whereas overweight (BMI > 25) and obesity (BMI > 30) were more prevalent in the liver metastasis group at the time of initial diagnosis (Table 1). For the liver metastasis cohort, there was significantly more moderate-poor or poorly differentiated PDAC's compared to patients with lung metastasis ($N = 40$ (40%) vs $N = 10$ (21%) respectively, $P = 0.047$). We observed a trend for more frequent tumor involvement in lymph nodes at the time of surgery in patients who had lung versus liver metastasis as the first site of recurrence (87% vs 75%, $P = 0.089$) (Table 2). Patients with initial liver recurrence were more likely to have a positive margin resection compared to lung recurrence cohort, however, this difference was not statistically significant (87% vs 77%, $P = 0.148$). We also observed a slightly increased rate of perineural invasion in the lung metastasis cohort compared to the liver metastasis cohort, although again not statistically significant (96% vs 88% $P = 0.226$). Sixty-eight percent of the lung metastasis cohort had a history of either social or daily-base alcohol use in

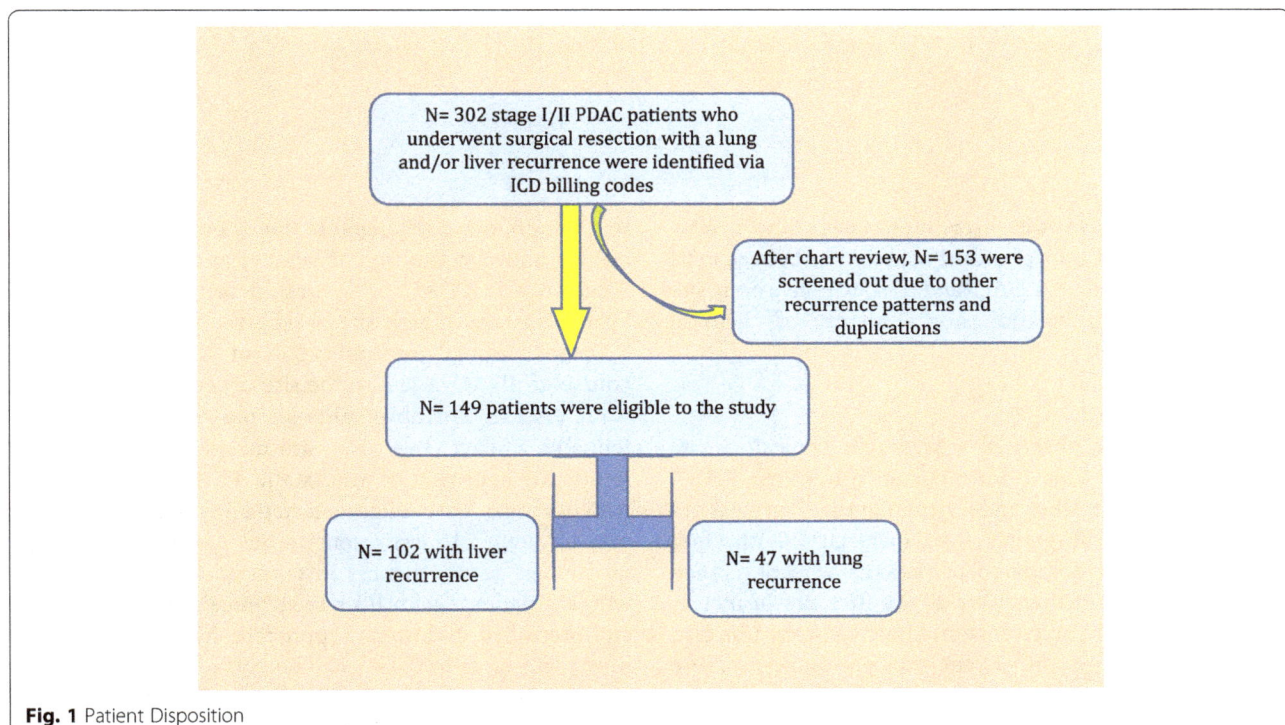

Fig. 1 Patient Disposition

Table 1 Demographics and treatment history by Recurrence Pattern

	Recurrence Pattern		p-value	Entire Cohort
	Liver Metastasis	Lung Metastasis		
Mean Age ±SD	64 ± 11 years	66 ± 10 years	0.43	
Gender			0.99	
Male	55 (54%)	25 (53%)		80 (54%)
Female	47 (46%)	22 (47%)		69 (46%)
Ethnicity			0.80	
Caucasian	86 (84%)	41 (87%)		127 (85%)
Hispanic	5 (5%)	1 (2%)		6 (4%)
African-American	1 (1%)	3 (6%)		4 (3%)
Asian	5 (5%)	1 (2%)		6 (4%)
Others	4 (4%)	–		4 (2%)
N/A	1 (1%)	1 (2%)		2 (2%)
BMI			0.050	
< 18.5	6 (6%)	5 (11%)		11 (8%)
18.5–24.9	40 (39%)	28 (60%)		68 (50%)
25–29.9	35 (34%)	11 (23%)		46 (28%)
30–34.9	15 (15%)	3 (6%)		18 (11%)
≥ 35	6 (6%)	–		6 (3%)
Adjuvant Therapy			0.17	
Gemcitabine-based	77 (75%)	43 (92%)		120 (84%)
Fluoropyrimidine- based	6 (6%)	1 (2%)		7 (4%)
5-FU/Gemcitabine	9 (9%)	2 (4%)		11 (6%)
N/A	10 (10%)	1 (2%)		11 (6%)
Treatment Metastatic Disease				
FOLFIRINOX	18 (18%)	5 (11%)	N/A	23 (15%)
Gemcitabine/Nab-paclitaxel	9 (9%)	1 (2%)		10 (5%)
Other: Single-agent	18 (18%)	11 (23%)		29 (20%)
Other: Multi-agent	31 (30%)	23 (49%)		54 (40%)
N/A (Unknown)	26 (25%)	7 (15%)		33 (20%)

contrast to 45% in the liver metastasis cohort ($P = 0.011$). There was no significant association between the recurrence pattern of PDAC and vascular invasion, site of primary tumor location nor a history of cigarette smoking (Table 2).

Discussion

In this study, we observed a favorable clinical course with a prolonged time from recurrence to death (TRD) in PDAC patients who underwent curative surgical resection and had subsequent lung metastasis as the first site of recurrence compared to patients who developed recurrent disease in their liver as the first site of metastasis ($P = 0.02$). The difference in clinical course was also supported by the 1 and 2-year survival outcomes. We also found that poorly differentiated PDAC was more likely to recur in the liver rather than lung ($P = 0.047$).

In addition, our data suggests that there may be an association between the use of alcohol and the first site of recurrence in PDAC, with lung metastasis compared to liver metastasis as first site of recurrence ($P = 0.011$).

These findings are indicative of a distinct clinical course of PDAC based on the site of recurrence in metastatic disease. The observations reported herein may potentially impact the risk stratification and standard treatment approach of metastatic PDAC. For example, patients who have oligometastatic disease in the lung may be subject to less intensive management, e.g., single or doublet agents therapy in contrast to triplet therapy) whereas patients with liver recurrence may benefit from an intensified treatment approach. Moreover, isolated lung metastases in PDAC can be considered for pulmonary resection with curative intent in a small number of selected patients [10]. The diverse behavior of PDAC

Table 2 Clinical and epidemiologic variables by Recurrence Pattern

	Recurrence Pattern		P value[*]	Entire Cohort
	Liver	Lung		
Tumor Differentiation[a]				
Well/well to moderate	1 (1%)	1 (2%)	P = 0.047	2 (1%)
Moderate	60 (59%)	36 (77%)		96 (65%)
Moderate- poorly/ Poorly	40 (40%)	10 (21%)		50 (34%)
Tumor Stage				
Stage I	3 (3%)	–	P = 0.194	3 (2%)
Stage IIA	23 (22%)	6 (13%)		29 (19%)
Stage IIB	76 (75%)	41 (87%)		117 (79%)
Lymph Node Status				
Positive	76 (75%)	41 (87%)	P = 0.089	117 (79%)
Negative	26 (25%)	6 (13%)		32 (21%)
Vascular Invasion[a]				
Positive	69 (68%)	34 (72%)	P = 0.703	103 (70%)
Negative	32 (32%)	13 (28%)		45 (30%)
Perineural Invasion				
Present	90 (88%)	45 (96%)	P = 0.226	135 (91%)
Absent	12 (12%)	2 (4%)		14 (9%)
Tumor Margin				
Negative	89 (87%)	36 (77%)	P = 0.148	125 (84%)
Positive	13 (13%)	11 (23%)		24 (16%)
Tumor Location				
Head	84 (83%)	38 (81%)	P = 0.942	132 (82%)
Body	7 (7%)	4 (8%)		11 (7%)
Tail	11 (10%)	5 (11%)		16 (11%)
Alcohol Use				
None	56 (55%)	15 (32%)	P = 0.011	71 (56%)
Social	29 (28%)	25 (53%)		54 (36%)
Daily/heavy	17 (17%)	7 (15%)		24 (16%)
Smoking				
None	55 (54%)	23 (49%)	P = 0.60	78 (52%)
Current/former	47 (46%)	24 (51%)		71 (48%)

Note: [*]p-value was calculated using Fisher's exact test, [a]Tumor differentiation and vascular invasion data was missing for one patient in liver group

based on recurrence pattern may also need to be taken into consideration for stratification in clinical trials including patients with prior surgical resection. Our findings should be further investigated in prospective analyses to confirm the observations.

In our study, we found that moderate to poor and poorly differentiated tumors were associated with an increased incidence of liver metastasis (Table 2). It is unclear, what molecular drivers in poorly differentiated tumors lead to liver metastasis. The relatively better outcomes we reported in regular alcohol users could be explained by the occurrence of different driver (founder) mutations in this patient population compared to the general population. Further genomic analyses based on epidemiological risk factors may shed light on different carcinogenesis pathways with different driver genes in PDAC. We further observed that there may be an increased incidence of liver metastasis in patients with a higher BMI. This association could be related to the direct metabolic effects of increased body weight on liver parenchyma such as fatty liver [11] and increased inflammation such as in non-alcoholic steatohepatitis (NASH) [12]. Given that chronic inflammation provides a safe haven for cancer cell proliferation [13], the liver may be a preferred site by cancer clones in patients with increased BMI. Further, prospective study is warranted to confirm these observations. Lastly, we observed a trend to the increased presence of lung metastasis in patients with lymph node positive disease putatively may be explained by lymphatic drainage of pancreatic lymph nodes into the thoracic duct which drains into the subclavian vein and eventually pulmonary arterial system. This circulatory system may provide a direct pathway for lung metastasis for cancer cells entering into the lymphatic system compared to cancer cells metastasizing via hematogenous spread. Further studies are needed to better understand the underpinnings of these findings.

The observations reported herein may be supported by multiple molecular mechanisms which are involved in the metastatic process. Metastasis is a very sophisticated process influenced by myriad factors such as the molecular behavior of cancer cells, the tumor microenvironment, the immune response to circulating cancer cells and the response of homing organs to the metastatic clones. Metastasis evolves via reprogramming of cancer cells, migration and invasion into stroma, evasion of the immune system, entry into the systemic circulation, colonization in a new tumor environment and homing [14]. This multistep progress may require an extended time period. A study by Yachida, et al., reported that the evolution of a PDAC cell with metastatic features requires considerable genetic modification and requires approximately 5 years from the birth of the parental cancer cell (non-metastatic founder cancer cell) [15]. In fact, throughout this complex process many cancer clones in the primary tumor site undergo either apoptosis or necrosis without achieving metastatic potential to disseminate and propagate in distant organs [16, 17]. Growing evidence suggests that metastatic disease in different distant organs may display varied molecular signatures and diverse clinical behavior. For example, one study explored genetic alterations in $N = 13$ PDAC patients with metastatic disease and found progressive genetic rearrangements in DNA leading to

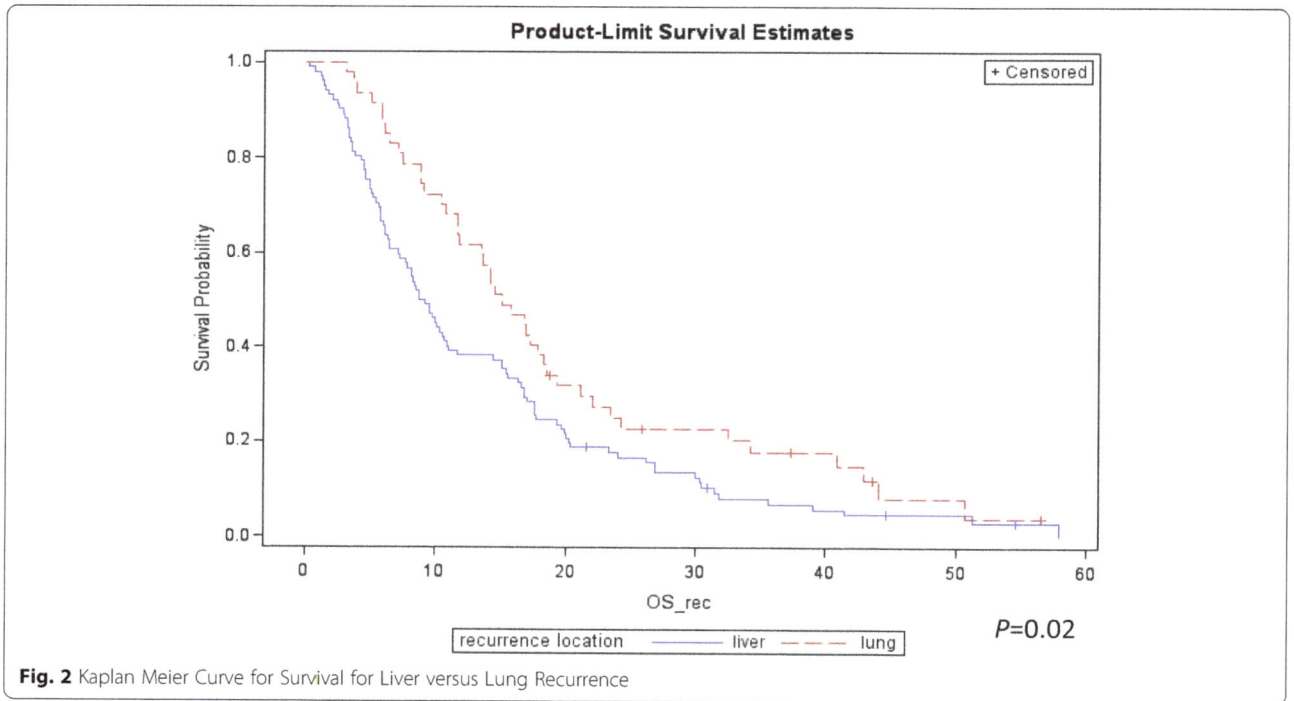

Fig. 2 Kaplan Meier Curve for Survival for Liver versus Lung Recurrence

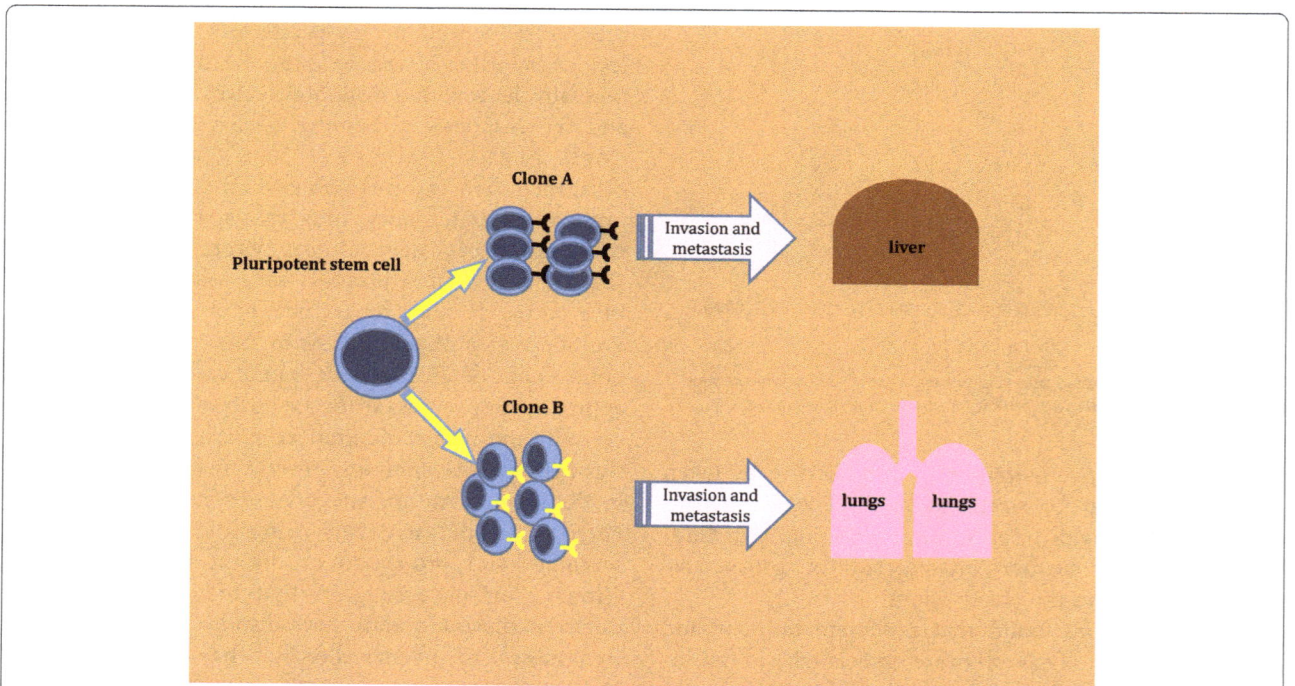

Fig. 3 Evolution of Metastasis. Stem cells give rise to new clones with differing features, including distinct chemokine receptors leading to diverse patterns of disease behavior

generation of distinct clones with unique mutational signatures among different metastases suggesting that tumor heterogeneity continuously evolves even after evolution of the metastatic process [18] (Fig. 3). Current evidence suggests that tissue hypoxia could be one of the important drivers of these genetic rearrangements that yields to multi-clonal expansion and activation of the metastasis process [19, 20]. Growth of cancer cells in the tumor environment is disproportionate to the nutritional and oxygen supply leading to changes in the metabolism of cancer cells including excessive use of glycolysis called the 'Warburg effect' [21]. These imbalances and dynamic changes within the microenvironment yield modifications in the gene expression profile of cancer cells [22]. It is likely that cancer cells continue to conform and modulate their gene expressions in distant metastatic organs including the liver and lungs [18]. The differences in clinical course of disease in liver versus lung metastasis observed in our study could be directly related to the degree of hypoxia in the distant organ along with other characteristics of the metastatic niche. Whether special characteristics of organ-specific homing [23] have an impact on progression of disease in the metastatic setting needs to be further investigated.

Conclusion

In summary, we observed a trend towards improved outcome in PDAC patients with lung metastasis as the first site of recurrence compared to patients with liver metastasis as the first site of recurrence following potentially curative resection. These observations are partly explained by the heterogeneity of PDAC, the distinct features of the homing microenvironment, and the impact of clonal selection by the chemokine receptor network and other processes. Our results also suggest that the epidemiologic context may be a determinant for disease behavior and recurrence pattern. Our study is limited by several factors including, the potential impact of adjuvant and subsequent treatment for metastasis, abstraction of data from a single institution database, the retrospective nature of cohort and the relatively small size of the patient cohort. Further prospective studies are warranted to interrogate our findings and to further characterize the biologic behavior of PDAC.

Abbreviations
BMI: Body-mass index; FOLFRINOX: 5-fluorouracil, oxaliplatin, irinotecan, leucovorin; IRB: Institutional Review and Privacy Board; NASH: Non-alcoholic steatohepatitis; PDAC: Pancreatic ductal adenocarcinoma; SD: Standard deviation; TRD: Time from relapse to death

Acknowledgements
The authors would like to acknowledge bioinformatic support at Memorial Sloan Kettering Cancer Center for their assistance in conducting the dataline search.

Funding
David M. Rubenstein Center for Pancreatic Cancer Research. NCI Cancer Center Support Grant: P30 CA008478 (PI Craig Thompson).

Authors' contributions
IHS and EOR designed the study and wrote the paper. IHS and HE extracted relevant clinical data. JFC and MC performed statistical analysis and IHS, EOR interpreted the statistical results. IHS, HE and EOR prepared the tables and figures. All authors have read and approved the final manuscript.

Competing interests
EOR has funding support and honoraria from Celgene. No other authors declare any competing interests.

Author details
[1]Emory University School of Medicine, Atlanta, USA. [2]New York University Langone Medical Center, New York, USA. [3]Memorial Sloan Kettering Cancer Center, 300 East 66th Street, Office 1021, New York, NY 10065, USA. [4]David M. Rubenstein Center for Pancreatic Cancer Research, 300 East 66th Street, Office 1021, New York, NY 10065, USA. [5]Weill Cornell Medical College, 300 East 66th Street, Office 1021, New York, NY 10065, USA.

References
1. Conroy T, Desseigne F, Ychou M, Bouché O, Guimbaud R, Bécouarn Y, Adenis A, Raoul J-L, Gourgou-Bourgade S, de la Fouchardière C. FOLFIRINOX versus gemcitabine for metastatic pancreatic cancer. N Engl J Med. 2011; 364(19):1817–25.
2. Von Hoff DD, Ervin T, Arena FP, Chiorean EG, Infante J, Moore M, Seay T, Tjulandin SA, Ma WW, Saleh MN. Increased survival in pancreatic cancer with nab-paclitaxel plus gemcitabine. N Engl J Med. 2013;369(18):1691–703.
3. Siegel RL, Miller KD, Jemal A. Cancer statistics, 2016. CA Cancer J Clin. 2016; 66(1):7–30.
4. Oettle H, Post S, Neuhaus P, Gellert K, Langrehr J, Ridwelski K, Schramm H, Fahlke J, Zuelke C, Burkart C. Adjuvant chemotherapy with gemcitabine vs observation in patients undergoing curative-intent resection of pancreatic cancer: a randomized controlled trial. JAMA. 2007;297(3):267–77.
5. Quail DF, Joyce JA. Microenvironmental regulation of tumor progression and metastasis. Nat Med. 2013;19(11):1423–37.
6. Peinado H, Lavotshkin S, Lyden D. The secreted factors responsible for premetastatic niche formation: old sayings and new thoughts. In: Seminars in cancer biology: 2011: Elsevier; 2011. p. 139–46.
7. Alderton GK. Metastasis: exosomes drive premetastatic niche formation. Nat Rev Cancer. 2012;12(7):447.
8. Grange C, Tapparo M, Collino F, Vitillo L, Damasco C, Deregibus MC, Tetta C, Bussolati B, Camussi G. Microvesicles released from human renal cancer stem cells stimulate angiogenesis and formation of lung premetastatic niche. Cancer Res. 2011;71(15):5346–56.
9. Costa-Silva B, Aiello NM, Ocean AJ, Singh S, Zhang H, Thakur BK, Becker A, Hoshino A, Mark MT, Molina H. Pancreatic cancer exosomes initiate premetastatic niche formation in the liver. Nat Cell Biol. 2015;17(6):816–26.
10. Arnaoutakis GJ, Rangachari D, Laheru DA, Iacobuzio-Donahue CA, Hruban RH, Herman JM, Edil BH, Pawlik TM, Schulick RD, Cameron JL. Pulmonary resection for isolated pancreatic adenocarcinoma metastasis: an analysis of outcomes and survival. J Gastrointest Surg. 2011;15(9):1611–7.
11. Wanless IR, Lentz JS. Fatty liver hepatitis (steatohepatitis) and obesity: an autopsy study with analysis of risk factors. Hepatology. 1990;12(5):1106–10.
12. Reddy JK, Sambasiva Rao M. Lipid metabolism and liver inflammation. II Fatty liver disease and fatty acid oxidation. Am J Physiol Gastrointest Liver Physiol. 2006;290(5):G852–8.
13. Coussens LM, Werb Z. Inflammation and cancer. Nature. 2002;420(6917):860.
14. Gupta GP, Massagué J. Cancer metastasis: building a framework. Cell. 2006; 127(4):679–95.
15. Yachida S, Jones S, Bozic I, Antal T, Leary R, Fu B, Kamiyama M, Hruban RH, Eshleman JR, Nowak MA, et al. Distant metastasis occurs late during the genetic evolution of pancreatic cancer. Nature. 2010;467(7319):1114–7.
16. Fidler IJ. Tumor heterogeneity and the biology of cancer invasion and metastasis. Cancer Res. 1978;38(9):2651–60.

17. Fidler IJ. The pathogenesis of cancer metastasis: the 'seed and soil' hypothesis revisited. Nat Rev Cancer. 2003;3(6):453–9.

18. Campbell PJ, Yachida S, Mudie LJ, Stephens PJ, Pleasance ED, Stebbings LA, Morsberger LA, Latimer C, McLaren S, Lin M-L. The patterns and dynamics of genomic instability in metastatic pancreatic cancer. Nature. 2010; 467(7319):1109.

19. Maxwell P, Dachs G, Gleadle J, Nicholls L, Harris A, Stratford I, Hankinson O, Pugh C, Ratcliffe P. Hypoxia-inducible factor-1 modulates gene expression in solid tumors and influences both angiogenesis and tumor growth. Proc Natl Acad Sci. 1997;94(15):8104–9.

20. Pouysségur J, Dayan F, Mazure NM. Hypoxia signalling in cancer and approaches to enforce tumour regression. Nature. 2006;441(7092):437–43.

21. Hsu PP, Sabatini DM. Cancer cell metabolism: Warburg and beyond. Cell. 2008;134(5):703–7.

22. Chan DA, Giaccia AJ. Hypoxia, gene expression, and metastasis. Cancer Metastasis Rev. 2007;26(2):333–9.

23. Joyce JA, Pollard JW. Microenvironmental regulation of metastasis. Nat Rev Cancer. 2009;9(4):239.

MicroRNA-29b-2-5p inhibits cell proliferation by directly targeting Cbl-b in pancreatic ductal adenocarcinoma

Ce Li[1,2], Qian Dong[3], Xiaofang Che[1,2], Ling Xu[1,2], Zhi Li[1,2], Yibo Fan[1,2], Kezuo Hou[1,2], Shuo Wang[1,2], Jinglei Qu[1,2], Lu Xu[1,2], Ti Wen[1,2], Xianghong Yang[4], Xiujuan Qu[1,2*] and Yunpeng Liu[1,2*]

Abstract

Background: MicroRNAs can be used in the prognosis of malignancies; however, their regulatory mechanisms are unknown, especially in pancreatic ductal adenocarcinoma (PDAC).

Methods: In 120 PDAC specimens, miRNA levels were assessed by quantitative real time polymerase chain reaction (qRT-PCR). Then, the role of miR-29b-2-5p in cell proliferation was evaluated both in vitro (Trypan blue staining and cell cycle analysis in the two PDAC cell lines SW1990 and Capan-2) and in vivo using a xenograft mouse model. Next, bioinformatics methods, a luciferase reporter assay, Western blot, and immunohistochemistry (IHC) were applied to assess the biological effects of Cbl-b inhibition by miR-29b-2-5p. Moreover, the relationship between Cbl-b and p53 was evaluated by immunoprecipitation (IP), Western blot, and immunofluorescence.

Results: From the 120 PDAC patients who underwent surgical resection, ten patients with longest survival and ten with shortest survival were selected. We found that high miR-29b-2-5p expression was associated with good prognosis ($p = 0.02$). The validation cohort confirmed miR-29b-2-5p as an independent prognostic factor in PDAC ($n = 100$, 95% CI $= 0.305–0.756$, $p = 0.002$). Furthermore, miR-29b-2-5p inhibited cell proliferation, induced cell cycle arrest, and promoted apoptosis both in vivo and in vitro. Interestingly, miR-29b-2-5p directly bound the Cbl-b gene, down-regulating its expression and reducing Cbl-b-mediated degradation of p53. Meanwhile, miR-29b-2-5p expression was negatively correlated with Cbl-b in PDAC tissues ($r = -0.33$, $p = 0.001$).

Conclusions: Taken together, these findings indicated that miR-29b-2-5p improves prognosis in PDAC by targeting Cbl-b to promote p53 expression, and would constitute an important prognostic factor in PDAC.

Keywords: PDAC, Prognosis, miR-29b-2-5p, Cbl-b, p53, Proliferation

Background

Pancreatic ductal adenocarcinoma (PDAC) is one of the most lethal solid tumors, with an exceedingly poor prognosis [1]. Despite great achievements in surgery, chemotherapy and radiotherapy, the 5-year survival rate of patients with PDAC remains low, less than 7% [2]. One of the reasons underlying poor prognosis in pancreatic cancer is that pancreatic cancer cells have a very strong proliferative capacity [3]. A wide range of prognostic factors are associated with proliferation, including vascular endothelial growth factor (VEGF) [4, 5], insulin-like growth factor(IGF) [6], nerve growth factor receptors (NGF) [7], transforming growth factor (TGF)-β [8]; however, their roles in PDAC have been assessed at the protein level. Increasingly, genetic and epigenetic, more recently, microRNA alterations are found in multiple tumors [9–11]. However, how miRNAs affect tumor progression or patient outcome is unclear, especially in PDAC.

MicroRNAs (miRNAs) are non-coding small RNAs, with a length of 20–23 nucleotides [12]. They bind specific target mRNAs in the 3′-untranslated region (UTR), resulting in target mRNA degradation or translation inhibition, which may affect cell proliferation [13]. Due

* Correspondence: xiujuanqu@yahoo.com; ypliu@cmu.edu.cn
[1]Department of Medical Oncology, the First Hospital of China Medical University, NO.155, North Nanjing Street, Heping District, Shenyang City 110001, China
Full list of author information is available at the end of the article

to high stability, small size, tissue specificity and simple isolation, miRNAs are more advisable as prognostic predictive biomarkers than mRNAs and proteins. Accumulating evidence strongly suggests that aberrant miRNA expression is a common and important feature of human malignancies, facilitating proliferation and promoting prognosis [14–17]. The expression levels of several miRNAs, including miR-125b, miR-199a, miR-100, let-7 g, miR-433 and miR-214, are associated with the progression and prognosis of gastric cancer [18]. A serum miRNA classifier (miR-21-5p, miR-20a-5p, miR-103a-3p, miR-106b-5p, miR-143-5p, and miR-215) is considered a stable prognostic tool for detecting disease recurrence in patients with stage II colon cancer [19]. However, studies assessing the prognostic significance of miRNAs in PDAC are scarce.

As an essential enzyme in the ubiquitin-proteasome system (UPS), Casitas B-lineage lymphoma (Cbl)-b functions as E3 ubiquitin ligase or multifunctional adaptor protein [20, 21]. In previous studies on solid tumors, Cbl-b is mostly focused on gastric cancer [22], breast cancer [23], and non-small-cell lung cells [24]. The function in those solid tumors are inhibiting the proliferation. But the relationship between Cbl-b and PDAC is less reported [25, 26]. We previously studies showed that silencing Cbl-b expression activated the Smad3/p21 axis and inhibited proliferation of PDAC cells [25]. However, the relationship between miRNA and Cbl-b as well as the Cbl-b related protein in PDAC is unclear. Whether Cbl-b plays a role in the prognosis of miRNA-expressing PDAC patients remains to be elucidated. Interfering with miRNA-Cbl-b expression or miRNA-Cbl-b signaling pathway may prolong the survival rate of PDAC patients, thereby elucidating potential therapeutic targets and prognostic biomarkers.

The present study demonstrated that miR-29b-2-5p was a good independent prognostic factor in resectable pancreatic cancer. Furthermore, miR-29b-2-5p negatively regulates Cbl-b to reduce Cbl-b-mediated ubiquitination and p53 expression, inhibiting the proliferation of PDAC cells.

Materials
Human tissue samples
Freshly isolated human PDAC tissues from 120 patients and adjacent pancreatic tissues were obtained with informed consent from the Department of Pathology, the affiliated Shengjing Hospital, China Medical University, between January 2009 to Feburary 2011. The clinic-pathologic characteristics and prognosis were available for 120 patients. The patients had not received chemotherapy or radiation therapy prior to surgery.

Each case diagnosis and histological grade, there are two pathologists confirmed based on the American joint committee on pathological diagnosis. Patient information included age, gender, location of tumor, Maximum tumor diameter, differentiation, surgical margins, pT category, pN category, vessel invasion, vascular tumor thrombus, adjacent organs invasion, pTNM category and Overall survival(OS). The maximal tumor size was defined as the maximum diameter on pathologic analysis. The tumor was staged according to the American Cancer Association (TNM's AJCC staging system) 2010. The final survival data were collected in 31 December 2014. During the 120 cases, 20 cases were analyzed with miRNA microarray. Because they were similar in clinic-pathologic features and treatment but were different in outcomes. The medium OS used as cut off value reference to previous studies [27, 28]. Half of the patients died within the first year of diagnosis were classified as "poor prognosis" with median OS of 6.3 months. Patients who survived more than 21 months had a median OS of 48.0 months, which classified as the "good prognosis" group. The background of the clinic-pathologic characteristics of the 20 patients has been published on our previous study [25]. This study was approved by the Human Ethics Review Committee of China Medical University (protocol #: 2015PS63K); informed consent was obtained from all patients in accordance.

Cell lines and culture conditions
The human pancreatic adenocarcinoma cell lines SW1990(#TCHu201), Capan-2(#SUER0449) were obtained from the Type Culture Collection of the Chinese Academy of Sciences (Shanghai, China) and Suer Biological Technology(Shanghai, China) respectively. Before the experiments, the two cell lines were authenticated on cell micrograph compared to the cell lines on ATCC. The cell lines were maintained in RPMI 1640 medium that contained 10% heat-inactivated foetal bovine serum (FBS), penicillin (100 U/ml) and streptomycin (100 mg/ml) under 5% CO_2 at 37 °C.

Transient transfection
MiR-29b-2-5p mimic and the negative control were obtained from RiboBio (Guangzhou, China). p3XFLAG—CMV9(NC) and p3XFLAG—CMV9 Cbl-b (OE Cbl-b) were obtained from Sigma(USA). The small interfering RNA sequences (Genepharma, Shanghai, China) for Cbl-b was 5'-CCUGAUGGGAGGAGUUAUAtt-3' (sense), 5'-UAUAACUCCUCCCAUCAGGtt – 3' (antisense). MiRNAs and siRNAs transfection was performed using Lipofectamine 2000 (Invitrogen) according to the manufacturer's instruction.

MicroRNA microarray
The levels of total human microRNAs' expression were quantified using a GenoSensor's GenoExplorerTM microRNA microarray (Tempe, AZ, USA). The hybridized miRNA chips were scanned and analyzed using an

Axon GenePix 4000B scanner and GenePix Pro software (Molecular Devices, CA, USA).

RNA extraction and quantitative reverse transcription real-time polymerase chain reaction (qRT-PCR)

Total RNA extracted as described above [25]. For miRNA detection, reverse transcription was performed using One Step PrimeScript® miRNA cDNA Synthesis kit (Takara, Japan), and real-time polymerase chain reaction (PCR) was carried out using SYBR® premix Ex Taq™ II (TaKaRa, Japan) with the ABI 7500 Sequence Detection System (Applied Biosystems, Foster, CA). The sequences (TaKaRa, Japan) for miR-29b-2-5p was 5′-CCTT CGACATGGTGGCTTAGAAA-3′, and U6 was 5′-GCTT CGGCAGCACATATACTAAAAT-3′(sense) and 5′-CGCT TCACGAATTTGCGTGTCAT-3′(anti-sense). The PCR conditions were 30 s at 95 °C, followed by 45 cycles at 95 °C for 5 s, and 58 °C for 25 s. Data were analyzed using the Applied Biosystems 7500 software program (version 2.3) with the automatic Ct setting for adapting baseline and threshold for Ct determination. The threshold cycle and $2^{-\Delta\Delta Ct}$ method were used for calculating the relative amount of the target RNA.

Reverse-transcription-polymerase chain reaction (RT-PCR)

For mRNA detection, reverse transcription was performed using the M-MLV Reverse Transcriptase System (Promega, USA). RT-PCR was performed with the following primer pairs for Cbl-b: forward (5′-CGCT TGACATCACTGAAGGA-3′); and reverse (5′-CTTG CCACACTCTGTGCATT-3′). GAPDH was used as a control: forward (5′-GTGGGGCGCCCCAGGCACC A-3′); and reverse (5′-CTCCTTAATGTCACGCACG ATTTC-3′). PCR conditions for Cbl-b were 95 °C for 5 min, 30 cycles at 95 °C for 30 s, 59 °C for 30 s, 72 °C for 30 s, and 1 cycle at 72 °C for 10 min. GAPDH were 95 °C for 5 min, 33 cycles at 95 °C for 30 s, 56 °C for 45 s, 72 °C for 45 s, and 1 cycle at 72 °C for 10 min. The amplified products were separated on 1% agarose gels, and stained with ethidium bromide and visualized under UV illumination.

Cell proliferation assay

To evaluate the effects of miR-29b-2-5p on cell growth, SW1990 and Capan-2 PDAC cells were incubated in the 6-well plates (3×10^5 cells per hole) in triplicate. The next day, the cells were transfected with miR-29b-2-5p mimics or negative control mimics (NC; Ribobio, China) or OE Cbl-b/NC(1.5 μg) using Lipofectamine 2000 (Invitrogen). The final concentration was kept constant (50 nmol/L). Measure the culture of cell proliferation, cell in 2 ml medium, counted manually after 24, 48, 72, and 96 h use the hemacytometer (Hawksley, West Sussex, UK) and bright field microscope. It combined

with Trypan blue staining method to determine growth state of dispersed cells.

Dual luciferase reporter assay

The 3′-UTR sequence of Cbl-b was obtained through gene synthesis (OriGene, Rockville, MD, USA), and then cloned into the vector pMirTarget through two restriction enzyme cutting sites (SgfI-MluI), resulting in the generation of SC209114. The reagents and methods are provided by OriGene Technologies (OriGene, Rockville, MD, USA). And the sequencing results were compared with the standard template sequences of the BLAST software on the PUBMED and CHROMAS software to identify the gene mutation *loci*. To generate the Cbl-b mutant reporter, the seed region was mutated to remove all complementary nucleotides to miR-29b-2-5p. PDAC cells were co-transfected with firefly luciferase reporter plasmids(0.5 μg), pRL-TK luciferase control vector(0.005 μg) and miR-29b-2-5p or NC(50 nmol) in the 24-well plates. Luciferase assays were performed 24 h after transfection, using the dual-luciferase reporter assay system (Promega, Madison, WI, USA) according to the manufacturer's protocol.

Western blotting analysis

Western blotting was performed as our previously described [29]. The primary antibodies, anti-Cbl-b, anti-b-actin, anti-p53, anti-Bax-2, anti-Bcl-1, anti-GAPDH, anti-UB were from Santa Cruz Biotechnology (Santa Cruz, CA); anti-IgG was from Cell Signaling Technology (Beverly, MA). Enhanced chemiluminescence reagent (SuperSignal Western Pico Chemiluminescent Substrate; Pierce, USA) were used to analysis proteins. The final result was analyzed by NIH Image J software.

Cell cycle analysis

Cells were fixed with 70% ice-cold ethanol overnight. Fixed cells were resuspended in PBS containing 10 μg/ml propidium iodide (PI, KeyGEN, China), 0.1% Triton, and 20 μg/ml RNase A (KeyGEN) and were incubated for 30 min in the dark. Finally, the samples were evaluated by flow cytometry and the data were analyzed with Flow Cytometry (BD Accuri C6; BD Biosciences, San Jose, CA, USA) and analyzed with WinMDI version 2.9 software (The Scripps Research Institute, La Jolla, CA, USA).

Cell apoptosis assay

Transfected cells were cultured in six-well plates. Samples were subsequently stained using an Annexin V-fluorescein isothiocyanate/propidium iodide apoptosis detection kit (cat no. BMS500FI-100; Invitrogen; Thermo Fisher Scientific, Inc.) and the number of apoptotic cells was determined by FACS Calibur flow cytometry (BD Biosciences, San Jose, CA, USA), according to the manufacturer's protocol. Finally, the results were analyzed with WinMDI v.2.9 software (The Scripps Research Institute, La Jolla, CA, USA).

In vivo tumor growth model

All in vivo studies were approved by the Institutional Review Board of China Medical University. These animals were cared of in accordance with institutional ethical guidelines of animal care. Female SPF BALB/c nude mice were bought from Vitalriver (Beijing, China). Mice were sacrificed in gas chamber and by cervical dislocation to confirm death according to the protocol filed with the Guidance of Institutional Animal Care and Use Committee of China Medical University. SW1990 cells (1×10^6) with 0.15 ml PBS subcutaneous injected into mice's right shoulder area. A week after the cells injected, randomly divided into two groups, each group of three mice, and mir-29-2b* agomir or mir-NC agomir (40 ul saline 5 nmol/L, Ribobio technology, Guangzhou, China) treatment by subcutaneous injection every 2 days. Every 2 days with a caliper measuring the volume of tumor, the calculation of tumor volume, use the following formula: V = 1/2 (width×length×height).Body weights were also recorded. With the protocol to the Animal Care and Use Ethnic Committee the China Medical University under the protocol number 16080 M, the tumor-bearing mice were sacrificed by cervical dislocation when the mice became moribund or on day 15.

Immunoprecipitation(IP)

SW1990 cells were seeded at 3×10^5 per well in six-well plates and incubated overnight; Cells were transfected with NC (1.5 μg), OE Cbl-b (1.5 μg) 24 h every six wells. The next day, the cells with OE Cbl-b treated with or without proteasome inhibitor PS341 (5 nM) for 24 h. After removal of the medium, cells were transferred to 1.5 ml EP tube for transient centrifugalization. Cell pellets were washed by ice-cold PBS for two times. For immunoprecipitation, cells were collected with denaturation buffer to separate protein complexes. Cell lysates were incubated with p53 antibody or immunoglobulin-G (1–4 μg, Cell Signaling Technology, MA) at 4 °C overnight followed by the addition of 20 μl of protein G-Sepharose beads (Santa Cruz Biotechnology) for an additional 2 h at 4 °C. The immunoprecipitated proteins with $3 \times$ sampling buffer were eluted by heat treatment at 100 °C for 5 min.

Immunofluorescence staining

Pancreatic cancer cells grew on Lab-Tek chamber slides (Nunc S/A, Polylabo, France). The following day, miR-29b-2-5p or NC (50 nmol/L) treated into cells for 48 h, 3.3% paraformaldehyde fixed for 15 min, 0.2% Triton X-100 permeabilized for 5 min, 5% bovine serum albumin (BSA) blocked for 1 h. And the cells incubated

with anti-Cbl-b and anti-p53 antibody (Santa Cruz, CA) at a dilution of 1:200 overnight at 4 °C. Blocking solution for 1 h at room temperature with Alexa Fluor 546-conjugated goat anti-mouse IgG and Alexa Fluor 488-conjugated goat anti-rabbit IgG (Molecular Probes) in the dark. Nuclei was stained by 4′-6-diamidino-2--phenylindole for 5 min. The cells were visualized by fluorescence microscopy (BX53, Olympus, Japan).

Immunohistochemistry(IHC)

One hundred of formalin-fixed, paraffin-embedded PDAC tissues were used for IHC. All sections were performed using the following antibodies: anti-Cbl-b (Santa Cruz Biotechnology) using S-P immunohistochemical kit (Fuzhou Maixin Biological Technology Ltd., Fujian, China) as described previously [30]. The scanning the entire tissue specimen evaluated the staining under low magnification (× 10) and confirmed under high magnification (× 20 and × 40). Visualized and classified the protein expression was based on the percentage of positive cells and the intensity of staining. Tumors with < 10% Cbl-b expression were regarded as negative or weak (0),10–70% were regarded as moderate (1) and ≥ 70% were considered positive (2). The cut off of weak-medium-strong is 10 and 70% respectively. Final scores were assigned by two independent pathologists.

Statistical analysis

Statistical analysis was performed using the GraphPad Prism software (La Jolla, CA, USA). Overall survival (OS) was defined as the time from the date of the surgery to the date of death or the last contact, i.e., the date of the last follow-up visit. Kaplan-Meier estimate was used to analyze the survival data and the statistical significance was evaluated by the log rank test. ROC curve from the point to cut off value is based on the previously study [31]. Multivariate analysis was performed using the multivariate Cox proportional hazards model (forward), which was fitted using all of the clinic-pathologic variables. Chi-square test was used to evaluated the correlation between miR-29b-2-5p expression levels and the clinical characteristics. The differences between groups were assessed by Student's t-test or Mann-Whitney U test. For correlation analysis, the non-parametric Spearman r tests were applied. All means were calculated from at least three independent experiments. Two-sided P values < 0.05 were considered to be statistically significant. SPSS software (version 13.0; SPSS, Inc. Chicago, IL, USA) was used for statistical analysis.

Results

MiR-29b-2-5p is correlated with good prognosis in pancreatic cancer

The flowchart of patient selection and schematic design were shown in Fig. 1a. We performed a comprehensive

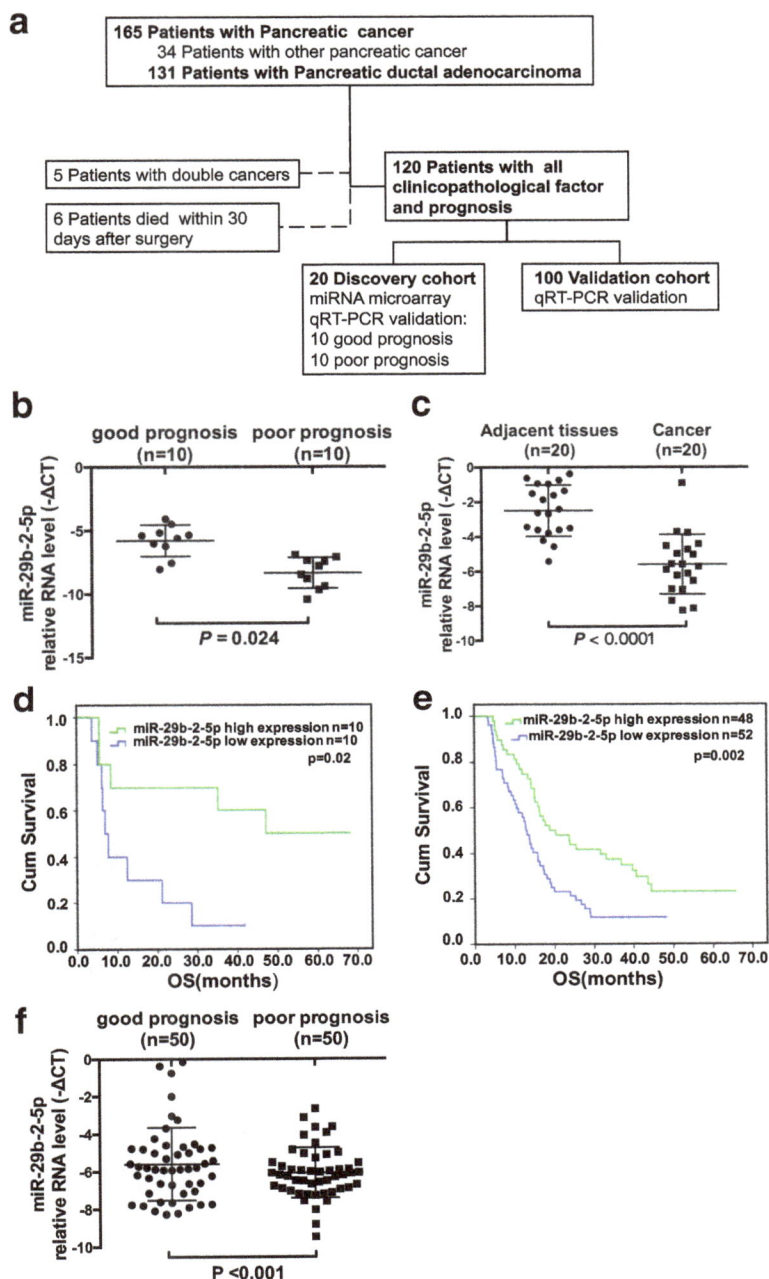

Fig. 1 miR-29b-2-5p has a positive correlation with the prognosis of pancreatic cancer and independently predicted better survival. **a** The flowchart of patient selection and schematic design. **b** Statistical analysis of miR-29b-2-5p expression in good and poor prognosis group, nonparametric Mann–Whitney test. All the bars represent SE. **c** Statistical analysis of miR-29b-2-5p expression in normal and cancerous pancreatic tissues, nonparametric Mann–Whitney test. All the bars represent SE. **d** In miRNA array cohort, miR-29b-2-5p high expression associated with a median survival of 35.2 months versus low expression of 6.4 months (log rank $x^2 = 21.837$, $p = 0.02$). **e** In miRNA validation cohort, patients with high or low miR-29b-2-5p expression associated with a median OS respectively time of 18.8 or 12.9 months. (log rank $x^2 = 9.296$, $p = 0.002$). **f** The good prognosis group levels of miR-29b-2-5p in these 100 validation cohort is higher than poor prognosis group. ($p < 0.001$)

microarray analysis to compare miRNA expression profiles in pancreatic tissues from two groups of participants. Our previous study showed that patients with good prognosis, median OS was 48.0 months, compared

to 6.3 months in those with poor prognosis. There was no statistically significant differences in the remaining clinical and pathological features between the two groups, corroborating previous findings [25]. The good prognosis group had 22 miRNAs significantly upregulated (miR-29b-2-5p, etc.) as demonstrated by miRNA microarray analysis [25]. Among these candidate miRNAs, 4 miRNAs are Dead miRNA Entry through miRbase which we cannot get the sequences. We used real-time PCR to test the result of miRNA array. In the rest of 18 candidate miRNAs, 2 miRNAs were opposite from the miRNA array, 16 were coherent with the miRNA array (see Additional file 1: Figure S2.A.B online). We tried to find targets which can be regulated by the miRNAs, and found 7 miRNAs had targets with softwares miRwalk and starBase. Among these candidate 7 miRNAs, miR-29b-5p, miR-891b and miR-490-5p could inhibit proliferation in cell lines, and miR-29b-2-5p was most stable in inhibiting PDAC tumor cell proliferation as well as the result of microarray (see Additional file 1: Figure S2.C online, Fig. 2a). Real-time PCR confirmed that miR-29b-2-5p was associated with better prognosis. MiR-29b-2-5p expression gradually increased from the poor to good prognosis groups (Fig. 1b), and from cancer to adjacent pancreatic

tissues (Fig. 1c). Furthermore, high miR-29b-2-5p expression was associated with a median OS of 35.2 months versus 6.4 months for the low expression group (log rank $x^2 = 21.837$, $p = 0.02$; Fig. 1d). A strong correlation between miR-29b-2-5p expression status and OS was demonstrated, confirming that miR-29b-2-5p was a prognostic factor in PDAC.

To verify the prognostic role of miR-29b-2-5p, the expression levels of this miRNA were assessed by qRT-PCR in 100 independent PDAC samples. This validation cohort contained stage I, II and III tumors. Other clinical pathologic features were not significantly different from those of the initial patient cohort (see Additional file 2: Table S1). We also evaluated the correlation between miR-29b-2-5p expression levels and the clinical characteristics using chi-square test (Table 1), found that Gender ($p = 0.028$), Maximum tumor diameter (cm) ($p = 0.11$), Differentiation ($p < 0.001$), Surgical margins ($p < 0.001$), pT category ($p = 0.002$), pN category ($p < 0.001$), Vascular tumor thrombus ($p < 0.001$),

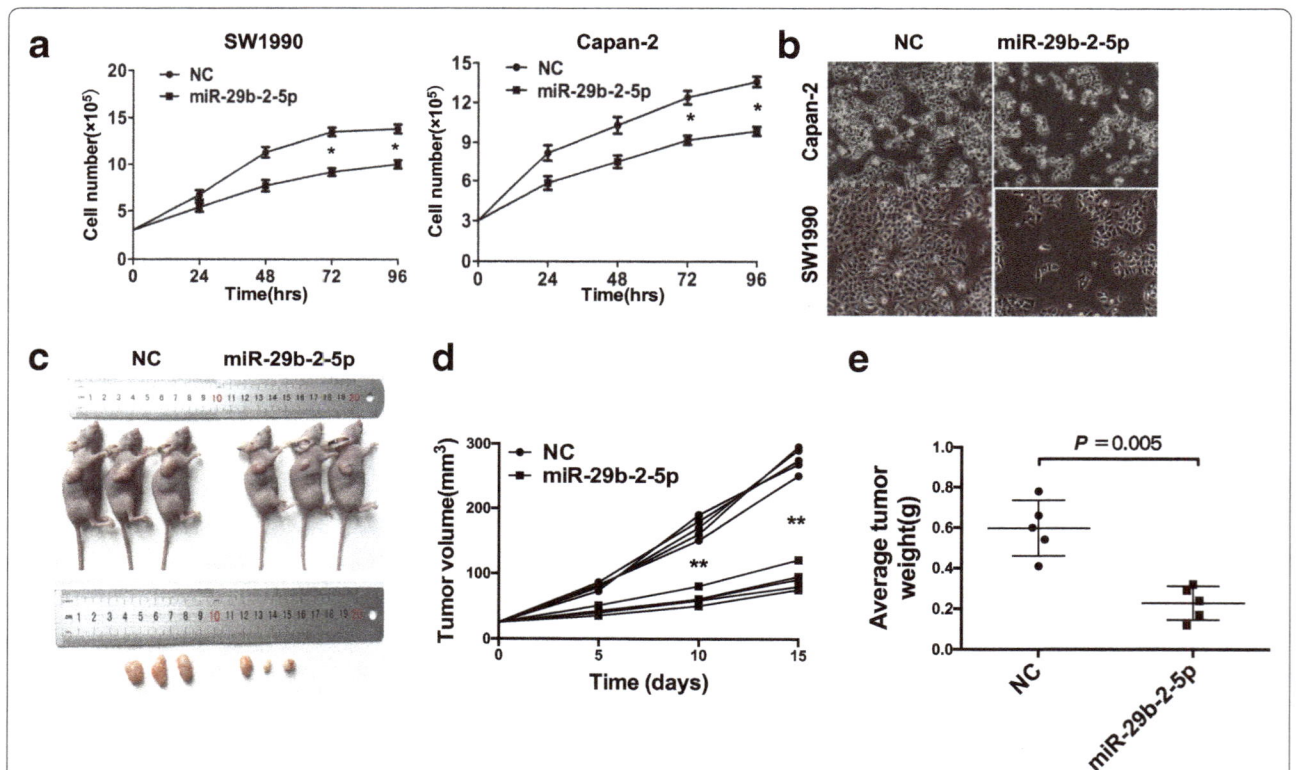

Fig. 2 miR-29b-2-5p inhibits PDAC cell proliferation in vitro and in vivo experiments systems. **a** PDAC cell lines, SW1990 and Capan-2, were transfected with miR-29b-2-5p or NC. Cells were collected at 48, 24, 72, and 96 h after transfection using Trypan blue staining method. The results suggested miR-29b-2-5p significantly inhibited the proliferation of PDAC cells (mean ± SD, results of three independent experiments, *$P < 0.05$). **b** Observation under microscope of the cells transfected with miR-29b-2-5p or NC 72 h after transfection. The number of cells in miR-29b-2-5p group was significantly decreased compared with that in NC group. **c** miR-29b-2-5p agomir was intratumorally injected after the tumor was formed. After 2 weeks, the size of the subcutaneous tumor treated with miR-29b-2-5p agomir significantly decreased compared with NC-treated tumor. **d** Quantification of tumor volume development in NC- and miR-29b-2-5p-bearing nude mice. **e** Subcutaneous tumors derived from SW1990 cells in the NC- or miR-29b-2-5p agomir-treated group were weighed after tumors were harvested in histogram, *$P < 0.05$, **$P < 0.001$

Table 1 The correlation between miR-29b-2-5p expression levels and the clinical characteristics

Characteristics	Cases	miR-29b-2-5p expression in PDAC		P value
		Low(%)	High(%)	
Age (years)				0.689
< 60	48	25(52.1)	23(47.9)	
≥ 60	52	27(51.9)	25(48.1)	
Gender				*0.028**
Male	61	33(54.1)	28(45.9)	
Female	39	19(48.7)	20(51.3)	
Location of tumor				0.072
Head	59	27(45.8))	32(54.2)	
Body or tail	41	25(61)	16(39)	
Type of operation				0.088
Pancreaticoduodenectomy	77	43(55.8)	34(44.2)	
Distal pancreatectomy	23	9(39.1)	14(60.9)	
Total pancreatectomy	0	0	0	
Maximum tumor diameter (cm)				0.11
< 4	42	28(66.7)	14(33.3)	
≥ 4	58	24(41.4)	34(58.6)	
Differentiation				*< 0.001**
Well	25	13(52)	12(48)	
Moderately	59	28(47.5)	31(52.5)	
Poor	16	11(68.8)	5(31.2)	
Surgical margins				*< 0.001**
Negative	97	51(52.6)	46(47.4)	
Positive	3	1(33.3)	2(66.7)	
pT category				*0.002**
pT1	11	7(63.6)	4(36.4)	
pT2	38	20(52.6)	18(47.4)	
pT3	24	12(50)	12(50)	
pT4	27	13(48.2)	14(51.8)	
pN category				*< 0.001**
pN0	73	37(50.7)	36(49.3)	
pN1	27	15(55.6)	12(44.4)	
Vessel invasion				0.841
No	51	32(62.8)	19(37.2)	
Yes	49	20(40.8)	29(59.2)	
Vascular tumor thrombus				*< 0.001**
No	97	49(50.5)	48(49.5)	
Yes	3	3(100)	0	
Adjacent organs invasion				*< 0.001**
No	83	43(51.8)	40(48.2)	
Yes	17	9(52.9)	8(47.1)	

Table 1 The correlation between miR-29b-2-5p expression levels and the clinical characteristics *(Continued)*

Characteristics	Cases	miR-29b-2-5p expression in PDAC		P value
		Low(%)	High(%)	
pTNM category				0.075
I	44	23(52.3)	21(47.7)	
II	29	15(51.7)	14(42.3)	
III	27	14(51.9)	13(48.1)	
CA19-9 (U/mL)				*< 0.001**
≥ 37	87	45(51.7)	42(48.3)	
< 37	13	7(53.9)	6(46.1)	

pT pathologic T, *pN* pathologic N, *pTNM* pathologic TNM
*Values shown in bold italics are statistically significant

Adjacent organs invasion ($p < 0.001$), CA19−9(($p < 0.001$) had correlation with miR-29b-2-5p. MiR-29b-2-5p was detected in all patients. Patients with high miR-29b-2-5p expression had median OS of 18.8 months (95% CI 10.4–27.3 months) versus 12.9 months (95% CI 10.6–15.1 months) for the low expression group (log rank $\chi^2 = 9.296$, $p = 0.002$; Fig. 1e). And scatter plot showed that the good prognosis group levels of miR-29b-2-5p in these 100 validation cohort is higher than poor prognosis group ($p < 0.001$, Fig. 1f). We also use ROC analyses based on clear cut-off values on which expression levels miRNA-29b-2-5p is prognostic relevant. The result is the same as Medium method. (see Additional file 3: Figure S1 online).

Multivariate Cox proportional hazard model (forward) was used to fit all 15 clinical pathological variables. MiR-29b-2-5p was included in the multivariate Cox proportional hazards model (forward) analysis of 100 patients along with prognostic clinic-pathologic factors. High miR-29b-2-5p expression (HR, 0.492; 95% CI, 0.300−0.807; $P = 0.005$), pT4 category (HR, 1.286; 95% CI 1.004−1.646; $P = 0.046$), serum CA19−9 level ≥ 37 U/ mL (HR, 3.47; 95% CI, 1.484−8.112; $P = 0.004$), and poorly differentiated tumor (HR, 1.472; 95% CI 1.016−2.133; $P = 0.041$) were significant independent prognostic factors associated with OS (Table 2). These data suggested that miR-29b-2-5p represented a tumor suppressor in PDAC.

MiR-29b-2-5p inhibits pancreatic cancer proliferation, and induces PDAC cell apoptosis and G1 phase cell cycle arrest

To assess whether miR-29b-2-5p plays a tumor suppressive role in PDAC development, we first evaluated the effect of miR-29b-2-5p on cell proliferation using the Trypan blue staining method in Capan-2 and SW1990 cells. MiR-29b-2-5p-treated Capan-2 and SW1990 cells exhibited significantly lower growth rates compared with

Table 2 Multivariate Cox regression analysis including miR-29b-2-5p expression levels and overall survival in 100 patients with PDAC

Variables	Univariable analysis			Multivariable analysis		
	HR	95% CI	P value	HR	95% CI	P value
miR-29b-5p(high/low)	0.503	0.32–0.788	0.003	0.492	0.300–0.807	0.005
pT category(T4/T3/T2/T1)	1.212	0975–1.508	0.084	1.286	1.004–1.646	0.046
pN category(N1/N0)	1.871	1.147–3.053	0.012			
CA 19-9(≥ 37 U/mL/<37 U/mL)	3.315	1.426–7.706	0.005	3.47	1.484–8.112	0.004
Tumor Differenciation (Poor/Moderately/Well)	1.45	1.014–2.074	0.042	1.472	1.016–2.133	0.041

The multivariate Cox proportional hazards model (forward) was fitted using all of the clinical and pathological variables, which included age (≥60 vs. <60 years old), gender (male vs. female), type of operation (pancreaticoduodenectomy vs. distal pancreatectomy vs. total pancreatectomy), surgical margins (positive vs. negative), location of tumor (head vs. body or tail), maximal tumor diameter, histological differentiation (poorly vs. moderately vs. well differentiated), pT category (pT4 vs. pT3 vs. pT2 vs. pT1), pN category (pN1 vs. pN0), vessel invasion (yes vs. no), vascular tumor thrombus (yes vs. no), adjacent organs invasion (yes vs. no), pTNM category (I vs. II vs. III), miR-29b-2-5p expression (high expression vs. low expression), and CA19–9 level (≥37 U/mL vs. < 37 U/mL)

control cells (Fig. 2a, b). Increased miR-29b-2-5p expression upon treatment of the two PDAC cell lines was confirmed by qRT-PCR (see Additional file 4: Figure S3 online). These results provided strong evidence that miR-29b-2-5p was a negative regulator of pancreatic cancer development and progression. To determine whether miR-29b-2-5p could have a potential therapeutic value in vivo, nude mice bearing subcutaneous SW1990 xenografts were treated with miR-29b-2-5p every other day for 14 days. After euthanasia, the tumors were removed from the animals for analysis (Fig. 2c–e). The results suggested that miR-29b-2-5p might have a therapeutic potential for the treatment of PDAC.

To further evaluate whether the miR-29b-2-5p-reduced cell proliferation was due to cell cycle arrest and/or apoptotic death, we first examined the effect of miR-29b-2-5p on cell cycle of SW1990 and Capan-2 cells. Compared with NC, the miR-29b-2-5p mimic significantly enhanced the G0/G1 subpopulation in SW1990 and Capan-2 cells (Fig. 3a). As shown in Fig. 3b, miR-29b-2-5p significantly promoted apoptosis in PDAC cells. In agreement, miR-29b-2-5p significantly reduced the levels of Bcl-2 and cyclinD1, and enhanced Bax2 amounts (Fig. 3c). These data suggested that miR-29b-2-5p up-regulation may promote cell cycle progression and inhibit cell apoptosis in PDAC cells.

Cbl-b is a direct target of miR-29b-2-5p and involved in miR-29b-2-5p-induced tumor suppression

We used predicted softwares to screen the target gene of miR-29b-5p. In the top three candidate genes, Cbl-b changed most significantly. Our previous study reported that Cbl-b plays an important role in PDAC. Silencing of Cbl-b expression inhibited proliferation in PDAC cells [25]. In this work, the relationship between miR-29b-2-5p and Cbl-b was assessed. As shown in Fig. 4a, the miRNA/mRNA comparative analysis showed that the 3′UTR of Cbl-b had the binding site for miR-29b-2-5p, at 611–617 nt. To assess whether Cbl-b is regulated by miR-29b-2-5p

through direct binding to its 3′UTR, we structured plasmids containing WT or mutant 3′UTR of human Cbl-b fused downstream of the firefly luciferase gene. WT and mutant plasmids were co-transfected into Capan-2 or SW1990 cells, respectively, with miR-29b-2-5p mimic or miR-NC. As shown in Fig. 4b, luciferase activity upon miR-29b-2-5p transfection was significantly reduced. Mutations of the Cbl-b 3′-UTR abrogated the suppressive effect of miR-29b-2-5p. RT-PCR showed that Cbl-b mRNA levels had no changes after miR-29b-2-5p treatment of both Capan-2 and SW1990 cells; miR-29b-2-5p repressed Cbl-b expression through post-transcriptional inhibition in human PDAC cells (Fig. 4c). These results suggested that Cbl-b serves as an actual target of miR-29b-2-5p.

To evaluate the effect of Cbl-b in PDAC cells, the overexpression plasmid targeting Cbl-b p3xFLAG-CMV9-cbl-b (OE Cbl-b) and control plasmid (NC) were transfected into SW1990 and Capan-2 cells. Cells with more than 50% of endogenous Cbl-b expression were used in subsequent experiments (Fig. 4d). The effect of Cbl-b on cell proliferation was assessed by the Trypan blue staining method. The results showed that Cbl-b could promote the proliferation of PDAC cells (Fig. 4e). To determine the impact of miR-29b-2-5p expression on PDAC biology, the levels of this miRNA in SW1990 cells were assessed after transfection with NC and miR-29b expression -2-5p, NC plus Cbl-b, or miR-29b-2-5p plus OE Cbl-b. The results showed that miR-29b-2-5p could effectively reverse the effect of Cbl-b on the proliferation of PDAC cells. (Fig. 4f).

MiR-29b-2-5p promotes p53 expression by suppressing Cbl-b, likely through ubiquitination-dependent proteasomal degradation of p53

It is well known that the tumor suppressor p53 induces G1 arrest in response to stress. The major downstream effectors of p53 include cyclin D1, Bcl-2 and Bax. Therefore, we further assessed the p53 response after miR-29b-2-5p treatment. As shown in Fig. 5a,

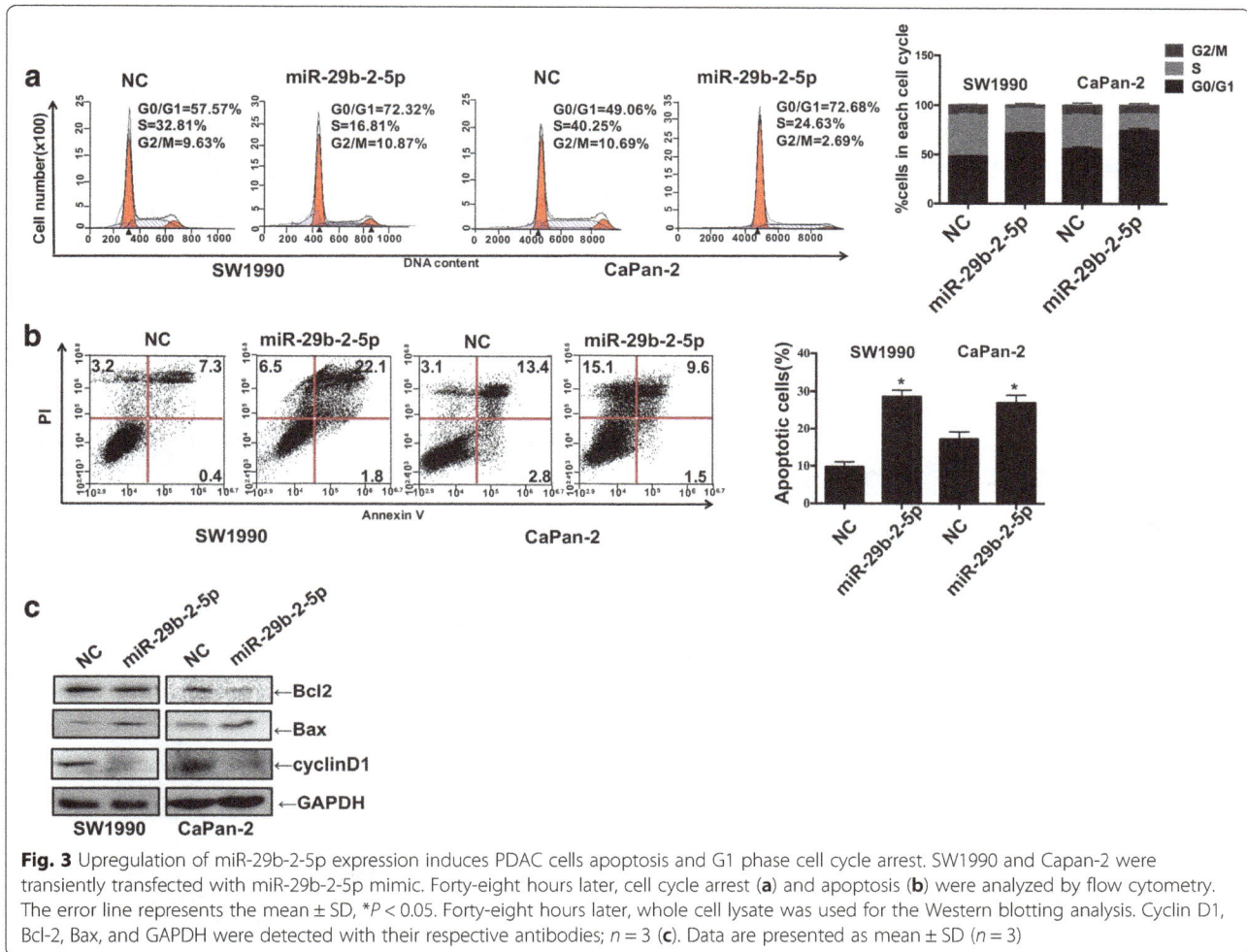

Fig. 3 Upregulation of miR-29b-2-5p expression induces PDAC cells apoptosis and G1 phase cell cycle arrest. SW1990 and Capan-2 were transiently transfected with miR-29b-2-5p mimic. Forty-eight hours later, cell cycle arrest (**a**) and apoptosis (**b**) were analyzed by flow cytometry. The error line represents the mean ± SD, *$P < 0.05$. Forty-eight hours later, whole cell lysate was used for the Western blotting analysis. Cyclin D1, Bcl-2, Bax, and GAPDH were detected with their respective antibodies; $n = 3$ (**c**). Data are presented as mean ± SD ($n = 3$)

miR-29b-2-5p significantly enhanced p53 and p-p53 expression after Cbl-b silencing. Multiple studies showed that p53 ubiquitination and degradation are largely controlled by Mdm2, an E3 ligase. Cbl-b, which is similar to Mdm2, is also an E3 ligase. However, the relationship between Cbl-b and p53 remains undefined. As shown in Fig. 5b, p53 was associated to Cbl-b, with which it could interact (immunoprecipitation, IP) (Fig. 5c). To valuate whether the ubiquitin-proteasome mediated p53 down-regulation, the proteasome inhibitor PS341 (5 nM) was incubated for 24 h with SW1990 cells. Interestingly, Cbl-b was associated with p53 in SW1990 cells (Fig. 5d). It is well known that p53 works in the cell nucleus to regulate proliferation. However, it remains unknown p53 is found after Cbl-b inhibition. As expected, miR-29b-2-5p reduced Cbl-b protein expression, while drastically inducing the expression of the nuclear form of p53. Immunofluorescent staining consistently confirmed the induced nuclear p53 expression (Fig. 5e). These findings strongly indicated that miR-29b-2-5p could promote

cellular p53 by suppressing Cbl-b, while promoting p53 translocation, from the cytoplasm to the nucleus.

The expression level of miR-29b-2-5p is negatively correlated with Cbl-b in patients with PDAC

The expression levels of the Cbl-b protein in tissue samples from 100 patients with PDAC were detected by immunohistochemistry. We first assessed the role of Cbl-b in pancreatic cancer; interestingly, Cbl-b amounts showed a significant negative correlation with prognosis in pancreatic cancer. Patients with high Cbl-b expression had a median survival of 13.1 months (95% CI 7.9–18.1 months); those with moderate expression had 22.0 months (95% CI 17.1–26.9 months), and the low expression group 32.4 months (95% CI 24.2–40.7 months; $P = 0.001$, Fig. 6A). Furthermore, the pancreatic tumor specimens were grouped according to Cbl-b expression levels as negative/weak, moderate, and strong as determined by immunohistochemical staining (Fig. 6B). The expression level of miR-29b-2-5p was negatively correlated

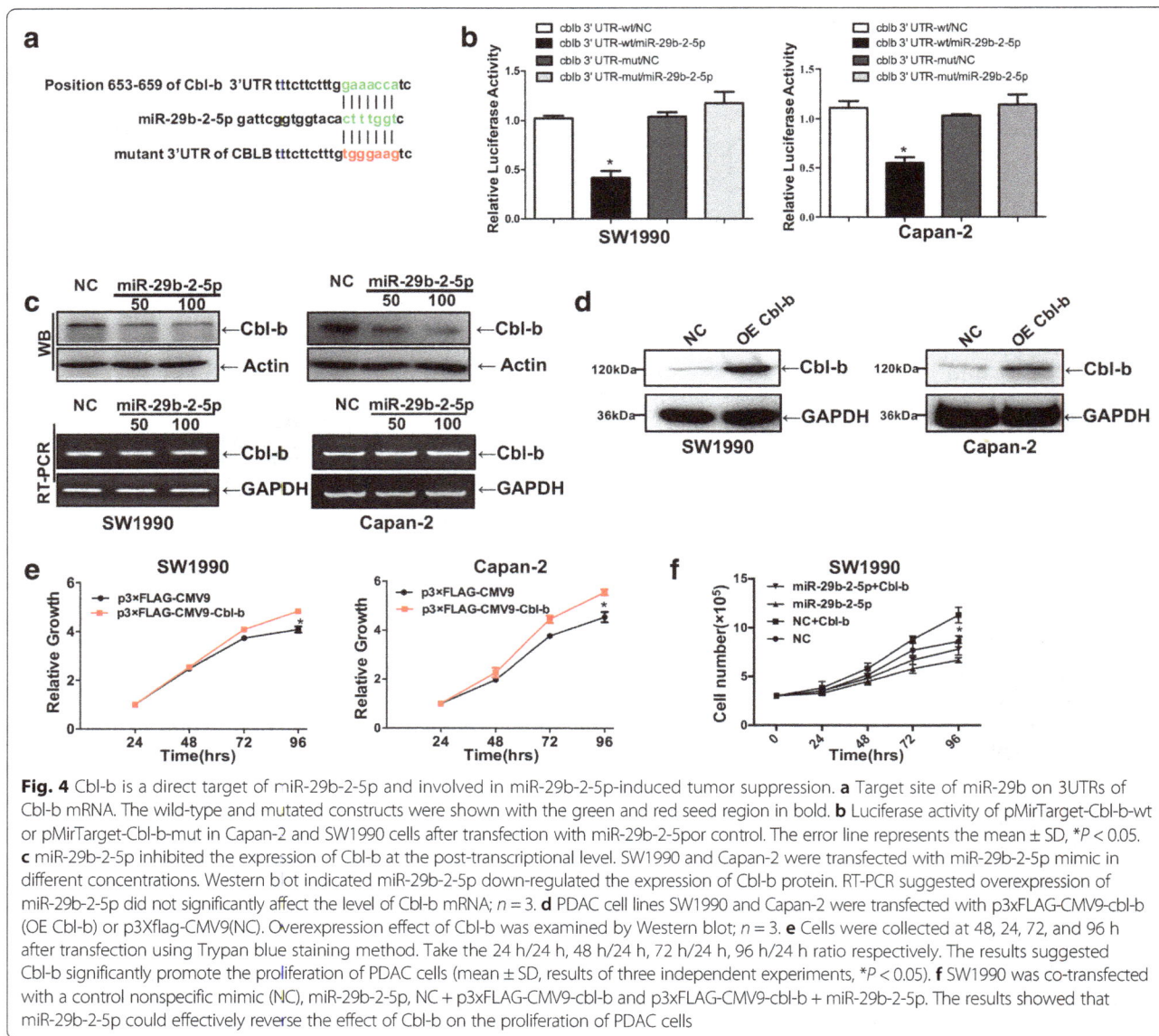

Fig. 4 Cbl-b is a direct target of miR-29b-2-5p and involved in miR-29b-2-5p-induced tumor suppression. **a** Target site of miR-29b on 3UTRs of Cbl-b mRNA. The wild-type and mutated constructs were shown with the green and red seed region in bold. **b** Luciferase activity of pMirTarget-Cbl-b-wt or pMirTarget-Cbl-b-mut in Capan-2 and SW1990 cells after transfection with miR-29b-2-5por control. The error line represents the mean ± SD, *P < 0.05. **c** miR-29b-2-5p inhibited the expression of Cbl-b at the post-transcriptional level. SW1990 and Capan-2 were transfected with miR-29b-2-5p mimic in different concentrations. Western blot indicated miR-29b-2-5p down-regulated the expression of Cbl-b protein. RT-PCR suggested overexpression of miR-29b-2-5p did not significantly affect the level of Cbl-b mRNA; n = 3. **d** PDAC cell lines SW1990 and Capan-2 were transfected with p3xFLAG-CMV9-cbl-b (OE Cbl-b) or p3Xflag-CMV9(NC). Overexpression effect of Cbl-b was examined by Western blot; n = 3. **e** Cells were collected at 48, 24, 72, and 96 h after transfection using Trypan blue staining method. Take the 24 h/24 h, 48 h/24 h, 72 h/24 h, 96 h/24 h ratio respectively. The results suggested Cbl-b significantly promote the proliferation of PDAC cells (mean ± SD, results of three independent experiments, *P < 0.05). **f** SW1990 was co-transfected with a control nonspecific mimic (NC), miR-29b-2-5p, NC + p3xFLAG-CMV9-cbl-b and p3xFLAG-CMV9-cbl-b + miR-29b-2-5p. The results showed that miR-29b-2-5p could effectively reverse the effect of Cbl-b on the proliferation of PDAC cells

with Cbl-b protein amounts in patients with SPSS (Table 3). Collectively, this clinical and experimental study strongly suggested that Cbl-b promotes PDAC growth.

Discussion

In recent years, significant advances in miRNA research have provided clues for understanding the occurrence and development of non-hereditary tumors [32]. Analysis of miRNA expression in clinical follow-up samples has provided valuable information for identifying tumor related prognostic factors [33–35]. However, the molecular regulatory mechanisms of miRNAs in PDAC occurrence and development are rarely studied. In most studies, samples were obtained from PDAC cell lines, PDAC tissues, and normal control tissues [36, 37]. In the present study, patients with similar clinicopathological parameters and treatments but completely different survival outcomes were selected. Among 120 patients with resectable pancreatic cancer, 10 cases with best prognosis and 10 with worst prognosis were selected for miRNA microarray analysis. Then, all cases were verified and a new prognostic model was established. This screening method could be more effective in identifying the potential prognostic values of miRNAs in PDAC.

The miR-29b-2 family has two members, including miR-29b and miR-29b-2-5p [38]. Multiple studies have previously assessed miR-29b as a prognostic factor in many cancers [39]. On the contrary, miR-29b-2-5p is rarely studied. Although miR-29b-2-5p is considered a promoter of bacterial binding to host cells in prokaryotes [40], its identity and function in pancreatic cancer remain unclear. In the current study, miR-29b-2-5p expression independently predicted good survival in PDAC as

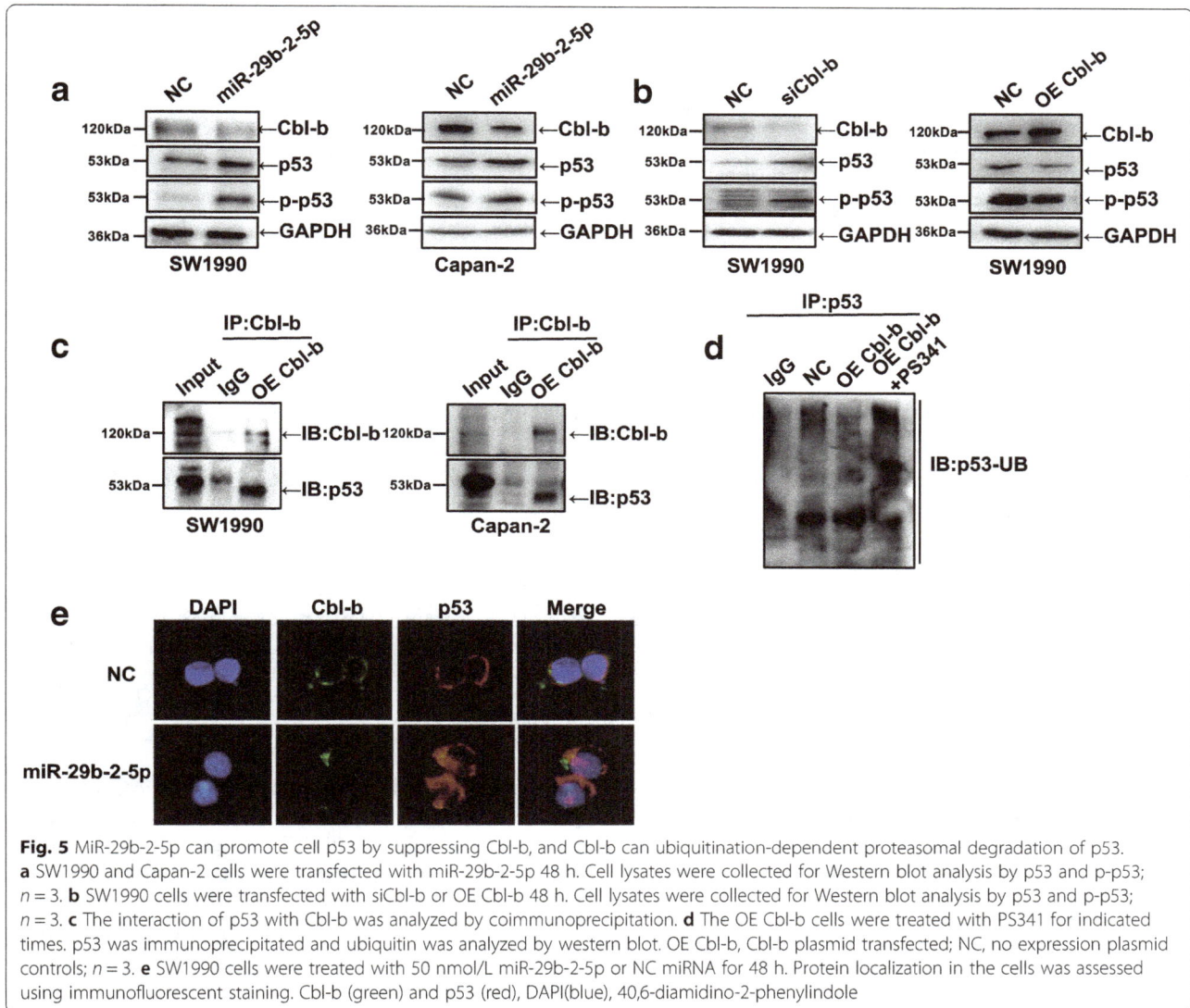

Fig. 5 MiR-29b-2-5p can promote cell p53 by suppressing Cbl-b, and Cbl-b can ubiquitination-dependent proteasomal degradation of p53. **a** SW1990 and Capan-2 cells were transfected with miR-29b-2-5p 48 h. Cell lysates were collected for Western blot analysis by p53 and p-p53; n = 3. **b** SW1990 cells were transfected with siCbl-b or OE Cbl-b 48 h. Cell lysates were collected for Western blot analysis by p53 and p-p53; n = 3. **c** The interaction of p53 with Cbl-b was analyzed by coimmunoprecipation. **d** The OE Cbl-b cells were treated with PS341 for indicated times. p53 was immunoprecipitated and ubiquitin was analyzed by western blot. OE Cbl-b, Cbl-b plasmid transfected; NC, no expression plasmid controls; n = 3. **e** SW1990 cells were treated with 50 nmol/L miR-29b-2-5p or NC miRNA for 48 h. Protein localization in the cells was assessed using immunofluorescent staining. Cbl-b (green) and p53 (red), DAPI(blue), 40,6-diamidino-2-phenylindole

evaluated by multivariate Cox regression analysis. In addition, miR-29b-2-5p inhibited cell proliferation both in vivo and in vitro, induced cell cycle arrest and promoted apoptosis in pancreatic cell lines. These findings clearly demonstrated for the first time that miR-29b-2-5p was associated with good prognosis and reduced proliferation in PDAC.

It is well known that a single miRNA can modulate multiple cellular signaling pathways by regulating the expression of target genes [41]. The expression and role of Cbl-b in different tissues are very controversial. Previous studies revealed that Cbl-b increases the sensitivity of gastric cancer cells by enhancing the epidermal growth factor receptor (EGFR) and mitochondria mediated signaling pathways in gastric cancer [42]. On the contrary, Cbl-b binds to Smad3 and promotes breast cancer proliferation by inhibiting the TGF-signaling pathway [43].

Our previous study revealed that Cbl-b is regulated by miRNA891b and promote proliferation of PDAC cells by inhibiting the Smad3/p21 pathway [25]. Therefore, the functions of Cbl-b on the proliferation of different cancer cells are absolutely tangled, it may be due to the varied proteins that interact with Cbl-b in different cancer cells.

In this study, the clinical data suggested that pancreatic cancer patients with low miR-29b-2-5p expression and high Cbl-b levels are more likely to have tumor proliferation. Consistently, we demonstrated that Cbl-b overexpression promoted pancreatic cancer cell proliferation both in vitro and in vivo. These findings indicated that Cbl-b is functionally involved in miR-29b-2-5p-mediated tumor growth inhibition in pancreatic cancer cells.

TP53, a classical gene in pancreatic cancer, is associated with apoptosis and G1 phase arrest [44]. Meanwhile, p53 is regulated by MDM2, another E3 ubiquitin ligase.

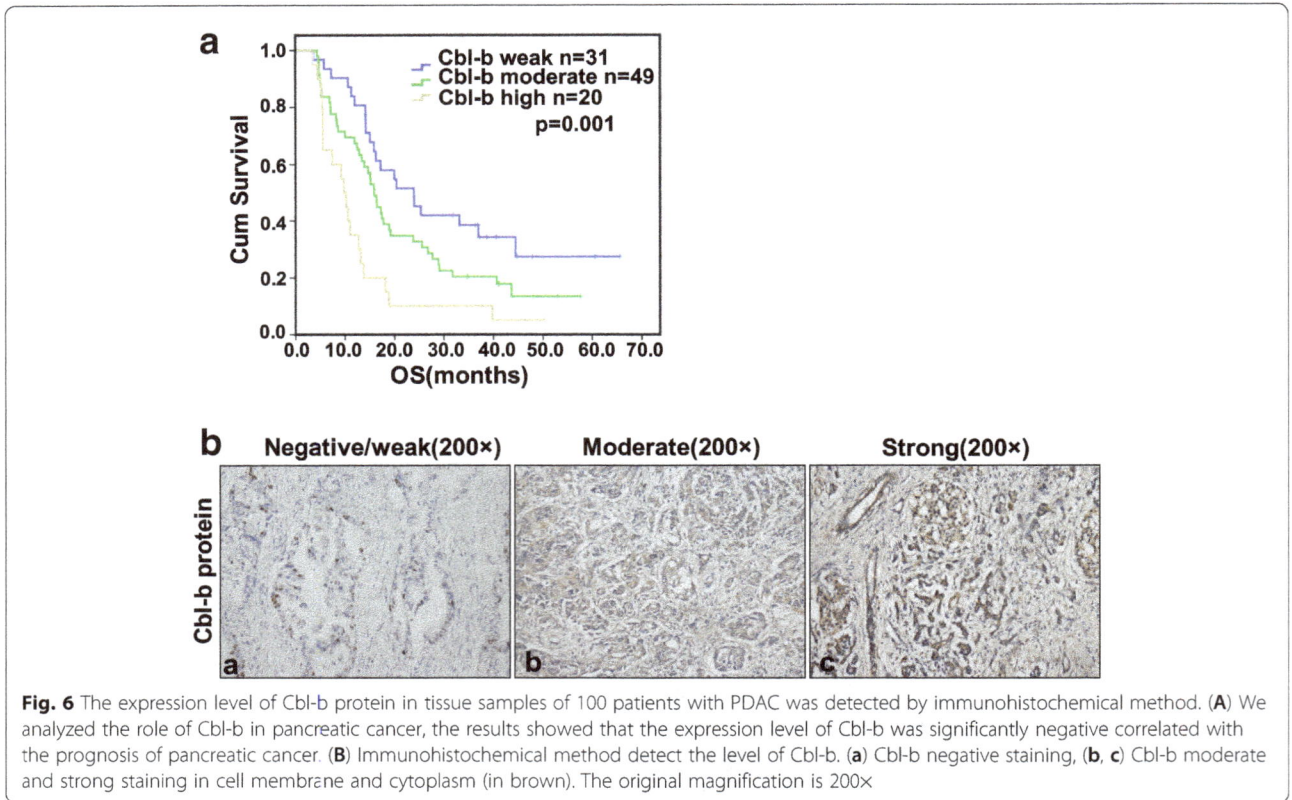

Fig. 6 The expression level of Cbl-b protein in tissue samples of 100 patients with PDAC was detected by immunohistochemical method. (**A**) We analyzed the role of Cbl-b in pancreatic cancer, the results showed that the expression level of Cbl-b was significantly negative correlated with the prognosis of pancreatic cancer. (**B**) Immunohistochemical method detect the level of Cbl-b. (**a**) Cbl-b negative staining, (**b**, **c**) Cbl-b moderate and strong staining in cell membrane and cytoplasm (in brown). The original magnification is 200×

MDM2 inhibits p53 activity in the cytoplasm, promotes p53 degradation and prevents p53 from entering the nucleus and exerts its function [45]. Moreover, previous studies reported that Cbl-b could target Siva 1 and upregulate p53 in lymphoma [46].

However, our results suggested that Cbl-b could bind p53, which in turn is degraded by ubiquitination. More interestingly, Cbl-b inhibition by miR-29b-2-5p resulted in overexpressed p53, which is translocated to the nucleus from the cytoplasm.

Conclusions

Therefore, the miR-29b-2-5p /Cbl-b/p53 signaling axis provides a basis for further understanding the occurrence and development of PDAC. In summary, miR-29b-2-5p

independently predicts better survival in PDAC, as an important tumor suppressor miRNA. Functionally, miR-29b-2-5p inhibits PDAC cell growth by negatively regulating the Cbl-b/p53 axis and reducing Cbl-b-mediated ubiquitination and degradation of p53. These findings provide important clues for understanding the development of PDAC, and suggest miR-29b-2-5p to be a potential biomarker for PDAC prognosis.

Additional files

Additional file 1: Figure S2. The identification of miRNAs. A. The flowchart of miRNA selection and schematic design. B. In the 18 candidate miRNAs, 2 miRNAs were opposite from the miRNA array, 16 were coherent with the miRNA array by Real-time PCR. Good prognosis group/poor prognosis. C. Among the candidate miRNAs, miR-891b and miR-490-5p could inhibit proliferation in cell lines.

Additional file 2: Table S1. Clinical characteristics of the PDAC patients.

Additional file 3: Figure S1. miRNA-29b-2-5p has a positive correlation with the prognosis of pancreatic cancer by Receiver operating characteristics (ROC) method. A. ROC curves for miR-29b-2-5p indicating the designated cut off points at 0.017. B. miRNA-29b-2-5p has a positive correlation with the prognosis as the cut off value is 0.017 in miRNA validation cohort with a median OS respectively time of 17.8 or 13.7 months. (log rank × 2 = 6.046, $p = 0.014$).

Additional file 4: Figure S3. Increased expression of miR-29b-2-5p upon infection in 2 PDAC cell lines was confirmed by qRT-PCR. (mean ± SD, results of three independent experiments, *$P < 0.05$).

Table 3 The expression level of miR-29b-2-5p was negatively correlated with the expression of Cbl-b protein in patients with SPSS

Cbl-b(n,%)	N(%)	miR-29b-2-5p(n,%)		R	P value
		Low	High		
Weak	31(31)	10(32)	21(68)	−0.33	0.001
Moderate	49(49)	26(53)	23(47)		
High	20(20)	16(80)	4(20)		
N(%)	100(100)	52(52)	48(48)		

Abbreviations
Cbl: Casitas B-lineage lymphoma; DAPI: 4',6-diamidino-2-phenylindole; IP: Immunoprecipitation; miR-29b-2-5p: microRNA-29b-2-5p; PDAC: Pancreatic ductal adenocarcinoma; pN: Pathologic N; pT: Pathologic T; pTNM: Pathologic TNM; TNM: Tumor node metastasis; UPS: Ubiquitin-proteasome system

Acknowledgements
The authors thank Yi Yang (Animal Center of China Medical University) for kindly providing technical support.

Funding
This work is supported by National Science and Technology Major Project of the Ministry of Science and Technology of China (No. 2017ZX09304025), and Science and Technology Plan Project of Liaoning Province (NO. 2014225013, 2014226033, 2016007010), The National Key Research and Development Program of China (NO.2017YFC1308900), and The general project of Liaoning province department of education (NO.LS201613), and Distinguished professor of Liaoning Province, and Project for clinical ability construction of Chinese medicine. The funding body had no role in the design of the study and collection, analysis, and interpretation of data and in writing the manuscript.

Authors' contributions
YL and XQ designed research; CL performed the data acquisition; QD and XC supervised the data and algorithms; YF, KH and ZL performed data analysis and interpretation; SW and TW carried out the statistical analysis; LX and JQ performed immunohistochemistry; XY and LX performed manuscript preparation; YL and XQ participated in manuscript editing and review. All authors read and approved the final manuscript.

Competing interests
The authors declare that they have no competing interests.

Author details
[1]Department of Medical Oncology, the First Hospital of China Medical University, NO.155, North Nanjing Street, Heping District, Shenyang City 110001, China. [2]Key Laboratory of Anticancer Drugs and Biotherapy of Liaoning Province, the First Hospital of China Medical University, Shenyang 110001, China. [3]Department of Oncology, Shengjing Hospital of China Medical University, Shenyang 110004, China. [4]Department of Pathology, Shengjing Hospital of China Medical University, Shenyang 110004, China.

References
1. Yonemori K, Kurahara H, Maemura K, Natsugoe S. MicroRNA in pancreatic cancer. J Hum Genet. 2017;62:33–40.
2. Siegel RL, Miller KD, Jemal A. Cancer statistics. CA Cancer J Clin. 2015;65:5–29.
3. Duffy JP, Eibl G, Reber HA, Hines OJ. Influence of hypoxia and neoangiogenesis on the growth of pancreatic cancer. Mol Cancer. 2003;2:12.
4. Niedergethmann M, Hildenbrand R, Wostbrock B, Hartel M, Sturm JW, Richter A, Post S. High expression of vascular endothelial growth factor predicts early recurrence and poor prognosis after curative resection for ductal adenocarcinoma of the pancreas. Pancreas. 2002;25:122–9.
5. Karayiannakis AJ, Bolanaki H, Syrigos KN, Asimakopoulos B, Polychronidis A, Anagnostoulis S, Simopoulos C. Serum vascular endothelial growth factor levels in pancreatic cancer patients correlate with advanced and metastatic disease and poor prognosis. Cancer Lett. 2003;194:119–24.
6. Hirakawa T, Yashiro M, Murata A, Hirata K, Kimura K, Amano R, Yamada N, Nakata B, Hirakawa K. IGF-1 receptor and IGF binding protein-3 might

7. predict prognosis of patients with resectable pancreatic cancer. BMC Cancer. 2013;13:392.
7. Dang C, Zhang Y, Ma Q, Shimahara Y. Expression of nerve growth factor receptors is correlated with progression and prognosis of human pancreatic cancer. J Gastroenterol Hepatol. 2006;21:850–8.
8. Javle M, Li Y, Tan D, Dong X, Chang P, Kar S, Li D. Biomarkers of TGF-β signaling pathway and prognosis of pancreatic cancer. PLoS One. 2014;9(1):e85942.
9. Habbe N, Koorstra JB, Mendell JT, Offerhaus GJ, Ryu JK, Feldmann G, Mullendore ME, Goggins MG, Hong SM, Maitra A. MicroRNA miR-155 is a biomarker of early pancreatic neoplasia. Cancer Biol Ther. 2009;8(4):340–6.
10. Caldas C, Hahn SA, da Costa LT, Redston MS, Schutte M, Seymour AB, Weinstein CL, Hruban RH, Yeo CJ, Kern SE. Frequent somatic mutations and homozygous deletions of the p16 (MTS1) gene in pancreatic adenocarcinoma. Nat Genet. 1994;8:27–32.
11. Tezel E, Hibi K, Nagasaka T, Nakao A. PGP9.5 as a prognostic factor in pancreatic cancer. Clin Cancer Res. 2000;6(12):4764–7.
12. Croce CM. Causes and consequences of microRNA dysregulation in cancer. Nat Rev Genet. 2009;10:704–14.
13. Bartel DP. MicroRNAs: genomics, biogenesis, mechanism, and function. Cell. 2004;116:281–97.
14. Li Y, Choi PS, Casey SC, Dill DL, Felsher DW. MYC through miR-17-92 suppresses specific target genes to maintain survival, autonomous proliferation, and a neoplastic state. Cancer Cell. 2014;26:262–72.
15. Valeri N, Braconi C, Gasparini P, Murgia C, Lampis A, Paulus-Hock V, Hart JR, Ueno L, Grivennikov SI, Lovat F, Paone A, Cascione L, Sumani KM, Veronese A, Fabbri M, Carasi S, Alder H, Lanza G, Gafa' R, Moyer MP, Ridgway RA, Cordero J, Nuovo GJ, Frankel WL, Rugge M, Fassan M, Groden J, Vogt PK, Karin M, Sansom OJ, Croce CM. MicroRNA-135b promotes cancer progression by acting as a downstream effector of oncogenic pathways in colon cancer. Cancer Cell. 2014;25:469–83.
16. Frampton AE, Castellano L, Colombo T, Giovannetti E, Krell J, Jacob J, Pellegrino L, Roca-Alonso L, Funel N, Gall TM, De Giorgio A, Pinho FG, Fulci V, Britton DJ, Ahmad R, Habib NA, Coombes RC, Harding V, Knösel T, Stebbing J, Jiao LR. MicroRNAs cooperatively inhibit a network of tumor suppressor genes to promote pancreatic tumor growth and progression. Gastroenterology. 2014;146:268–77.
17. Slattery ML, Herrick JS, Mullany LE, Wolff E, Hoffman MD, Pellatt DF, Stevens JR, Wolff RK. Colorectal tumor molecular phenotype and miRNA: expression profiles and prognosis. Mod Pathol. 2016;29:915–27.
18. Ueda T, Volinia S, Okumura H, Shimizu M, Taccioli C, Rossi S, Alder H, Liu CG, Oue N, Yasui W, Yoshida K, Sasaki H, Nomura S, Seto Y, Kaminishi M, Calin GA, Croce CM. Relation between microRNA expression and progression and prognosis of gastric cancer: a microRNA expression analysis. Lancet Oncol. 2010;11:136–46.
19. Zhang JX, Song W, Chen ZH, Wei JH, Liao YJ, Lei J, Hu M, Chen GZ, Liao B, Lu J, Zhao HW, Chen W, He YL, Wang HY, Xie D, Luo JH. Prognostic and predictive value of a microRNA signature in stage II colon cancer: a microRNA expression analysis. Lancet Oncol. 2013;14:1295–306.
20. Liu Q, Zhou H, Langdon WY, Zhang J. E3 ubiquitin ligase Cbl-b in innate and adaptive immunity. Cell Cycle. 2014;13(12):1875–84.
21. Liyasova MS, Ma K, Lipkowitz S. Molecular pathways: cbl proteins in tumorigenesis and antitumor immunity-opportunities for cancer treatment. Clin Cancer Res. 2015;21(8):1789–94.
22. Xu L, Zhang Y, Qu X, Che X, Guo T, Cai Y, Li A, Li D, Li C, Wen T, Fan Y, Hou K, Ma Y, Hu X, Liu Y. E3 ubiquitin ligase Cbl-b prevents tumor metastasis by maintaining the epithelial phenotype in multiple drug-resistant gastric and breast Cancer cells. Neoplasia. 2017;19(4):374–82.
23. Vennin C, Spruyt N, Dahmani F, Julien S, Bertucci F, Finetti P, Chassat T, Bourette RP, Le Bourhis X, Adriaenssens E. H19 non coding RNA-derived miR-675 enhances tumorigenesis and metastasis of breast cancer cells by downregulating c-Cbl and Cbl-b. Oncotarget. 2015;6(30):29209–23.
24. Li P, Wang X, Liu Z, Liu H, Xu T, Wang H, Gomez DR, Nguyen QN, Wang LE, Teng Y, Song Y, Komaki R, Welsh JW, Wei Q, Liao Z. Single nucleotide polymorphisms in CBLB, a regulator of T-cell response, predict radiation pneumonitis and outcomes after definitive radiotherapy for non-small-cell lung Cancer. Clin Lung Cancer. 2016;17(4):253–62.
25. Dong Q, Li C, Che X, Qu J, Fan Y, Li X, Li Y, Wang Q, Liu Y, Yang X, Qu X. MicroRNA-891b is an independent prognostic factor of pancreatic cancer by targeting Cbl-b to suppress the growth of pancreatic cancer cells. Oncotarget. 2016;7(50):82338–53.

26. Dong Q, Ma Y, Zhang Y, Qu X, Li Z, Qi Y, Liu Y, Li C, Li K, Yang X, Che X. Cbl-b predicts postoperative survival in patients with resectable pancreatic ductal adenocarcinoma. Oncotarget. 2017;8(34):57163–73.

27. Hansen TF, Sørensen FB, Lindebjerg J, Jakobsen A. The predictive value of microRNA-126 in relation to first line treatment with capecitabine and oxaliplatin in patients with metastatic colorectal cancer. BMC Cancer. 2012;12:83.

28. Wen F, Xu JZ, Wang XR. Increased expression of miR-15b is associated with clinicopathological features and poor prognosis in cervical carcinoma. Arch Gynecol Obstet. 2017;295(3):743–9.

29. Xu L, Zhang Y, Liu J, Qu J, Hu X, Zhang F, Zheng H, Qu X, Liu Y. TRAIL-activated EGFR by Cbl-b-regulated EGFR redistribution in lipid rafts antagonises TRAIL-induced apoptosis in gastric cancer cells. Eur J Cancer. 2012;48:3288–99.

30. Li H, Xu L, Li C, Zhao L, Ma Y, Zheng H, Li Z, Zhang Y, Wang R, Liu Y, Qu X. Ubiquitin ligase Cbl-b represses IGF-I-induced epithelial mesenchymal transition via ZEB2 and microRNA-200c regulation in gastric cancer cells. Mol Cancer. 2014;13:136.

31. Hajian-Tilaki K. Receiver operating characteristic (ROC) curve analysis for medical diagnostic test evaluation. Caspian J Intern Med. 2013;4(2):627–35.

32. Rupaimoole R, Slack FJ. MicroRNA therapeutics: towards a new era for the management of cancer and other diseases. Nat Rev Drug Discov. 2017;16:203–22.

33. Liu B, Ding JF, Luo J, Lu L, Yang F, Tan XD. Seven protective miRNA signatures for prognosis of cervical cancer. Oncotarget. 2016;7:56690–8.

34. Kong W, He L, Richards EJ, Challa S, Xu CX, Permuth-Wey J, Lancaster JM, Coppola D, Sellers TA, Djeu JY, Cheng JQ. Upregulation of miRNA-155 promotes tumour angiogenesis by targeting VHL and is associated with poor prognosis and triple-negative breast cancer. Oncogene. 2014;33:679–89.

35. Iqbal J, Shen Y, Liu Y, Fu K, Jaffe ES, Liu C, Liu Z, Lachel CM, Deffenbacher K, Greiner TC, Vose JM, Bhagavathi S, Staudt LM, Rimsza L, Rosenwald A, Ott G, Delabie J, Campo E, Braziel RM, Cook JR, Tubbs RR, Gascoyne RD, Armitage JO, Weisenburger DD, McKeithan TW, Chan WC. Genome-wide miRNA profiling of mantle cell lymphoma reveals a distinct subgroup with poor prognosis. Blood. 2012;119:4939–48.

36. Li L, Li Z, Kong X, Xie D, Jia Z, Jiang W, Cui J, Du Y, Wei D, Huang S, Xie K. Down-regulation of microRNA-494 via loss of SMAD4 increases FOXM1 and β-catenin signaling in pancreatic ductal adenocarcinoma cells. Gastroenterology. 2014;147:485–97.

37. Zheng J, Huang X, Tan W, Yu D, Du Z, Chang J, Wei L, Han Y, Wang C, Che X, Zhou Y, Miao X, Jiang G, Yu X, Yang X, Cao G, Zuo C, Li Z, Wang C, Cheung ST, Jia Y, Zheng X, Shen H, Wu C, Lin D. Pancreatic cancer risk variant in LINC00673 creates a miR-1231 binding site and interferes with PTPN11 degradation. Nat Genet. 2016;48:747–57.

38. Liston A, Papadopoulou AS, Danso-Abeam D, Dooley J. MicroRNA-29 in the adaptive immune system: setting the threshold. Cell Mol Life Sci. 2012;69:3533–41.

39. Chou J, Lin JH, Brenot A, Kim JW, Provot S, Werb Z. GATA3 suppresses metastasis and modulates the tumour microenvironment by regulating microRNA-29b expression. Nat Cell Biol. 2013;15:201–13.

40. Sunkavalli U, Aguilar C, Silva RJ, Sharan M, Cruz AR, Tawk C, Maudet C, Mano M, Eulalio A. Analysis of host microRNA function uncovers a role for miR-29b-2-5p in Shigella capture by filopodia. PLoS Pathog. 2017;13:e1006327.

41. Eulalio A, Huntzinger E, Izaurralde E. Getting to the root of miRNA-mediated gene silencing. Cell. 2008;132:9–14.

42. Feng D, Ma Y, Liu J, Xu L, Zhang Y, Qu J, Liu Y, Qu X. Cbl-b enhances sensitivity to 5-fluorouracil via EGFR- and mitochondria-mediated pathways in gastric cancer cells. Int J Mol Sci. 2013;14:24399–411.

43. Kang JM, Park S, Kim SJ, Hong HY, Jeong J, Kim HS, Kim SJ. CBL enhances breast tumor formation by inhibiting tumor suppressive activity of TGF-β signaling. Oncogene. 2012;31:5123–31.

44. Makohon-Moore A, Iacobuzio-Donahue CA. Pancreatic cancer biology and genetics from an evolutionary perspective. Nat Rev Cancer. 2016;16:553–65.

45. Wade M, Li YC, Wahl GM. MDM2, MDMX and p53 in oncogenesis and cancer therapy. Nat Rev Cancer. 2013;13:83–96.

46. Park IK, Blum W, Baker SD, Caligiuri MA. E3 ubiquitin ligase Cbl-b activates the p53 pathway by targeting Siva1, a negative regulator of ARF, in FLT3 inhibitor-resistant acute myeloid leukemia. Leukemia. 2017;31:502–5.

23

Impact of tumor size on survival of patients with resected pancreatic ductal adenocarcinoma

Debang Li[1†], Bin Hu[2†], Yanming Zhou[3*] ⓘ, Tao Wan[3] and Xiaoying Si[3]

Abstract

Background: The impact of tumor size on prognosis for surgically treated patients with pancreatic ductal adenocarcinoma (PDAC) remains controversial. A systematic review and meta-analysis was performed to evaluate this issue.

Methods: Relevant studies published from January 2000 to June 2017 were identified through EMBASE and PUBMED. Data were pooled for meta-analysis using Review Manager 5.3.

Results: Twenty eight observational studies involving a total of 23,945 patients were included. Tumors > 2 cm was associated with poor prognosis: the pooled hazard ratio (HR) estimate for overall survival was 1.52 (95% confidence interval [CI]: 1.41–1.64; $P < 0.0001$) by univariate analysis and 1.61 (95% CI: 1.35–1.91; $P < 0.0001$) by multivariate analysis; the pooled HR estimate for disease-free survival was 1.74 (95% CI: 1.46–2.07; $P < 0.0001$) by univariate analysis and 1.38 (95% CI: 1.12–1.68; $P = 0.002$) by multivariate analysis. When compared with patients with tumors ≤2 cm, those with the tumors > 2 cm had higher incidences of lymph node metastasis, poor tumor differentiation, lymph vessel invasion, vascular invasion, perineural invasion, and positive intraoperative peritoneal cytology.

Conclusion: These data demonstrate that PDAC size > 2 cm is an independent predictive factor for poor prognosis after surgical resection and associated with more aggressive tumor biology.

Keywords: Pancreatic ductal adenocarcinoma, Resection, Size, Prognosis

Background

Pancreatic ductal adenocarcinoma (PDAC) represents 90% of pancreatic cancers and is the fifth leading cause of cancer-related death in Western countries. Complete surgical resection is the only option that can offer hope of prolonged survival; however, the long-term survival remains unsatisfactory with a 5-year survival rate around 20% because of the high frequency of postoperative disease recurrence [1]. Therefore, it is necessary to identify prognostic factors to help stratify patients for appropriate management categories. Tumor specific factors, such as the margin status, histological differentiation, lymph node metastasis, and vascular invasion, have been shown to predict poor clinical outcomes [2, 3]. Tumor size is also a significant prognostic factor and is included in tumor node metastasis system (TNM) classification. According to the American Joint Committee on Cancer (AJCC) staging system for PDAC, the optimum tumor size cutoff value distinguishing T1 and T2 disease is 2 cm [4]. Despite the availability of many publications, the impact of PDAC size on prognosis remains controversial [5, 6]. A systematic review and meta-analysis of the literature was therefore undertaken to investigate this issue.

* Correspondence: zhouymsxy@sina.cn
†Debang Li and Bin Hu contributed equally to this work.
3Department of Hepatobiliary & Pancreatovascular Surgery, First affiliated Hospital of Xiamen University, Xiamen, China
Full list of author information is available at the end of the article

Methods

Study selection

The present study was performed by following the recommendations of the Preferred Reporting Items for Systematic Reviews and Meta-Analyses (PRISMA) Statement [7]. An electronic search of the PUBMED and EMBASE databases from January 2000 to June 2017 were performed to identify relevant citations. The following keywords were used: "pancreatic cancer", "pancreatic ductal adenocarcinoma", and "prognosis". The reference lists of all retrieved articles were manually reviewed in order to identify additional studies.

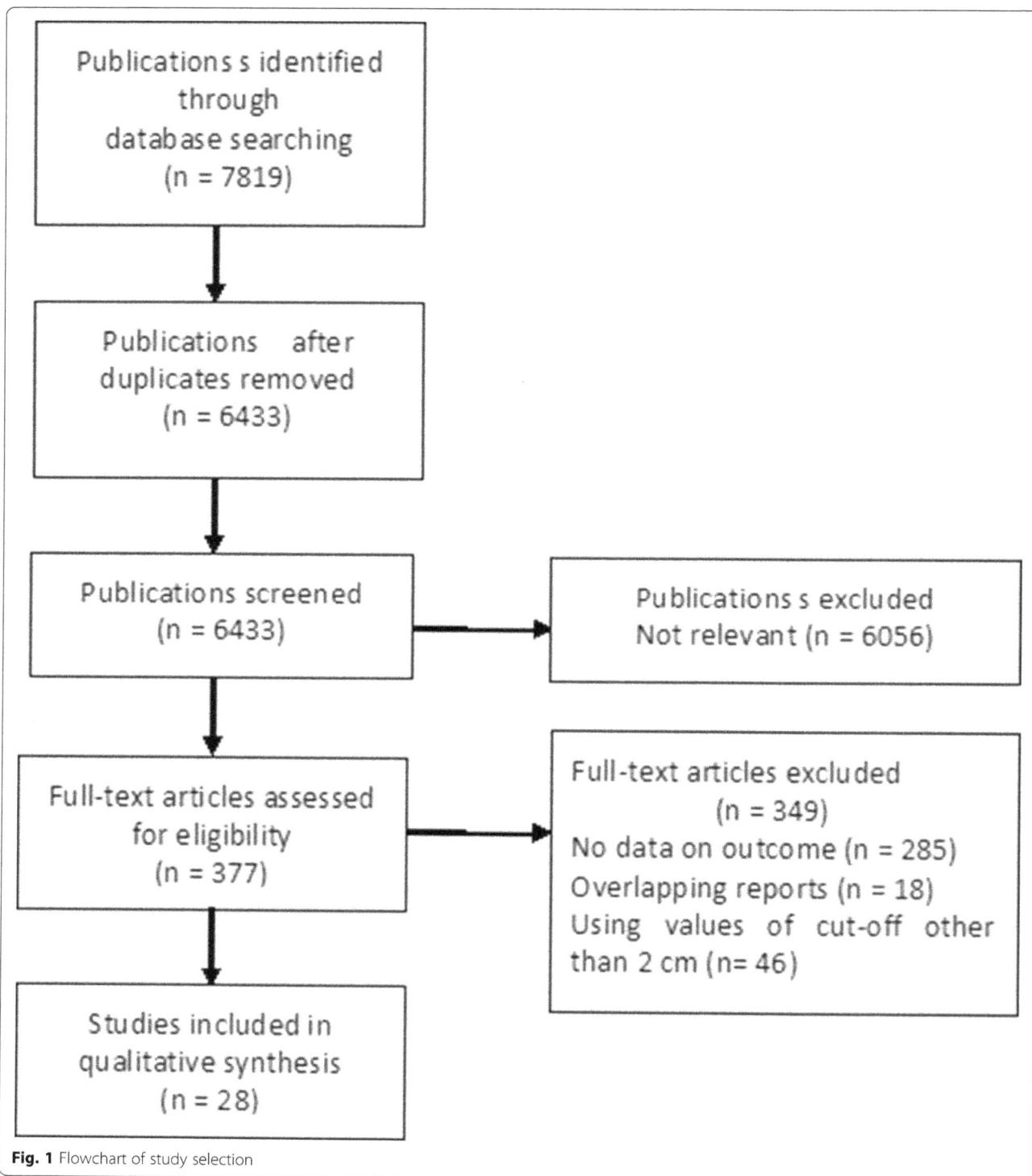

Fig. 1 Flowchart of study selection

Criteria for inclusion and exclusion

All original full-text articles reporting the impact of tumor size using a cut-off of 2 cm on overall survival (OS) or disease-free survival (DFS) in patients with PDAC after resection were considered eligible. Abstracts, letters, editorials and expert opinions, reviews without original data, case reports, non-human studies, non-English language studies, studies using values of cut-off other than 2 cm for tumor size, and studies that included other periampullary carcinomas (ampullary, duodenal, and biliary) in the same study cohort without separate assessments were excluded.

Data extraction and methodological assessment

All selected studies were evaluated independently by two investigators (ZY and SX) for data extraction and quality

assessment. Disagreement in the evaluation of studies was resolved by discussion and consensus. Parameters extracted included first author, study origin, year of publication, study design, type of resection, pathology, available long-term outcomes, and univariate and multivariate hazard ratios (HR) for OS and DFS.

The level of evidence of each study was categorized according to the Evidence-Based Medicine Levels of Evidence [8].

Statistical methods

Data for OS and DFS were analyzed using HR with 95% confidence intervals (CI), and a HR >1 represents a worse outcome. Between-study heterogeneity was assessed with I^2 statistics, and a value of > 50% was considered significant heterogeneity. A funnel plot based on the OS

Table 1 The main characteristics of included studies

Reference	Year	Country	N	TS > 2.0 cm, n (%)	TRPD/DP/TP	R0 R, n (%)	LNM, n (%)	PNI, n (%)	PTD, n (%)	MOS (Months)	5-yr OS (%)
Meyer [9]	2000	Germany	91	67/86 (77.9)	–/–/–	93 (100)	66 (72.5)	41 (45.1)	14 (16.3)	16.8	10.5
Ahmad [10]	2001	USA	116	70/94 (74.4)	–/–/–	88 (75.8)	73 (62.9)	–	61 (52.5)	16	19
Kim [11]	2006	USA	70	50 (71.4)	68/2/0	–	40 (57.1)	46 (65.7)	26 (37.1)	21	19
Smith [12]	2008	UK	109	81 (74.3)	109/0/0	80 (73.3)	88 (80.7)	–	36 (33.0)	13.9	–
Chiang [13]	2009	Taiwan,	159	123 (77.3)	–/–/–	114 (71.6)	95 (59.7)	–	32 (20.1)	–	12.5
Chang [14]	2009	Australia	365	281 (76.9)	295/70/0	233 (63.8)	217 (59.5)	256 (70.1)	98 (26.8)	16.8	11.4
Kato [15]	2009	Japan	176	148 (84.1)	176/0/0	115 (65.3)	123 (69.8)	145 (82.3)	11 (6.2)	9.9	12.3
Massucco [16]	2009	Italy	77	60 (77.9)	63/0/14	59 (76.6)	59 (76.6)	58 (75.3)	50 (64.9)	16.5	–
Bhatti [17]	2010	UK	84	78 (92.8)	84/0/0	49 (58.3)	56 (66.6)	–	24 (28.5)	22	13
de Jong [5]	2011	USA	1697	1279 (75.4)	1640/0/57	1213 (71.8)	1280 (75.4)	1126 (66.3)	649 (38.2)	18.3	21.2
Cannon [18]	2012	USA	245	213 (86.9)	220/20/0	184 (75.1)	–	–	72 (29.4)	18.3	–
Petermann [19]	2013	Switzerland	86	76 (88.3)	86/0/0	89 (68.6)	72 (83.7)	–	–	16.8	–
Yamada [20]	2013	Japan	390	312 (80.0)	288/71/31	–	277 (71.0)	–	–	–	–
Buc [21]	2014	France,	306	–	242/45/19	195 (72.5)	214 (71.3)	212 (83.8)	–	34	32
Elberm [22]	2015	UK	1070	–	1070/0/0	482 (45.9)	757 (70.7)	–	–	18.5	–
Iwagami [23]	2015	Japan	39	27 (69.2)	–/–/–	–	14 (35.9)	34 (87.2)	3 (7.6)	–	–
Liu [24]	2015	USA	411	242 (58.9)	411/0/0	379 (92.2)	223 (54.3%)	–	150 (36.5)	–	–
Okumura [25]	2015	Japan	230	–	155/66/9	190 (82.6)	135 (58.7).	–	33 (14.3)	–	–
Yamamoto [26]	2015	Japan	195	156 (80.0)	123/61/11	138 (70.7)	145 (74.3)	108 (55.3)	–	27.1	34.5
Lin [27]	2016	China	233	189 (81.1)	233/0/0	196 (84.1)	161 (69.1)	–	147 (63.1)	–	19.0
Abe [28]	2017	Japan	355	273 (76.9)	215/98/22	282 (79.4)	223 (62.8)	282 (79.4)	137 (38.5)	–	–
Ansari [29]	2017	USA	15,398	12,725 (82.6)	–/–/–	–	–	–	–	–	16.1
Chikamoto [30]	2017	Japan	138	66 (47.8)	138/0/0	–	46 (33.3)	–	10 (7.2)	–	–
Marchegiani [6]	2017	Italy, USA	1507	1183 (78.5)	1179/268/59	840 (55.7)	1149 (76.2)	1376 (91.3)	468 (31.1)	26.0	–
Kurata [31]	2017	Japan	90	41 (45.6)	–/–/–	–	31 (34.4)	–	–	–	–
Le [32]	2017	USA	93	70/86 (81.3)	93/0/0	–	78 (84.7)	–	50 (53.8)	40.6	–
Watanabe [33]	2017	Japan	122	98 (87.5)	73/47/2	122 (100)	62 (55.3)	–	6 (4.9)	21	27
Yu [34]	2017	China	93	32 (34.4)	–/–/–	89 (96.6)	49 (52.6)	52 (55.9)	36 (38.7)	–	–

UK United Kingdom, *PNI* peri-neural invasion, *TS* tumor size, *LNM* lymph node metastasis, *PTD* poor tumor differentiation, *MOS* median overall survival, *TR* type of resection, *PD* pancreaticoduodenectomy, *DP* distal pancreatectomy, *TP* total pancreatectomy, *R0 R* R0 resection

outcome was conducted to evaluate the presence of publication bias. The differences in clinicopathologic features were estimated as a pooled odds ratio (OR) with 95% CI. All analyses were performed using the Review Manager 5.3 (Cochrane Collaboration, Software Update, Oxford). A value of $P < 0.05$ was considered statistically significant.

Results

Selection of studies

A total of 28 studies comprising 23,945 individuals were identified for inclusion (Fig. 1). The summary characteristics of the included studies are shown in Table 1 [5, 6, 9–34]. There were no randomised controlled trials (RCT). All these studies were observational in nature and classified as level-4 evidence. There were 18 single-center [5, 9, 10, 12, 13, 15, 17, 19–21, 23–28, 32, 33] and 10 multicenter studies [6, 11, 14, 16, 18, 22, 29–31, 34].

Meta-analysis

The impact of PDAC size on OS was evaluated in 26 studies [5, 6, 9–13, 15–18, 20–34], among which univariate HR was reported in 14 [5, 6, 10, 11, 21–25, 28, 30, 31, 34] and multivariate HR was reported in 20 [5, 6, 12, 14–18, 20, 22, 23, 25–29, 31–33]. Both univariate and multivariate HR were reported in 8 studies [5, 6, 20, 22, 23, 25, 28, 31]. The pooled HR estimate for OS was 1.52 (95% CI: 1.41–1.64; $P < 0.0001$) by univariate analysis and 1.61 (95% CI: 1.35–1.91; $P < 0.0001$) by multivariate analysis (Figs. 2-3). In sensitivity analysis, exclusion of any single study from the analysis did not alter the results significantly (data not shown). Also, the results from three

subgroup analysis were in line with those from overall analyses (Table 2).

The impact of PDAC size on DFS was evaluated in 6 studies [18, 23–25, 28, 33], among which univariate HR was reported in 4 [23–25, 27] and multivariate HR was reported in 5 [18, 23, 25, 28, 33]. Both univariate and multivariate HR were reported in 3 studies [23, 25, 28]. The pooled HR estimate for DFS was 1.74 (95% CI: 1.46–2.07; $P < 0.0001$) by univariate analysis and 1.38 (95% CI: 1.12–1.68; $P = 0.002$) by multivariate analysis (Fig. 4a-b). Sensitivity and subgroup analyses were not performed due to the small number of studies.

Nine studies compared the clinicopathological factors between tumors > 2 cm and tumors ≤ 2 cm groups [5, 6, 9, 13, 15, 19, 20, 23, 28]. Pooled analysis showed that patients with tumor > 2 cm had higher incidences of lymph node metastasis (79.1% vs. 64.2%, OR 2.24, 95% CI: 1.43–3.51; $P < 0.001$), poor tumor differentiation (36.2% vs. 28.4%, OR 1.45, 95% CI: 1.22–1.73; $P < 0.001$), perineural invasion (80.8% vs. 67.1%, OR 1.89, 95% CI: 1.22–2.92; $P = 0.004$), vascular invasion (39.8% vs. 27.7%, OR 1.78, 95% CI: 1.41–2.24; $P < 0.001$), positive resection margins (36.9% vs. 27.2%, OR 1.56, 95% CI: 1.31–1.87; $P < 0.001$), and positive intraoperative peritoneal cytology (14.2% vs. 2.6%, OR 5.66, 95% CI: 2.15–14.93; $P < 0.001$), as compared with patients with tumors ≤ 2 cm.

Publication bias

No significant funnel plot asymmetry was observed in the meta-analysis of univariate and multivariate OS (Fig. 5a-b).

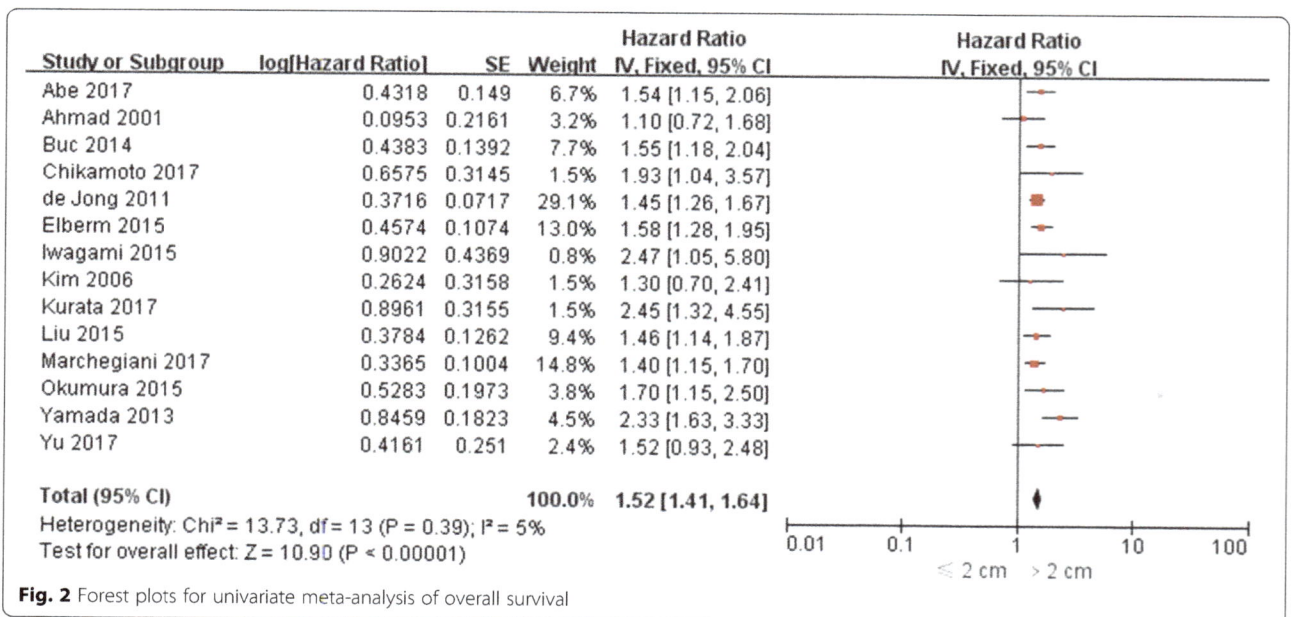

Study or Subgroup	log[Hazard Ratio]	SE	Weight	Hazard Ratio IV, Fixed, 95% CI
Abe 2017	0.4318	0.149	6.7%	1.54 [1.15, 2.06]
Ahmad 2001	0.0953	0.2161	3.2%	1.10 [0.72, 1.68]
Buc 2014	0.4383	0.1392	7.7%	1.55 [1.18, 2.04]
Chikamoto 2017	0.6575	0.3145	1.5%	1.93 [1.04, 3.57]
de Jong 2011	0.3716	0.0717	29.1%	1.45 [1.26, 1.67]
Elberm 2015	0.4574	0.1074	13.0%	1.58 [1.28, 1.95]
Iwagami 2015	0.9022	0.4369	0.8%	2.47 [1.05, 5.80]
Kim 2006	0.2624	0.3158	1.5%	1.30 [0.70, 2.41]
Kurata 2017	0.8961	0.3155	1.5%	2.45 [1.32, 4.55]
Liu 2015	0.3784	0.1262	9.4%	1.46 [1.14, 1.87]
Marchegiani 2017	0.3365	0.1004	14.8%	1.40 [1.15, 1.70]
Okumura 2015	0.5283	0.1973	3.8%	1.70 [1.15, 2.50]
Yamada 2013	0.8459	0.1823	4.5%	2.33 [1.63, 3.33]
Yu 2017	0.4161	0.251	2.4%	1.52 [0.93, 2.48]
Total (95% CI)			100.0%	1.52 [1.41, 1.64]

Heterogeneity: Chi² = 13.73, df = 13 (P = 0.39); I² = 5%
Test for overall effect: Z = 10.90 (P < 0.00001)

Fig. 2 Forest plots for univariate meta-analysis of overall survival

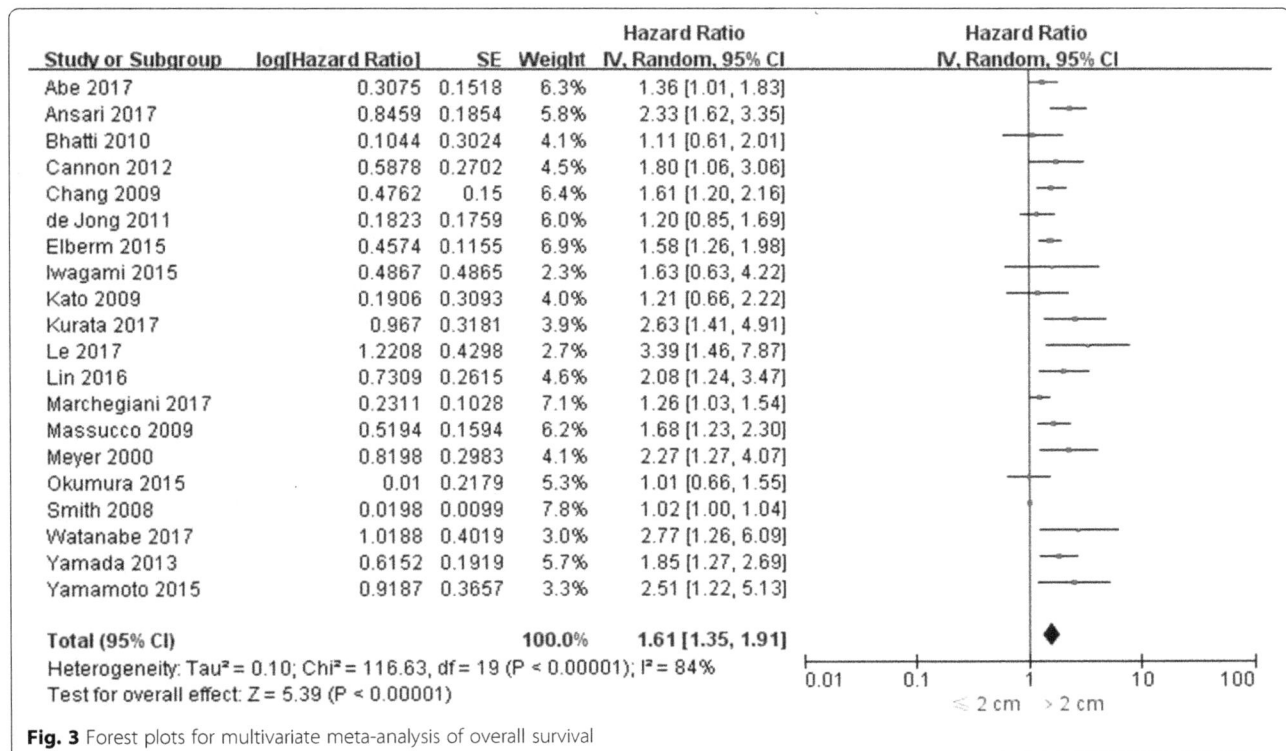

Study or Subgroup	log[Hazard Ratio]	SE	Weight	Hazard Ratio IV, Random, 95% CI	Hazard Ratio IV, Random, 95% CI
Abe 2017	0.3075	0.1518	6.3%	1.36 [1.01, 1.83]	
Ansari 2017	0.8459	0.1854	5.8%	2.33 [1.62, 3.35]	
Bhatti 2010	0.1044	0.3024	4.1%	1.11 [0.61, 2.01]	
Cannon 2012	0.5878	0.2702	4.5%	1.80 [1.06, 3.06]	
Chang 2009	0.4762	0.15	6.4%	1.61 [1.20, 2.16]	
de Jong 2011	0.1823	0.1759	6.0%	1.20 [0.85, 1.69]	
Elberm 2015	0.4574	0.1155	6.9%	1.58 [1.26, 1.98]	
Iwagami 2015	0.4867	0.4865	2.3%	1.63 [0.63, 4.22]	
Kato 2009	0.1906	0.3093	4.0%	1.21 [0.66, 2.22]	
Kurata 2017	0.967	0.3181	3.9%	2.63 [1.41, 4.91]	
Le 2017	1.2208	0.4298	2.7%	3.39 [1.46, 7.87]	
Lin 2016	0.7309	0.2615	4.6%	2.08 [1.24, 3.47]	
Marchegiani 2017	0.2311	0.1028	7.1%	1.26 [1.03, 1.54]	
Massucco 2009	0.5194	0.1594	6.2%	1.68 [1.23, 2.30]	
Meyer 2000	0.8198	0.2983	4.1%	2.27 [1.27, 4.07]	
Okumura 2015	0.01	0.2179	5.3%	1.01 [0.66, 1.55]	
Smith 2008	0.0198	0.0099	7.8%	1.02 [1.00, 1.04]	
Watanabe 2017	1.0188	0.4019	3.0%	2.77 [1.26, 6.09]	
Yamada 2013	0.6152	0.1919	5.7%	1.85 [1.27, 2.69]	
Yamamoto 2015	0.9187	0.3657	3.3%	2.51 [1.22, 5.13]	
Total (95% CI)			**100.0%**	**1.61 [1.35, 1.91]**	

Heterogeneity: Tau² = 0.10; Chi² = 116.63, df = 19 (P < 0.00001); I² = 84%
Test for overall effect: Z = 5.39 (P < 0.00001)

Fig. 3 Forest plots for multivariate meta-analysis of overall survival

Discussion

Assessment of tumor size for prognostication had better reproducibility for both clinical and pathologic staging [35]. Indeed, many studies investigating the prognostic factors in PDAC have shown that tumor size is one of the most important parameters in predicting the clinical outcome of cancer patients. The cut-off point for PDAC size in the published reports varies from 2, 2.5, 3, 4, and 5 cm [6]. Generally, tumors ≤2 cm in the greatest dimension are defined as small PDAC [36]. Some authors noted that tumors > 2 cm have prognostic implications after resection [6, 12, 14, 16], while others failed to confirm this finding [5, 10, 11]. Meta-analysis provides a way to increase statistical power and resolves inconsistencies. Our pooling data have shown that tumors > 2 cm have negative impact on the survival of patients with PDAC. These findings affirm the validity of the T-stage of the current AJCC classification, in which the cut-off value of 2 cm is proposed to be the sole factor determining whether a pancreatic tumor is staged as T1 or T2 disease [4]. When the clinicopathologic findings in the two groups were compared, patients with tumors > 2 cm showed higher incidences of lymph node metastasis, poor tumor differentiation, lymph vessel invasion, vascular invasion, perineural invasion, positive resection margin, and positive intraoperative peritoneal cytology, implying that tumors > 2 cm intrinsically have more aggressive tumor biology that contributes to worse prognosis. Marchegiani et al. speculated that tumor size could be considered a surrogate of neoplastic progression, knowing that it is an expression

Table 2 Subgroup analysis for the influence of tumor size on overall survival after pancreatic ductal adenocarcinoma resection

Subgroup	No. of studies	HR	95% CI	P-value	I² (%)
Single centre studies					
Univariate analysis	8	1.52	1.39, 1.67	< 0.001	29
Multivariate analysis	13	1.53	1.22, 1.91	< 0.001	76
Multicentre studies					
Univariate analysis	7	1.54	1.36, 1.74	< 0.001	0
Multivariate analysis	7	1.67	1.41, 1.99	< 0.001	51
Western studies					
Univariate analysis	8	1.46	1.34, 1.59	< 0.001	0
Multivariate analysis	11	1.55	1.25, 1.92	< 0.001	87
Eastern studies					
Univariate analysis	7	1.82	1.55, 2.15	< 0.001	0
Multivariate analysis	10	1.62	1.40, 1.87	< 0.001	35

CI confidence interval, HR hazard ratio

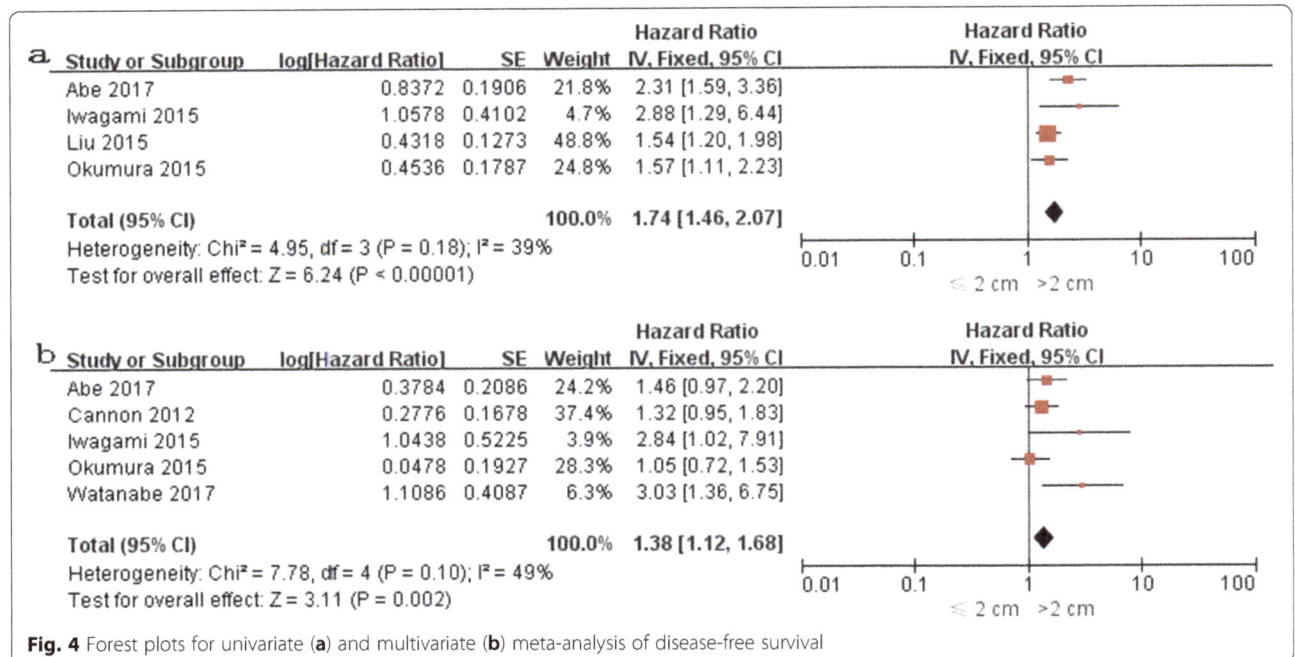

Fig. 4 Forest plots for univariate (**a**) and multivariate (**b**) meta-analysis of disease-free survival

of time passing from its original development. Therefore, a tumor with bigger dimensions often implies a relatively delayed diagnosis and therefore has a higher likelihood of being associated with other adverse pathologic factors [6].

The PDAC size also has impact on operative outcomes. Patients with tumors > 2 cm were found to be associated with more intra-operative blood loss and a greater need for packed red blood cell transfusion [5], knowing that the latter variable may lead to worse oncologic outcomes via transfusion-related immune modulation [37].

There is growing evidence that neoadjuvant therapy is associated with a statistically significant reduction in the

tumor positive margin status, tumor stage and grade, lymph node metastasis, and perineural invasion, thereby resulting in improved survival in patients with initially resectable PDAC [38]. However, identification of patients who will benefit from neoadjuvant therapy remains challenging. Unlike other malignant pathological features of PDAC, tumor size can be diagnosed by preoperative imaging and therefore may be able to guide clinical decision making. Our results show that tumors > 2 cm are characterized by the presence of other relevant poor prognostic factors and therefore can be considered as an indication for neoadjuvant therapy. The potential aim is to achieve dual purposes of attenuating malignant pathological features

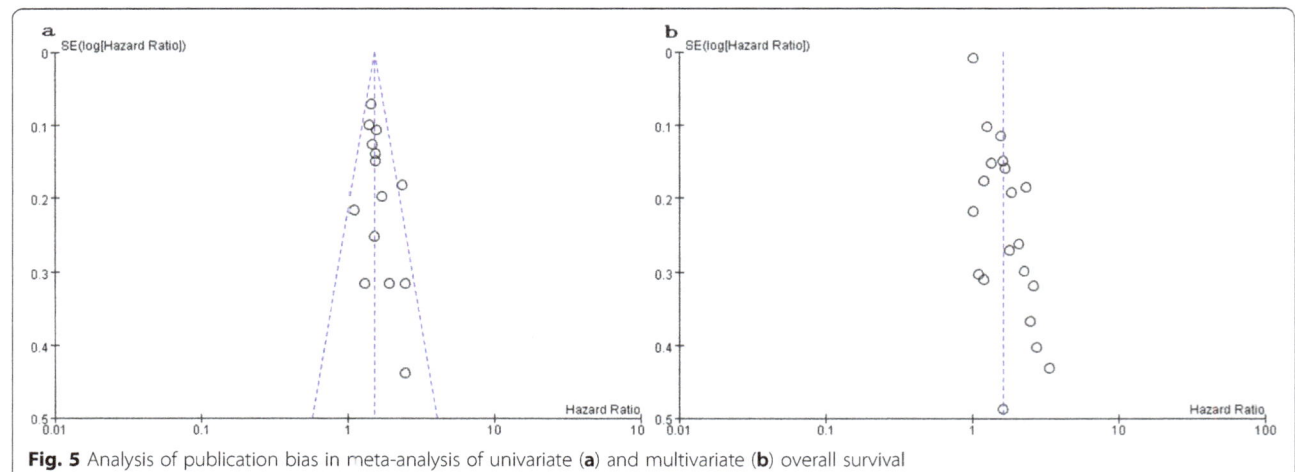

Fig. 5 Analysis of publication bias in meta-analysis of univariate (**a**) and multivariate (**b**) overall survival

on the one hand and improving the surgical outcome on the other. Randomized controlled trials are necessary to confirm this preliminary recommendation.

This review is limited by the low quality. All included studies were retrospective in nature and classified as level-4 evidence, which underlines the validity of the analyzed outcomes. Ansari et al. [29] found that the association between survival and PDAC size was linear in patients with localized tumors but stochastic in patients with regional and distant stages. Unfortunately, none of the included studies analysed the stage-dependent relationship between PDAC size and survival. Similarly, subgroup analysis based on anatomic location of the PDAC could not be performed due to insufficient data.

The strength of our findings is that it represents a variety of clinical settings, including Eastern and Western data rather than the sole experience of a single institution. In addition, these pooled results based on multivariate analysis do not differ essentially from those of analyses based on univariate analysis. These findings indicate that tumors > 2 cm, per se rather than a confounder, have a prognostic implication. Finally, there is no evidence of publication bias.

Conclusion

The current evidence demonstrates that PDAC size > 2 cm is an independent predictive factor for poor prognosis after surgical resection and associated with more aggressive tumor biology. Future trials are necessary to evaluate the survival benefit of neoadjuvant therapy in this subset of patients.

Abbreviations

95% CI: 95% confidence interval; DFS: Disease-free survival; DM: Diabetes mellitus; HR: Hazard ratio; OR: Odds ratio; OS: Overall survival; PDAC: Pancreatic ductal adenocarcinoma; PRISMA: Preferred reporting items for systematic reviews and meta-analyses; WMD: Weighted mean difference

Acknowledgements

We thank Doctor Yanfang Zhao (Department of Health Statistics, Second Military Medical University, Shanghai, China) for her critical revision of the meta-analysis section.

Funding

The project was supported by Natural Science Foundation of Fujian province (2015 J01561) and Major Diseases Joint Research Program of Xiamen City (3502Z20170943).

Authors' contributions

LD, HB and ZY participated in the design and coordination of the study, carried out the critical appraisal of studies and wrote the manuscript. HB, WT, and XS developed the literature search, carried out the extraction of data, assisted in the critical appraisal of included studies and assisted in writing up, WT and YZ carried out the statistical analysis of studies. All authors read and approved the final manuscript.

Competing interest

The authors declare that they have no competing interests.

Author details

Department III of General Surgery, First Hospital of Lanzhou University, Lanzhou, China. ²Department of Clinical Laboratory Medicine, First affiliated Hospital of Xiamen University, Xiamen, China. ³Department of Hepatobiliary & Pancreatovascular Surgery, First affiliated Hospital of Xiamen University, Xiamen, China.

References

1. Strobel O, Hinz U, Gluth A, Hank T, Hackert T, Bergmann F, et al. Pancreatic adenocarcinoma: number of positive nodes allows to distinguish several N categories. Ann Surg. 2015;261:961–9. https://doi.org/10.1097/SLA.0000000000000814.
2. Wagner M, Redaelli C, Lietz M, Seiler CA, Friess H, Büchler MW. Curative resection is the single most important factor determining outcome in patients with pancreatic adenocarcinoma. Br J Surg. 2004;91:586–94. https://doi.org/10.1002/bjs.4484.
3. Crippa S, Partelli S, Zamboni G, Barugola G, Capelli P, Inama M, et al. Poorly differentiated resectable pancreatic cancer: is upfront resection worthwhile? Surgery. 2012;152:S112–9. https://doi.org/10.1016/j.surg.2012.05.017.
4. Allen PJ, Kuk D, Castillo CF, Basturk O, Wolfgang CL, Cameron JL, et al. Multi-institutional validation study of the American joint commission on Cancer (8th edition) changes for T and N staging in patients with pancreatic adenocarcinoma. Ann Surg. 2017;265:185–91. https://doi.org/10.1097/SLA.0000000000001763.
5. de Jong MC, Li F, Cameron JL, Wolfgang CL, Edil BH, Herman JM, et al. Re-evaluating the impact of tumor size on survival following pancreaticoduodenectomy for pancreatic adenocarcinoma. J Surg Oncol. 2011;103:656–62. https://doi.org/10.1002/jso.21883.
6. Marchegiani G, Andrianello S, Malleo G, De Gregorio L, Scarpa A, Mino-Kenudson M, et al. Does size matter in pancreatic Cancer?: reappraisal of tumour dimension as a predictor of outcome beyond the TNM. Ann Surg. 2017;266:142–8. https://doi.org/10.1097/SLA.0000000000001837.
7. Moher D, Liberati A, Tetzlaff J, Altman DG. PRISMA group: preferred reporting items for systematic reviews and meta-analyses: the PRISMA statement. BMJ. 2009;339:b2535.
8. Zhu JC, Yan TD, Morris DL. A systematic review of radiofrequency ablation for lung tumors. Ann Surg Oncol. 2008;15:1765–74. https://doi.org/10.1245/s10434-008-9848-7.
9. Meyer W, Jurowich C, Reichel M, Steinhäuser B, Wünsch PH, Gebhardt C. Pathomorphological and histological prognostic factors in curatively resected ductal adenocarcinoma of the pancreas. Surg Today. 2000;30:582–7. https://doi.org/10.1007/s005950070096.
10. Ahmad NA, Lewis JD, Ginsberg GG, Haller DG, Morris JB, Williams NN, et al. Long term survival after pancreatic resection for pancreatic adenocarcinoma. Am J Gastroenterol. 2001;96:2609–15. https://doi.org/10.1111/j.1572-0241.2001.04123.x.
11. Kim J, Reber HA, Dry SM, Elashoff D, Chen SL, Umetani N, et al. Unfavourable prognosis associated with K-ras gene mutation in pancreatic cancer surgical margins. Gut. 2006;55:1598–605. https://doi.org/10.1136/gut.2006.098814.
12. Smith RA, Bosonnet L, Ghaneh P, Raraty M, Sutton R, Campbell F, et al. Preoperative CA19-9 levels and lymph node ratio are independent predictors of survival in patients with resected pancreatic ductal adenocarcinoma. Dig Surg. 2008;25:226–32. https://doi.org/10.1159/000140961.
13. Chang DK, Johns AL, Merrett ND, Gill AJ, Colvin EK, Scarlett CJ, et al. Margin clearance and outcome in resected pancreatic cancer. J Clin Oncol. 2009;27:2855–62. https://doi.org/10.1200/JCO.2008.20.5104.
14. Chiang KC, Yeh CN, Lee WC, Jan YY, Hwang TL. Prognostic analysis of patients with pancreatic head adenocarcinoma less than 2 cm undergoing resection. World J Gastroenterol. 2009;15:4305–10. https://doi.org/10.3748/wjg.15.4305.
15. Kato K, Yamada S, Sugimoto H, Kanazumi N, Nomoto S, Takeda S, et al. Prognostic factors for survival after extended pancreatectomy for pancreatic head cancer: influence of resection margin status on survival. Pancreas. 2009;38:605–12. https://doi.org/10.1097/MPA.0b013e3181a4891d.

16. Massucco P, Ribero D, Sgotto E, Mellano A, Muratore A, Capussotti L. Prognostic significance of lymph node metastases in pancreatic head cancer treated with extended lymphadenectomy: not just a matter of numbers. Ann Surg Oncol. 2009;16:3323–32. https://doi.org/10.1245/s10434-009-0672-5.

17. Bhatti I, Peacock O, Awan AK, Semeraro D, Larvin M, Hall RI. Lymph node ratio versus number of affected lymph nodes as predictors of survival for resected pancreatic adenocarcinoma. World J Surg. 2010;34:768–75. https://doi.org/10.1007/s00268-009-0336-4.

18. Cannon RM, LeGrand R, Chagpar RB, Ahmad SA, McClaine R, Kim HJ, et al. Multi-institutional analysis of pancreatic adenocarcinoma demonstrating the effect of diabetes status on survival after resection. HPB (Oxford). 2012;14: 228–35. https://doi.org/10.1111/j.1477-2574.2011.00432.x.

19. Petermann D, Demartines N, Schäfer M. Is tumour size an underestimated feature in the current TNM system for malignancies of the pancreatic head? HPB (Oxford). 2013;15:872–81. https://doi.org/10.1111/hpb.12052.

20. Yamada S, Fujii T, Kanda M, Sugimoto H, Nomoto S, Takeda S, et al. Value of peritoneal cytology in potentially resectable pancreatic cancer. Br J Surg. 2013;100:1791–6. https://doi.org/10.1002/bjs.9307.

21. Buc E, Couvelard A, Kwiatkowski F, Dokmak S, Ruszniewski P, Hammel P, et al. Adenocarcinoma of the pancreas: does prognosis depend on mode of lymph node invasion? Eur J Surg Oncol. 2014;40:1578–85. https://doi.org/10.1016/j.ejso.2014.04.012.

22. Elberm H, Ravikumar R, Sabin C, Abu Hilal M, Al-Hilli A, Aroori S, et al. Outcome after pancreaticoduodenectomy for T3 adenocarcinoma: a multivariable analysis from the UK vascular resection for pancreatic Cancer study group. Eur J Surg Oncol. 2015;41:1500–7. https://doi.org/10.1016/j.ejso.2015.08.158.

23. Iwagami Y, Eguchi H, Wada H, Tomimaru Y, Hama N, Kawamoto K, et al. Implications of peritoneal lavage cytology in resectable left-sided pancreatic cancer. Surg Today. 2015;45:444–50. https://doi.org/10.1007/s00595-014-0964-7.

24. Liu L, Katz MH, Lee SM, Fischer LK, Prakash L, Parker N, et al. Superior mesenteric artery margin of Posttherapy Pancreaticoduodenectomy and prognosis in patients with pancreatic ductal adenocarcinoma. Am J Surg Pathol. 2015;39:1395–403. https://doi.org/10.1097/PAS.0000000000000491.

25. Okumura S, Kaido T, Hamaguchi Y, Fujimoto Y, Masui T, Mizumoto M, et al. Impact of preoperative quality as well as quantity of skeletal muscle on survival after resection of pancreatic cancer. Surgery. 2015;157:1088–98. https://doi.org/10.1016/j.surg.2015.02.002.

26. Yamamoto T, Yagi S, Kinoshita H, Sakamoto Y, Okada K, Uryuhara K, et al. Long-term survival after resection of pancreatic cancer: a single-center retrospective analysis. World J Gastroenterol. 2015;21:262–8. https://doi.org/10.3748/wjg.v21.i1.262.

27. Lin JY, Zhang XM, Kou JT, Fa H, Zhang XX, Dai Y, He Q. Analysis of prognostic factors for pancreatic head cancer according to Para-aortic lymph node. Cancer Med. 2016;5:2701–7. https://doi.org/10.1002/cam4.853.

28. Abe T, Ohuchida K, Endo S, Ookubo F, Mori Y, Nakata K, et al. Clinical importance of intraoperative peritoneal cytology in patients with pancreatic cancer. Surgery. 2017;161:951–8. https://doi.org/10.1016/j.surg.2016.10.035.

29. Ansari D, Bauden M, Bergström S, Rylance R, Marko-Varga G, Andersson R. Relationship between tumour size and outcome in pancreatic ductal adenocarcinoma. Br J Surg. 2017;104:600–7. https://doi.org/10.1002/bjs.10471.

30. Chikamoto A, Inoue R, Komohara Y, Sakamaki K, Hashimoto D, Shiraishi S, et al. Preoperative high maximum standardized uptake value in association with glucose transporter 1 predicts poor prognosis in pancreatic Cancer. Ann Surg Oncol. 2017;24:2040–6. https://doi.org/10.1245/s10434-017-5799-1.

31. Kurata M, Honda G, Murakami Y, Uemura K, Satoi S, Motoi F, et al. Multicenter study Group of Pancreatobiliary Surgery (MSG-PBS): retrospective study of the correlation between pathological tumor size and survival after curative resection of T3 pancreatic adenocarcinoma: proposal for reclassification of the tumor extending beyond the pancreas based on tumor size. World J Surg. 2017 Jun 15. https://doi.org/10.1007/s00268-017-4077-5.

32. Le AT, Huang B, Hnoosh D, Saeed H, Dineen SP, Hosein PJ, Durbin EB, et al. Effect of complications on oncologic outcomes after pancreaticoduodenectomy for pancreatic cancer. J Surg Res. 2017;214:1–8. https://doi.org/10.1016/j.jss.2017.02.036.

33. Watanabe Y, Nishihara K, Matsumoto S, Okayama T, Abe Y, Nakano T. Effect of postoperative major complications on prognosis after pancreatectomy for pancreatic cancer: a retrospective review. Surg Today. 2017;47:555–67. https://doi.org/10.1007/s00595-016-1426-1.

34. Yu R, Li C, Lin X, Chen Q, Li J, Song L, et al. Clinicopathologic features and prognostic implications of MYBL2 protein expression in pancreatic ductal adenocarcinoma. Pathol Res Pract. 2017;213:964–8. https://doi.org/10.1016/j.prp.2017.04.024.

35. Morganti AG, Brizi MG, Macchia G, Sallustio G, Costamagna G, Alfieri S, et al. The prognostic effect of clinical staging in pancreatic adenocarcinoma. Ann Surg Oncol. 2005;12:145–51. https://doi.org/10.1245/ASO.2005.02.021.

36. Agarwal B, Correa AM, Ho L. Survival in pancreatic carcinoma based on tumor size. Pancreas. 2008;36:e15–20. https://doi.org/10.1097/mpa.0b013e31814de421.

37. Dusch N, Weiss C, Ströbel P, Kienle P, Post S, Niedergethmann M. Factors predicting long-term survival following pancreatic resection for ductal adenocarcinoma of the pancreas: 40 years of experience. J Gastrointest Surg. 2014;18:674–81. https://doi.org/10.1007/s11605-013-2408-x.

38. Schorn S, Demir IE, Reyes CM, Saricaoglu C, Samm N, Schirren R, et al. The impact of neoadjuvant therapy on the histopathological features of pancreatic ductal adenocarcinoma - a systematic review and meta-analysis. Cancer Treat Rev. 2017;55:96–106. https://doi.org/10.1016/j.ctrv.2017.03.003.

Permissions

The contributors of this book come from diverse backgrounds, making this book a truly international effort. This book will bring forth new frontiers with its revolutionizing research information and detailed analysis of the nascent developments around the world.

We would like to thank all the contributing authors for lending their expertise to make the book truly unique. They have played a crucial role in the development of this book. Without their invaluable contributions this book wouldn't have been possible. They have made vital efforts to compile up to date information on the varied aspects of this subject to make this book a valuable addition to the collection of many professionals and students.

This book was conceptualized with the vision of imparting up-to-date information and advanced data in this field. To ensure the same, a matchless editorial board was set up. Every individual on the board went through rigorous rounds of assessment to prove their worth. After which they invested a large part of their time researching and compiling the most relevant data for our readers.

The editorial board has been involved in producing this book since its inception. They have spent rigorous hours researching and exploring the diverse topics which have resulted in the successful publishing of this book. They have passed on their knowledge of decades through this book. To expedite this challenging task, the publisher supported the team at every step. A small team of assistant editors was also appointed to further simplify the editing procedure and attain best results for the readers.

Apart from the editorial board, the designing team has also invested a significant amount of their time in understanding the subject and creating the most relevant covers. They scrutinized every image to scout for the most suitable representation of the subject and create an appropriate cover for the book.

The publishing team has been an ardent support to the editorial, designing and production team. Their endless efforts to recruit the best for this project, has resulted in the accomplishment of this book. They are a veteran in the field of academics and their pool of knowledge is as vast as their experience in printing. Their expertise and guidance has proved useful at every step. Their uncompromising quality standards have made this book an exceptional effort. Their encouragement from time to time has been an inspiration for everyone.

The publisher and the editorial board hope that this book will prove to be a valuable piece of knowledge for researchers, students, practitioners and scholars across the globe.

List of Contributors

Dannel Yeo, Hong He, Oneel Patel, Graham S. Baldwin and Mehrdad Nikfarjam
Department of Surgery, Austin Health, University of Melbourne, Heidelberg, VIC, Australia

Andrew M. Lowy
Department of Surgery, Division of Surgical Oncology, University of California at San Diego, Moores Cancer, La Jolla, CA, USA

Haiyan Song and Yuxiang Zhang
Department of Biochemistry and Molecular Biology, Cancer Institute, Beijing Key Laboratory for Cancer Invasion and Metastasis Research, Capital Medical University, No. 10 Xitoutiao, You An Men, Fengtai District, Beijing 100069, People's Republic of China

M. Buchholz, B. Majchrzak-Stiller, W. Uhl, C. Braumann and A. M. Chromik
Division of Molecular and Clinical Research, St. Josef-Hospital, Ruhr-University Bochum, Bochum, Germany

S. Hahn
Department of Molecular Gastrointestinal Oncology, Ruhr-University Bochum, Bochum, Germany

R. W. Pfirrmann
Geistlich Pharma AG, Wolhusen, Switzerland

D. Vangala
Department of Molecular Gastrointestinal Oncology, Ruhr-University Bochum, Bochum, Germany
Department of Internal Medicine, Knappschaftskrankenhaus, Ruhr-University Bochum, Bochum, Germany

Hui Wang
Department of Nuclear Medicine, Xinhua Hospital Affiliated to Shanghai Jiaotong University School of Medicine, Shanghai 200092, China

Guorong Jia and Changjing Zuo
Department of Nuclear Medicine, Changhai Hospital, Second Military Medical University, Shanghai 200433, China

Jian Zhang
Department of Nuclear Medicine, Xinhua Hospital Affiliated to Shanghai Jiaotong University School of Medicine, Shanghai 200092, China
Department of Nuclear Medicine, Changhai Hospital, Second Military Medical University, Shanghai 200433, China

Ningyang Jia
Department of Radiology, Eastern Hepatobiliary Surgery Hospital, Second Military Medical University, Shanghai 200433, China

Monika Bauden, Bodil Andersson, Roland Andersson and Daniel Ansari
Department of Surgery, Clinical Sciences Lund, Lund University, Skåne University Hospital, SE-221 85 Lund, Sweden

Theresa Kristl and György Marko-Varga
Clinical Protein Science and Imaging, Department of Biomedical Engineering, Lund University, Biomedical Center, Lund, Sweden

Agata Sasor
Department of Pathology, Skåne University Hospital, Lund, Sweden

Andrew J. Scott, Amanda S. Wilkinson and John C. Wilkinson
Department of Chemistry and Biochemistry, North Dakota State University, Dept. 2710, Fargo, ND 58108-6050, USA

Toshinori Ozaki
Laboratory of DNA Damage Signaling, Chiba Cancer Center Research Institute, Chiba 260-8717, Japan

Meng Yu
Department of Laboratory Animal of China Medical University, Shenyang 110001, People's Republic of China

Danjing Yin and Meixiang Sang
Research Center, Fourth Hospital of Hebei Medical University, Shijiazhuang, Hebei 050017, People's Republic of China

Dan Sun and Yuyan Zhu
Department of Urology, First Hospital of China Medical University, Shenyang 110001, People's Republic of China

Youquan Bu
Department of Biochemistry and Molecular Biology, Chongqing Medical University, Chongqing 400016, People's Republic of China

Shi Wen, Weize Hu, Xianchao Lin, Jianxi Bai and Heguang Huang
Department of General Surgery, Fujian Medical University Union Hospital, Fuzhou 350001, China

Bohan Zhan and Jianghua Feng
Department of Electronic Science, Fujian Provincial Key Laboratory of Plasma and Magnetic Resonance, Xiamen University, Xiamen 361005, China

Chaobin He, Yize Mao, Jun Wang, Fangting Duan, Xiaojun Lin and Shengping Li
Department of Hepatobiliary and Pancreatic Surgery, State Key Laboratory of Oncology in South China, Collaborative Innovation Center for Cancer Medicine, Sun Yat-sen University Cancer Center, Guangzhou, Guangdong 510060, People's Republic of China

Sibylle Baechmann and Steffen Ormanns
Institute of Pathology, Ludwig-Maximilians University of Munich, Munich, Germany

Michael Haas, Stephan Kruger, Dominik Paul Modest and Stefan Boeck
Department of Internal Medicine III and Comprehensive Cancer Center, Klinikum Grosshadern, Ludwig-Maximilians University of Munich, Marchioninistr. 15, 81377 Munich, Germany

Anna Remold
Institute of Pathology, Ludwig-Maximilians University of Munich, Munich, Germany
Department of Internal Medicine III and Comprehensive Cancer Center, Klinikum Grosshadern, Ludwig-Maximilians University of Munich, Marchioninistr. 15, 81377 Munich, Germany

Jens Werner
Department of General, Visceral, Vascular and Transplantation Surgery, Klinikum Grosshadern, Ludwig-Maximilians-University of Munich, Munich, Germany

Thomas Kirchner and Andreas Jung
Institute of Pathology, Ludwig-Maximilians University of Munich, Munich, Germany
DKTK, German Cancer Consortium, German Cancer Research Center (DKFZ), Heidelberg, Germany

Volker Heinemann
Department of Internal Medicine III and Comprehensive Cancer Center, Klinikum Grosshadern, Ludwig-Maximilians University of Munich, Marchioninistr. 15, 81377 Munich, Germany
DKTK, German Cancer Consortium, German Cancer Research Center (DKFZ), Heidelberg, Germany

Ye-Tao Wang, Ya-Wen Gou, Wen-Wen Jin, Mei Xiao and Hua-Ying Fang
Department of gastroenterology, Anhui provincial hospital, NO.17, Lujiang Road, Hefei City, Anhui Province 230001, China

Lucia Moletta, Nicola Passuello, Michele Valmasoni and Cosimo Sperti
Department of Surgery, Oncology and Gastroenterology, 3rd Surgical Clinic, University of Padua, Padua, Italy

Sergio Bissoli
Department of Nuclear Medicine, Castelfranco Veneto General Hospital, Castelfranco Veneto, Treviso, Italy

Alberto Fantin
Gastroenterology Unit, University of Padua, Padua, Italy

Morten Lapin
Department of Haematology and Oncology, Stavanger University Hospital, N–4068 Stavanger, Norway
Laboratory for Molecular Biology, Stavanger University Hospital, N–4068 Stavanger, Norway
Department of Mathematics and Natural Sciences, University of Stavanger, N–4036 Stavanger, Norway

Kjersti Tjensvoll, Satu Oltedal, Rune Smaaland, Bjørnar Gilje and Oddmund Nordgård
Department of Haematology and Oncology, Stavanger University Hospital, N–4068 Stavanger, Norway
Laboratory for Molecular Biology, Stavanger University Hospital, N–4068 Stavanger, Norway

Milind Javle
Department of Gastrointestinal (GI) Medical Oncology, Division of Cancer Medicine, MD Anderson Cancer Center, The University of Texas, Houston, TX, USA

Thalia M. Rebelo, Carryn J. Chetty, Eloise Ferreira and Stefan F. T. Weiss
School of Molecular and Cell Biology, University of the Witwatersrand, Johannesburg, Republic of South Africa (RSA)

Ruihua Xu
Sun Yat-sen University Cancer Center, 651 Dongfeng East Road, Guangzhou 510060, China

Xianjun Yu
Fudan University Shanghai Cancer Center, No 270, Dongan Road, Shanghai 200032, China

Jihui Hao
Tianjin Cancer Hospital, Huan-Hu-Xi Road, Tianjin 300060, China

Liwei Wang
Renji Hospital, Shanghai Jiaotong University, 160 Pujian Lu, Shanghai 200127, China

Hongming Pan
Sir Run Run Shaw Hospital, Zhejiang University, 3 East Qingchun Road, Hangzhou City 310016, China

Guohong Han
Xijing Hospital, W Rd, Xi'an, Changle 127, China

Jianming Xu
307 Hospital of the People's Liberation Army, Beijing 100021, China

Yanqiao Zhang
Harbin Medical University Cancer Hospital, Haping Road No.150, Harbin, China

Shujun Yang
Henan Cancer Hospital, Zhengzhou 450003, China

Jia Chen
Jiangsu Provincial Tumor Hospital, 300 Guangzhou Road, Nanjing 210029, China

Jieer Ying
Zhejiang Cancer Hospital, 38 Guangji Road, Banshan Bridge, Hangzhou City 310022, China

Guanghai Dai
Chinese People's Liberation Army General Hospital No.28, Fuxing Road, Beijing, China

Mingyu Li, Damir Begic and Brian Lu
Celgene Corporation, Summit, NJ, USA

Lin Shen
Peking University Cancer Hospital and Institute, No. 52 Fucheng Road, Haidian District, Beijing 100142, China
Department of Gastrointestinal Oncology, Peking University Cancer Hospital and Institute, No. 52 Fucheng Road, Haidian District, Beijing 100142, China

Yuanyuan Xiao
Department of Biostatistics, School of Public Health, Fudan University, 130 Dong'an Road, Shanghai, China
School of Public Health, Kunming Medical University, Kunming, Yunnan, China

Wen Chen, Zhihui Xie, Zhenyi Shao and Hua Xie
Information Center, Shanghai Municipal Commission of Health and Family Planning, Shanghai, China

Guoyou Qin and Naiqing Zhao
Department of Biostatistics, School of Public Health, Fudan University, 130 Dong'an Road, Shanghai, China
Key Lab of Health Technology Assessment, Ministry of Health (Fudan University), Shanghai, China

Daniel Seoane-Mato
Research Unit, Spanish Society of Rheumatology, Madrid, Spain

Olivier Nuñez, Nerea Fernández-de-Larrea, Beatriz Pérez-Gómez, Marina Pollán, Gonzalo López-Abente and Nuria Aragonés
Cancer and Environmental Epidemiology Unit, National Center for Epidemiology, Carlos III Institute of Health, Madrid, Spain
Consortium for Biomedical Research in Epidemiology and Public Health (CIBER Epidemiología y Salud Pública, CIBERESP), Madrid, Spain

Mu Xu, Xiaoman Jung, Aune Moro, Caroline Ei Ne Chou, Jonathan King and O. Joe Hines
Departments of Surgery, David Geffen School of Medicine, University of California, Los Angeles, 10833 Le Conte Ave, CHS 72-236, Los Angeles, CA 90095, USA

Hui-Hua Chang and Guido Eibl
Departments of Surgery, David Geffen School of Medicine, University of California, Los Angeles, 10833 Le Conte Ave, CHS 72-236, Los Angeles, CA 90095, USA
Digestive Diseases Research Center, University of California at Los Angeles, Los Angeles, USA

James Sinnett-Smith and Enrique Rozengurt
Departments of Medicine, David Geffen School of Medicine, University of California, Los Angeles, Los Angeles, CA, USA
CURE: Digestive Diseases Research Center, University of California at Los Angeles, Los Angeles, USA

Erin L. Young and Russell Bell
Department of Oncological Sciences, University of Utah School of Medicine, Salt Lake City, United States

Amanda Gammon, Cathryn Koptiuch and Wendy K. Kohlmann
Huntsman Cancer Institute, University of Utah School of Medicine, Salt Lake City, United States

Sean V. Tavtigian
Department of Oncological Sciences, University of Utah School of Medicine, Salt Lake City, United States
Huntsman Cancer Institute, University of Utah School of Medicine, Salt Lake City, United States

Bryony A. Thompson
Huntsman Cancer Institute, University of Utah School of Medicine, Salt Lake City, United States
Centre for Epidemiology and Biostatistics, School of Population and Global Health, University of Melbourne, Melbourne, Australia

Deborah W. Neklason
Huntsman Cancer Institute, University of Utah School of Medicine, Salt Lake City, United States

Division of Genetic Epidemiology, Department of Internal Medicine, University of Utah, Salt Lake City, United States

Matthew A. Firpo and Sean J. Mulvihill
Huntsman Cancer Institute, University of Utah School of Medicine, Salt Lake City, United States
Department of Surgery, University of Utah School of Medicine, Salt Lake City, United States

Theresa Werner
Huntsman Cancer Institute, University of Utah School of Medicine, Salt Lake City, United States
Division of Oncology, Department of Medicine, University of Utah, Salt Lake City, United States

Justin Berger and Alison Fraser
Population Sciences, Huntsman Cancer Institute, University of Utah, Salt Lake City, United States

Leigh Neumayer
Department of Surgery and Arizona Cancer Center, University of Arizona, Tucson, United States

David E. Goldgar
Huntsman Cancer Institute, University of Utah School of Medicine, Salt Lake City, United States
Department of Dermatology, University of Utah School of Medicine, Salt Lake City, United States

Lisa A. Cannon-Albright
Huntsman Cancer Institute, University of Utah School of Medicine, Salt Lake City, United States
Division of Genetic Epidemiology, Department of Internal Medicine, University of Utah, Salt Lake City, United States
George E. Wahlen Department of Veterans Affairs Medical Center, Salt Lake City, United States

Johannes Betge, Jing Chi-Kern, Nadine Schulte, Sebastian Belle, Tobias Gutting, Elke Burgermeister, Ralf Jesenofsky, Matthias P. Ebert and Nicolai Haertel
Department of Medicine II, Medical Faculty Mannheim, University Hospital Mannheim, Heidelberg University, Theodor-Kutzer-Ufer 1-3, 68167 Mannheim, Germany

Martin Maenz
AIO-Studien gGmbH, Berlin, Germany

Ulrich Wedding
Department of Medicine II, University Hospital Jena, Jena, Germany

Ibrahim H. Sahin
Emory University School of Medicine, Atlanta, USA

Harold Elias
New York University Langone Medical Center, New York, USA

Joanne F. Chou and Marinela Capanu
Memorial Sloan Kettering Cancer Center, 300 East 66th Street, Office 1021, New York, NY 10065, USA

Eileen M. O'Reilly
Memorial Sloan Kettering Cancer Center, 300 East 66th Street, Office 1021, New York, NY 10065, USA
David M. Rubenstein Center for Pancreatic Cancer Research, 300 East 66th Street, Office 1021, New York, NY 10065, USA
Weill Cornell Medical College, 300 East 66th Street, Office 1021, New York, NY 10065, USA

Ce Li, Xiaofang Che, Ling Xu, Zhi Li, Yibo Fan, Kezuo Hou, Shuo Wang, Jinglei Qu, Lu Xu, Ti Wen, Xiujuan Qu and Yunpeng Liu
Department of Medical Oncology, the First Hospital of China Medical University, NO.155, North Nanjing Street, Heping District, Shenyang City 110001, China
Key Laboratory of Anticancer Drugs and Biotherapy of Liaoning Province, the First Hospital of China Medical University, Shenyang 110001, China

Qian Dong
Department of Oncology, Shengjing Hospital of China Medical University, Shenyang 110004, China

Xianghong Yang
Department of Pathology, Shengjing Hospital of China Medical University, Shenyang 110004, China

Debang Li
Department III of General Surgery, First Hospital of Lanzhou University, Lanzhou, China

Bin Hu
Department of Clinical Laboratory Medicine, First affiliated Hospital of Xiamen University, Xiamen, China

Yanming Zhou, Tao Wan and Xiaoying Si
Department of Hepatobiliary and Pancreatovascular Surgery, First affiliated Hospital of Xiamen University, Xiamen, China

Index

www.ingramcontent.com/pod-product-compliance
Lightning Source LLC
Chambersburg PA
CBHW080516200326
41458CB00012B/4228